BROWSING COLLECTION
14-DAY CHECKOUT
No Holds • No Renewals

HOW NOT TO AGE

Also by Michael Greger, M.D.

How Not to Die
The How Not to Die Cookbook
How Not to Diet
The How Not to Diet Cookbook
How to Survive a Pandemic

HOW NOT TO AGE

THE SCIENTIFIC APPROACH TO GETTING HEALTHIER AS YOU GET OLDER

MICHAEL GREGER, M.D.

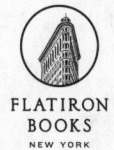

FLATIRON
BOOKS
NEW YORK

HOW NOT TO AGE. Copyright © 2023 by NutritionFacts.org Inc. All rights reserved. Printed in the United States of America. For information, address Flatiron Books, 120 Broadway, New York, NY 10271.

www.flatironbooks.com

Graphs and charts by Caroline Garriott, NutritionFacts.org

Designed by Jen Edwards

Library of Congress Cataloging-in-Publication Data

Names: Greger, Michael, author.
Title: How not to age : the scientific approach to getting healthier as you get older / Michael Greger, M.D., FACLM.
Description: First edition. | New York : Flatiron Books, 2023. | Includes index.
Identifiers: LCCN 2023026352 | ISBN 9781250796332 (hardcover) | ISBN 9781250796325 (ebook)
Subjects: LCSH: Longevity—Nutritional aspects. | Aging—Nutritional aspects. | Aging—Prevention.
Classification: LCC RA776.75 .G744 2023 | DDC 612.6/8—dc23/eng/20230830
LC record available at https://lccn.loc.gov/2023026352

Our books may be purchased in bulk for promotional, educational, or business use. Please contact your local bookseller or the Macmillan Corporate and Premium Sales Department at 1-800-221-7945, extension 5442, or by email at MacmillanSpecialMarkets@macmillan.com.

First Edition: 2023

10 9 8 7 6 5 4 3 2 1

For my great-aunt Pearl
(1911–2015)

Contents

PREFACE 1

INTRODUCTION 9

I. SLOWING ELEVEN PATHWAYS OF AGING 13

INTRODUCTION 13

AMPK 14

AUTOPHAGY 23

CELLULAR SENESCENCE 38

EPIGENETICS 44

GLYCATION 54

IGF-1 66

INFLAMMATION 78

mTOR 101

OXIDATION 109

SIRTUINS 130

TELOMERES 136

CONCLUSION 148

II. THE OPTIMAL ANTI-AGING REGIMEN 151

DIET 151

BEVERAGES 162

WHAT DO CENTENARIANS EAT? 173

THE MEDITERRANEAN DIET 180

THE OKINAWAN DIET 187

THE RED, WHITE, AND BLUE ZONE 197

PLANT-BASED EATING 202

LIFESTYLE 212

EXERCISE 214

WEIGHT CONTROL 219

SLEEP 223

STRESS MANAGEMENT 229

SOCIAL TIES 230

III. PRESERVING FUNCTION 233

PRESERVING YOUR BONES 233

PRESERVING YOUR BOWEL AND BLADDER FUNCTION 245

PRESERVING YOUR CIRCULATION 262

PRESERVING YOUR HAIR 278

PRESERVING YOUR HEARING 287

PRESERVING YOUR HORMONES 294

PRESERVING YOUR IMMUNE SYSTEM 319

PRESERVING YOUR JOINTS 342

PRESERVING YOUR MIND 357

PRESERVING YOUR MUSCLES 404

PRESERVING YOUR SEX LIFE 418

PRESERVING YOUR SKIN 439

PRESERVING YOUR TEETH 464

PRESERVING YOUR VISION 470

PRESERVING YOUR DIGNITY 480

IV. DR. GREGER'S ANTI-AGING EIGHT 485

INTRODUCTION 485

NUTS 489

GREENS 492

BERRIES 499

XENOHORMESIS AND microRNA MANIPULATION 507

PREBIOTICS AND POSTBIOTICS 530

CALORIC RESTRICTION 551

PROTEIN RESTRICTION 566

NAD$^+$ 583

CONCLUSION 597

REFERENCES 603

ACKNOWLEDGMENTS 605

INDEX 607

HOW NOT
TO AGE

Preface

I turned fifty in the process of writing this book, so the subject has a certain salience lacking from my last nutrition book, *How Not to Diet*, which covered weight loss. There is, however, a clear parallel between the two topics: Both are tainted with the same corrupting influence of commercial interests. The diet[1] and anti-aging[2] industries are both multibillion-dollar behemoths. With so much money in the mix, the temptation to promote products purporting all sorts of preposterous claims is apparently irresistible.

Even an educated layperson seeking basic, practical advice in either arena, living lighter or longer, is faced with an inscrutable barrage of pills and potions. Even as a physician with the luxury of wading neck deep through the peer-reviewed medical literature, it's been a challenge to tease out the naked truth from the emperor's clothing. But that makes the endeavor all the more important. If it took me three years to sift through all the science on aging, I'm afraid the casual observer would have little hope in separating facts from farce. A former president of the Gerontological Society of America wrote that "few subjects . . . have been more misleading to the uncritical and more profitable to the unscrupulous."[3]

The anti-aging field is said to be a "fertile ground for cons, scams and get-rich-quick schemes,"[4] with the popular literature on the subject harboring a "huge amount of misinformation."[5] Marketers often target older people with quack remedies for aging.[6] Their wares are hawked pervasively on the internet as well as brick-and-mortar "anti-aging" clinics.[7] These schemes have been the subject of multiple Senate and congressional inquiries with names like "Swindlers, Hucksters and Snake Oil Salesmen"[8] and "Quackery: A $10 Billion Scandal."[9] These days, the anti-aging industry in America may be worth more like $88 billion,[10] with the global industry valued at $292 billion.[11] This encompasses everything from wrinkle creams to televangelist Pat Robertson offering "Pat's Age-Defying Protein Pancakes." Aging may not be good for health, one economics editorial put it, "but it certainly is good for business."[12]

BLINDED BY SCIENCE

According to one industry group, 60 percent of Americans sixty-five and older are pursuing anti-aging interventions,[13] yet, according to the director of the Institute for Biomedical Aging Research, in almost all instances, these interventions are not supported by science.[14] They sound like they are, though. Scientific breakthroughs exploited by the sensationalist press have long been opportunistically repackaged by profiteers.

Nineteenth-century advances in magnetism led to ads asserting, "[t]here need not be a sick person in America . . . if our Magneto-Conservative Underwear would become a part of the wardrobe of every lady and gentleman, as also of infants and children." Less comically, more tragically, public interest in Marie Curie's work led to a range of radioactive products said to "revitalize" and "energize."[15] As one *Wall Street Journal* headline read, "The Radium Water Worked Fine Until His Jaw Came Off."[16]

Today, this so-called scienceploitation is evident in hundreds of rogue "stem cell" clinics concentrated in California and Florida,[17] using the language of science to give a veneer of legitimacy to their unproven therapies.[18] In their *Scientific American* feature "No Truth to the Fountain of Youth," three noted aging researchers concluded that the "public is bombarded by hype and lies."[19]

One of those researchers was sued for more than $200 million by the cofounders of the American Academy of Anti-Aging Medicine[20] for presenting the organization with a Silver Fleece Award, a mock prize shaming "the most ridiculous, outrageous, scientifically unsupported or exaggerated assertions about intervening in ageing or age-related diseases."[21] The American Academy of Anti-Aging Medicine countered that it "does not promote or endorse any specific treatment nor does it sell or endorse any commercial product."[22] However, looking back at its website, it has actively solicited and displayed a whole catalog of advertisements in its "Find an Anti-Aging Product or Service" directory whose development, it justifies, was "prompted by the numerous inquiries received each day."[23,24]

The "gerontological establishment" has been accused of trying to wantonly sabotage upstarts like the American Academy of Anti-Aging Medicine,[25] whose cofounder claims to be fighting the "old-line philosophy" that "aging is inevitable, nothing can be done, get used to it, grow old and die."[26] I see merit on both sides of this culture clash, with the field of gerontology (the study of old age) struggling to retain hard-fought gains in public funding for basic aging research versus the

more ambitious anti-aging crusaders who appear to more fundamentally question underlying assumptions. "Simply put," the American Academy of Anti-Aging Medicine's official response to the criticism read, "the death cult of gerontology desperately labors to sustain an arcane, outmoded stance that aging is natural and inevitable."[27]

The anti-aging medicine movement would have more credibility had it been started by those steeped in the research rather than "entrepreneurial businessmen responding to market opportunities,"[28] but the backlash against the anti-aging new wave may have pushed the pendulum too far in the other direction. Yes, as noted by the founding editor in chief of *Biogerontology*, the history of anti-aging research is undoubtedly "replete with fraud, pseudoscience, quackery and charlatanism,"[29] but the (admirable!) crusade against any whiff of impropriety seems to have led to a knee-jerk "all hype, no hope" position that belies the genuine scientific advances that have been made in the feasibility of intervening in the aging process.[30]

I know in some circles today, "science" is a dirty word. After years of COVID craziness, colleagues I once respected for their intellect seemed to have abandoned their critical thinking skills. If you have been similarly sucked down some rabbit hole of cabalistic conspiracies, this may not be the book for you. It is true that the pandemic revealed glaring institutional flaws that even encroached on the scholarly literature. Two of the most prestigious medical journals were forced to retract papers over concerns of data integrity.[31,32] But scientific journals remain the gold standard for establishing the best approximation of truth about our shared reality. To paraphrase Winston Churchill's quote about democracy as a form of governance, the peer-reviewed medical literature is the worst way to establish facts about our health—except for all the others.

SHOWING MY WORK

An editor in chief of a leading gerontology journal claims that most anti-aging scientists "widely known to the public are unscrupulous purveyors of useless nostrums."[33] It is easy to be swayed by charismatic gurus, but when it comes to something as life-and-death important as the health and well-being of ourselves and our families, we should rely not on anecdote but on evidence. That's why I cite everything to the teeth. *How Not to Die* had about 2,000 citations. *How Not to Diet*, 5,000. This book ended up with more than 13,000, which turned out to be a problem.

I promised the publisher a book with no more than about 600 pages, but when all was said and done, my manuscript was closer to 2,150 pages. Yikes. I didn't want to lose any content, so my first stab at trimming was to put the 995 pages of citations online. On page 603, there's a web address (see.nf/citations) and QR code for the full list of searchable citations referenced throughout this book.

Over the last three years, my team and I read more than 20,000 papers on aging so you don't have to—but you're certainly welcome to! The advantage of presenting the citations online is that it allows me to hyperlink each one to take you directly to the source. That way, you can download the PDFs and access the original research yourself.

Nevertheless, that still left me with a manuscript with a quadruple-digit page count. I needed to figure out how to essentially halve the book to meet the publisher's printing specifications. The problem is there wasn't any chaff to chop. Too many popular physician authors recycle rehashed content from their prior works to cash in on another publication. I try to do the opposite, featuring all-new material, which is why, throughout the text, I refer you to sections in my previous books where I covered relevant concepts. (Search worldcat.org to find print copies, e-books, or audiobooks of all my works at your local public library.) So, the only way I could think of to meet the target page count was to turn *How Not to Age* into a full audiovisual experience.

You'll see I've sprinkled video links throughout the book. My team and I produced hundreds of bite-sized videos, each about five minutes long, to cover the hundreds of thousands of words of additional information I had to cut from this manuscript. Don't worry, all the actionable takeaways are self-contained within this text. I just never want anyone to take my word for anything. I always strive to justify exactly how I arrive at each recommendation. Unfortunately, space limitations didn't always allow me to do that in this book, so even though I still relay the bottom-line conclusions, you may want to follow the links to take a deeper dive into the supporting evidence.

AGING IS THE ACTUAL LEADING CAUSE

There may be no such thing as dying from old age. From a study of more than 42,000 consecutive autopsies, centenarians—those who lived at least to one hundred—were found to have succumbed to diseases in 100 percent of the cases examined. Though most were perceived, even by their physicians, to have been healthy just prior to death, not one "died of old age." They died from disease, most commonly heart attacks.[34] Similar results were found from other autopsy series of centenarians[35] and those over eighty-five, an age bracket referred to in the medical literature as the "oldest old."[36,37,38]

If aging kills via diseases,[39] why wasn't my *How Not to Die* the only longevity book anyone needs? In it, I ran through what we can do to prevent, arrest, and reverse each of our fifteen leading causes of death, starting with heart disease, not only the number one killer of centenarians but of people in general.[40] In the United States, heart disease has been the leading cause of death every year since 1900, with the exception of 1918 when pandemic flu ruled the roost.[41] (In contrast, as I detail in *How to Survive a Pandemic*, COVID only made it to number three.[42]) Heart disease has been the leading cause of death and disability around the world for most of this century[43] and is projected to remain that way in the decades to come.[44] But is it *really*?

Because old age is the greatest risk factor for most of our killer diseases,[45] one could argue that the leading cause of death is actually aging.[46] The rate of death increases exponentially for age-related diseases, such as heart disease, cancer, stroke, and dementia.[47] So, yes, in the same age bracket, having high cholesterol can increase your risk of heart disease as much as twentyfold,[48] but an eighty-year-old may have *five hundred* times the risk of having a heart attack[49] compared to someone in their twenties.[50] Eating a plant-based diet may reduce the risk of dementia as much as threefold,[51] but the difference in dementia rates between those older than eighty-five compared to younger than sixty-five is *three hundredfold*.[52] The reason we focus on things like cholesterol is that it is a *modifiable* risk factor, but what if the rate of aging was modifiable, too?

Instead of our current, piecemeal approach of focusing on individual degenerative diseases, what about slowing down the aging process itself? I remember as a nerdy kid I wanted to cure cancer when I grew up. Even if all forms of cancer were eliminated, the average life expectancy in the United States would only go up about three years.[53] Why? Because dodging cancer would just mean delaying death from something like a heart attack or stroke. If one age-related ailment doesn't get us, another will. Rather than playing "whack-a-mole" by tackling each disease separately, progress in decelerating aging could address all these issues simultaneously.[54]

Imagine if there was an intervention that didn't just reduce your risk of the leading killers but also arthritis, dementia, osteoporosis, Parkinson's disease, and sensory impairments. Because such risks tend to double every seven years, even just slowing aging, such that the average sixty-five-year-old, for example, would have the health profile and disease risk of today's fifty-eight-year-old, would be expected to cut *in half* everyone's risk of death, frailty, and disability.[55]

This is why I wrote *How Not to Age*.

Is Aging Itself a Disease?

For decades, one of the most contested questions in gerontology has been whether or not aging itself should be considered a disease.[56] Aging is natural, yes, but so is getting an infection and we call that a disease. Aging is universal. Yes, but everybody gets the common cold, too.[57] If you're interested, I dive deeper into the discussion in my video see.nf/agingdisease. What does it matter what we call it? A rose by any other name wilts just as fast. The hope is that disease classification would lead to greater resource allocation for aging research, just as the recent declaration of obesity as a disease did for obesity research.[58]

You'd think Big Pharma would invest in what would certainly be a blockbuster drug. But why spend the money on research when it can be spent on marketing all the unproven anti-aging products they already sell? Many of the leading lines of dietary supplements are owned by drug companies.[59,60] They're the ones selling "cosmeceuticals"[61] and "age reverse" skin creams.[62] Drug maker Sanofi even partnered with Coca-Cola to come up with a "beauty drink."[63] They're already making money hand over fist preying on the public's gullibility and desperation for anti-aging products.[64] Why waste money on proving anything actually works?

ALIVE AND WELL

When asked, *How long do you wish to live?* and offered the choice of 85, 120, or 150 years, or indefinitely, about two-thirds said they'd prefer to live to be eighty-five. But, when the question was reframed as *How long do you wish to live in guaranteed mental and physical health?*, the most popular answer switched to an unlimited lifespan.[65] It's not just how long we live, but how well, embodied in the Greek myth of Tithonus, to whom Zeus granted eternal life, but not eternal youth, so he shriveled with age and began to babble continuously (before eventually transforming into a cicada).[66]

Longevity is indeed a Pyrrhic victory if those additional years are characterized by inexorable decline.[67] Only about 18 percent of people can be described as undergoing "successful aging."[68] Studies have found the prevalence of multimorbidity, the coexistence of multiple chronic diseases, ranges between 55 percent and 98 percent among older individuals.[69] By age eighty-five, more than 90 percent may have at least one disease and, on average, about four diseases.[70] And just like 85 percent of cancer patients tend to overestimate their survival,[71] so, too, do those with other chronic diseases. Those suffering from heart failure or chronic obstructive lung diseases like emphysema are about three times more likely to die within the subsequent year than they predicted. Ninety-six percent of outpatient dialysis patients thought the odds were in their favor that they'd be alive five years later, but nearly half were dead in fewer than two years.[72]

This raises the concept of healthspan, the period of life spent in good health, free from chronic disease and disability.[73] No wonder people are skeptical about longevity interventions as we see our lifespans expand but our healthspans contract. "Everyone wants to live forever," to paraphrase Jonathan Swift, "but no one wants to grow old."

In the United States, for example, we're living longer in sickness, not in health. A twenty-year-old in 1998 could expect to live about fifty-eight more years, while a twenty-year-old in 2006 could look forward to fifty-nine more years. However, the twenty-year-old from the 1990s might live ten of those years with chronic disease, whereas now it's more like thirteen years. So it feels like one step forward, three steps back. The researchers also noted that we're living two fewer *functional* years—that is, years we're no longer able to perform basic life activities, such as walking a quarter of a mile, standing or sitting for two hours without having to lie down, or standing without special equipment.[74] In other words, we're living longer, but we're living *sicker*.

That is why this book addresses both lifespan and healthspan. What's the point of living longer if you can't enjoy it vibrantly? It is my sincere hope this book adds not just years to your life but life to your years.

Introduction

My earlier book, *How Not to Die*, was not about living forever. It was not *How to Not Die*. Instead, it was how not to die prematurely, in pain after a long, chronic, disabling illness. The good news I shared is that we have tremendous power over our health destiny, in that the vast majority of premature death and disability is preventable with a healthy enough diet and lifestyle. *How Not to Age* has a similar premise. This book is not about immortality but rather how to age with grace and vitality rather than suffering from the ravages of infirmity and decrepitude. But why can't we stop aging and go on forever?

"MAN WILL NEVER BE CONTENTED UNTIL HE CONQUERS DEATH." ——BERNARD STREHLER

From the Epic of Gilgamesh more than 4,000 years ago[75] to the recent quincentennial of Ponce de León's pursuit for the fountain of youth, humankind has yearned for the mythical elixir of life that would remedy the scourges of aging.[76] And why not? It's not like aging is some immutable constant in nature. Evolution has produced lifespans in animals that vary more than a millionfold, from mayflies whose adult lives may last only a few minutes to clams clocking in at over five hundred years.[77] Just like the Wright brothers may have taken inspiration from birds, we can take inspiration from animals that age slowly, if at all.[78]

Why can't we live forever? Some animals do, and I'm not talking about a two-hundred-year-old whale or even a thousand-year-old tree. There are actually species (with names like the immortal jellyfish) who apparently do not age and could technically go on forever.[79] In a sense, humans are immortal, in that a few of our cells live on—the sperm or egg cells lucky enough to find each other. Each of our kids grows out of one of our cells, and that alone—I mean, the fact that a single cell can grow into a person—should make, in comparison, the notion of keeping our body going indefinitely seem biologically trivial. One little fertilized microscopic blob can turn into perhaps the most complex object in the known universe, the human brain, with its 100,000 miles[80] of 86 billion neurons[81] making 150 trillion connections.[82] If that's possible in biology, then what isn't?

Still, there is much skepticism in the scientific community, where many believe aging is an irreversible process.[83] "Anti-aging" is compared to "anti-gravity."[84] Vocal critics in the gerontology community have accused those suggesting the possibility of greatly extended human lifespans as being "contemptible . . . for duping the public" and claim that "anything past 130 [years of age] is ridiculous."[85] Such doubts are reliably countered by proponents who quote preeminent scientists of yore making similarly absolutist claims that did not age well.[86] Nobel Prize–winning physicists spoke of the prospect of nuclear power as "talking moonshine," a "completely unscientific Utopian dream, a childish bug-a-boo."[87] Lord Kelvin, considered one of the greatest scientists of his time, notoriously asserted, "Heavier-than-air flying machines are impossible,"[88] doubling down on their impracticality in 1902, just one year before the first flight at Kitty Hawk.[89]

Already in the laboratory, genetic mutations can affect a tenfold increase in lifespan, at least in a species of tiny worm.[90] In mice, dietary and genetic manipulation yields more like a 70 percent increase.[91] Single tweaks, such as methionine restriction, incorporated into one of my Anti-Aging Eight (see page 485), can extend the average and maximum lifespans of rats by about 40 percent,[92] which could translate to boosting human lifespan to an average of about 110, with the rare "centenarian" hitting 140 years of age.[93] These results have yet to be replicated in people, but if we discovered interventions not only to slow aging but to actively repair the accumulated damage, the sky could be the limit.

Starry-eyed scientists in the field imagine that time could be effectively melted away, like that surrealist painting of drooping clocks,[94] a "rejuvenation of your body leading ultimately to an endless summer of literally perpetual youth."[95] A "longevity escape velocity" is envisaged in which we would just have to live long enough for innovations to add more time than is passing, the tipping point at which each year we can add at least one extra year of life expectancy.[96] This could theoretically enable humanity to have an essentially unlimited lifespan. Imagine dying the year before the critical juncture! I remain agnostic as to whether such a breakthrough is possible, but I hope this book will help regardless, whether you're striving to live long enough to live forever[97] or just trying to die young as old as possible.

FOUR BOOKS IN ONE

When I sat down to write (or rather stood up and started walking, typing at my treadmill desk), I needed to make a decision. What should I focus on? The more superficial signs of aging that everybody wants to know about, like wrinkles and graying hair, or the clinical aspects, like declining cognition? Or should I address how we might slow the aging process itself? I decided, as you can probably guess by the heft if you're reading a printed copy old-school style, all of the above.

My inspiration for writing *How Not to Age* was a consensus document titled "Interventions to Slow Aging in Humans" that was compiled by the top researchers in anti-aging medicine, the likes of Drs. Fontana, Longo, Sinclair, and dozens of others—nearly everyone who's anyone in the field. Brought together to identify the most promising strategies for developing drugs to combat aging, they identified a list of "essential pathways," for example, the pharmacological inhibition of the hormone IGF-1 or drugs to block the enzyme mTOR. As I looked through the list, I realized: *Every single one of these pathways could be regulated through diet.* That became the opening section of this book.

PART I: SLOWING ELEVEN PATHWAYS OF AGING

The science of aging has been called "the most dynamic and provocative in modern biology."[98] An attempt to classify the theories of aging published more than thirty years ago identified more than three hundred such theories, and the number has only grown since then.[99] In Part I, I identify the eleven most promising pathways for slowing the sands of time, ending each with practical proposals for targeting them naturally with diet and lifestyle changes. Part I is the nerdy section, and it contains critical concepts and terms that will be used throughout the book.

PART II: THE OPTIMAL ANTI-AGING REGIMEN

The odds of living to age one hundred have risen from approximately one in twenty million to as high as one in fifty.[100] Why do some make it to their hundredth birthday but others don't? It's not just a matter of picking better parents. Studies following identical twins suggest that no more than 20 to 30 percent of the variance in lifespan is explained by gene inheritance.[101] The media loves stories about hard-living centenarians who attribute their longevity to some combination of lard, vodka, and their favorite brand of cigarette, but how do centenarians and supercentenarians (those older than 110) really eat and live?

In Part II, I delve deep into the behaviors that those in the five longevity hot spot "blue zones" around the world share in common. In constructing the optimal anti-aging regimen, I explore the best and worst foods and beverages. Is red wine deserving of its symbolic status for longevity? What about coffee? I cover the "longevity vitamin" ergothioneine, the vegetarian's Achilles' heel, and the best exercise and sleep routine for the longest, healthiest life.

PART III: PRESERVING FUNCTION

Then, in Part III, I get to the nitty-gritty. What can you do to preserve your bones, bowels, and circulation? Your hair, hearing, and hormone balance? Your immune function and joint health? Your mind and your muscles? Your sex life and skin? Your teeth, your vision, and, finally, your dignity in death? There are chapters on each. Sneak peeks can be had at see.nf/trailer.

PART IV: DR. GREGER'S ANTI-AGING EIGHT

My Anti-Aging Eight is the final section of the book, an actionable checklist to complement the Daily Dozen I established in my earlier book *How Not to Die*. In addition to the wealth of recommendations throughout *How Not to Age*, this last part highlights specific foods, supplements, or behaviors that have the potential to offer some of the best opportunities to slow aging or improve longevity. My aim is to cover every possible angle for developing the optimal diet and lifestyle for the longest, healthiest lifespan based on the best available balance of evidence.

I. Slowing Eleven Pathways of Aging

INTRODUCTION

It has long been said that the best hope for a long life is to choose your parents wisely.[102] Doesn't longevity just run in the family? Siblings of centenarians, people who live to be at least one hundred, are certainly more likely to become centenarians themselves, and their parents are more likely to have lived to be at least ninety.[103] On the other hand, the lifespans of spouses sometimes correlate as much as—or even more than—those of genetic relatives.[104] Your partner may have as much of an impact as your parent. After all, we don't only pass down genes. Perhaps Grandma's healthy recipes or even a lifelong love of running runs in the family, too.

HOW IMPORTANT ARE YOUR GENES?

To tease out the role of genetics, researchers often turn to twin studies, comparing differences between identical twins and fraternal twins.[105] Check out see.nf/genes to understand exactly how this ingenious method works to estimate heritability and what this and other methods have found. In short, only about 15 to 30 percent[106] or less[107] of our lifespan appears determined by our genes, which means *how* we live our lives may determine the bulk of our destiny.

To leverage the lifespan leeway we have beyond the relatively small genetic component, we must first understand the various aging pathways. The term "anti-aging" has been much abused in popular culture, attached to all manner of unproven products and procedures. The term should probably be reserved for things that can delay or reverse aging through the targeting of one or more of the established aging mechanisms.[108] In a landmark paper cited more than 7,000 times in the biomedical literature,[109] "The Hallmarks of Aging" identified nine common denominators of the aging process. I expound on them in see.nf/genes and address each one in this book.

There's a Fly in My Aging Research!

There are numerous ways to try to unlock the mysteries of aging. You could study long-lived individuals like centenarians and supercentenarians (people who reached the age of 110), for instance, or particularly long-lived smokers to uncover the secrets to their resilience.[110] Or, you could strike out in the opposite direction and study short-lived people, investigating tragic accelerated aging syndromes like progeria, where children age at eight to ten times the normal rate,[111] wrinkling, balding, and then typically dying around age thirteen of a heart attack or stroke.[112] Or, you could study long-lived animals. There's a clam called the ocean quahog, whose heart can beat more than a billion times over its five-century lifespan.[113]

In my video see.nf/models, I talk about both the opportunities and difficulties of extrapolating from the "model organisms" used in aging research, such as yeast, worms, flies, and mice,[114] as well as citizen science initiatives in which family dogs are enrolled in noninvasive studies to investigate why some "Methuselah dogs" reach ages of twenty-five or more, but 99.9 percent of other dogs do not.[115] Aged pooches suffer many of the same ravages of aging that we do, such as arthritis, cancer, cataracts, kidney problems, and muscle loss.[116] Advances made in canine longevity might not only be applicable to human aging but have the intrinsic value of enhancing the quality and quantity of life for the more than seventy million canine companions with whom we share our homes in the United States alone.[117]

AMPK

In my book on everything evidence-based in weight loss, *How Not to Diet*, there is a section titled Amping AMPK. AMPK (AMP-activated protein kinase) is an enzyme that acts as a sensor for plants and animals, similar to a fuel gauge in a car. It revs up when it detects a depletion of the universal fuel, just as a light may blink on your dashboard when you're almost out of gas. AMPK flips the switch in your body from storing fat to burning it to restore energy balance. That's why AMPK is known not only as the *master energy sensor*[118] in our body but also the *fat controller*.[119] That's why it played a starring role in *How Not to Diet*. But it doesn't affect only weight control. It can also control aging.[120]

In times of plenty, our cells can plow full steam ahead. However, when times are lean—when there isn't enough food for an animal or enough light for a plant (darkness is essentially plant starvation)[121]—AMPK kicks in to reorient the cell into conservation mode and start tapping into energy stores, like burning off body fat. Our cells can also institute a recycling program called autophagy.

Autophagy is a housekeeping process by which defective cellular components, such as misfolded proteins that had been allowed to build up wastefully in times of surplus, are broken down and scrapped for spare parts. As I discuss in detail in the Autophagy chapter, autophagy doubles as both salvage operation and garbage disposal unit, scavenging raw materials in scarce supply while clearing away some of the built-up damaged debris that is implicated in the aging process. This is one of the reasons AMPK is increasingly recognized as a pro-longevity factor.[122] AMPK induces autophagy, which cleans house, sweeps away accumulated waste, and effectively institutes a sort of cellular reset.[123]

There are three main ways longevity researchers establish an aging pathway: Does the factor worsen with age? If you amplify it, does it accelerate aging? And, if you dampen it, does it slow aging and thereby extend lifespan?[124] The loss of AMPK activity as we age fits all three criteria. As we grow older, AMPK levels drop and it gets harder to activate, harder to flip the switch to recharge our batteries.[125] When this decline is exacerbated, aging is hastened (at least in mice),[126] but when this process is reversed and AMPK activation is boosted, lifespan is extended in model organisms[127]—by as much as 38 percent in *C. elegans*,[128] a roundworm I profile in see.nf/models.

Up and down the evolutionary tree of life, the most reliable way to extend lifespan may be long-term food restriction.[129] AMPK activation is thought to be one of the mechanisms for this longevity boost. What was remarkable about the AMPK-boosting experiments, though, is that the animals' lives were extended even though they were allowed to eat as much as they wanted.[130] AMPK activators can effectively fool the body into thinking it is starving, switching it into protective housecleaning mode without causing any pangs of deprivation. In this way, AMPK activators can be considered dietary restriction *mimetics*, or imitators. That's why AMPK is considered a "druggable" target for longevity, with pharmaceutical companies producing a variety of AMPK activators.[131]

EXERCISE IN A PILL

Is there a way we can naturally boost AMPK activation to slow aging without starving ourselves? Since AMPK is activated by a fuel shortage, if we don't want to limit the amount of energy going in through our mouths, then we have to ramp up the amount of energy going out through our muscles. If you put people on bikes and take muscle biopsies while they cycle, a near tripling of AMPK activity can be detected within twenty minutes.[132] That's one way exercise can result in weight loss.

AMPK activation also leads to mitochondrial biogenesis, the formation of extra mitochondria, the power plants where fat is burned.[133] So, AMPK doesn't just shovel more fat into the furnace—it also builds more furnaces to burn that fat. This helps explain why endurance training enables us to run faster and farther over time. So, might an AMPK activator be "exercise in a pill"? Indeed, when sedentary mice were given an AMPK-activator drug for a month, it boosted their running endurance by 44 percent.[134] After one such drug was discovered at the famed Tour de France,[135] AMPK activators were banned by the World Anti-Doping Agency.[136]

So, are we talking about not only fasting in a pill but an exercise mimetic, too? A way to trick our body into thinking it's starving without suffering from hunger, while also amping up our physical prowess? Obese individuals are often "unwilling to perform even a minimum of physical activity," wrote a group of pharmacologists, "thus, indicating that drugs mimicking endurance exercise are highly desirable."[137] The "mass appeal" of such a pill may tempt Big Pharma to "view physical inactivity as a market to be medicalized for profit,"[138] but that pales in comparison to the *universal* market for an anti-aging remedy.

POWER PLANT MAINTENANCE

In his book *On Youth and Old Age*, the Greek philosopher Aristotle described death as the loss of inner heat.[139] Well, the progressive loss of function of the estimated ten million billion mitochondria spread throughout our body[140] is considered a core tenet of the biology of aging,[141] one of the nine established hallmarks.[142] Mitochondrial dysfunction isn't just a consequence of aging, though, but also one of its causes. Dysfunctional mitochondria are thought to actively contribute to the aging process,[143] an insight illustrated by a pioneering experiment published in the early 1990s.[144]

If you inject mitochondria from a young rat into a human cell, nothing happens. The cell doesn't appear to notice. Each human skin cell averages about three hundred mitochondria, and adding ten to fifteen extra mitochondria from a rat pup doesn't appear to have any effect. But if you add the same number of mitochondria from an old rat—a centenarian in human years[145]—the human cells start to show signs of degeneration within just a few days.[146] Even just having a few percent of those old mitochondria was enough to drive the human cells to an early grave. So, age-impaired mitochondria don't just become less efficient—they may become actively harmful. That's where AMPK comes in.

With age, our mitochondrial function declines,[147] but building new cellular power plants, expanding existing ones, and decommissioning old ones (so-called *mitophagy*) are ways in which AMPK could promote survival.[148] AMPK is said to serve as a "mitochondrial guardian" and in that role may help protect against the ravages of age-related disease.[149]

If an AMPK-activating drug really could help us reap the fat-burning and health-promoting benefits of fasting and exercise without the hunger and sweat, one could imagine how it would become one of the best-selling drugs on the planet.

And it is.

METFORMIN

Sold originally as Glucophage (meaning "sugar eater"), metformin is now prescribed more than eighty-five million times a year in the United States alone.[150] Despite all the strides in biotechnology, Big Pharma has yet to come up with a safer, more effective, first-line treatment for type 2 diabetes than an AMPK-boosting drug that retails at pennies per pill.[151] In see.nf/metformin, I talk about its interesting origin story and all the other upsides, including the mind-blowing revelation that diabetics placed on metformin may live longer lives than those who never got diabetes in the first place.[152] From a longevity standpoint, it's as if their diabetes diagnoses were beneficial, because they then had access to this lifespan-enhancing drug. If metformin is so powerful as to more than offset such a dreaded diagnosis as diabetes, should everyone be taking it?

In see.nf/metformindownsides, I cover its common but mild symptoms and the rare but potentially fatal one.[153] Another adverse consequence of metformin is less side effect than main effect. The way metformin boosts AMPK is by impairing our body's ability to produce energy by acting as a mild mitochondrial poison, so, not surprisingly, it may undercut physical fitness achievements from exercise, including aerobic capacity[154] and muscle gains.[155]

The only way to determine if metformin's benefits outweigh its risks for expanding the healthspan and lifespan of nondiabetics is to put it to the test. Enter the upcoming TAME trial, Targeting Aging with Metformin, which I profile in see .nf/tame. The bottom line is that there may be reason to temper our expectations. Though it can increase the average lifespan of certain mice by 5 percent, at a higher dose, metformin actually shortens lifespan.[156] Further reservations about its panacean prospects arise from the landmark Diabetes Prevention Program study in which the drug only appeared to benefit those at highest risk.[157] One small study even found that despite metformin alleviating the insulin resistance of diabetics, the drug actually made things worse for nondiabetic obese individuals without the family history of diabetes.[158] So, healthier individuals may not reap the benefits of metformin that we try to extrapolate from longevity studies on diabetics.

FOODS THAT MAY IMPAIR AMPK

There's a type of saturated fat called palmitic acid that suppresses AMPK.[159] Although originally discovered in palm oil, palmitic acid is most concentrated in meat and dairy fat.[160] Of all saturated fats, palmitic acid appears particularly pathogenic when it comes to metabolic disease, cardiovascular disease, cancer, neurodegenerative diseases, and inflammation,[161] which is at least partly attributable to AMPK inhibition. This may be why saturated fat can be so toxic to the liver.[162]

SATURATING YOUR LIVER

Nonalcoholic fatty liver disease has become the leading cause of chronic liver disease in the world.[163] Studies now estimate seventy-five to one hundred million people in the United States already have it—about one in three American adults.[164] The overaccumulation of fat in the liver is caused by the overconsumption of calories,[165] but not all calories are equally liver-fattening. Excess sugar is often framed as the main culprit, but saturated fat is even worse. See my video see .nf/liver for details, but basically, overfeeding sugary foods, like candy and soda, can increase liver fat by 33 percent, whereas overfeeding the same amount of saturated fat (butter and cheese) increased liver fat by 55 percent.[166] Overfeeding unsaturated fats, like pecans and olive oil, only caused a 15 percent increase in liver fat,[167] presumably because unsaturated fats don't impair AMPK as potently as do saturated fats.[168]

What makes saturated fat particularly insidious is that it can increase liver fat even without enforced overeating. *Excess* sugar calories can foie gras your liver with fat, but even if you have people swap twenty-five spoonsful of sugar in the form of candy and soda into their diets each day, liver fat remains unchanged as long as they keep overall calorie intake steady. But, if you do that with a fraction of the amount of saturated fat in the form of meat and dairy, even without being made to overeat, study subjects marbled their livers with 39 percent more fat within four weeks.[169]

FOODS THAT MAY BOOST AMPK

We know of more than a hundred plant products that can activate AMPK,[170] but many of them are toxic, to defend against noshing nibblers. Take nicotine, for example. Fat biopsies show that, compared to nonsmokers, those who light up have more than five times the AMPK activation.[171] Unsurprisingly, smokers often gain weight when they quit,[172] and nicotine gum can blunt that phenomenon.[173] Although smoking cigarettes may be one of the worst things you can do to yourself, it's one of the most reliable ways to lose weight, thanks to AMPK.[174] Is there any way to get the AMPK-boosting benefits without the risks of dying a gruesome death from lung cancer?

BARBERRIES

Because AMPK activation leads to weight loss, I cover a number of natural AMPK activators in my book on the subject, including berberine, found in barberries. Rather than reiterate it here, allow me to refer you to the Raising the Barberries section of my Amping AMPK chapter in *How Not to Diet*.

In short, barberries, which can be found inexpensively priced at Middle Eastern groceries in dried form, have been shown to successfully lower LDL cholesterol levels an average of fourteen points (mg/dL),[175] as well as improve acne,[176] artery function,[177] triglycerides, blood sugars, and insulin resistance.[178] One could achieve the dose of berberine used widely in China for diabetes management,[179] which is presumably AMPK-enhancing, by eating as few as two teaspoons of barberries three times a day or a single tablespoon twice a day.[180] Eating the whole food is preferable, especially since an analysis of berberine supplements on the market found that 60 percent failed to match what was claimed on their labels.[181]

A word of caution: Barberries are classified as unsafe to eat during pregnancy and are not recommended for consumption while breastfeeding.[182] The reason so many different plants produce compounds that activate AMPK may be for self-preservation; they may be trying to fend off herbivores by producing compounds that impair animal metabolism. These functions can be harnessed for our benefit but could potentially be harmful for developing fetuses and infants. Cyanide is another AMPK activator and can kill by completely blocking energy production, whereas compounds like berberine and metformin are thought to just impair our mitochondrial function, making energy production less efficient.[183]

BLACK CUMIN

Black cumin is another plant traditionally used in Middle Eastern cuisines that can boost AMPK.[184] Please see the Black Cumin section in my Appetite Suppression chapter in *How Not to Diet*. In summary, from the more than one thousand papers published in the medical literature about the spice, daily black cumin consumption has been found in systematic reviews and meta-analyses of randomized controlled trials to significantly improve weight loss,[185] cholesterol, triglycerides,[186] blood pressure,[187] and blood sugar control.[188] Typical doses used in studies are just 1 or 2 g of black cumin a day, which is about a quarter teaspoon.[189] Using such small amounts allows researchers to conduct randomized, double-blind, placebo-controlled trials by putting the whole-food spice into capsules rather than extracting out just a few components.

The spice also lowers markers of inflammation, such as C-reactive protein,[190] and has favorable effects on inflammatory conditions, such as asthma,[191] rheumatoid arthritis,[192] and a common cause of hypothyroidism called Hashimoto's thyroiditis.[193] Black cumin also appears to help get rid of kidney stones[194] and help with the symptoms of menopause.[195] The dose used in most of these studies would cost about three cents a day.

HIBISCUS AND LEMON VERBENA TEA

Another AMPK-boosting zinger is hibiscus,[196] which delivers the tart cranberry-like flavor and bright red color of Red Zinger tea. Also known as *roselle* or *jamaica*, hibiscus tea has been enjoyed around the world for millennia as both a delicious hot or cold drink and an ancient medicinal remedy.[197] In *How Not to Die*, I covered its blood pressure benefits, working as well as,[198] or even beating out, some antihypertensive medications in head-to-head clinical trials.[199] In *How Not to Diet*, in the Flower Power section of my Fat Blockers chapter, I describe its role in AMPK activation[200] and in improving blood sugars, LDL cholesterol,[201] artery function,[202] and weight loss,[203] with or without another herbal tea, lemon verbena. See page 470 for my note about tooth enamel and sour beverages, though.

VINEGAR

Hibiscus[204] and black cumin[205] bump up AMPK the same way barberry's berberine and metformin do—by interfering with cellular energy production. Can we activate AMPK without mucking with our mitochondria?

Alcohol is yet another plant product that activates AMPK, but it does so by a totally different mechanism. Our body detoxifies alcohol into acetic acid but has to use energy to then metabolize it.[206] So AMPK is activated naturally in response to this fuel expenditure.[207] Before alcohol gets fully converted into acetic acid, though, there is a toxic intermediate called *acetaldehyde*, which is a known carcinogen. That may be why alcohol consumption has been found to increase the risks of at least half a dozen cancers,[208] including breast cancer, even among light drinkers.[209] Is there any way to skip over the toxic step and take in acetic acid directly?

Upon reviewing AMPK's role in burning off excess body fat, a researcher determined that "it is crucial that oral compounds with high bioavailability are developed to safely induce chronic AMPK activation . . . [for] long-term weight loss and maintenance."[210] Why develop such a compound when you can already buy it at any grocery store? It's called vinegar.

Acetic derives from the Latin word *acetum*, meaning "vinegar." By definition, vinegar is merely a dilute solution of acetic acid in water.[211] When we consume vinegar, the acetic acid is absorbed and metabolized, giving us a natural boost in AMPK at the dose you might typically get dressing a salad.[212]

In the Take an Acid Trip section of my Amping AMPK chapter in *How Not to Diet*, I cover how vinegar can diminish both visceral and superficial body fat[213] and reduce blood sugars in diabetics on par with antidiabetic drugs[214] by improving the uptake of blood sugar by our muscles.[215] That's an AMPK effect also seen with exercise.[216] Surprisingly, vinegar plus metformin worked better to control blood sugars than metformin alone, suggesting either additive benefits to further AMPK stimulation (the metformin dose was relatively low) or vinegar benefits above and beyond AMPK.[217]

Vinegar has also been shown to improve artery function[218] and to have other AMPK-activation benefits, such as decreasing blood cholesterol and triglyceride levels.[219] Can it make you live longer? In *C. elegans*, vinegar has a "prominent lifespan-extending effect,"[220] but it's never been tested in people. The Harvard Nurses' Health Study did find that women who consumed at least one tablespoon of oil and vinegar salad dressing five or more days a week had fewer than half the fatal heart attacks compared to women who hardly ever used the dressing. Even after taking the extra vegetable intake into account, they found a 54 percent lower risk of dying from the number one killer of women.[221]

FIBER-RICH FOODS

Don't like the taste of vinegar? Instead of delivering acetic acid through your mouth, you can also supply it to your bloodstream from the opposite direction. You know how vegetables and grains turn sour when they're fermented? Think sauerkraut or sourdough. That's because there are good bacteria like *Lactobacillus* that produce organic acids like lactic acid. Acetic acid is a type of short-chain fatty acid made by the friendly flora in our gut from the fiber and resistant starch we eat. These prebiotics are concentrated in legumes (beans, split peas, chickpeas, and lentils) and whole grains, but fiber can be found throughout the plant kingdom.

When we eat whole plant foods, our gut flora can make acetic acid from scratch inside our colons by fermenting fiber. Then, that acetic acid can get reabsorbed back into our bloodstreams. So, we can use the top-down approach to activate AMPK by consuming vinegar or the bottom-up approach by eating fiber.[222]

How much fiber are we talking about? Even eating just the measly minimum recommended intake of fiber of about 30 g a day can result in the production of more than four tablespoons' worth of vinegar in our colon.[223,224] Some inevitably get flushed, so only about 40 percent of the acetic acid produced in the colon gets absorbed,[225] but if we eat enough healthful foods, it could potentially have a substantial impact on our AMPK status. The sparking of AMPK by colon-produced acetic acid is suspected to play a role in some of the metabolic benefits of a high-fiber diet.[226]

Based in part on studies of human coprolites[227]—fossilized feces (paleopoo!)—our ancient ancestors may have consumed in excess of 100 g of fiber a day.[228] That's more than five times that of the average American today.[229] So, we evolved to be AMPK-activating machines, not only because we were often hungry and active but because our guts were churning out spoonfuls of vinegar every day from all the plants we ate. And, before you ask, no, you can't just take a fiber supplement like psyllium (Metamucil) because it's nonfermentable, meaning our gut bacteria can't eat it. So, although such fiber supplements can improve bowel regularity, they cannot be used to make the key ingredients for AMPK activation.[230]

Food for Thought

The discovery of AMPK is considered to be one of the most important break-throughs in biomedicine in the last few decades.[231] Because this enzyme is involved in the functioning of the majority of aging-associated regulators, including autophagy, which I discuss next, the importance of AMPK in anti-aging interventions is hard to overestimate.[232]

The drug metformin activates AMPK but carries adverse side effects and may not benefit healthy individuals. AMPK is an energy sensor, so it's activated when we eat less or move more. Some food components, like saturated fat, can suppress AMPK, whereas others, like fiber, can boost it. There are also specific AMPK-activating compounds in barberries, black cumin, hibiscus tea, and vinegar.

To help boost this anti-aging pathway, at each meal, consider:
- reducing consumption of saturated fat (concentrated in meat, dairy, and desserts)

- increasing consumption of fiber (concentrated in legumes and whole grains)
- taking each of the following:
  - ° 2 teaspoons of barberries
  - ° a dash (¹⁄₁₂ teaspoon) of ground black cumin
  - ° ¾ cup hibiscus tea mixed with ¼ cup of lemon verbena tea
  - ° 2 teaspoons of vinegar (though *never* taken straight; sprinkle on food or dilute it in the tea)

AUTOPHAGY

When food is scarce, our body shifts into conservation mode, slowing down cell division and turning on the process of autophagy,[233] from the Greek *auto* meaning "self" and *phagy* meaning "to eat." Autophagy means, quite literally, "eating yourself."

TAKING OUT THE TRASH

Upon realizing there isn't much food around, our body starts rummaging through our cells in a salvage operation, looking for anything we don't need—defective proteins, malfunctioning mitochondria, and other stuff that isn't working anymore. It clears out the junk and upcycles it, turning it into fuel or new building materials, thereby renewing our cells. So, autophagy plays two major roles: nutrient recovery and quality control. The conservation of autophagy machinery over a billion years of biological evolution underscores the importance of this universal recycling program,[234] recognized in 2016 with a Nobel Prize awarded for teasing out its secrets.[235]

At any given time, most of our cells are producing and assembling more than 10,000 distinct proteins.[236] Each of them can become misfolded or damaged at any moment and require a cleanup on aisle three. We evolved in a context of scarcity, though, where food was hard to come by. When we'd get to eat next was unpredictable. So, our body expects we'll fall back on hard times any day—maybe even tomorrow—and figures it can put off cleaning up until then. But, these days, those lean times hardly ever come. Most of us live in nutrient excess, so our body figures, *why bother?* We can just toss the defective protein or broken-down mitochondrion in the corner and make another. So, our cells end up continually hoarding junk.

The buildup of cellular detritus isn't merely wasteful but harmful, too. Out with the old and in with the new doesn't just restock the pantry; it also clears away decay. Our ancient ancestors often ate only once a day or went for several days without any food, so our autophagy switches were constantly getting tripped.[237] Today, in our three-meals-a-day world, our cells no longer need to look under the couch cushions for sustenance, and the trash heaps just pile higher.

In the modern context of not only having relatively easy access to sufficient nutrients but to food in excess, our baseline rate of autophagy is low[238] and slips down even lower as we get older. A decline in autophagic capacity with age has been described in nearly all animals analyzed.[239] This can lead to more accumulation of cellular debris, which can then further impair our aging cells. This may be why inadequate autophagy is not just a consequence of aging but is considered to be one of its causes.

Autophagy is critical for most lifespan-enhancing interventions. Whether through diet, drugs, or genetic manipulations, if autophagy pathways are blocked, so, too, are many pro-longevity effects. What's more, autophagy appears to be not only necessary for life extension but also, in some cases, sufficient.[240] Boosting autophagy alone can lengthen lifespan in mice by an average of 17 percent, as well as improve healthspan.[241] No wonder autophagy is at the forefront of so much longevity research.[242]

FAST OR GO FAST

The most commonly cited inducer of autophagy is dietary restriction, which gives new meaning to the term fasting "cleanse,"[243] but autophagy doesn't really maximally ramp up until twenty-four to forty-eight hours of fasting, which is too long to go unsupervised.[244] (See page 563, Don't Try This at Home.) However, moderate dietary restriction over the long term may also work, based on muscle biopsies taken from volunteers of the Calorie Restriction Society. See details in see.nf/fast.

Dietary restriction has been called the "safest way" to stimulate autophagy,[245] but that distinction probably belongs to exercise, though it may take sixty minutes or more of moderate to vigorous aerobic exercise (55 to 70 percent VO_2 max).[246] Again, more details in the video. High-intensity interval training didn't seem to make a difference,[247] and to date, data are insufficient to characterize the autophagy response to resistance exercise.[248]

FOODS THAT MAY IMPAIR AUTOPHAGY

As I discussed in the last chapter, we know that the enzyme AMPK activates autophagy. So, anything that suppresses AMPK activation, like saturated fat intake, may also suppress autophagy. Inversely, the enzyme mTOR (see the chapter on mTOR) deactivates autophagy,[249] so anything that activates mTOR, like animal protein,[250] may also suppress the autophagy process. When study participants completely fasted for thirty-six hours and were then given a whey protein drink, their autophagy levels were suppressed significantly more than if they were given even more calories of straight carbohydrate.[251] Some carbohydrate-rich foods, though, notably french fries and potato chips,[252] may inhibit autophagy through another mechanism, acrylamide.

Watch see.nf/acrylamide for details, but basically, acrylamide is a chemical formed when carbohydrates are exposed to particularly high temperatures that can inhibit autophagy, at least in cells in a petri dish.[253] This may explain why high acrylamide exposure is associated with increased mortality.[254] A diminished lifespan among frequent eaters of fast food and salty snacks isn't exactly a revelation, but an experiment I profile in the video comparing the effects of potato chips to boiled potatoes mixed with the same fat and salt does seem to implicate the chemical,[255] though acrylamide isn't the only potentially harmful by-product of deep frying. As one of the earliest geriatric medicine textbooks presciently concluded in 1849, "frying is an abomination."[256]

FOODS THAT MAY BOOST AUTOPHAGY

Any food that activates AMPK should also activate autophagy, so any of the AMPK-boosting foods in the previous chapter should fit the bill. However, autophagy can also be activated directly in pathways independent of AMPK. The most reliable way to kick autophagy into high gear may be to eat less food altogether, but there is a downside to dietary restriction: Starving yourself, as was understated in a major review, "generates discomfort."[257] There is, however, something we can consume that induces autophagy that many find comforting: coffee.

COFFEE

We've long known that alcohol consumption is associated with liver inflammation, but a group of Norwegian researchers made an unexpected finding back in 1986: Coffee consumption is associated with *less* liver inflammation.[258] Subsequent studies conducted around the world replicated their results. In the United States, for example, researchers looked at people at high risk for liver disease—those who were overweight or drank alcohol in excess, for instance—and found that those who drank more than two cups of coffee a day appeared to have less than half the risk of developing chronic liver problems as those who drank less than one cup.[259] The fact that regular coffee consumption seems protective against the development of fatty liver disease[260] gave researchers an idea.

Since autophagy plays such an important role in clearing fat out of the liver,[261] they tested whether caffeine might have cell-cleansing properties. Indeed, it was found to be a potent autophagy stimulant.[262] So, does coffee or caffeine extend the lifespan of model organisms like yeast and worms? Yes[263] and yes.[264] Mice, too. In mice, coffee rapidly triggered autophagy within hours at a human-equivalent dose. Moreover, the autophagy-promoting properties of coffee were independent of the caffeine content—decaffeinated coffee worked just as well.[265] Both regular and decaf also had similar anti-aging effects on another aging pathway (mTOR)—in mice.[266] What about in people?

Good Until You Last Drop

A systematic review of the health impacts of coffee concluded that "daily coffee consumption should be encouraged" in patients with chronic liver disease.[267] If coffee enhances autophagy, shouldn't its benefits extend to a wide range of diseases? Yes. Intake is also associated with lower risk of kidney disease,[268] along with reduced risk of conditions as varied as gout, type 2 diabetes, skin cancer, and Parkinson's disease. Decaf was also associated with a range of health benefits.[269] The results are all the more remarkable because many of the studies failed to adequately control for smoking and unhealthy food intake, both of which tend to accompany coffee drinking.[270] So, coffee drinkers appeared to be healthier in spite of their tendency for less wholesome habits. Does all this translate into them living longer? Apparently so.

Interventional studies on rats showing that coffee can improve lifespans go back to the 1940s.[271] We only have observational research on coffee and mortality in humans, but, to date, more than twenty studies following more than ten million individuals over time have found that, overall, those drinking three cups of coffee a day had 13 percent lower risk of death from any cause.[272] If practiced throughout adulthood, that would be expected to translate into approximately an extra year of life.[273]

Three cups of decaf appeared to be just as protective, so it's not the caffeine.[274] This is supported by data showing the longevity link extended similarly to those who were genetically slow caffeine metabolizers and others who metabolize caffeine more quickly.[275] If it's not the caffeine, then what is it? Coffee contains more than a thousand bioactive compounds. The polyphenol chlorogenic acid is the most abundant antioxidant in coffee beans,[276] so researchers started there and indeed found that it was able to enhance autophagy in cultured human cells.[277]

How to Brew the Most Healthful Cup

More than a hundred coffees have been tested, and the levels of chlorogenic acids varied by more than thirtyfold. Interestingly, the major contributor widening the range was the coffee purchased from Starbucks, which had an extremely low chlorogenic acid content, averaging ten times lower than the others.[278] This may be because Starbucks roasts its beans so dark.[279] Caffeine is relatively stable to heat, but a dark roast may wipe out nearly 90 percent of the chlorogenic acid in the beans.[280] The difference between a medium light roast and a medium roast did not appear to matter, though—at least when it came to boosting the total antioxidant status in people's bloodstreams after drinking the coffees.[281]

Don't be fooled by "low acid" coffee. It doesn't help with the acid reflux, heartburn, or stomach upset that plagues some coffee drinkers. The low acid is a reference to low *chlorogenic* acid—which is exactly what we don't want. Low-acid coffee producers use a slow roasting process that destroys the autophagy-activating compound. That's like an orange juice company going out of its way to destroy the vitamin C and then branding its OJ as "low acid." Technically true, since vitamin C is ascorbic acid, but the OJ maker would be bragging about de-stroying some of the nutrition, and that's exactly what low-acid coffee companies are doing.[282]

Save Room for Milk in Your Coffee?

Adding dairy milk or creamer may undercut some of coffee's benefits. The milk protein casein binds to chlorogenic acid and thereby may block its absorption in the digestive tract.[283] Based on human urine studies, drinking coffee with milk cuts bioavailability of chlorogenic acid, dropping it from 68 percent (in black coffee) down to 40 percent (in a latte).[284] Milk protein can also undercut the benefits of tea,[285] berries,[286] and chocolate.[287]

What about soymilk? In a test tube, phytonutrients in coffee not only bind to proteins in dairy but also in eggs and soy.[288] Eggs haven't been put to the test yet in humans, so the jury's still out on whether having an omelet with black coffee would impair absorption, but soy appears to have been given the all-clear. Soy proteins initially bind up the coffee compounds in the small intestine, but our good bacteria release them so they can be absorbed down in the lower intestine.[289] Other nondairy milks, such as almond-, rice-, oat-, and coconut-based milks, have so little protein that I'd assume there wouldn't be a binding issue, but they have yet to be directly tested.

The freeze-drying and spray-drying processes used to make instant coffee don't seem to significantly affect levels of chlorogenic acids, but the preparation method used to make fresh coffee does. Brewed coffee has higher chlorogenic acid content than espresso, presumably due to the longer contact time between water and coffee grounds, as well as the greater ultimate volume.[290]

The brewing method also affects the impact of coffee on our cholesterol. Watch see.nf/cafestol to see why paper-filtered is preferable. A study out of Norway following half a million men and women for an average of twenty years appeared to corroborate the cholesterol concern on a population scale. Those drinking paper-filtered coffee had even lower mortality rates than those drinking unfiltered coffee.[291] These findings led some to bemoan the growing popularity of "unfiltered" brews from capsule coffee machines,[292] but the little plastic cups, like K-cups, actually have a paper filter inside. Capsule coffee does end up with more estrogen-like chemicals in it,[293] as one would expect from heating nearly any sort of plastic (BPA-free or not),[294] but the levels found were low compared to established safety guidelines.[295]

Grounds for Concern?

Coffee is not for everyone. People with glaucoma[296] or perhaps even merely a family history of it[297] may want to stay away from caffeinated coffee. Consumption is also associated with urinary incontinence in women[298] and men.[299] There are case reports of individuals with epilepsy having fewer seizures after laying off coffee, so avoiding it is certainly worth a try if you have a seizure disorder.[300] Coffee may also worsen acid reflux disease.[301] Finally, it almost goes without saying that if you have trouble sleeping, you might not want to drink too much caffeine. Just a single cup of caffeinated coffee at night can cause a significant deterioration in sleep quality.[302]

There are also consistent associations between drinking coffee and certain adverse outcomes during pregnancy, including miscarriage, early preterm birth, and low birth weight. Coffee consumption has not been linked to birth defects, but it may increase the risk of childhood leukemia.[303]

Also, don't stick it up your butt. A recent review on the questionable safety of coffee enemas warned against their use, citing reports of colitis, electrolyte imbalance, rectal burns, and perforation.[304]

Keep in mind that daily consumption of caffeinated beverages can lead to physical dependence. It's no coincidence that Americans alone spend nearly $75 billion annually on the stuff.[305] Caffeine withdrawal symptoms can include days of headache, fatigue, difficulty concentrating, and mood disturbances.[306] Ironically, coffee's tendency to be habit-forming could turn out to be a good thing. If coffee is indeed confirmed to induce autophagy and increase longevity, then a daily habit may ultimately prove to be an advantage.[307]

SPERMIDINE

In 1676, Antonie van Leeuwenhoek, the father of microscopy, was the first person in history to see bacteria. The following year, he saw his own sperm,[308] and a year after that, in 1678, he discovered tiny crystals forming in the semen he had left sitting around.[309] Centuries later, this compound would be recognized as spermine. It and its precursor spermidine are actually found throughout the body, so their names are just an accident of history. It was independently discovered in brain tissue in 1885 and named "neuridine," but when it was revealed to be the same as spermine, naming rights defaulted to the indelicate original.[310]

Spermidine plays a key role in regulating cell growth.[311] It is positively charged, so it naturally binds to negatively charged molecules like DNA.[312] Spermidine fits neatly in both the major and minor grooves of the DNA helix.[313] Most spermidine in our body is actively bound to our genetic material,[314] stabilizing our genetic code for proper translation.[315] Spermidine is also a potent activator of autophagy.

The spermidine in our tissues is obtained from three sources. Our cells can make it from scratch from an amino acid called arginine, as can certain bacteria in our gut, or we can get it preformed directly through our diet.[316] Certain foods are naturally rich in it. Once ingested, dietary spermidine is rapidly absorbed and circulates throughout our body to contribute to cellular pools.[317] Feed extra spermidine to mice, and they live up to 25 percent longer and have more healthful lives.[318] Similar lifespan and healthspan benefits were also found across other tested species, as detailed in the landmark paper "Induction of Autophagy by Spermidine Promotes Longevity."[319]

The problem is that spermidine levels decline with age. Ours tend to drop by more than half by the time we reach our fifties.[320] This decline is seen across the biological spectrum, but there is a remarkable exception.[321]

The naked mole rat (sometimes referred to by its cuddly nickname, sand puppy) lives an astonishing ten to twenty times longer than other rodents of a similar size without showing any signs of visible aging.[322] They can live for decades without exhibiting typical indications of deterioration, such as loss of fertility or muscle mass. The naked mole rat is considered a "non-aging mammal." This amazing feat may have to do with the maintenance of consistently high levels of spermidine throughout their lifetime, because the same has been found in human centenarians.[323]

Researchers in Italy found that by the time most people reached their sixties and seventies, their spermidine levels had already fallen to about a third of what they measured in middle age. But those living into their nineties and beyond were somehow able to maintain their youthful spermidine levels, presumably by just making more of it internally. However, we could also replenish declining levels *externally* with a spermidine-rich diet. The researchers suggested foods like soybeans and mushrooms,[324] but, as we'll learn, wheat germ is an even more concentrated natural source.

What's particularly encouraging about the rodent studies is that the extra dietary spermidine extended lifespans even when started late in life in older mice,[325] the human equivalent of changing your diet when you're already in your fifties.[326] Significant anti-aging effects were also found throughout vital organs—in the heart, kidneys,[327] and liver—and in boosted autophagy in the brain.[328]

Wheat Germ vs. Dementia

In see.nf/wheatgermdementia, I review all the trials of spermidine for cognition, including a remarkable study in which those with mild dementia randomized to eat rolls made with added wheat germ (versus wheat bran) experienced cognitive improvements "way beyond all available antidementia treatments so far."[329]

Letting Your Hair Down

Our hair follicles, as one of the most highly active tissues in all of mammalian biology, are like little spermidine-generating machines. In see.nf/spermidinehair, I show how taking the amount of spermidine in a daily half teaspoon of wheat germ[330] can significantly reduce hair shedding (as determined by the so-called pull test) compared to placebo even months after the study ended.[331]

Out-of-Antibody Experience

Long-term immunity requires the maintenance of Methuselahian antibody-producing cells, yet the level of spermidine in our cells drops as we age, a decline in autophagy follows, and the ability of our immune cells to function declines.[332] As I show in see.nf/immuneheart, a restoration of youthful spermidine levels can improve antibody production in immune cells taken from older adults,[333] suggesting that spermidine may help "reverse immune aging."[334]

For the Faint of Heart

In see.nf/immuneheart, I also review the evidence that led to the medical journal editorial "Spermidine to the Rescue for an Aging Heart."[335] The reason people who eat more spermidine tend to have less cardiovascular disease[336] may be that spermidine can restore autophagy in the cells lining our blood vessels that are responsible for healthy artery function.[337]

Spermidine as an "Anti-Aging Vitamin"

Higher levels of dietary spermidine were found to correlate with reduced blood pressure and a lower combined incidence of heart attack, stroke, and death from vascular disease. Okay, but the top sources of spermidine in the population studied were whole wheat, apples, pears, and salad.[338] How do we know spermidine intake wasn't just a proxy for a more healthful diet in general? Only recently did we discover that not only do the apparent benefits appear to be independent of dietary quality but the magnitude of the effect seems unprecedented.

Eight hundred men and women in their forties through eighties were followed for twenty years. Researchers looked at 146 different nutrients in their diet, and the component most predictive of longevity was spermidine. Those who consumed the most spermidine didn't just have lower risk of dying from cardiovascular disease; spermidine intake was associated with a lower risk of *all* major causes of death, which is what we'd expect from an anti-aging agent. Critically, this survival advantage persisted even after controlling for dietary excellence, meaning it didn't appear to be just because they were eating more healthful foods in general.[339]

How big of an effect are we talking about? The mortality rate of those in the top third of spermidine intake (consuming more than about 12 mg a day) was compared to those in the bottom third (consuming less than 9 mg a day). The difference in death rate was as if those eating more spermidine were 5.7 years younger.[340] By eating more of certain foods, it's as if they had effectively turned back the clock nearly six years.

The findings were so extraordinary that, before publication, the researchers sought to replicate their results in an entirely separate cohort of individuals. And, indeed, they arrived at the same conclusion.[341] This led some to propose that, as we age, spermidine approaches the status of a vitamin.[342] When we're younger, we seem to be able to make enough ourselves, but, as we get older, we need to start ensuring that we're getting enough through our diet to maintain autophagy into old age. If spermidine is going to be considered an anti-aging vitamin, where is that "vitamin" found?

Sources of Spermidine

In developed countries, the average intake of spermidine is approximately 10 mg a day.[343] Some countries in Asia and Europe, especially around the Mediterranean,[344] achieve a per capita daily intake closer to 13 mg or higher,[345] while the United States is down at 8 mg,[346] which may not be surprising since vegetables are the main source.[347]

Swedish researchers calculated that a healthy diet would include 25 mg of spermidine for women and 30 mg for men.[348] If those of us in the United States need to bump up our average daily intake from 8 mg, where are we going to find another 20 mg? Rich spermidine sources fall into three main categories: "unprocessed plant-derived foods" (including mushrooms, though they're technically fungi), certain fermented foods[349] (some bacteria can make it, too, if you recall), and select animal viscera (internal organs).

Which are the best sources? There are a number of different ways that you can rank nutrients in food. You could order them by spermidine per calorie to see which has the best bang for your caloric buck. Or you could sort by spermidine per dollar to see which has the best bang for your actual buck. In the medical literature, the most common ranking is by weight, so you can see which foods are most concentrated with spermidine, ounce for ounce. However, this can be misleading for practical purposes. By this measure, dill, for example, has been singled out for its high spermidine content, ranking as high as chickpeas on a pound-for-pound basis,[350] but one serving of

TOP SPERMIDINE SOURCES

(MILLIGRAM PER 100-GRAM SERVING UNLESS OTHERWISE SPECIFIED)

1. 9.7 mg: tempeh[351,352]
2. 9.2 mg: mushrooms[353,354]
3. 9.2 mg: pig pancreas (1 oz)[355]
4. 8.2 mg: natto (1 oz)[356]
5. 6.1 mg: mango (one, 210 g)[357,358]
6. 5.9 mg: edamame[359,360]
7. 5.8 mg: green peas[361,362]
8. 5.7 mg: cheddar (aged one year, 1 oz)[363]
9. 5.5 mg: lentil soup (1 cup)[364]
10. 5.1 mg: soybeans[365]
11. 4.4 mg: lettuce[366]
12. 4.3 mg: polenta[367]
13. 4.3 mg: corn[368,369]
14. 3.8 mg: soymilk (1 cup)[370]
15. 3.8 mg: mussels[371]
16. 3.7 mg: broccoli[372,373]
17. 3.4 mg: cow intestine[374]
18. 2.9 mg: chickpeas[375]
19. 2.8 mg: cauliflower[376,377]
20. 2.7 mg: celeriac[378]
21. 2.6 mg: yellow peas[379]
22. 2.5 mg: wheat germ (1 Tb)[380]
23. 2.5 mg: french fries[381]
24. 2.4 mg: oysters[382]
25. 2.4 mg: lentils[383]
26. 2.4 mg: adzuki beans[384,385,386]
27. 2.3 mg: eel livers (1 oz)[387]
28. 2.2 mg: salad[388]
29. 2.1 mg: popcorn (50 g)[389]
30. 2.0 mg: kidney beans[390]

low, averaging 0.4 mg per 3-oz serving and only 0.2 mg in fish.[426] The meat with the most is mussel muscle. Scallops and clams don't seem to have as much,[427] but oysters and mussels make the chart.[428]

If one wanted to extend the chart down to 1.5 mg per serving, the next entries would be 1.9 mg in a potato (170 g),[429,430,431] 1.8 mg in rabbit liver (1 oz),[432] 1.8 mg in pine nuts (1 oz),[433] 1.7 mg in asparagus,[434] 1.6 mg in peanuts (1 oz),[435] 1.6 mg in cucumber,[436] 1.5 mg in rabbit spleen (1 oz), 1.5 mg in pig lung (1 oz),[437] and 1.5 mg in black-eyed peas.[438,439] Although separate components may not make the cut, a composite food like a PB&J could, with its 1.6 mg in the ounce of peanuts (about 2 tablespoons) and 1.3 mg found in two slices of whole-wheat bread.[440] That's in quarter-can-of-chickpeas territory. A hummus sandwich could score even higher.

Hard to Swallow

This line in a medical journal gave me a double take: "Spermidine is also contained in fruits, such as mango, in semen, and especially in red wine."[441] That's quite the spunky cocktail! Mangos finish cum laude, but wine doesn't actually have much at all. And semen?

You can imagine how giddy headline writers were to the news that spermidine boosts longevity. *Cosmo* ran a column.[442] Provocative titles included "Drinking Semen Might Help You Live Longer."[443]

Since there's only about one calorie per teaspoon of semen,[444] on a spermidine-per-calorie basis, even lentil soup is no match. But, based on an average of five dozen men, each "serving" only contains 0.1 mg, so, nope. Semen doesn't make the chart.[445]

Wheat Germ

The spermidine in semen is a testament (from the Latin *testis*, but for "witness," not "testicles")[446] to its DNA-protective effects. The same is true for wheat germ, which is the tiny plant embryo within the whole-wheat kernel. Though it falls relatively far down the chart in spermidine per serving, you'll notice it has the smallest serving size, just one tablespoon or 7 g.[447] So, on a volume or weight basis, wheat germ reigns supreme.

It's also the cheapest source of spermidine, as low as two cents per mg. Wheat germ is a by-product of the white flour milling industry and typically just discarded, which may account for its reasonable price.[448] You know something's a bargain when it can even beat out dried beans in nutrient per dollar.

Pop a Spermidine Supplement?

I was surprised to read that spermidine supplements were not commercially available.[449] That couldn't be true. I searched online and *poof*—there it was, a bottle plastered with the word SPERMIDINE. But, if you read the label, you can see it's just wheat germ stuffed into capsules. Not even an extract. Literally straight wheat germ.

On the one hand, it's nice to see supplement manufacturers not trying to concoct some proprietary formula. For example, to meet the turmeric quota in my Daily Dozen (see *How Not to Die*), I often just take the spice in capsule form since I don't always want to curry up my meals. It may be harder to find straight turmeric spice in capsules, as opposed to some patented extract, but if you can, the price premium for convenience is steep.

Unlike turmeric, the taste of wheat germ is pretty neutral, and I've found I can just sprinkle it onto foods. (I mix it with ground flaxseeds, also from my Daily Dozen.) You can buy wheat germ in bulk for as low as $3 a pound. In capsule form, wheat germ comes out to more than $200 per pound, which is at least a dollar per teaspoon as opposed to just a penny or two.

With a Little Help from Our Little Friends

At sufficient doses, wheat germ can also help control cholesterol, triglycerides,[450] diabetic blood sugars,[451] and pain, fatigue, headache, and mood swings associated with painful periods.[452] (Details in see.nf/wheatgerm.) It can also boost *Bifidobacteria* in the gut. A common constituent of commercial probiotics, *Bifidobacteria* are considered one of the proxies for a beneficial balance of good bugs in general[453] and may even have the knock-on effect of adding extra spermidine to the system.

Our good gut flora produce spermidine that can then get absorbed into our bloodstream from our colon and circulate throughout the body.[454] Eating tempeh or sprinkling wheat germ onto dishes can provide periodic bumps at meals, but even better if your microbiome were making it 24/7.[455] In fact, our good gut bacteria probably churn out more spermidine than most of us eat.[456] So, we may be getting less spermidine from the top down than the bottom up, though this may change as we age.

Spermidine levels don't just decline in our bloodstream as we get older but in our stool, too.[457] Feces of thirty-year-olds have more than twice the spermidine concentration of those of eighty-year-olds,[458] and this decline has been linked to changes in our microbiome.[459]

Give people a strain of probiotic *Bifidobacteria*, and you can increase spermidine levels in their stool.[460] The same strain given to mice had the same effect. Enough to prolong their lives? Yes. A boost in spermidine-producing friendly flora was shown to improve the healthspan and lifespan of the mice[461]— even protection from age-induced memory impairment.[462] What about in people?

A symbiotic combination of prebiotics and spermidine-producing *Bifidobacteria* was able to increase spermidine levels in people's blood. This then translated in a randomized, double-blind, placebo-controlled trial to improve endothelial function,[463] thought due to a boost of autophagy.[464] Spermidine-producing bacteria are fiber-feeding,[465] so prebiotics alone would likely foster the growth of more spermidine producers. Then, even if you miss a day, your colonic colleagues can pick up the slack. Since beans and whole grains are leading sources of spermidine and also the fiber and resistant starch our good bugs eat, they may offer a double dose of cellular spring cleaning.

Who Shouldn't Up Their Spermidine?

The lack of reported side effects[466] is not surprising, given that our own body makes so much of it and spermidine's found naturally in some of the very foods associated with health and longevity.[467] But, is it safe for everyone? I note in see.nf/spermidinedownsides who might want to be cautious about attempting to restore youthful spermidine levels. Though spermidine may reduce the risk of getting cancer,[468] because autophagy's nutrient replenishment action could potentially help sustain tumor viability,[469] perhaps people with cancer shouldn't go out of their way to increase their spermidine intake.[470] The other group I would advise caution for are those with kidney failure.[471]

Spermidine Bottom Line

Given the safety and efficacy of spermidine to induce autophagy at achievable dietary doses, it is one of the most promising anti-aging compounds. DrugAge is an extensive online database[472] of more than five hundred lifespan-extending compounds.[473] Among the small subset with the fewest side effects, spermidine had the largest documented lifespan extension.[474] A "predominantly plant-based diet" has therefore been recommended to help counteract the decline in spermidine as we age.[475] Certain foods have more than others, though. While some have suggested the genetic engineering of high-spermidine transgenic potatoes,[476] there are already a plethora of naturally spermidine-rich foods.

Food for Thought

Autophagy is considered the "primary system for cleaning the body" from the inside out.[477] Some food components, like acrylamide, may suppress autophagy, whereas others, like spermidine, can boost the process. Chlorogenic acids in coffee can also help your cells take out the trash. What's more, autophagy can be boosted indirectly by amping AMPK or quelling mTOR.

To help boost this anti-aging pathway, on a daily basis, consider:
- 60 minutes of moderate to vigorous aerobic activity
- minimizing your intake of french fries and potato chips
- trying to consume at least 20 mg of spermidine by incorporating foods such as tempeh, mushrooms, peas, and wheat germ into your diet
- drinking three cups of regular or decaffeinated coffee
- instituting the recommendations to activate AMPK (see the AMPK chapter)
- following the recommendations to suppress mTOR (see the mTOR chapter)

CELLULAR SENESCENCE

Fifty years ago, microbiologist Leonard Hayflick demonstrated that, contrary to what was believed, human cells in a petri dish do not continue to double forever.[478] They only grow and divide about fifty times before entering an irreversible state of arrested replication, known as cellular senescence.[479] Senescence comes from the Latin word *senex*, meaning "growing old."[480] We always have immortal stem cells that can create new cells with a fresh start, but, once they form, they only have about fifty divisions before they, too, are dead in the water. This is a good thing.

This natural "Hayflick limit" helps protect the body against cancer by blocking the proliferation of damaged cells.[481] That's great for successfully getting us through reproductive age and passing along our genes, but what happens when the "natural" human lifespan of about thirty years gets extended to eighty years or more by miracles like sanitation? Our body ends up littered with senescent cells.[482]

ZOMBIE CELLS

Hayflick figured that these nondividing cells might contribute to aging simply because they had lost their capacity to participate in tissue repair and regeneration.[483] Instead, it turns out they *actively damage* surrounding tissues, earning them the moniker "zombie cells."[484] The problem with zombies isn't only that they are no longer productive members of society. They also want to eat your brains.

When we are younger, senescent cells are cleared by our immune system. When our cells reach their limit and are ready to retire, they are programmed to start releasing a cocktail of inflammatory chemicals called the senescence-associated secretory phenotype, or SASP. Inflammation, a process that often carries negative connotations, can sometimes be a benefit. Just like inflammation caused by a splinter draws immune cells out of circulation to a puncture wound, senescent cells make their own funeral arrangements by releasing inflammatory factors to flag themselves for immune clearance.[485] There's a problem, though. As we age, more and more senescent cells are piling up at the very same time that our immune systems are falling into disarray. So, the localized transient inflammation that is usually beneficial, like in the splinter scenario, develops into a detriment—the chronic systemic inflammation that characterizes aging and disease.

Even though the senescent cell burden in aged tissues represents just a small fraction of total cells,[486] they can have an outsized impact through SASP secretion, which can disrupt local tissue architecture and spill out into circulation.[487] What is frequently the largest organ in the human body? Is it the liver? The skin? No. In a growing number of people, it's our adipose tissue—that is, body fat. The inflammation related to obesity, which tends to worsen with age,[488] has been tied to the buildup of SASP-producing senescent fat cells.[489] SASP inflammation may even account for some of the most dreaded side effects of chemotherapy. Chemo works by successfully driving cancer cells senescent, but the ensuing SASP storm can drive bone marrow suppression and heart toxicity.

With all this SASP inflammation, it is no surprise that senescent cells are connected to a spectrum of age-related diseases, including Alzheimer's, Parkinson's, osteoarthritis, osteoporosis, herniated discs, spinal curvature, and loss of muscle mass and kidney function.[490,491] Even cancer, ironically. Although cellular senescence likely evolved as an anticancer mechanism, late in life the excess inflammation can actively feed tumor growth—as in feed quite literally via angiogenesis, the sprouting of new blood vessels into the tumor.[492] But, how do we know cellular senescence is the cause rather than the consequence of disease?

Young Blood

In see.nf/parabiosis, I detail a macabre set of experiments showing that old animals surgically conjoined like "Siamese twins" to young animals grow healthier, stronger, and smarter,[493] and live significantly longer.[494] To determine if this was due to transmissible bloodborne factors rather than just shared organ capacity, researchers turned to transfusing old animals with young blood. I explore those vampire 2.0 experiments in see.nf/bloodboy.

Yes, the injection of blood from young mice into old improves cognition, for example, suggesting there's some sort of restorative factor in youthful blood, but the injection of blood from old mice into young can make things worse, suggesting there's some sort of debilitating factor in older blood.[495] Or, maybe the old blood is just diluting the revitalizing factor in the young mouse? For that matter, maybe the young blood is diluting the debilitating factor in the old mouse.[496] Amazingly, the latter seems closer to what's happening, as the simple dilution of blood in older animals can replicate much of the regeneration found in the parabiotic and transfusion studies.[497] And indeed, patients with moderate Alzheimer's randomized to blood dilution experienced about 60 percent less cognitive and functional decline over a period of fourteen months compared to a sham, placebo procedure.[498] The advantage over blood transfusions, as the director of the University of Zurich's Institute of Biomedical Ethics put it: "There is something peculiar about the old literally feeding on the young."[499]

OUT WITH THE OLD

Researchers proved cause and effect by transplanting senescent cells from older mice into younger ones, and all it took were a few to cause persistent age-related physical dysfunction and a quintupling of their mortality.[500] Conversely, clearing even a fraction of senescent cells can profoundly delay tumor development and age-related organ deterioration.[501] The marked extension of healthspan and lifespan through senescent cell clearance sparked a gold rush to identify *senolytics*, compounds that can eliminate senescent cells.[502] In my video see.nf/senolytics, I review both drug and lifestyle approaches.

In short, cellular senescence can be thwarted by preventing our DNA from becoming damaged beyond repair in the first place (see page 109). Senescent cells can then be eliminated by exercise[503] and caloric restriction[504] (details in see.nf /senolytics), as well as a variety of dietary components.

QUERCETIN

In 1936, Albert Szent-Györgyi, who won the Nobel Prize the following year for discovering vitamin C, suggested that a class of phytonutrients called flavonols should also be considered a vitamin. (He suggested "vitamin P.")[505] The most common flavonol in the diet is quercetin,[506] which is found concentrated in onions, kale, and apples.[507] It's what gives apple peels their bitter taste.[508] Researchers had been testing dozens of different compounds on cells scraped from umbilical cords and then irradiated to force senescence. In 2015, they announced their results: Quercetin was a natural senolytic.[509]

More details in see.nf/quercetin, but, bottom line, quercetin doses as low as the human equivalent of one small apple a week reduced cellular senescence and improved the healthspan of aging mice. For example, they experienced less hair loss, had enhanced heart function, and gained greater athletic endurance into the equivalent of their sixties.[510] So, we may want to share a few kale stems with our pet mouse, but what about people?

Sources of Quercetin

Quercetin can also be found in its namesake—oak trees, from the Latin *quercus*[511]—but it is considered "widespread in plant-based foods."[512] In fact, quercetin is so pervasive in the plant kingdom that it can even be found in iceberg lettuce.[513] (Lettuce is the fifth leading source of quercetin in the American diet.[514]) Onions have between 20 mg[515] and 100 mg[516] each, apples between 4 mg and 20 mg,[517] a one-pound bunch of kale may have 50 mg, and a cup of tea about 5 mg.[518] Capers have 20 mg per tablespoon, but stay away from high-sodium brands.[519] (I've seen capers in the market with anything between 0 and 200 percent of your entire daily sodium limit per serving.)

Although quercetin supplements procured online tend to be accurately labeled[520] and there are safety data to suggest no significant adverse effects to taking as much as 1,000 mg for as long as twelve weeks, I recommend sticking to dietary sources,[521] as does the Mayo Clinic team who established the field.[522]

Apples and Onions

It's hard to tease out the effects of quercetin from the range of salutary effects attributed to quercetin-rich foods, such as apples and onions. I note in see.nf/applesonions how the wisdom of *an apple a day keeps the doctor away*, a public health aphorism dating back to 1866, seems to have borne fruit.[523] It appears to be less the apple of one's eye than the apple of one's arteries. Significantly better improvement in artery function within hours of eating unpeeled apples than after eating apples that had been peeled[524] is consistent with a quercetin effect, and indeed, even isolated quercetin supplements can lower blood pressure,[525] cholesterol,[526] and inflammation.[527] Unfortunately, quercetin-rich onion powder failed to improve cognition in elderly with[528] or without[529] Alzheimer's disease. (Details in see.nf/onionpowder.)

Although most of the quercetin supplement studies used doses not easily achievable through diet, even just three-quarters of a teaspoon of fresh onion can acutely improve blood pressure and fluidity compared to placebo,[530] helping to explain why those who consume more quercetin appear to have less than half the risk of dying from heart disease.[531] A modeling study even suggested that prescribing an apple a day could prevent about as many deaths from vascular disease on a population scale as prescribing everyone a cholesterol-lowering statin drug—and with fewer side effects.[532] (Ironically, now that drugs like Lipitor are available in generic form, the drug would likely be cheaper than the fruit.)

A New Wrinkle

The disappointing interventional cognition data were met in 2018 by a report questioning quercetin's senolytic activity. The original quercetin studies in people had been performed on cells from the lining of umbilical cord blood vessels, a convenient source of human tissue. When the experiment was repeated with cells from adult donors, though, quercetin didn't seem to have the same senescent cell–killing effect.[533] However, in 2019, quercetin was found to do something even better.

Werner syndrome is a rare genetic disease characterized by a mutation of a DNA repair enzyme that results in premature aging. When senescent Werner cells were exposed to the levels of quercetin one could get in the bloodstream by eating quercetin-rich foods,[534] they seemed to be rehabilitated rather than eradicated.[535] It appeared as though the senescence was reversed, like waking the living dead. What about aging cells that aren't mutated? A "rejuvenating effect" on senescent cells was found there as well. In the journal *Experimental Gerontology*, researchers in Greece claimed to have put quercetin to the test topically on volunteers and reported "positive results as regards to [skin] elasticity, moisturization and depth of wrinkles,"[536] but their data do not appear to have been published, which raises concerns about the veracity of the claims.

FISETIN

Given the senolytic success of a quercetin cocktail, researchers started screening other flavonoids.[537] In doing so, they found one that was nearly twice as potent: fisetin.[538] It can increase the lifespan of yeast by 55 percent and fruit flies by 23 percent. Fisetin can also increase the lifespan of mice even when begun later in life.[539] When started at an age roughly equivalent to seventy-five years in humans, fisetin extended the average and maximum lifespans of older mice by about 75 percent. Markers of cellular senescence and SASP were significantly reduced in all analyzed tissues in conjunction with a reduction in age-related pathology.[540] A separate study found that fisetin can also increase long-term memory in mice.[541] What about us?

Like quercetin, fisetin has been shown to have anti-inflammatory effects in clinical trials,[542] but what about senolytic effects? When human fatty tissue that had been removed during routine surgery was exposed to fisetin, there was indeed a reduction of senescence and SASP markers. Given that fisetin is naturally found in the diet, has no reported side effects, and is already sold over the counter in dietary supplements, researchers immediately started designing studies to put fisetin's anti-aging potential to the test.[543] Currently, there are more than a dozen trials in the works, pitting fisetin against a range of age-related conditions, including osteoarthritis, osteoporosis, frailty, kidney disease, cognitive decline, and even COVID-19 complications.[544] The fact that there is so much clinical interest in a natural product that lacks the financial incentives that traditionally drive so much of biomedical research speaks to its promise.

Berried Treasure

Though first isolated from Venetian sumach, fisetin is concentrated in strawberries, the richest known dietary source.[545] This may help explain why strawberries, but not blueberries (despite having even more antioxidants), were able to more effectively rescue rats exposed to radiation.[546] I run through all the landmark strawberry studies in see.nf/fisetin. In short, randomized controlled trials show that strawberries can improve cognition,[547] cholesterol, inflammation,[548] and osteoarthritis,[549] as well as boost beneficial gut bugs, including *Christensenellaceae*,[550] a newly discovered[551] bacterial family found associated with longevity based on studies of centenarians and supercentenarians.[552] In the video, I also explain why fisetin supplements are not recommended.

PIPPALI

A third natural senolytic compound has been discovered: piperlongumine,[553] found concentrated in a spice commonly sold in Indian grocery stores as pippali (*Piper longum*, also known as pibo in China and long pepper in Europe).[554] I detail what it is and what it can do in <u>see.nf/pippali</u>. I was convinced enough to add it to my daily spice regimen alongside amla (see page 503), black cumin (see page 19), and turmeric (see page 97). Note that the use of pippali during pregnancy and breast-feeding is not recommended.[555]

Food for Thought

Cellular senescence is considered to be one of the foundational hallmarks of aging.[556] The inflammatory SASP, secreted by senescent cells, is thought to be a main driver of tissue deterioration and disease.[557] To prevent cellular senescence in the first place, we can avert DNA damage by following the recommendations in the Oxidation chapter, and, to potentially help clear such cells and their SASP, there are natural senolytic compounds in foods—quercetin, fisetin, and piper-longumine. Although it is not yet clear whether sufficient levels can be reached by eating foods rich in these compounds, such foods are healthful in their own right.

To help slow this aging pathway, on a daily basis, consider:
- consuming quercetin-rich foods, beverages, and seasonings, such as onions, apples, kale, tea, and salt-free capers
- eating fresh, frozen, or freeze-dried strawberries
- seasoning meals with pippali (long pepper)

EPIGENETICS

Until recently, the aging process was considered to be an inexorable decline characterized by the cumulative buildup of molecular damage to key cellular components, particularly our very DNA.[558] Just as the various components of a car eventually break down with time, so do the components of our body. Challenging this assumption were life-forms that could seemingly defy aging by attaining a sort of state of suspended animation, such as date pits unearthed during archaeological digs germinating after thousands of years,[559] plants regenerating from fruits buried by Arctic squirrels 30,000 years before,[560] and bacterial spores viable after tens of millions of years encased in amber or hundreds of millions of years preserved in salt crystals. However, one need not seek exotic examples to demonstrate the uncoupling of biological aging with chronological ("calendar") aging. Instances of the aging clock not only being halted but actively reversed and even reset to zero happen every day.[561]

THE GREAT RESET

Think about it. A baby girl is born with all the eggs she will ever have. It may be decades before one of those eggs is fertilized. That egg could be sitting in her ovaries for twenty, thirty, forty years—all the while, aging just like every other cell in her body. Let's say she gets pregnant at thirty. Upon fertilization, if that egg doesn't somehow rewind its aging clock to zero, then that thirty-year-old egg could lead to the birth of another baby girl with ovaries that are then thirty years and nine months old. By the time she gave birth decades later, the eggs would be more than fifty years old and they would continue to age and accumulate molecular damage with every successive generation. This is why, necessarily, all manifestations of aging in egg cells must be erased.[562] Otherwise, the eggs in women's ovaries would be millions of years old!

In 1996, we learned that eggs aren't the only cells that can undergo a complete reversal of aging. That was the year a sheep named Dolly was born. The nucleus of an unfertilized egg was removed and, in its place, the nucleus of an udder cell was inserted. ("Dolly is derived from a mammary gland cell," one of the key researchers said unabashedly while explaining her namesake, "and we couldn't think of a more impressive pair of glands than Dolly Parton's.")[563] Then, with a little electric shock, the cell started dividing—no sperm required—and Dolly, the first animal cloned from an adult cell, was born. (Previously, a frog had been cloned from a tadpole cell, earning the researcher the Nobel Prize, but Dolly was the first animal cloned from the cell of an adult.[564])

The world marveled that a genetically identical duplicate of an animal could be created. Since Dolly, thousands of clones have been made of mice, goats, pigs, rats, cows, horses, ferrets, wolves, deer, buffalo, camels, and dogs. Cats, too, the first one predictably named "Copycat."[565] The implications, however, go far beyond replicating particularly productive farm animals or generating Fido 2.0. Hidden within that one mature, specialized cell dedicated to milk production, taken from a sheep's udder, was the full genetic blueprint for the entire animal we'd come to know as Dolly.[566] Furthermore, the cell's age appeared to have rewound back to zero.

There is a lingering misconception that Dolly was beset by some sort of premature aging syndrome. After all, sheep live to be about twelve years old, the mammary cell was taken from a six-year-old,[567] and Dolly died at age six, suggesting that the aging clock had just kept ticking without resetting. But, Dolly died from a viral illness, not old age,[568] and subsequent experience shows clones can have normal lifespans.[569] In fact, mice have been serially recloned—meaning there have been clones made from clones made from clones going out twenty-five generations—and they have all aged normally with respect to lifespan.[570] So, not only can adult cells be dialed back to an embryonic state, but they can effectively be rejuvenated by having any traces of aging wiped clean.[571]

Welcome to epigenetics.

GENES LOAD THE GUN, LIFESTYLE PULLS THE TRIGGER

The term "epigenetics" was coined in the 1940s before we even knew the physical nature of genes, a full decade before Watson and Crick (and Wilkins and Franklin) solved the structure of DNA.[572,573] Epigenetics, which literally means "above genetics," layers an extra level of information on top of the DNA sequence, which on its own is only about 750 megabytes of data[574] encoding 50,000 genes.[575] All our dividing cells are genetically identical, carrying a full complement of our DNA, but each cell doesn't need to express all our tens of thousands of genes. Our nerve cells don't need to be pumping out liver enzymes, and our heart cells don't need to be growing hair. That's where epigenetics comes in—in effect, it's what switches genes on and off. There are a multitude of ways our body does this.[576] I'll talk about sirtuins and microRNAs in their own chapters, but the best-known epigenetic regulator is DNA methylation.[577]

We have enzymes that can strategically add methyl groups directly onto our DNA to silence gene expression. A methyl group is a simple, stable configuration of carbon that can be added to flag stretches of DNA as skippable. It's one of more than a dozen ways DNA can be tagged.[578] We have a separate set of enzymes that can remove these tags to turn the gene back on. There are approximately twenty-eight million common methylation sites along our genetic code, most of which are methylated at any one time.[579] The pattern of methylation is conserved when our cells divide—so a liver cell splits into two new liver cells rather than a bone or muscle cell, for example—and, in this way, methylation patterns in sperm and eggs can be passed down through the generations.[580]

We used to think that once cells matured and had their DNA appropriately methylated to lock them into their specialized functions, that was it.[581] But we now know that our "epigenome," the pattern of methyl markings in our cells, is a dynamic system and responsive to external stimuli. Epigenetics allows organisms to more rapidly adapt to changing environmental conditions.

It can take eons for large-scale shifts in the genetic code to happen, but the genes we already have can be switched on or off within a matter of hours. Epigenetics is how green grasshoppers can turn themselves black after a grassland fire to better camouflage against the charred soil[582] and how our body determines the number of active sweat glands we have in our skin based on whether we're born in the tropics or in a colder setting.[583] Epigenetics is good news. It means our DNA is not our destiny. No matter our family history, the lifestyle choices we make can effectively turn on and off some of our genes, not only affecting us individually but also our kids and maybe even our grandkids.[584]

In the Gene Expression Modulation by Intervention with Nutrition and Lifestyle (GEMINAL) study, Dr. Dean Ornish and colleagues took tissue biopsies before and after subjects adopted intensive lifestyle changes for three months that included a whole food, plant-based diet. Beneficial changes in gene expression were noted for five hundred different genes. The expression of disease-preventing genes was boosted, and the oncogenes that promote breast and prostate cancer, for example, were suppressed.[585] No matter the genes we may have inherited from our parents, we can affect how those genes affect our health with what we eat and how we live. That's the power of epigenetics. Same DNA, but with different results.

The most striking example of the epigenetic effect of diet on lifespan involves the humble honeybee. Queen bees and worker bees are genetically identical, yet queens may live for three years and lay up to 2,000 eggs a day, while worker bees may live for only three weeks and are functionally sterile.[586] How can this be if there is no difference between them genetically? They have a different diet. When the hive's queen is dying, a larva is picked by nurse bees to be fed a secreted substance called royal jelly. (The workers just get mostly a mixture of honey and pollen adorably named *beebread*.)[587] When the chosen larva eats this jelly, the enzyme that had been silencing the expression of royal genes is turned off and a new queen is born.[588] The queen bee has the exact same genes as any of the worker bees, but simply because of what she ate, different genes are expressed, resulting in dramatic alterations to her life and lifespan. A fiftyfold increase in longevity, thanks to epigenetics.

Live Like a Queen?

If royal jelly can turn a simple larva into a queen who can live more than fifty times longer, should we consider eating royal jelly ourselves? I review the available evidence in <u>see.nf/royaljelly</u>. Spoiler alert: While it may be the bee's knees for bees, given rare cases of hemorrhagic (bloody) colitis attributed to royal jelly supplements,[589] eating PB&RJs could just end up being a royal pain in the butt.

THE EPIGENETIC CLOCK

There are certain DNA sites on our chromosomes that so predictably methylate or demethylate as we age that it's like clockwork, presenting a potential "molecular crystal ball for human aging."[590] In a remarkable triumph of Big Data, out of the millions of methylation sites in our DNA, a tiny subset so dependably shifts over time that you can predict someone's age within a few years[591] just by strategically measuring the methylation pattern in a few hundred—or even just a few dozen— sites[592] in someone's three-billion-letter genome.[593]

Over the last few years, these "epigenetic clocks" have become established as robust measures of chronological age, surpassing telomere length (see the Telomeres chapter) as the best age predictor.[594] Why invent some costly Rube Goldberg approach to divining someone's age when you can simply ask them? Well, you can imagine forensic applications, the determination of an unidentified victim's age with a blood or tissue sample, but that just scratches the surface.[595] The kicker is that epigenetic clocks don't just track our chronological age but appear to measure our true biological age.[596] In other words, our epigenetic age can better predict our remaining life expectancy than our calendar age.[597] Check out see.nf/clock for the whole wild story.

It's like science fiction.[598] Feed a drop of your blood into some futuristic machine that scans the placement of chemical markers on a strand of DNA and out pops your true age, reflecting a lifetime of lifestyle choices.[599] In addition to predicting time-to-death, epigenetic clocks also appear to foretell healthspan indicators, such as cognitive decline, frailty,[600] arthritis, and the progression of diseases like Alzheimer's and Parkinson's.[601] As you can imagine, the insurance industry has jumped on this, and your premiums may soon be determined by your epigenetic age.[602] But it's not some set-in-stone fortune teller's curse. You can change the rate at which you age and may soon be able to use epigenetic clocks to track your progress, potentially presenting a radically faster and cheaper way to test anti-aging interventions.[603]

SPEEDING AND SLOWING BIOLOGICAL AGING

Studies of centenarians show that some age so slowly that a 105-year-old may have a DNA methylation age of a 60-year-old.[604] No wonder they lived so long! What can we do to decelerate our epigenetic clocks and slow down aging? Epigenetic clock analyses show that women age more slowly than men,[605] which makes sense since women tend to live longer,[606] a pattern so robust that one demographer quipped, "to be a male is a genetic disease."[607] To catch up, men have to make even healthier changes to their diet and lifestyle.

Cigarette smoke is linked to accelerated biological aging, with marked effects evident even at low levels of exposure.[608] In contrast, both exercise frequency and intensity are associated with a deceleration of aging.[609] What about meditation? Two months of daily practice failed to significantly affect aging rates,[610] and long-term meditators appear to have the same aging rates as nonmeditating controls, though practitioners racking up an average of 6,000 hours of meditation may blunt the increase in epigenetic age acceleration over time.[611]

Until recently, caloric restriction had yet to be tested in people, but it had been shown to slow epigenetic aging in mice and monkeys. Over about a fifteen- to twenty-one-year period of 30 percent dietary restriction, middle-aged rhesus monkeys appeared to epigenetically age seven years less. Even more dramatically, mice at a 40 percent calorie restriction seemed to age only about one year over a period of about three years.[612] In 2018, an aging analysis was published of the CALERIE study, the first major randomized trial of calorie restriction in humans. Using nonepigenetic estimates of biological aging, the control group continued to age at a rate of about one year per year, but in that time, the dietary restriction group only seemed to age by about one *month*. And they achieved this with only a 12 percent calorie restriction, which is like skipping just one donut a day.[613]

Aging rates were slowed in the dietary restriction group independent of weight loss,[614] but obesity has been associated with epigenetic age acceleration in samples of liver tissue[615] and deep abdominal fat.[616] However, even about a hundred pounds of weight loss due to bariatric surgery did not appear to wind back the clock.[617] Maybe we don't just have to eat less, but better.

The lifestyle factor most closely associated with slowing aging—even more than exercise—is a marker of fruit and vegetable intake, blood levels of carotenoid phytonutrients like beta-carotene.[618,619] So, an "epigenetic diet" would focus on consuming more fruits and vegetables.[620] On the other hand, the food most con- sistently linked to accelerating aging is meat.[621,622] Perhaps this is partly due to the fact that blood levels of by-products of banned pesticides like DDT are themselves associated with both accelerated aging[623] and meat consumption.[624] Long-term ex- posure to air pollution may also be associated with accelerated aging,[625] but the data are mixed.[626]

WINDING BACK THE CLOCK

The fact that our epigenetic age is a better predictor of lifespan and several diseases of old age than our chronological age is powerful evidence that DNA methylation is inexorably linked with some fundamental cause of age-related decline.[627] Could it be what's actually driving human aging,[628] or is it merely a passive marker of age?[629]

Is our epigenetic clock the cause of aging or just the result? If it's an active driver, it's a driver that can go in reverse.

Remember how, in cloning, an adult cell could be reprogrammed to revert it into an embryonic state? Not only were methylation marks erased to free up the whole genome, but all vestiges of aging appeared to vanish. We obviously don't want to reset the clock so far back that we dissolve into an amorphous blob, but might we be able to rewind the clock a little and rejuvenate our cells?

In a Nobel Prize–winning discovery,[630] stem cell researcher Shinya Yamanaka identified what we now refer to as Yamanaka factors, a small handful of DNA-binding proteins responsible for cellular reprogramming that serve, in essence, to return a cell to factory settings.[631] With these tools in hand, an international team of researchers set out to turn back the clock by reestablishing the regenerative properties of nerve tissue. For example, young kids can actually regrow an entire amputated fingertip, bone and all, but we gradually lose such capacities as we age.[632] The cells that make up the optic nerves that connect our eyes to our brain similarly lose their regenerative properties. With a little Yamanaka factor manipulation, however, the researchers were able to successfully reset the methylation marks to a more youthful state, restoring vision in old mice and rejuvenating human neurons in a petri dish. The cells seemed to have retained a faithful copy of the epigenetic map from earlier in life that could serve as directions to reverse aging.[633]

METHYLATION CALIBRATION

Increasing our access to exercise, fruits, and vegetables while reducing our consumption of tobacco and meat may help slow aging, as evidenced by a deceleration of the epigenetic clock, but what about directly changing DNA methylation? A lot of things affect methylation patterns, but the modifications are hard to interpret. For example, in one study, a high-fat diet caused widespread DNA methylation changes in men within just five days, affecting more than 6,000 genes that were able to only partially reverse six to eight weeks after the participants returned to their usual diets.[634] And, overeating saturated fat causes different methylation changes than overeating polyunsaturated fat, but to what effect?[635] We don't know. Do the epigenetic changes play a role in the ensuing physiological effects, or are they incidental?

We are just starting to tease out the consequences of the epigenetic changes induced by diet and lifestyle. We know now, for instance, that among the consistent methylation differences in vegans compared to omnivores is hypomethylation (less methylation) of a tumor suppressor gene and a gene that encodes a DNA repair enzyme.[636] Since methylation silences genes, unmuzzling them may help account for the lower overall cancer rates among those eating plant-based diets.[637,638] Similarly, in vegetarians, the superoxide dismutase enzyme is less often methylated. That's an antioxidant enzyme that can squelch a million free radicals *per second*.[639] The hypomethylation is associated with a threefold increase in the expression of that detoxifying enzyme used to explain the "higher protection against chronic diseases in vegetarians."[640]

Beyond tweaking the volume knob of individual genes, there is evidence that large-scale methylation shifts can have health and longevity implications. If you boost the enzyme that actually does the methylating in fruit flies, you can prolong their average lifespan by more than 50 percent. Suppress the enzyme, and you cut short their lifespan. However, this strategy has yet to be shown to work in mammals.[641]

Human DNA methylation is much more complicated. But the fruit fly findings suggest that increasing global methylation capacity may positively affect longevity.

TURN OVER A NEW LEAF

The nutritional factor most widely studied for its epigenetic effects is folic acid.[642] That's the supplemental form of folate, a B vitamin concentrated in beans and greens that is converted into a methyl donor. (Folate comes from the same word root as foliage—*folium*, the Latin word for "leaf.")[643] The methyl group that ends up on your DNA may originate from the folate in your salad, for instance, or the folic acid in a supplement or enriched flour. The recommended daily allowance for most adults is 400 micrograms (µg),[644] yet the average daily intake of older men and women is less than 300 µg and a third don't even get 200 µg.[645] What are the epigenetic implications?

Postmenopausal women had their folate levels moderately depleted by being placed on a relatively low-folate diet to study the epigenetic effects. Even though folate levels didn't fall enough to show clinical signs of deficiency (such as anemia), within two months, the subjects suffered a genome-wide DNA hypomethylation across the board. It was reversed within three weeks, though, upon resuming healthy levels of folate intake.[646] A subsequent study of even older individuals resulted in the same undermethylation but took longer to reverse, underscoring the importance of maintaining adequate levels in the first place.[647]

Even without depletion, a meta-analysis of randomized controlled trials of folic acid supplementation using the most sophisticated methods of laboratory analysis found an increase in global methylation, suggesting that most of us may not be getting enough in our diet.[648] There's no real benchmark for a "normal" level of methylation, so terms like "hypomethylation" are used in a relative sense,[649] making these changes hard to interpret functionally.[650] But, our ancient ancestors ate a lot more leaves. They likely got twice as much folate as we do today,[651] so the fact that our body puts the extra methyl group availability to use when we get a bump in folic acid levels suggests to me that our folate status may be suboptimal. This is easy to fix, though. For example, just meet my Daily Dozen recommendations for legumes and dark green leafy vegetables. (*Dr. Greger's Daily Dozen* is available as a free app for iPhone and Android.)

Hard as a MTHFR?

So-called MTHFR mutations are a popular scapegoat often used by alternative medicine practitioners[652] to prescribe special supplements (that they not-so-coincidentally may also sell) for a variety of common ailments.[653] MTHFR is an enzyme our body makes to activate folate. A common variant of the MTHFR gene, which has DNA code letter T rather than the more common C at the 677th position, makes for a less functional enzyme. This can have epigenetic implications, as those who got the T variants from both parents (about 10 percent of the global population)[654] have diminished DNA methylation, but only when their folate intake is low.[655] If you get enough folate, your methylation levels are the same regardless of whether you have the T variants. Similarly, those with two of the T variant genes may have higher risk of cancer, but, again, it's only among those not getting enough folate.[656] You don't need a special kind of folate either. The folate in foods and folic acid in supplements and enriched foods are perfectly usable, irrespective of which gene type you have.[657]

Since everyone should be striving to get enough folate, there is no benefit to routine genetic testing to see which variant you have, which is why major medical organizations in the field recommend against MTHFR testing.[658] The only thing you might do differently if you knew you had a double dose of the less functional enzyme is to be especially careful about alcohol intake. Acetaldehyde, the breakdown product of alcohol, can destroy the folate in our body,[659] so those with double T variants should consider restricting their consumption to less than one drink a day.[660] As everyone should probably be trying to minimize alcohol intake,[661] I agree there's little value in knowing your MTHFR genetics.

FOLIC ACID IS NOT THE SAME AS FOLATE

A review of more than a hundred meta-analyses of population studies shows that those who get more folate in their diet tend to live longer and are protected against cardiovascular disease, several cancers, and a wide range of other chronic diseases.[662] But some randomized controlled trials of folic acid supplements found *increased* cancer risk.[663] As I explore in see.nf/folic, the mystery appears to have been solved when scientists figured out that we aren't rats.

Natural folate isn't shelf-stable, but there's an enzyme in our liver that can convert the stable synthetic folic acid found in supplements into an active form of folate in our body.[664] The original experiments were done on rats, though, and it turns out that their livers are fifty times more efficient at this conversion than ours,[665] so we can end up with unmetabolized folic acid circulating throughout our body,[666] which may impair our anticancer defenses.[667] For example, randomized controlled trials have shown that men taking folic acid supplements significantly increase their risk of developing prostate cancer. Randomized trials have also found that those taking folic acid supplements for more than three years are more likely to develop colorectal polyps.[668] So, natural sources of folate, like beans and greens, may be best, though women who want to get pregnant are still advised to take folic acid supplements, given their proven efficacy for reducing birth defects.[669]

Beyond food and supplements, the third way to improve your folate status is to contract out some of the production to your microbiome. A folate transporter in our colon appears to be specially designed to absorb folate[670] produced by good bacteria like *Bifidobacterium* when we feed them fiber.[671] Increasing your fiber intake can bolster the growth of little folate factories in your gut.

Food for Thought

Our epigenome, characterized by the pattern of DNA methylation, can be thought of as a lens through which our genetic information is filtered.[672] Unfortunately, it's a lens that can become cloudy as it deteriorates with age. Thankfully, epigenetic changes are reversible, so we may be able to polish it back into focus. Caloric restriction, as well as diet and lifestyle improvements, including physical activity, smoking cessation, and shopping more in the produce aisle than at the meat counter, may all slow the epigenetic clock. Getting sufficient levels of methyl-donor nutrients, such as folate, can also affect global methylation capacity.

To help boost this anti-aging pathway, on a daily basis, consider:
  • restricting calories by 12 percent, which would be cutting about

(continued)

250 calories out of a 2,000-calorie diet (e.g., skipping a piece of pie or cake every day)

- meeting the 400 µg recommended daily allowance of folate, which could be achieved with about a cup of cooked lentils or edamame, a cup and a half of cooked spinach or asparagus, or two and a half cups of broccoli, for example

GLYCATION

You may have heard of the Maillard reaction if you're a foodie or watch cooking shows. It's what gives seared steaks, panfried dumplings, toasted marshmallows, or freshly baked cookies their distinctive browned look, feel, and flavor. In 1912, the French chemist Louis Camille Maillard discovered, rather by chance, that mixtures of proteins and sugars turn brown upon heating. In the century since, more than 50,000 scientific papers have been published on this "Maillard reaction," in which proteins can become irreversibly glycated, or bonded with sugar.[673] The same reaction can occur at body temperature, leading to an accumulation of advanced glycation end products (AGEs),[674] which we now know are one of the main factors contributing to the aging process.[675]

ADVANCED GLYCATION END PRODUCTS

If you are diabetic, you're familiar with HbA1c, a test that measures blood sugar control, reflecting average blood sugar levels over the prior two to three months. The blood test just reflects the percentage of hemoglobin in your blood that has been glycated. (Hemoglobin is the protein in red blood cells that carries oxygen.) The higher your blood sugars are, the more your proteins are glycated. Since red blood cells last about a hundred days, the test gives you a rolling average over that time.[676]

Diabetes can be diagnosed with an HbA1c of 6.5 percent or higher, meaning 6.5 percent or more of the hemoglobin in the blood has been glycated. A percentage of 5.7 to 6.4 gives a diagnosis of prediabetes, and less than 5.7 is considered normal.[677] So, even if you have normal blood sugars, some proteins and other molecules in your body are being irrevocably glycated. This isn't such an issue for short-lived proteins like hemoglobin, which are rapidly recycled and created anew, but what about long-lived proteins, like the crystallins in the lens of your eye?[678]

Hemoglobin's half-life, the rate at which half gets renewed, is about fifty days.

The collagen in your skin has a half-life of more like fifteen years,[679] and the half-life of collagen in the intervertebral discs in your spine is estimated to be at least *ninety-five years*. Similarly, elastin, another connective tissue protein, is formed in infancy and has to last your whole lifespan. Glycation causes proteins to cross-link together, which stiffens our tissues—most critically, our arteries and the heart muscle itself. This impaired elasticity can result in high blood pressure, peripheral artery disease, heart disease, and even cancer. (Stiffness of breast tissue is associated with an increased risk of cancer.)[680] The acronym for advanced glycation end products was chosen intentionally, to emphasize their role in the aging process.[681]

RAGE OUT OF CONTROL

There are AGEs and then there's RAGE. Advanced glycation end products not only stick our proteins together, they trigger chronic, systemic inflammation. In the search for the mechanism for this response, researchers discovered receptors for AGEs in our body that spark the inflammatory cascade and named them RAGE: receptors for advanced glycation end products.[682] RAGE can function as a master switch. When AGE sparks RAGE, a whole host of inflammatory genes are triggered, along with a promotion of further RAGE expression, which leads to a vicious, cyclical feedback loop that can have profound pathological effects.[683]

As AGEs accumulate in our bones, joints, and muscles, they may contribute to osteoporosis, arthritis, and muscle wasting, the weakening, shrinking, and loss of muscle mass with age.[684] AGEs are implicated in age-related memory decline, impaired wound healing, skin aging, cataracts, Alzheimer's disease, and erectile dysfunction (where the stiffening of penile arteries evidently results in penile unstiffening).[685] AGEs have been found to adversely affect virtually all tissues and organs.[686] As one pathologist put it, "It is hard to find an age-related disease that AGEs are not involved."[687]

The toxicity of AGE accumulation is underscored by the number of defense mechanisms our body employs to prevent their formation.[688] Once they have been formed, though, they're hard to get rid of, so they gradually accumulate and wreak havoc.[689] Over five to six decades, AGE levels in our tissues roughly double.[690] The reason this is seen as not only a marker of aging but an active *driver* of the aging process is that AGE inhibitors have been shown to extend the lifespan of model animals, whereas AGE augmentation can cut lives short.[691] The preferred laboratory animal model of accelerated aging uses *galactose* (a major breakdown product of the milk sugar lactose)[692] to fast-track AGE accumulation.[693] Across the animal kingdom, the slower the rate of AGE formation, the longer species tend to live. The bowhead whale, for example, who, by living more than two centuries, is probably the longest-living mammal, has exceptionally low rates of AGE accumulation.[694] How can we best keep our levels low?

AGE formation is heat-dependent. At body temperature, the Maillard reaction is exceedingly slow, taking weeks, months, or even years to generate sugar-protein cross-linking.[695] Imagine what would happen if our body, instead of an internal temperature of about 100°F (38°C), hit 200°F, 300°F, or 400°F (93°C, 149°C, or 204°C)? That's what happens when we put meat in the oven. Calling the yellowish then brownish discoloration of cataracts the "AGE food colors of roasted turkey"[696] is not just poetic license. The same AGEs that cloud the pristine clear quality of the lens proteins in your eyes over a period of decades can be formed within minutes on the stove.[697] The burden of AGEs in our tissues appears to be less a matter of how much we make and more a matter of how many AGEs we eat.[698]

DIETARY AGE SOURCES

About a million years ago, our ancestors harnessed fire.[699] When muscle cells are exposed to the high temperatures of flames, they rupture and out spill highly reactive amino acids that combine with blood and body sugars to form AGEs.[700] Like us, animals we eat also have AGEs naturally in their tissues, but high-heat cooking can radically ramp up production.[701] Different cooking methods expose tissues to different amounts of heat and moisture. Poached or steamed chicken, for example, had less than one-fourth of the AGEs of roasted or broiled chicken that had been prepared in drier conditions and at higher temperatures.[702]

Research on rats performed in the 1970s found that diet-derived AGEs weren't absorbed very well, so dietary sources were dismissed as irrelevant—that is, until a quarter century later, when AGE absorption was finally tested in people.[703] The landmark paper, published in the *Proceedings of the National Academy of Sciences*, demonstrated that diet-derived AGEs were indeed absorbed into the human body.[704] Further research showed that dietary AGEs contribute more to the toxic pool of AGEs in our body than our own endogenous production. In other words, our AGE exposure is more from what we eat than what we make.[705] As a result, dietary AGEs have emerged as a burning concern in the food industry.[706] The investigators suggest eliminating high-AGE foods and high-AGE cooking methods to reduce the body's burden of these toxins.[707]

Researchers got to work testing AGE levels in more than five hundred foods, everything from Big Macs and Hot Pockets to Frosted Flakes and Pop-Tarts.[708] They identified the highest levels in "high-heat-treated meat" and, more generally, in "[a]nimal-derived foods that are high in fat and protein," and determined that the lowest levels are found in vegetables, fruits, whole grains, and milk[709,710] (with the exception of dairy milk–based infant formula Enfamil, which has nearly a hundred times more AGEs than human breast milk).[711] Meat averages about 20 times more AGEs than highly processed foods like breakfast cereals and about 150 times more than fresh fruits and vegetables. Poultry was the worst, containing about 20 percent more AGEs than beef in general.[712]

Based on the most extensively cited[713] AGE food database,[714] which includes hundreds of nonmeat items, the majority of the top fifteen single most AGE-contaminated sources per serving were poultry products, led by oven-fried chicken breast.

Researchers were rather surprised that high-fat and protein-rich foods created more AGEs than starchy and sugary high-carbohydrate foods.[715] After all, AGEs are called "glycotoxins" for a reason.[716] They involve glycation reactions, like the Maillard reaction I mentioned earlier in which sugars bind to proteins. Sugars alone can brown at high heat in a way that may superficially look, smell, and taste similar to products of the Maillard reaction, but that's the result of an entirely different chemical process called caramelization. By definition, Maillard reaction AGEs are created only when amino acids from proteins are involved.[717] For a deeper dive into other AGE rankings, see see.nf/agerank.

HOW TO REDUCE TOXIC AGE INTAKE

Most of the largest AGE food databases used a single AGE (carboxymethyllysine) as a marker for total AGE content,[718] but more than forty individual AGEs have been identified[719] and not all of them are toxic.[720] Some may even be beneficial. A component in roasted coffee beans called melanoidin, for example, may even act as an antioxidant.[721] AGEs from animal-derived foods appear to produce more toxic effects than AGEs from plant-derived foods.[722] Not only may plant foods average thirty times fewer AGEs; even if you expose proteins to the same amount of AGEs from plant versus animal sources, there are twenty-five times fewer cross-linkages and forty times fewer when compared to poultry AGEs. Plant-derived AGEs also produce less inflammation and fewer free radicals.[723] The AGEs created by the curing of tobacco may be an exception, as the AGEs from cigarettes are implicated in the deleterious effects of smoking.[724]

Even without cutting down on meat, you can significantly cut down on AGE intake by using different cooking methods. High dry-heating methods create the most AGEs, with oven-frying meat worse than deep-frying, which is worse than broiling, which is worse than roasting. Given that there is no threshold temperature, the general recommendation is that the lower the heat, the better when it comes to combating AGE generation.[725] The safest ways of cooking meat are lower temperature moist methods, such as boiling, poaching, stewing, and steaming.[726] Boiled beef has three times fewer AGEs than broiled beef,[727] boiled chicken has five times fewer AGEs than broiled chicken, and boiled eggs have nearly six times fewer than fried eggs. Microwaving from scratch is also relatively safe, found to be on par with boiling.[728]

Much of the focus on reducing dietary AGEs has to do with these kinds of culinary changes.[729] Cooking methods do matter. A raw apple has three times fewer AGEs than one that's been baked, and a boiled hot dog has less than one that's been broiled. But don't lose perspective: A raw apple has 13 units of AGEs compared to a baked apple's 45 units, while a boiled hot dog has 6,736 units compared to a broiled hot dog's 10,143. So, a baked apple still has 150 times fewer AGEs than a boiled frankfurter,[730] and vegetables, even when grilled, have but a fraction of the AGEs of raw meat.[731]

Researchers recommend cooking meat using moist-heat methods like steaming or stewing, but even boiled fish has in excess of ten times more AGEs than a sweet potato roasted for an hour. Even deep-fried potatoes have less than boiled meat. The researchers concluded that daily AGE intake could realistically be cut in half just by modestly reducing meat intake.[732]

Marinating meat with an acidic ingredient, like lemon juice or vinegar, before cooking can significantly decrease the amount of dietary AGEs produced.[733] This works with both broiling and boiling. Boiling chicken with lemon may decrease AGE content by 15 percent compared to boiling in water alone.[734] Another way to cut down on AGE absorption is to reduce fat content. A high-fat meal increases blood levels of AGEs more than a low-fat meal with the same AGE content and prepared with nearly the same foods but, for example, with reduced-fat cheese in place of a full-fat variety.[735]

CASTING LIGHT ON AGEs

What evidence do we have that cutting down on dietary AGEs will benefit us? Population studies have found that those with elevated AGEs in their blood are at greater risk for anemia, artery and cartilage stiffness, cardiovascular disease, chronic kidney disease,[736] osteoarthritis,[737] and osteoporosis,[738] but most of the studies have focused on the adverse effects of AGEs on our muscles, mortality, and minds. For a run-through, see my video see.nf/ages.

There's a noninvasive way to assess the accumulation of AGEs over time that circumvents the problem of the day-to-day variability in blood levels based on the curious fact that some AGEs that build up in our skin are fluorescent.[739] Using a special detector, long-term AGE exposure can be correlated with frailty,[740] premature death,[741] and accelerated brain shrinkage.[742] In the influential paper "Oral Glycotoxins Are a Modifiable Cause of Dementia . . . [in] Humans," the reduction of food-derived AGEs is suggested as a feasible, effective strategy to combat our dementia epidemic.[743]

AGEs may help explain why those who eat the most meat were found to have triple the risk of becoming demented compared to longtime vegetarians,[744] but other factors may be contributing. For example, high intake of saturated fat, found mostly in meat, dairy, and junk food, is associated with a 40 percent increased risk of cognitive impairment and a nearly 90 percent higher risk of Alzheimer's disease.[745] Even just a few days on a high-fat, low-carb diet has been shown to cause cognitive dysfunction.[746] There is a problem with all these studies, though. Maybe the correlation between AGEs and chronic disease is just a correlation between high-AGE foods like processed meat and chronic disease. The only way to prove cause and effect is to put it to the test through interventional trials.

THE AGE DIET TRIALS

Journal articles with titles like "Extended Lifespan in Mice Exposed to a Low Glycotoxin Diet"[747] exemplify the studies that show that lowering dietary AGE intake can improve longevity, whereas increasing AGE intake can impair learning and memory,[748] as well as cut lives short in rodents[749] and other model animals.[750] In one study, for instance, while 76 percent of the mice fed a low-AGE diet lived at least fifty-six weeks, not a single one of the mice fed an AGE-rich diet survived after forty-four weeks.[751]

The negative effect of AGEs is so great it can even trump the benefits of calorie restriction. While lifelong calorie restriction predictably prolongs the lifespan of mice, when they're fed high-AGE food pellets, they not only die sooner than mice eating regular chow but they also do worse in every category tested—inflammation, oxidative stress, insulin resistance, and marked heart and kidney fibrosis (scar tissue buildup).[752] The benefits of reducing food quantity can be undone by reductions in food quality. We'll see this in the next chapter, where the well-being enjoyed by members of the Calorie Restriction Society may be constrained by their relatively high protein intake.

I review the human AGE trials in see.nf/agetrials, but basically, a single meal of broiled chicken causes a "profound impairment" of artery function within hours compared to eating the same amount of boiled chicken. Boiled chicken still impaired arterial function, but significantly less than when the chicken was broiled.[753] This difference was attributed to AGEs, but other heat-generated toxins are also created when meat is cooked, such as heterocyclic amines, which originate mainly from the creatine in the muscle, so it's impossible to say with absolute certainty what caused the difference.[754]

GLYCEMIC LOAD

Even though the majority of AGEs in the body come externally through our diet, AGEs are also formed internally. This normally happens at a slow, continuous rate, but it is sped up in the context of high blood sugars.[755] In my previous books, I explore the prevention, arrest, and reversal of prediabetes and type 2 diabetes.

However, even people with normal fasting blood sugars can get spikes that are too high after eating meals with a high glycemic load.

TAKE A LOAD OFF

In my Low Glycemic Load chapter in *How Not to Diet*, I take a deep dive into the impact different carbohydrate-rich foods have on our blood sugars, focusing on a measure called glycemic load. The higher the glycemic load, the higher our blood sugars tend to spike when we eat them. Here's a breakdown of some common sweet and starchy foods:[756]

Glycemic Load Per Serving

Low ≤ 10	Medium 11–20	High ≥ 20
Beans	Oatmeal	Breakfast Cereals
Chickpeas & Split Peas	Spaghetti	Dates
Fruits	Brown Rice	White Rice
Lentils	Sweet Potato	White Potato
Whole-Grain Bread	White Bread	Raisins

PUTTING LOWER-GLYCEMIC EATING TO THE TEST

In the boiled versus broiled chicken study, even the boiled chicken meal led to some artery dysfunction, whereas a low-glycemic, high-fiber meal can actually improve artery function in the subsequent four hours after consumption.[757] Like AGE studies involving meat reduction, though, it can be difficult to separate out the specific effects of glycemic changes. Many high-glycemic foods are fiber-depleted and highly processed, so you're doing more than just changing glycemic load when you swap them out for beans, fruits, or other low-glycemic foods.[758] A constant challenge with diet studies is that it's hard to change just one thing. It's simple with drug trials because researchers can just give the drug or a sugar pill. Then, if there's a change, they know it was caused by the drug. If only we could somehow stuff a change in glycemic load into a pill. Well, it turns out, we can.

The drug acarbose partially blocks our starch- and sugar-digesting enzymes in the digestive tract, which slows carbohydrate absorption into our body.[759] When we take the drug with a meal, a high-glycemic meal is effectively transformed into a low-glycemic one—without changing the foods at all.[760] Acarbose is how researchers were able to show that lowering dietary glycemic load leads to weight loss independent of fiber intake,[761] and it can do the same with AGE reduction.

Acarbose has been shown to lower blood AGE levels in diabetics by about 30 percent within twelve weeks.[762] No wonder acarbose has been found to improve the healthspan and longevity of mice, increasing their maximum lifespan by about 10 percent. As drugs go, acarbose has an outstanding safety record.[763] However, flatulence, bloating, and diarrhea are commonly reported.[764] We can reap the upsides of the drug without its downside side effects by simply choosing lower glycemic load carbs, such as legumes (beans, chickpeas, split peas, and lentils), fruits, and intact whole grains.

BE FULL OF BEANS

By 1980, it had already been shown that beans cause an "exceptionally" low blood sugar response, half that of other common foods.[765] But two years later, an extraordinary discovery was published: Legumes can benefit your metabolism hours after consumption[766] or even the following day. If you eat lentils for dinner, your body reacts differently to breakfast eleven hours later.[767] Even if you drink straight sugar water the next morning, your body is better able to handle it if you had lentils the night before. Researchers initially dubbed it the "lentil effect," but when subsequent studies found that chickpeas appeared to work, too, they changed the name to the "second meal effect."[768]

How does it work? We scratch our gut bacteria's backs, and they scratch ours. Good gut flora take fiber we eat and produce short-chain fatty acids for us that get absorbed into our bloodstreams and circulate throughout our systems. So, if we eat a bean burrito for dinner, by morning, our gut bacteria are eating that same burrito and the by-products they create may affect how we digest our breakfast. This helps explain why diabetics randomized to a cup a day of beans, chickpeas, or lentils successfully improved their blood sugar control.[769]

WHY NOT JUST A LOW-CARB DIET?

Contrary to popular belief, eating a piece of fruit with a meal would be expected to lower, rather than raise, our blood sugar response,[770] which is why type 2 diabetics are no longer encouraged to restrict fruit intake.[771] A half dozen randomized controlled trials swapped in fruits for other foods, like higher glycemic carbs, and found, on average, a significant improvement in blood sugar control.[772] In fact, those who eschew fruits and go on a ketogenic diet to lower blood sugars may actually make things worse in the long run.

Those going on ketogenic diets may nearly quadruple their saturated fat intake,[773] and saturated fat can impair the action of the blood sugar–lowering hormone insulin. We've known for nearly a century that a high-fat diet can double blood sugar reactions to the same carbohydrate challenge within a matter of days.[774]

Even a single meal can do it. Eating a stick of butter,[775] for example, or drinking a milkshake can dramatically increase insulin resistance within hours.[776] But, what if keto dieters stick with the program and avoid carbohydrates to stay in a state of ketosis? AGE levels can skyrocket.

One reason diabetics suffer nerve and artery damage is due to *methylglyoxal*, an inflammatory metabolic toxin that forms at high blood sugar levels. Methylglyoxal is the single most potent creator of AGEs.[777]

Since AGEs are concentrated in high-fat and high-protein animal-based foods, it makes sense that we'd expect high exposure to preformed ones on a keto diet. Similarly, it follows that we'd expect less internal, *new* AGE formation due to presumably low levels of methylglyoxal, given low blood sugars.[778] Surprisingly, Dartmouth researchers found *more* methylglyoxal. After just two to three weeks on the Atkins diet, subjects had a significant increase in methylglyoxal levels and those in active ketosis did even worse, experiencing a doubling of glycotoxin in the bloodstream.[779]

High sugars may not be the only way to create methylglyoxal. One of the ketones you make on a ketogenic diet is acetone. Sound familiar? It's a primary ingredient in nail polish remover. But acetone does more than strip paint and make keto dieters develop "rotten apple breath"[780] and fail Breathalyzer tests.[781] It can oxidize in the blood to acetol, which may be a precursor for methylglyoxal. This may be why nondiabetic keto dieters can end up with methylglyoxal levels as high as those with uncontrollable diabetes.[782]

What About Natural and Artificial Sweeteners?

When people were randomized to drink beverages sweetened with aspartame, monk fruit, or stevia instead of sixteen spoonsful of sugar[783] (the amount of added sugar in a 20 oz bottle of Coke[784]), they were all found to be equally bad when it came to calorie intake, blood sugars, or insulin spikes throughout the day.[785] Similar results were found for Splenda (sucralose).[786] How is that possible? The mystery is solved in my video see.nf/sweeteners.

HOW TO REDUCE THE GLYCEMIC IMPACT OF GRAINS

In my Wall Off Your Calories chapter in *How Not to Diet*, I explore how the same foods in different forms can have different effects. Steel-cut oatmeal is considered to be a low-glycemic-index food, averaging under 55, whereas the glycemic index of instant oatmeal is 79, which makes it a high-glycemic-index food. Instant oatmeal isn't as bad as some breakfast cereals, though, which can get into the 80s or 90s—even zero-sugar cereals like shredded wheat.[787] How can this be? Modern industrial methods used to manufacture breakfast cereals, like explosion puffing and extrusion cooking, accelerate starch digestion and absorption, which cause exaggerated blood sugar responses.[788] Shredded wheat and spaghetti have the same ingredients—straight wheat—but shredded wheat has twice the glycemic index.[789]

From a glycemic-index standpoint, breads made from sprouted grains[790] with added cracked wheat,[791] whole wheatberries,[792] or rye berries,[793] or made with stone-ground flour are preferable.[794] If you simply just can't live without white bread, toasting it,[795] using sourdough fermentation if you bake your own,[796] and freezing and defrosting it all lower the blood sugar response.

When starch is cooked, then cooled, some of it crystallizes into "resistant" starch—starch that is resistant to being broken down into sugars by the enzymes in our digestive tract, which lowers its glycemic impact.[797] This is why pasta salad can be more healthful than hot pasta, and potato salad better than a baked potato. Some grains—notably sorghum[798] and millet—inherently contain resistant starch, resulting in a 20 to 25 percent lower blood sugar response compared to other grains, such as rice,[799] wheat,[800] or corn.[801]

HOW TO REDUCE THE GLYCEMIC IMPACT OF POTATOES

If you look at most whole plant foods—legumes, nuts, vegetables, and fruits—increased consumption is associated with living a longer life, with about 25 percent less chance of dying prematurely from all causes put together. There appears to be no such protective association with white potatoes, though. Now, potatoes aren't like meat, which may actively shorten your life, but there is an opportunity cost to eating white potatoes, since every bite of a potato is a lost opportunity to put something even more healthful into your mouth that may actively make your life longer.[802]

The reason the consumption of white potatoes may just have a neutral impact on mortality risk is that their fiber, vitamin C, and potassium might be counterbalanced by the detrimental effects of their high glycemic index.[803] Can we have our potatoes and eat them, too, by somehow lowering their glycemic index? There is that cool crystallization trick. By consuming potatoes as chilled potato salad, for instance, it's possible to get nearly a 40 percent lower glycemic impact. To minimize the glycemic index of potatoes, simply precook them and either eat them cold or reheated in the microwave.[804] (I call it the nip-and-nuke method.) The vinegar in that potato salad may even have an additional benefit.

STRIKE A SOUR NOTE

Randomized controlled trials involving both diabetic and nondiabetic subjects suggest that blood sugar control may be improved by adding two teaspoons of vinegar to a meal, effectively blunting the post-meal blood sugar spike by about 20 percent.[805] So, the effects of these high-glycemic foods may be blunted by adding vinegar to rice (like the Japanese do to make sushi) or dipping bread in balsamic vinegar, for example. The combination of chilling before eating and adding vinegar to make potato salad was found to have an additive effect.[806] See see.nf/lemony for a comparison to the effects of lemon juice.

SPICE THINGS UP

As you can see in the Glycemic Load Per Serving chart (see page 60), the simplest way to stick to a lower glycemic diet is to try to stick to foods that were grown, not made. If you are going to eat high-glycemic foods, vinegar isn't the only way to help blunt the blood sugar surge. For example, if you eat berries with your meals, they can act as starch blockers by inhibiting the starch-digesting enzyme.[807] This then slows the absorption of blood sugars into your system. So, if you're preparing a high-glycemic breakfast, add blueberries to your pancakes or top your bowl of Franken Berry with actual berries.

On the other end of the culinary spectrum, onions can do the same thing. When subjects downed about three tablespoons of corn syrup, their blood sugars shot up over the next hour and a half from their baseline of about 90 mg/dL up to around 130 mg/dL before their bodies were able to tamp them back down. However, when they ate a quarter of an onion with that corn syrup, their sugars only went up to about 115 mg/dL.[808] After eating a whole onion, their blood sugars only reached 105 mg/dL, and two onions resulted in only about a five-point increase to 95 mg/dL. Simply by eating onions, their blood sugars hardly went up at all, similar to what one might experience on an antidiabetes drug.

Spices can also be helpful. An Indian curry with 6 g of spices (about one tablespoon) cut the blood sugar response to white rice by 19 percent, compared to no added spices, and 12 g of spices cut the glycemic impact by 32 percent.[809] You can also drink your spices. Have some ginger tea with two slices of refined flour white bread, and you drop the bread's glycemic index by nearly 30 percent. Cinnamon tea works even better, with nearly a 40 percent drop in glycemic response. Even regular unsweetened green tea cuts the glycemic impact by about 20 percent.[810] Of course, not eating white bread in the first place would work even better.

What about drinking herbs? Chamomile is one of the most widely used medicinal plants in the world—and for good reason.[811] When type 2 diabetics drank a small cup of chamomile tea after their meals for a few months, they got significant improvement in long-term blood sugar control compared to drinking the same volume of warm water[812] or when pitted head-to-head against black tea.[813] And the side effects? All good—lower LDL cholesterol and triglycerides,[814] a decrease in inflammation,[815] and improved sleep, mood,[816] and antioxidant status.[817] Chamomile tea and green tea appear to share the same mechanisms for blood sugar control: blocking the transport of sugars through the intestinal wall.[818]

Slave to the Rhythm

In my Chronobiology chapter in *How Not to Diet*, I explore how our ability to keep our blood sugars under control deteriorates as the day progresses.[819] Thanks to our circadian rhythm, a meal eaten at 8:00 at night can cause twice the blood sugar response as an identical meal eaten at 8:00 in the morning.[820] Even eating lunch earlier, rather than later, can make a significant difference.[821] So, if you simply have to have refined grains and sugary foods, giving in to your craving might be less detrimental in the morning.[822]

WALK IT OFF

Since active muscles can siphon off excess blood sugars, exercise timing can complement meal timing. When type 2 diabetics were randomized to a leisurely twenty-minute stroll (about 2 mph) either before or after dinner, researchers found that after-dinner walking can comparatively blunt blood sugar spikes by 30 percent.[823] Thanks to some tactical timing, the same meal and the same amount and intensity of exercise can give us a significant bonus effect on blood sugar control. Exercising after a meal can bring down blood sugars just as effectively as some blood sugar–lowering drugs,[824] and even just a short ten-minute walk after eating may make a difference.[825] See my Exercise Tweaks section in *How Not to Diet* for specifics on optimal timing.

Food for Thought

AGEs are considered "gerontotoxins,"[826] meaning aging agents (from the Greek *geros* for "old age," as in *geriatric*), and are implicated in a wide spectrum of age-related diseases. In a sense, we are all slowly being cooked alive. AGEs are formed endogenously at body temperature, especially with high blood sugars, but their buildup in our tissues is largely determined by the AGEs we eat (or smoke), which are formed at much higher temperatures when some foods are cooked at high heat (or tobacco is cured).

(continued)

Rather than addressing dietary change, however, the medical field has focused on inventing drugs to combat AGEs. Lifestyle approaches are said to have "zero commercial value,"[827] and an argument is made that "stewed chicken would be less tasty than fried chicken. . . ."[828] Why not have your KFC and eat it, too, by taking Kremezin, the drug that blocks AGE absorption every time you eat to reduce the absorption of the toxins?[829] It turns out the drug is just a preparation of activated charcoal,[830] like what's used for drug overdoses and when people are poisoned. I'm sure chasing your KFC with some ipecac would lower your AGE levels, too! A safe level of dietary AGE intake has yet to be established, but animal studies show even cutting intake just by 50 percent can lead to a longer life.[831]

The best way to reduce absorption of AGEs is to reduce your exposure in the first place.

To help slow this aging pathway, on a daily basis, consider:
- stopping smoking[832]
- avoiding the very worst foods, such as bacon and hot dogs[833]
- eating an "AGE Less" diet by emphasizing lower AGE foods, such as fruits and vegetables[834]
- cooking high-protein foods using relatively low heat and high humidity methods, such as boiling or steaming rather than broiling or frying
- favoring raw nuts and seeds over roasted or toasted
- choosing lower-glycemic-load foods

IGF-1

A major breakthrough in our thinking about aging happened in the early 1990s. Aging was generally considered to be a hopelessly intractable problem.[835] We just wear out, the thinking went, in a haphazard and passive process of wear and tear. Then, in 1993, a single genetic mutation was found to double the lifespan of *C. elegans*,[836] the roundworm oft used in aging research. Instead of all worms being dead by thirty days, some lived for sixty days or longer in one experiment. As principal investigator Cynthia Kenyon recalled, the "mutants were the most amazing things I had ever seen. They were active and healthy and they lived more than twice as long as normal. It seemed magical but also a little creepy: they should have been dead, but there they were, moving around."[837]

This lifespan extension was the largest reported to date in any organism. These Methuselahian worms were touted as medical marvels, "the equivalent of a healthy 200-year-old human,"[838] all because of a single mutation. That was particularly surprising. Presumably, aging is caused by multiple processes affected by many genes. How could knocking out a single gene double lifespan?

DON'T GEAR THE REAPER

What is this so-called Grim Reaper gene—one that so accelerates aging that, if it's knocked out, the animals live twice as long? It is the worm equivalent of the receptor to human insulin-like growth factor 1 (IGF-1),[839] a potent growth hormone structurally similar to insulin. Mutations of that same receptor in humans may help explain why some people live to be a hundred and others don't.[840] It was a stunning discovery, the first life-extension pathway to be defined. We learned that aging is controlled by hormone signals conserved evolutionarily from tiny worms all the way up to us.[841]

Interference with the signaling in the IGF-1 pathway has since been shown to extend the lives of a variety of species.[842] Mice that have had IGF-1 disrupted live 42 to 70 percent longer.[843] Marveled Kenyon, "Some of these long-lived mutants are breathtaking; in human terms, they look like forty-year-olds when they are actually eighty or even older." The dialing down of growth-hormone signaling is thought to shift the body's priorities from growth to maintenance and repair, thereby extending survival.[844] The decline in IGF-1 levels as we get older may even be nature's way of sustaining us into old age.[845]

CENTENARIAN SECRETS

The majority of long-lived rodent models have lower levels of IGF-1.[846] What about people? Centenarian humans have lower IGF-1 levels in their blood, but is it cause or effect? IGF-1 levels decline as we age, so did the growth hormone cause centenarians to live long lives, or did living long lives cause the low IGF-1 level?[847] It's not as if you can compare them to controls of the same age who *aren't* centenarians. This led researchers to look at the IGF-1 levels of the offspring of centenarians so they could compare them to age-matched controls, and, indeed, the children have lower IGF-1 levels, too.[848] This suggests that lower IGF-1 levels may have given the centenarians the advantage.

Hundreds of different common human genetic variants have been studied, and this same pathway consistently implicated in extending lifespans in other animals is the very one associated with longevity and reduced risk of the major causes of death.[849] There is a single IGF-1-lowering gene variant that adds as much as ten years or so to life expectancy if you inherit it from both parents.[850]

Those lucky enough to be born with genetically lower IGF-1 levels are more likely to live to be nonagenarians.[851] Then from age ninety, low IGF-1 levels[852] and activity[853] have been found to subsequently predict their future survival. Interestingly, there are two mutations linked to centenarianism in Ashkenazi Jews—my heritage—that lead to *elevated* IGF-1 levels, but the mutations are in the IGF-1 receptor, so the elevated levels are presumably due to their body's futile attempt to overcome the enfeebled receptor.[854] Either way, the dampening of IGF-1 signaling appears to be a human-longevity mechanism.[855]

Is it just the luck of the draw whether we're born with good genes? Regardless of what our genetically determined baseline level of IGF-1 activity is, we can ramp it up or tamp it down, depending on what we eat.

The Taller Live Shorter

Dog lovers may know that smaller breeds tend to live longer than larger ones.[856] Tiny toy poodles average nearly twice the lifespan of the Great(est) Dane.[857] This makes sense when you realize that a major determinant of the difference in breed size is IGF-1.[858] The same phenomenon is observed in other species.[859] Asian elephants are smaller than their African cousins and typically live longer, and smaller horses, rodents, and cows generally outlive larger ones, too. What about people?

Bigger used to be better. Taller height was once an indicator of socioeconomic status and superior childhood living conditions, which translated into improved longevity.[860] However, now that relatively few kids are stunted by malnutrition, that baseline welfare allows inborn factors to shine through. These days, shorter stature predicts a longer lifespan.[861] In fact, this may help explain the gender differential in life expectancy. Men, on average, are about 8 percent taller than women and have about an 8 percent shorter lifespan.[862]

The relationship between a taller stature and a shorter life is driven mainly by increased cancer rates. That could help explain why, in general, men have more than a 50 percent increased risk of developing cancer compared to women.[863] Each additional inch in height is associated with about a 6 percent increased risk in dying from cancer.[864] This could just be because bigger people simply have more cells to potentially turn malignant.[865] After all, those with more skin might have a greater chance of developing skin cancer.[866] But the connection between height and cancer could also be because of cancer-promoting growth hormones like IGF-1.[867]

The Ashkenazi centenarians with the IGF-1 mutation were, on average, about an inch shorter, but the difference in height was not statistically significant.[868] This suggests we may be able to enjoy all the longevity benefits of dampening IGF-1 while still having a shot at the NBA.

CANCER BOOSTER

Each year, you are reborn. You destroy and create anew nearly your entire body weight in cells every year. About fifty billion of your cells die each day, but about fifty billion new cells are born.[869] Of course, there are times that you need to grow, such as during infancy or puberty, but your cells don't grow in size as you mature—they grow in number. As an adult, you may have around forty trillion cells, four times more than when you were a child.

During periods of growth like puberty, you need a net growth of cells, creating more than you retire, but that's not the case in your later years. Of course, you still need your cells to grow and divide, but extra cell growth in adulthood can mean the development of tumors.

How does your body maintain its balance? It sends hormones—chemical signals—to all your cells. IGF-1 is one of those key signals for regulating cell growth. When you're a child, the growth hormone's levels go up to power your development, but they decline when you reach adulthood, cueing your body to stop producing more cells than it puts out to pasture.

If your IGF-1 levels stay elevated after you're old enough to vote, your cells will continue to get the message to continue to grow and divide. As you might expect, the higher the IGF-1 in your bloodstream, the higher your risk for developing some cancers, such as breast,[870] colorectal,[871] and prostate.[872] (That doesn't seem to be the case, though, with lung,[873] ovarian,[874] or pancreatic cancer.[875]) In the Harvard Nurses' Health Study, premenopausal women younger than fifty in the upper third of IGF-1 levels had nearly five times the risk of developing breast cancer compared to those in the lower third.[876] In fact, before there was successful chemotherapy, surgeons would treat advanced breast cancer cases by not only removing the ovaries but operating on the brain to remove the patient's pituitary gland, which orchestrates growth hormone production in the body.[877]

Those with a tendency to have lower IGF-1 levels are less likely to get cancer in the first place,[878] and cancer survivors with lower levels are more likely to survive longer.[879] It's not the original tumor that tends to kill you; it's the metastases.[880] As a growth factor, IGF-1 doesn't just make tumors grow;[881] it helps cancer cells separate from the main tumor, infiltrate surrounding tissues, and invade the bloodstream.[882] IGF-1 is what helps breast cancer get into the bone,[883] liver, lung, brain, and lymph nodes.[884] It's involved every step of the way, facilitating the transformation of normal cells into cancer cells to begin with, then nurturing them to survive, proliferate, self-renew, grow, migrate, invade, and, finally, stabilize into new tumors. It even helps new tumors hook up their blood supply.[885]

Centenarians, however, seem to be endowed with a peculiar resistance to cancer.[886] As you age, your risk of developing and dying from cancer grows every year—until you hit eighty-five or ninety. Interestingly, that's when your cancer risk begins to drop.[887] At age sixty-five, we are a hundred times more likely to have a tumor than we are at age thirty-five, but if you don't get a cancer diagnosis by a certain age, you may never get one.[888] Centenarians appear ten times less likely to die from malignant tumors than people in their fifties and sixties (4 percent versus 40 percent, respectively).[889] What appears to account, at least in part, for this relative resistance to cancer among centenarians? Less IGF-1.[890] So, lowering IGF-1 activity could have the dual benefit of decreasing cancer risk while increasing longevity.

Cancer-Proofing Mutation

The primacy of IGF-1's role in tumor biology is demonstrated by a natural experiment involving a genetic defect that causes severe, lifelong, IGF-1 deficiency called Laron syndrome. The first case of this syndrome was reported in the *Israel Journal of Medical Sciences*,[891] but the largest affected population is in a remote area of Ecuador.[892] Jews fleeing the Spanish Inquisition in the fifteenth century escaped to South America and brought the gene mutation with them, causing this disparate geographic distribution.[893]

Lifelong IGF-1 deficiency not only gives people with Laron syndrome a small stature but it also appears to make them effectively cancer-proof.[894] Only a single case of (nonlethal) cancer was described among nearly five hundred affected individuals.[895] That's a cancer rate one hundred times lower than people without Laron syndrome, and without a single cancer death.[896] Most malignant tumors are covered in IGF-1 receptors. Without any IGF-1 around, the tumors may not be able to grow and spread.[897]

When we're kids, we need growth hormones to grow, but what if, as a child, we could get all of the growth hormones we needed to grow to a typical height and then downregulate hormones like IGF-1 once we reach adulthood? Turning off excess growth signals could potentially keep our cellular life-and-death balance sheets balanced to prevent cancer and settle us into repair-and-maintenance mode to prolong our lives. It turns out that we can do just that. We can suppress IGF-1 activity—not with surgery or medication but through simple dietary choices.

HOW TO REDUCE IGF-1 LEVELS WITH DIET

Unsurprisingly, drug companies have come up with a variety of IGF-1-blocking chemo agents, including ones with cute names like *figitumumab* and not-so-cute side effects like "early fatal toxicities."[898]

How can we reduce IGF-1 levels naturally?

Complete fasting can do it. Consuming nothing but water for five days can temporarily cut your levels in half.[899] (Don't try this at home, though. See page 563.) This is why cancer patients often fast for a few days before and after chemotherapy. The reduction in IGF-1 makes cancer cells more vulnerable to being killed off. How do we know that the fasting benefit is due to the IGF-1 reduction? Because restoring IGF-1 eliminates the starvation-induced vulnerability of cancer cells.[900]

Fasting is the poster child of unsustainability, though. If you fast long enough, you're guaranteed to stop aging—because you'll be dead. Avoiding the finality of long-term fasting fatality is the impetus behind creating fasting-*mimicking* diets designed to lower IGF-1 levels by eliminating the key dietary component that drives them up to begin with: animal protein.[901]

In rodents, calorie restriction alone reduces IGF-1 levels,[902] but in humans, unless protein consumption is also reduced, even severe caloric restriction doesn't work. Researchers were only able to get subjects' IGF-1 levels to budge after the protein intake of calorie-restriction practitioners was cut from typical American quantities down closer to the recommended daily allowance.[903]

At intakes far exceeding recommended consumption, protein from plants and animals equally raises IGF-1 levels,[904] but at more reasonable levels, animal protein appears to be the main culprit. Men[905] and women who avoid meat, egg, and dairy proteins have significantly lower IGF-1 levels even when moderately exceeding protein recommendations.[906] When people switch to a plant-based diet, their IGF-1 levels can drop significantly in less than two weeks.[907] However, just adding more plant foods,[908] cutting out meat,[909,910] or switching to fish may not help.[911,912] It's not all or nothing, though. A study of women carrying the BRCA mutation who are at high risk for breast cancer found that IGF-1 levels could be lessened by simply reducing, but not completely eliminating, animal product consumption across the board.[913]

Even a single serving of chicken breast a day would be expected to significantly raise IGF-1 levels in the blood.[914] When it comes to aggravating IGF-1, chicken may be worse than beef, but that's based on rat studies and has yet to be tested in people.[915] More than a half dozen randomized controlled trials have shown that dairy consumption increases IGF-1 in as little as a week.[916] Perhaps the strangest was a study out of Denmark in which IGF-1 levels were lowered successfully by switching people from two-thirds of a gallon of milk every day for ten days to two-thirds of a gallon of Coca-Cola.[917] I do believe that's the only study where people show a benefit from drinking twenty-five liters of Coke!

The relationship between milk consumption and IGF-1 is so consistent that the link has reached a P value of 10^{-27}.[918] In science, *P value* refers to the chance of getting a result that extreme if in fact there really was no such effect. It's used to determine how likely you would be to get the same results by random chance. How small of a chance is 10^{-27}? The probability that the association between milk consumption and IGF-1 is just a fluke is less than the chances of winning the lottery not once, not twice, but three times in a row, then subsequently getting struck and killed by lightning.[919]

IGF-1 may help explain the relationship between dairy consumption and prostate cancer,[920] but the reason those who drink the most milk appear to live shorter lives on average and are more likely to die from cancer may have more to do with the animal fat rather than the animal protein, since those findings were absent for low-fat milk.[921]

The bump in IGF-1 from dairy intake may be partly due to the absorption of preformed IGF-1 already in the milk.[922] After all, the whole point of milk is to put a few hundred pounds onto a calf in a matter of months,[923] so it shouldn't be surprising that it has high levels of growth-stimulating hormones.[924] Bovine IGF-1, which is identical to human IGF-1,[925] isn't affected by pasteurization.[926] While oral consumption of IGF-1 has been shown to be absorbed into the circulation of rats, pigs,[927] and presumably calves, similar studies have yet to be done on humans. Regardless, the protein in dairy can cause a surge in our own IGF-1 production, something less likely to happen when consuming protein from plants.[928]

ANIMAL VS. PLANT PROTEIN

The varying effects of animal versus plant protein appear to be due to different profiles of amino acids, the building blocks of proteins.[929] When you were a kid, did you love Tinker Toys as much as I did? I still remember how excited I was unwrapping a huge Tinker Toy set on my sixth birthday. I dumped out the new load of raw building materials onto the floor in front of me and couldn't wait to start scaling up. Our liver responds with just as much excitement when faced with a bunch of protein building blocks.

Although some IGF-1 is made locally in various tissues, our liver is responsible for approximately 75 percent of the IGF-1 that circulates throughout our body.[930] So, what happens when we consume a load of protein? Our liver starts pumping out IGF-1 to tell all the cells in our body that it's time to grow to use up the excess. With so much extra protein to work with, our liver sends the signal to our cells to be fruitful and multiply.

The problem is that tumors may be some of the new additions spurred by this growth hormone. When you're a fully grown adult, cell growth is something we want to slow down, not accelerate. The goal, therefore, would be to maintain adequate, but not excessive, protein intake. But animal protein appears to send a different signal to our livers than most plant proteins. Why is protein from an animal associated with increased levels of IGF-1, but not protein from a plant?[931] Let's go back to Tinker Toys.

Let's say you want to build a really big cube, and a pile of little cubes is dumped in front of you. Nice, right? You start stacking them together and are done in no time. What if, instead, you got a bunch of pyramid shapes? Each of the pyramids can certainly be broken down into the constituent sticks and connectors. You'd still have all the essential elements to construct your big cube, but you probably wouldn't be as excited to dive into the pile of pyramids because so much more work would be involved breaking them down first. Basically, it's the same with your liver and IGF-1.[932]

All plant proteins and nearly all animal proteins are complete proteins, containing all nine essential amino acids.[933] (The only incomplete protein in the food supply is the animal protein collagen [gelatin], which is missing tryptophan.[934]) So, while you couldn't live on Jell-O and marshmallows, all other dietary proteins, whether from plants or animals, contain all the essentials you need. When you hear about high- versus low-quality proteins, that's referencing the relative proportions of the different essential amino acids. The more closely the proportion matches our own proteins, the higher quality it's considered to be.

In a sense, there's only one truly "perfect protein" for us—human flesh. Failing that, any flesh will do. We don't practice species cannibalism, but by practicing kingdom cannibalism (Animalia) or, if we eat our fellow mammals, class cannibalism (Mammalia), we're getting protein that more closely mirrors our own than, say, a kidney bean. This is not necessarily a good thing.[935]

When a big load of incoming animal proteins hits our liver, it's analogous to the head start with the pile of Tinker Toy cubes: The protein's meat and we're meat, so we start pumping out IGF-1 to speed up cell division to use up the excess. When we get plant proteins, though, they're like the pyramids. Our body can break them down into all the essential amino acids we need, but they just don't stimulate the same kind of real estate boom that animal protein does. This phenomenon doesn't appear to affect muscle mass, as those afflicted with acromegaly (a form of high-IGF-1 giantism) aren't disproportionately muscular,[936] and people injected with IGF-1 twice a day for a year don't experience an increase in lean mass or muscle strength.[937] But the IGF-1 surge associated with animal protein consumption may very well affect lifespan and cancer risk.[938]

What About Soy Protein?

What about the few plant proteins that have amino acid profiles similar to animal proteins, like soy? One of soy's selling points is that it has "high-quality" protein, but when it comes to IGF-1, so-called higher quality may mean higher risk. Is that the case with soy-based protein?

We know that the consumption of animal protein is associated with significantly higher levels of IGF-1, while the consumption of non-soy plant protein is associated with significantly lower levels.[939] Soy protein falls in the middle, with no significant association with IGF-1 levels either way. This suggests that if we simply replace animal protein with soy protein, we may not see as dramatic a drop in IGF-1 as achieved by replacing meat, eggs, and dairy with a variety of proteins from plants other than soybeans. This was confirmed in a Stanford study: Switching from regular beef, pork, and chicken to plant-based (Beyond Meat) beef, pork, and chicken analogs made from soy and pea protein only caused an insignificant (3 percent) drop in IGF-1.[940]

Interventional studies showed that adding large quantities of soy protein supplements (40 g a day) increased IGF-1 levels,[941,942] but eating a couple of daily servings of actual soy *foods* did not.[943] The cutoff appears to be about 25 g of soy protein a day.[944] Of course, the main reasons we care about IGF-1 are cancer and longevity, and, if anything, soy consumers appear to be protected from cancer. A recent systematic review and meta-analysis found a 12 percent reduction in breast cancer death associated with each daily 5 g increase in soy protein intake, such as three-quarters of a cup of soymilk or two tablespoons of soy nuts.[945] Soy food intake also seems to be protective against prostate cancer.[946] And, in terms of longevity, as we'll explore in Part II, the two longest-lived formally studied populations on Earth, the Okinawa Japanese[947] and the vegetarian Seventh-day Adventists in California, tend to eat soy foods on a daily basis.[948]

QUIT COLD TURKEY

IGF-1 may help explain why people's lives appear to be cut short when they eat some low-carb diets but not others.[949] Twin Harvard cohorts found that vegetable-based low-carb diets were associated with lower mortality rates, while those based on animal sources increased the risk of premature death by 23 percent and the risk of dying specifically from cancer by 28 percent.[950] Even just substituting 5 percent of calories of animal protein with protein from plants, such as beans or nuts, may be associated with a 14 percent lower risk of dying prematurely (and a 19 percent lower risk of dying specifically from dementia).[951] Egg protein (found mostly in the egg white) appears to be the worst. Replacing just 3 percent of egg protein with plant protein may be associated with a 24 percent lower risk of premature death in men and a 21 percent lower risk in women.[952]

When a dream team of longevity researchers, including Luigi Fontana and Valter Longo, followed a nationally representative sample of thousands of Americans over age fifty for an average of eighteen years, they found that those under sixty-five with high protein intakes had a 75 percent increase in overall mortality and a fourfold increase in the risk of dying from cancer. When the protein sources were split up into plant versus animal, however, the overall mortality risk was found to be limited to the consumption of animal protein.[953] The sponsoring university described the study with a memorable opening line: "That chicken wing you're eating could be as deadly as a cigarette."[954]

The researchers explained that, compared to someone on a low-protein diet, the quadrupling of risk for cancer death from eating a diet rich in animal proteins during middle age is a mortality risk comparable to smoking. And when they say "low protein," that is just compared to what most people eat. The "low protein" group was actually getting the *recommended* amount of protein, 0.8 g per kg of healthy body weight, or about 50 g a day for someone weighing about 140 pounds—preferably from plants to keep IGF-1 activity low.[955] Overall, the amount of life lost from each burger is estimated to equate to smoking two cigarettes.[956]

Two Risks Don't Make a Right

What was the response in the scientific community to the revelation that, as the *Guardian* headline put it, "Diets high in meat, eggs, and dairy could be as harmful to health as smoking"? One nutrition scientist said that it was "potentially dangerous" to compare the effects of smoking with the effects of animal foods because a smoker might think, "Why bother quitting smoking if my cheese and ham sandwich is just as bad for me?"[957]

(continued)

This reminds me of a famous Philip Morris cigarette ad that tried to downplay the risks of smoking. It argued that if you think secondhand smoke is bad (increasing the risk of lung cancer by 19 percent), drinking one or two glasses of milk every day may be three times as bad (a 62 percent higher risk of lung cancer). So, it concluded, "Let's keep a sense of perspective." The ad went on to say that the risk of cancer from secondhand smoke may be "well below the risk reported . . . for many everyday items and activities."[958]

That's like saying we shouldn't worry about getting stabbed, because getting shot is so much worse. (Note: Philip Morris stopped throwing dairy under the bus after it acquired Kraft Foods.)

CANCELING CANCER

One of the ways our body tries to protect us from cancer is by releasing a binding protein into our bloodstream to tie up any extraneous IGF-1. Think of it as our emergency brake. Let's say you've managed to downregulate production of new IGF-1 through diet. What about all that excess IGF-1 still circulating from the bacon and eggs you may have eaten the day before? No problem: The liver releases a snatch squad of binding proteins to help take it out of circulation.

The release of IGF-1 triggered by animal protein consumption may explain why you can so dramatically bolster the cancer-fighting power of your bloodstream within weeks of switching to a plant-based diet. After only eleven days of cutting back on animal protein, your IGF-1 levels can drop by 20 percent and your levels of IGF-1 *binding protein* can jump by 50 percent. After study subjects ate plant-based for less than two weeks, researchers dripped their blood onto some cancer cells growing in a petri dish and found that it suppressed cancer growth 30 percent better than before. This has been demonstrated on both prostate cancer and breast cancer cells.[959] The remarkable strengthening of cancer defenses is attributed to the dietary changes in IGF-1. How do we know? If you add back to the cancer cells the amount of IGF-1 that had been banished by plant-based eating, the cancer cell growth comes surging back.[960] Participants in this intervention also added a walking component to their routines, but when it comes to IGF-1 binding and killing off cancer cells, even 3,000 hours in the gym appear to be no match against some walking plant-eaters.[961]

The cancer-suppressing effect seems so powerful that, in a randomized controlled trial, Dr. Ornish and colleagues appeared to be able to slow, stop, and even reverse the progression of early-stage, non-aggressive prostate cancer without chemotherapy, surgery, or radiation—just a plant-based diet and lifestyle program. After one year, the subjects' bloodstream was nearly eight times better at suppressing the growth of cancer cells.[962] Biopsies showed a downregulation of critical cancer genes, effectively the switching off of the expression of cancer growth genes at a genetic level.[963] If you instead eat a lot of dairy after a prostate cancer diagnosis, for example, you may suffer a 76 percent higher risk of death overall and a 141 percent increased risk of dying specifically from your cancer.[964] The reduction in IGF-1 from the reduction of animal protein intake may explain why vegans—those who don't eat meat, eggs, dairy, or other animal products—have been found to have lower rates of all cancers combined.[965]

A Food That Lowers IGF-1

Are there any foods that actively lower IGF-1? A retrospective[966] and snapshot-in-time study suggested that tomato consumption may be associated with lower IGF-1 levels.[967] One fruitful trial (funded by a lycopene supplement company) of colon cancer patients and lycopene, the red pigment in tomatoes, got people's hopes up.[968] Six other such studies done to date, however, fell flat on their face.[969] There appears to be no overall effect of lycopene supplementation on IGF-1 levels.

Flaxseed reduces IGF-1 levels in rats[970] but failed to do so when it was put to the test in people.[971] Similarly, green tea worked in mice,[972] but neither green tea[973] nor green tea supplements did the same in us.[974] Seaweed may help, though. Giving postmenopausal women just 5 g a day of alaria (*Alaria esculenta*) cut the IGF-1 bump caused by a 67 g protein load by 40 percent.[975]

IGF-1 AND LONGEVITY

Epidemiological studies have found both high *and* low IGF-1 concentrations associated with a shorter lifespan,[976] prompting editorial titles such as "IGF-I: Panacea or Poison?"[977] I take a deep dive into the data in see.nf/igf1, showing how the correlation between low IGF-1 levels and mortality can be a case of reverse causation, as both acute and chronic illness can lower IGF-1 levels to create the spurious appearance of harm.[978] Mendelian randomization methods can help tease this out, studying what happens when people are effectively randomized at birth to genetically have lower or higher lifelong IGF-1 set points. Such studies show that IGF-1 may indeed causally increase the risks of age-related ailments such as heart disease,[979] osteoarthritis,[980] and diabetes.[981] This may help explain why type 2 diabetes risk appears to be increased by animal protein intake but decreased by consumption of plant protein.[982]

As we'll see in the Anti-Aging Eight section, protein restriction alone can improve longevity, but it is possible to separate out the effects of IGF-1 and protein intake. As I noted earlier in the chapter, those who won the genetic lottery to have lower IGF-1 levels without even having to work at it are more likely to survive into their nineties[983] and even live through that decade,[984] and have a longer lifespan overall.[985]

Beyond genetics, there are interventional studies showing a reduction of total protein intake down to recommended levels[986] and/or switching from animal to plant protein sources has a variety of metabolic benefits.[987] However, the prospective study by Longo and colleagues that found the positive association between decreased protein intake and decreased mortality in middle age appeared to flip at around age sixty-five into a negative relationship. This could be due to reverse causation—for example, frail adults may be more likely to be malnourished. Nevertheless, the researchers recommended a protein intake of at least 10 percent of calories after age sixty-five, which would be 50 g on a 2,000-calorie-a-day diet, preferably from plants.[988]

Food for Thought

Insulin-like growth factor 1 is considered to be of cardinal importance for cancer expansion,[989] so downregulating IGF-1 activity not only has the potential to slow the aging process[990] but may be a way to turn anti-aging genes against cancer.[991] IGF-1 is cranked up on high-protein diets and by animal protein in particular. This helps explain the benefits of more plant-oriented eating,[992] as well as why consuming a diet with a relatively low proportion of protein is considered critical for lifelong health.[993]

To help slow this aging pathway, on a daily basis, consider:
- striving to stick to the recommended daily intake of protein of 0.8 g per healthy kg of body weight (0.36 g per pound), which translates to about 45 g a day for the average-height woman and about 55 g a day for the average-height man
- choosing plant-based protein sources whenever possible

INFLAMMATION

In recent years, one of the most medically important discoveries was recognizing the potential role of inflammation in many chronic diseases, including at least eight of the top ten leading causes of death.[994] The magnitude of this new understanding has been compared to the discovery of the germ theory centuries ago, which revolutionized how we prevent and treat infectious diseases.[995]

For most of our time on Earth, infections were a primary cause of death and disease. Without soap, sanitation, or water purification, we were under constant barrage, racked with chronic parasitic infestations from within and attacked on all sides by microbial threats. Without antibiotics, a scraped knee could end up being a mortal wound, which is why our immune systems evolved to be on high alert, erring on the side of overreaction rather than under-reaction.[996] Sometimes, though, that can do us more harm than good. For example, head trauma may kill hundreds of thousands of brain cells, but the ensuing inflammatory response may kill millions of brain cells or the patient themself.[997]

META-INFLAMMATION

Inflammation evolved to be beneficial. When you get a splinter in your finger, for example, and the digit turns red and gets warm, painful, and swollen, that inflammation is your body's natural reaction to tissue damage or irritation. Its purpose is to trigger the healing process, not a disease process.

Your body's reaction to that splinter is an example of acute inflammation, a localized, temporary, direct response to infection or injury focused on resolving a problem. Chronic inflammation, also called *metabolic inflammation*, or *meta-inflammation* for short, on the other hand, is systemic, persistent, and nonspecific and appears to perpetuate disease.[998] It has a low-grade, smoldering quality that can be picked up on blood tests showing abnormally high levels of inflammatory markers like C-reactive protein (CRP).

Ideally, CRP levels in the blood are under 1 mg/L,[999] but, in the presence of infection, it can skyrocket within hours up to 100 mg/L or more.[1000] Today, our highly sensitive CRP blood tests can measure levels to a fraction of a point, which has led the medical community to recognize that having baseline levels of just 2 or 3 mg/L may place us at increased risk of catastrophes like heart attacks and strokes. Baseline CRP levels below 1 mg/L denote lower risk, but most middle-aged Americans have levels that exceed this level,[1001] suggesting that most suffer from chronic inflammation—chronic inflammation that tends to worsen with age.

INFLAMMAGING

As we get older, our immune system gradually deteriorates in a process known as immunosenescence.[1002] This plays a part in explaining why pneumonia, for example, moves up from being the tenth leading cause of death when we're in our fifties and early sixties to being the eighth leading cause when we're sixty-five and older.[1003] It's why latent viruses can reemerge, like chickenpox erupting as shingles after lying dormant for a half century. It also explains why vaccines don't work as well as we age. The annual flu vaccine is only about 50 percent effective among those who need it most.[1004]

On the flip side, the activated immune cells of eighty-year-olds produce significantly *more* pro-inflammatory signals.[1005] This suggests the worst of both worlds—a decline in the part of the immune system that fights specific infections and an aggravation of nonspecific overreactions that can lead to inflammation.[1006] This progressive increase in pro-inflammatory status is now recognized as a major feature of the aging process, formalized in 2000 into a concept called "inflammaging," a chronic low-grade inflammation that may be responsible for the further decline and onset of disease in the elderly.[1007,1008]

CRP levels rise as we age and are associated with reduced survival, poorer physical and cognitive performance,[1009] diminished feelings of vitality,[1010] and a range of age-related diseases, including Alzheimer's, Parkinson's, cardiovascular disease, diabetes, and chronic kidney disease.[1011] Inflammaging is also thought to play a key role in degenerative disc disease in our spine[1012] and the loss of muscle mass and strength as we age.[1013]

CRP is the most widely studied inflammatory biomarker for predicting remaining lifespan.[1014] Having higher CRP levels in your blood may increase your risk of dying prematurely by 42 percent. However, interleukin 6 (IL-6), the most important trigger for CRP production, may be an even better predictor.[1015] Interleukins are chemical messengers used to communicate between (*inter-*) white blood cells (-*leuko*cytes).

In our youth, blood levels of IL-6 are typically low or may even be undetectable, but they begin to increase when we're around fifty to sixty. As a potent pro-inflammatory agent, elevated levels are considered to be one of the most powerful predictors of disease and death in the elderly.[1016] Researchers looked at single blood samples from healthy individuals aged sixty-five and older and found that if their IL-6 levels were in the highest quarter of values, their risk of dying may be 40 percent over the next five years, compared to less than 10 percent among those with values in the lowest quarter.[1017] IL-6 even seems predictive at extreme ages. Centenarians with an IL-6 level in the lowest third of values are three times more likely to be alive nearly five years later, compared to the highest third.[1018] IL-6 appears to be a cause, rather than just a consequence, of life-threatening disease since those born genetically predisposed to higher IL-6 levels are less likely to survive to old age.[1019]

Save Your Skin

Which organs do you think are our largest? Maybe our lungs, liver, or intestines? Those weigh about five pounds each. Our skin, on the other hand, weighs about twenty pounds.[1020] How might our skin contribute to inflammaging?

As young as age forty-five, we start to lose hydration in the outermost layer of our skin, as our skin's barrier function starts to deteriorate.[1021] Barrier breaches can then trigger inflammation that can spill over into the bloodstream. Would topical application of some kind of skin cream be able to lock in moisture and prevent this inflammation? When aged mice were rubbed with petroleum jelly three times a day for ten days, the inflammatory markers went down not only in their skin but throughout their bodies.[1022] This prompted a 2019 study in which researchers put it to the test in people.

Elderly men and women (average age seventy-eight) were randomized to a twice-daily application of 3 mL (about two-thirds of a teaspoon) of an emollient to their skin for a month. Remarkably, not only did the blood levels of inflammatory markers like IL-6 drop significantly compared to elderly controls who didn't moisturize their skin but they dropped down to levels close to that of younger individuals (average age thirty-two).[1023] This suggests that applying skin lotion may be a simple way to dampen systemic inflammation.

HOT AND HEAVY

Inflammation is considered to be an important indicator and driver of aging,[1024] but where is all this inflammaging coming from? Some have suggested chronic infections, such as Epstein-Barr virus or cytomegalovirus (CMV), but preindustrial populations of forager-horticulturalists and hunter-gatherers don't appear to have suffered from inflammaging despite large infectious exposures. We've already covered two implicated sources of inflammaging: the buildup of dietary advanced glycation end products[1025] (the Glycation chapter) and senescent cells spewing SASP[1026] (the Cellular Senescence chapter). Our age-related decline in autophagy machinery (the Autophagy chapter) can also lead to what's been dubbed "garbaging."[1027]

Our immune system may start reacting to the cellular detritus that can build up as we age, and that has led some to speculate that inflammaging—and even part of the aging process itself—may be an elaborate autoimmune, autoinflammatory reaction.[1028] This would be consistent with the fact that two years of modest caloric restriction cut inflammation markers such as CRP by 40 percent. This dramatic anti-inflammatory effect could have been due to a boost in autophagy that cleared out inflammatory cellular debris or simply as a consequence of their weight loss.[1029]

Dozens of studies have found that obesity is strongly associated with increased levels of inflammatory markers, such as CRP, in the blood.[1030] But is the inflammation a cause or a consequence of obesity? We once thought that fatty tissue was simply a passive depot for the storage of excess fat, but we now know that it plays an active role in secreting inflammatory chemicals. Fatty tissue is able to expand so rapidly that it may even outpace its own blood supply and become starved of oxygen.[1031] (An electrode can be inserted directly into an obese belly to measure how low oxygen levels may fall compared with individuals at a healthy weight.[1032]) This oxygen deprivation is thought to contribute to the death of fat cells. But this is not a good thing; fat cell death draws out inflammatory cells like macrophages, a type of roaming white blood cell found in pus, to try to clean up the debris. Indeed, belly biopsies from obese individuals show macrophages swarming throughout the fat.[1033] Then, the macrophages appear to get stuck and fuse together into giant cells, which are a hallmark of chronic inflammation seen in resistant infections like tuberculosis or around foreign bodies our body can't clear.[1034] All this is occurring while inflammatory compounds spill out into general circulation.[1035] As such, obesity appears to lead to systemic inflammation, rather than the other way around.[1036,1037]

Unsafe at Any Feed

Dietary cholesterol may also contribute to inflammation in body fat that can spill over into our bloodstream.[1038] Body fat is a major site for cholesterol storage in humans.[1039] Our fat cells can accumulate high levels of free cholesterol, which cannot be broken down by our cells and is toxic at high concentrations.[1040]

We've known since 2014 that dietary cholesterol promotes the swelling of fat cells and belly fat inflammation in monkeys,[1041] but there weren't any human studies until 2019, when researchers took biopsies from vegetarians and meat eaters. Vegetarians generally consume significantly less cholesterol than do omnivores. Although eggs are the single largest source of cholesterol in the American diet, more than any individual type of meat, the number one overall source of cholesterol is meat in general (with twice as much cholesterol coming from white meat as from red).[1042] So, researchers expected to find less inflammation in the biopsies from vegetarians than from meat eaters, and they did. Not only did the vegetarians' thigh fat average fewer than half of the pro-inflammatory macrophages compared to biopsies taken from omnivores, the meat eaters had 80 percent greater expression of tumor necrosis factor, a potent inflammatory marker, in their abdominal fat.[1043]

Preeminent Harvard nutrition professor Mark Hegsted once wrote that if cholesterol were introduced as a new food additive, the conclusion would almost certainly be that it could not be considered safe at any level,[1044] if only because any intake of dietary cholesterol above zero increases the risk of our number one killer, heart disease.[1045]

As we get older, we experience an increase in visceral fat, the deep abdominal fat that coils around and infiltrates our internal organs, bulging out our belly. The increase in fat mass alone may contribute to inflammaging,[1046] but, as they age, even *individual* fat cells spill out more pro-inflammatory mediators like IL-6 compared to younger fat cells.[1047] So, loss of body fat with chronic caloric restriction may play a role independent of autophagy induction, though it appears to work disproportionally better than weight-loss surgery at reducing inflammation over the same general time frame. Bariatric surgery alone causes about a 60 percent drop in both excess body weight[1048] and CRP,[1049] whereas just a 10 percent drop in body weight in the nonsurgically calorie-restricted group was associated with a 40 percent drop in CRP.[1050]

Visceral fat isn't the only place in the gut that can spill out inflammatory factors. As we age, our microbiome changes. We start to take on opportunistic pro-inflammatory bacteria at the same time that our gut permeability ("leakiness") is increasing, which leads to the seepage of bacterial components into our bloodstream.[1051] Thankfully, as we'll see, all these contributors to inflammaging can be mediated by diet.

THE DIETARY INFLAMMATORY INDEX

The widespread meta-inflammation that occurs throughout our lives appears in part to be the reaction by our immune system to many unhealthy aspects of daily living—from environmental factors, like traffic pollution and toxic chemicals, to our everyday lifestyle choices, including factors such as cigarettes, sleep, chronic stress, and level of physical activity.[1052] However, we may introduce into our body the *primary* driver of meta-inflammatory chronic disease multiple times a day— every time we eat.[1053]

How can we tell if a food is pro-inflammatory or anti-inflammatory? Simple. We can just watch what happens to the levels of C-reactive protein and other inflammation markers after someone eats it. By doing so, we can also assess the impact of individual nutrients, whole foods, meals, or entire dietary patterns.

Researchers scoured thousands of such experiments and developed a scoring system called the Dietary Inflammatory Index.[1054] It's very straightforward: The more pro-inflammatory foods we eat on a daily basis, the higher our score, and the more anti-inflammatory foods we eat, the lower our score. Our goal is an overall negative score, which we can achieve if we eat more anti-inflammatory foods than pro-inflammatory ones. In other words, an anti-inflammatory diet.

Generally, components of animal products and processed foods, like saturated fat, trans fat, and cholesterol, were found to be pro-inflammatory, while constituents of whole plant foods, such as fiber and phytonutrients, came up strongly anti-inflammatory.[1055] It shouldn't be a surprise, then, that the Standard American Diet (SAD) scores as pro-inflammatory. This reached a peak in the early aughts during the Atkins craze, but we still run hot[1056] and have the elevated disease rates to show for it.

Higher Dietary Inflammatory Index scores have been linked to impaired kidney,[1057] lung,[1058] and liver function[1059] and a higher risk of cardiovascular disease.[1060] Those eating more inflammatory diets also appear to experience faster aging at a cellular level.[1061,1062] Pro-inflammatory diets are also associated with the development of frailty[1063] and increased risk of falls in the elderly.[1064]

Pro-inflammatory diets don't only impact our physical health. A recent review concluded that every study that looked at the Dietary Inflammatory Index and cognitive performance found that diets with higher inflammatory potential were linked to impaired memory and cognitive dysfunction.[1065] Inflammatory diets have also been associated with worse mental health, including higher rates of depression, anxiety, and impaired well-being,[1066] as well as lower sleep quality.[1067]

What about cancer? Eating more pro-inflammatory foods has been tied to higher risk of prostate,[1068,1069,1070] breast,[1071,1072] endometrial,[1073] and ovarian cancers.[1074] Higher Dietary Inflammatory Index scores are also associated with heightened risk of esophageal,[1075] stomach,[1076] liver,[1077] pancreatic,[1078] colorectal,[1079] kidney,[1080] and bladder[1081] cancers, as well as non-Hodgkin's lymphoma.[1082]

Overall, eating a more inflammatory diet has been associated with 75 percent increased odds of having cancer and 67 percent increased risk of dying from it.[1083] Not surprisingly, those eating more *anti*-inflammatory diets appear to live longer lives[1084,1085,1086,1087] with less functional disability.[1088] A meta-analysis of a dozen cohort studies, where populations are followed over time, found that those scoring at the higher end of the Dietary Inflammatory Index had a 23 percent higher risk of dying prematurely compared to those at the lower end.[1089]

You've Got to Move It Move It

Lifelong, voluntary wheel-running dampens inflammaging in mice,[1090] but what about in men and women? There have been more than twenty controlled interventional studies on the effect of exercise on inflammation in older adults, and they've consistently shown a beneficial, anti-inflammatory effect.[1091] The IL-6 levels of active older adults may be about 30 percent lower than sedentary age-matched individuals.[1092] Sadly, nearly eight out of ten American adults fail to meet the national physical activity guidelines.[1093]

PRO-INFLAMMATORY FOODS

The food components that rate as most pro-inflammatory are saturated fat and trans fat. In the United States, the top five sources of saturated fat are essentially cheese (including pizza), desserts like cake and ice cream, chicken dishes, pork, then burgers.[1094] With the ban on added trans fat, the only remaining sources in the food supply are the small amounts found naturally in meat and dairy and what's created during the refining of vegetable oils.[1095]

HOW TO REDUCE YOUR ENDOTOXIN EXPOSURE

The inflammatory effects of saturated fat can manifest after a single meal. We've known for nearly twenty years that within hours of eating a high-fat meal (Sausage and Egg McMuffins were used in the original study), your arteries can stiffen, cutting in half their ability to relax normally.[1096] Unhealthy meals don't just cause damage decades down the road but right here and now, within hours of going into your mouth. How do we know it was the fat and not the junky refined carbs in the English muffin? Because you can also cause a spike in inflammation by drinking straight cream, which has zero carbs and is mostly saturated butter fat.[1097] And, just as this inflammatory state starts to calm down five or six hours later, it's time for lunch, when we may once again whack our arteries with another load of saturated fat. This cycle leaves many Americans trapped in a dangerous pit of chronic, low-grade inflammation. It's no wonder dietary saturated fat has been considered an "accelerator of the aging process."[1098]

After just one meal high in saturated fat, IL-6 levels can double within six hours,[1099] approaching levels associated with twice the risk of premature death.[1100] Why is saturated fat so pro-inflammatory?

Palmitic acid, the predominant saturated fat in the American diet[1101] and concentrated in meat and dairy,[1102] directly induces an inflammatory response. Drip some onto human white blood cells in a petri dish, and they start spewing out inflammatory chemicals.[1103] But, saturated fat may also help endotoxins leak through the gut wall into your circulation.[1104] Endotoxins are highly pro-inflammatory structural components of certain types of bacteria, like *E. coli*. As such, the highest levels of these endotoxins are found in foods with high bacterial loads, like meat.[1105] (Fresh hamburger, for example, has been shown to contain approximately a hundred million bacteria per quarter pound.[1106]) Endotoxin activity can be detected in your bloodstream just one hour after eating a high-fat meal.[1107] It's no wonder your body reacts so strongly!

The theory has its critics, though, who argue that since we already have so many bacteria and their endotoxins living in our large intestine, ingesting a few more endotoxins from our food shouldn't matter much in terms of causing systemic inflammation.[1108] After all, we have about two pounds of pure bacteria down where the sun don't shine, so we may already have a whole ounce or so of endotoxin in us. Given that a lethal dose of intravenously injected endotoxin can be just a few millionths of a gram, we could theoretically have a million lethal doses inside our body. The apparent paradox, though, is explained by compartmentalization.[1109] It's all about location, location, location.

Poop is harmless in our colon, but feces shouldn't be injected into our bloodstream, or eaten, for that matter, particularly with fat, as that can promote the absorption of endotoxins high up in the small intestine.[1110] The palmitic acid in animal fat can both disrupt the barrier function of the gut lining, which, in effect, makes it leakier,[1111] and directly ferry endotoxins into our lymph vessels, which eventually dump into our bloodstream.[1112] The same goes even if the poop is well cooked.

You can boil endotoxins for two straight hours with no detriment to their ability to induce inflammation.[1113] Yes, you can kill off any bacteria if you boil your poop soup long enough, but that doesn't destroy their endotoxins. In other words, even when you cook the crap out of meat, you can't really cook the crap out of meat.

Ironically, even when slaughterhouse workers trim off visible fecal contamination, which can occur when the animal's digestive tract is ruptured during the evisceration process,[1114] the trimming can lead to an increase in certain fecal bacteria, thought to be caused by cross-contamination from one carcass to the next.[1115] Then, even when properly stored in refrigeration, endotoxins start accumulating along with the bacterial growth.[1116]

Bust Your Chops

The highest levels of endotoxins have been found in meat and dairy, and the lowest levels in fresh fruits and vegetables—but that was testing *whole* fruits and vegetables.[1117] Most spoilage organisms cannot penetrate the plant's surface barrier to then go on to spoil its inner tissues. That's why fruits and veggies can be out in the orchards and fields all day in the hot sun. Once you cut them open, though, and bacteria can gain access to the inner tissues, the produce can start to spoil within a matter of days.[1118] What does that mean for the prechopped veggies conveniently stocked in grocery stores?

Watch see.nf/precut for details, but basically, endotoxins can build up in refrigerated prechopped vegetables to the point of neutralizing their anti-inflammatory benefits.[1119] The prechopped veggies did not cause inflammation, like in the meat, eggs, and dairy studies, but they did appear to extinguish some of the plant's anti-inflammatory effects.[1120] It's still better to eat prechopped vegetables than no veggies at all, but chopping your own might be the more healthful option.[1121]

BLUNTING THE ENDOTOXIN SURGE

Not all high-fat foods cause inflammation. More than a dozen studies have shown that nuts, for example, don't increase inflammatory markers,[1122] even if you eat handfuls of them a day.[1123] Spreading half an avocado on a beef burger may even blunt some of the inflammation caused by the meat.[1124]

Some reviews purport to show a drop in inflammatory markers when consuming wild game,[1125] which is about as lean as you can get, but that's only compared to store-bought meat. If you eat some really fatty meat, all the common markers of inflammation—CRP, IL-6, and tumor necrosis factor alpha (TNF-α)—shoot up within hours of consumption. What if you instead eat a kangaroo steak, which is extremely low-fat, on the order of elk or moose?[1126] The same thing happens—a rise in all three inflammatory markers—but to a significantly lesser extent.[1127] This would suggest that venison, for example, would cause less inflammation than chicken, which, these days, contains two to three times more calories from fat than from protein and ten times more calories from fat than it had a century ago.[1128] (Note that this may depend on how the deer was shot. Standard rifle bullets can disperse millions of microscopic lead fragments into wild game,[1129] and lead exposure may also be pro-inflammatory.[1130])

"[T]he most obvious solution to this metabolic endotoxinemia appears to be to reduce saturated fat intake," concluded endotoxin scientists.[1131] In the United States, that would mean prioritizing cutting down on the top three sources: cheese, desserts, and chicken.[1132] However, "the Western diet is not conducive to this mode of action," the scientists wrote, "and it is difficult for patients to comply with this request." If that's the case, there is a way to blunt some of the endotoxin surge: Eat fiber-rich foods with your meals.

Researchers randomized people to eat the same McDonald's Sausage and Egg McMuffin breakfast bomb with or without a high-fiber breakfast cereal. The fiber seemed to glom onto the endotoxins, preventing that bump of endotoxemia three hours after the meal. The fiber also reduced the oxidative stress, the free radicals generated by such a meal. Of course, the best way to mediate the impact is to skip past the golden arches altogether, but adding fiber-rich foods may at least make your sad meal a little happier.[1133]

Don't Get Hyper

Animal fat can be inflammatory, but so can animal protein. Check out my *How Not to Die* kidney disease chapter. I describe in detail how a high intake of animal protein can profoundly influence normal human kidney function by inducing *hyperfiltration*, a dramatic increase in our kidneys' workload. Within hours of consuming meat, our kidneys rev up into that hyperfiltration mode. Beef, chicken, and fish all appear to have similar effects.[1134] An equivalent amount of plant protein, though, causes virtually no noticeable stress on the kidneys,[1135] which can translate into the preservation of ailing kidney function.[1136] Why does protein from animals cause that overload reaction while protein from plants doesn't? Because of inflammation. Researchers found that the hyperfiltration response disappeared when study participants were given a powerful anti-inflammatory drug along with animal protein.[1137]

NEU5GC

There's even an inflammatory animal *sugar*. Watch my video see.nf/neu5gc to learn how an acidic sugar called Neu5Gc could be a "Trojan horse" in meat and dairy contributing to the higher rates of cancer, heart disease, and autoimmune diseases.[1138] To quell the inflammation caused by this foreign sugar, the researchers suggest "reduction of dietary Neu5Gc intake and accumulation through simple diet-based interventions."[1139]

Since humans and plants don't make Neu5Gc, does that mean we can only choose between cannibalism and veganism if we want to avoid exposure? No. Already, transgenic pigs have been engineered without Neu5Gc for organ transplants, so one suggestion is that we could use "genetically modified livestock as a source of red meat."[1140] Or, we could stick to eating animals that naturally don't express it in the first place. Neu5Gc is found in most mammals, amphibians, and fish,[1141] with the highest levels in caviar,[1142] but it is rare in birds and reptiles.[1143] Among mammals, the highest levels were found in goat meat,[1144] but, in terms of "potential candidates for human consumption,"[1145] levels were low in venison and missing entirely from the muscles of kangaroos and dogs (but not cats).[1146] Another suggestion would be to take some kind of Neu5Gc-blocker every time we eat meat. The researchers acknowledge that "[i]n practice, it would be hard to arrange for such an antidote to be easily available as part of every meal. . . ."[1147]

POURING SALT ON THE WOUND

Excess sodium raises not only your blood pressure[1148] but also the level of inflammation in your body. It's hard to control people's food intake long-term to study the effects—unless, of course, you can lock people in a space capsule. Mars520 was a 520-day space flight simulation designed so we could see how people might do on the way to Mars and back. For up to months at a time, the nascent astronauts were put on different levels of salt, and the findings clearly showed that a drop in sodium intake leads to a drop in inflammation.[1149] This has implications for inflammatory diseases such as asthma,[1150] multiple sclerosis,[1151] psoriasis,[1152] lupus,[1153] and arthritis.[1154] For more details, see my video see.nf/saltinflammation.

ANTI-INFLAMMATORY FOODS

In the Dietary Inflammatory Index, the spice turmeric is the single most anti-inflammatory food, followed by ginger and garlic, and tea, green or black, is the most anti-inflammatory beverage. In terms of the most anti-inflammatory food *components*, the top two are fiber and flavones.[1155] Dietary fiber, found in all whole plant foods, is most highly concentrated in whole grains and legumes, such as chickpeas, beans, lentils, and split peas.[1156] Flavones are plant compounds concentrated in fruits, herbs, and vegetables,[1157] with apples, oranges, parsley, celery, and bell peppers the leading sources in the American diet,[1158] while chamomile tea is the most flavone-filled beverage.[1159]

FIBER SOOTHES THE SAVAGE BEAST

How and why is fiber so anti-inflammatory? Check out see.nf/fiber for the full story, but basically, we feed the good bacteria in our gut with prebiotics like fiber, and they feed us right back with short-chain fatty acids like butyrate, the primary fuel of the cells lining our colon. The good bacteria in our gut feed us and try to keep us healthy because they have a pretty good thing going. Our guts are warm and moist, and food magically keeps coming down the pipe. If we die, though, they lose all that. If we die, they die, so it's in their best evolutionary interest to keep us happy.[1160] But there are bad bugs, too, like cholera that causes diarrhea. They have a different strategy: The *sicker* they can make us, the more explosive the diarrhea, for example, the better their chances of spreading to other people and into other colons. They don't care if we die, because they don't intend on going down with the ship.[1161]

So, how does the body keep the good bacteria around while getting rid of the bad? Think about how tricky this is. We have literally trillions of bacteria in our gut, so our immune system must constantly maintain a balance between tolerating good bacteria and attacking bad. Wouldn't there need to be a way for our good bacteria to signal to our immune system that they're the good guys? Yes, and there is. That signal is the fiber breakdown product butyrate. Researchers found that butyrate suppresses the inflammatory reaction and tells our immune system to stand down, saying in effect, "The good guys are on board, so all's well."[1162] (This does not apply to fiber supplements like Metamucil, which are nonfermentable, that is, inedible, to our good bacteria.[1163])

We're not just talking about intestinal inflammation. If you eat some whole grain barley for supper, by the next morning, your good gut bacteria are having it for breakfast, releasing butyrate into the bloodstream[1164] to exert broad anti-inflammatory activities throughout the body.[1165] This may explain why those eating fiber-rich foods are less likely to develop inflammatory conditions from knee pain[1166] and osteoarthritis[1167] to lung inflammation and respiratory diseases like COPD (chronic obstructive pulmonary disease).[1168] Most important, those who eat more fiber-rich foods live longer lives.

ALL IN ONE PIECE

An analysis of ten studies encompassing more than ten million person-years of data found that higher intake of dietary fiber compared to lower intake was associated with a 15 percent lower risk of premature death from all causes combined.[1169]

But since fiber is concentrated in some of the most healthful foods on the planet—fruits, vegetables, whole grains, beans, and nuts—how do we know that fiber intake isn't just a proxy for a healthy diet in general and the survival benefit isn't merely due to the myriad other beneficial components in whole plant foods? If you remember, we ran into a similar conundrum trying to tease out the benefits of eating foods with lower glycemic loads. The solution we turned to was acarbose, the starch-blocking drug that slows the digestion of carbohydrates.

Fiber is just a carbohydrate chain we can't digest, so acarbose can effectively turn some of the regular starch we eat into fiber. Indeed, those taking acarbose end up with more starch in their stool, which provides a bounty for our good gut bacteria.[1170] That's why acarbose can increase the level of good bugs like *Bifidobacterium*,[1171] *Lactobacillus*, and *Prevotella*.[1172] This all means more anti-inflammatory butyrate entering the bloodstream,[1173] and it also gives researchers a tool to test out the fiber–inflammation–longevity connection.

Just as you can enable rats to live longer by feeding them fiber,[1174] you can enable mice to live longer by feeding them acarbose while keeping their diets the same. Why do we suspect the survival benefit is not just a blood-sugar effect? Because the lifespan enhancement correlated with fecal concentrations of butyrate. A single fecal sample taken several months before death (the equivalent of several years for humans) could predict the mouse's likely lifespan.[1175] How can we replicate the effects of acarbose without taking a drug?

Switching from refined grains to whole grains would ferry more fiber down to our colon, but taking the next step and switching to *intact* whole grains (groats) wouldn't only give us more fiber but also sneak down a load of starch. To see why powdered grains can starve our microbial selves, check out my video see.nf/intact. Researchers found that subjects fed the same amount of the same foods doubled their stool size when fed intact versus ground grains.[1176] Our stool is not primarily composed of undigested food. Most of it—about 75 percent—is pure bacteria,[1177] more than a trillion per tablespoon.[1178] No matter how well we chew intact plant foods, when we eat the way nature intended, we transport an array of starch and other prebiotic nutrients down to our good bacteria, who get fruitful and multiply. Production of short-chain fatty acids increases, and we get to bask in all the anti-inflammatory benefits of butyrate.

Centenarian *Anti*-Inflammaging

Since inflammation has a critical role in aging, wouldn't you expect centenarians to have somehow escaped inflammaging? That isn't the case, though. As expected, at their advanced age, people more than a hundred years old have high blood levels of inflammatory compounds. So, what sets them apart? A counterbalance of an equally high blood level of *anti*-inflammatory compounds.[1179] This response is known as *anti-inflammaging*. "[I]f inflammaging is a key to understand aging," an Italian research team suggested, "anti-inflammaging may be one of the secrets of longevity."[1180]

(continued)

Interleukin 10 (IL-10) may be the most potent anti-inflammatory cellular messenger in our blood. Is there a way to boost IL-10 levels?[1181] Eat more fiber. Butyrate "massively" enhances secretion of IL-10,[1182] so raising IL-10 blood levels is as easy as swapping out refined grains in favor of whole grains.[1183] A type of fiber called *beta-glucan* in brewer's, baker's, and nutritional yeasts has been found to boost IL-10. The amount found in two daily tablespoons of nutritional yeast triples IL-10 levels within four weeks.[1184] However, if you have Crohn's disease[1185] or the skin condition known as *hidradenitis suppurativa*,[1186] I caution against the use of nutritional yeast due to potential immune reactivity (see see.nf/crohns for details).

Based on three decades of studying more than a thousand centenarians, researchers identified "a provegetarian diet, rich in vegetables and legumes" as a common denominator. Part of the centenarians' aging success may have been due to an anti-inflammatory boost from all that fiber, but their diets also contained "relatively little meat and animal fat,"[1187] so it's hard to tease out the decisive dietary factors.

PLANT YOURSELF

Given that saturated fat ranks as the single most pro-inflammatory food component and fiber as the single most anti-inflammatory food component,[1188] an anti-inflammatory diet would be one centered around whole plant foods.[1189] See details in see.nf/plantshift, but basically, dozens of interventional trials that put different diets to the test in thousands of individuals have shown that more plant-based diets were more effective in lowering systemic inflammatory markers such as C-reactive protein.[1190]

A completely plant-based diet can help lower CRP levels by 30 to 40 percent within just a few weeks in both adults[1191] and children,[1192] but it need not be all or nothing. Simply swapping out a few servings a week of meat for beans, split peas, chickpeas, or lentils can lower your CRP, IL-6, and TNF-α by about a third within two months.[1193] What if you just add plant foods to your regular diet? Five a day aren't enough. Five daily servings of fruits and veggies don't appear to be sufficient to make a difference, but if you get eight servings a day, you can significantly drop your CRP levels compared to those who eat close to the American average,[1194] a paltry two servings a day.[1195] That's one of the reasons my Daily Dozen recommends a minimum of nine daily servings.

Of course, not all plant-derived foods are anti-inflammatory. If all you do is boost your intake of vegan junk like white bread, soda, and cake, you can end up even more inflamed.[1196] Are any plants particularly potent?

What About Fish?

First and foremost, an anti-inflammatory diet in clinical practice "focuses on eating whole, plant-based foods."[1197] But just as all plant-derived foods are not anti-inflammatory, all animal foods are not necessarily pro-inflammatory. Omega-3 fatty acids found in fish, for example, score as an anti-inflammatory component in the Dietary Inflammatory Index,[1198] even though they only appear to help among those with chronic disease.[1199] When healthy people were given fish oil supplements equivalent to eating about a serving of salmon, one can of tuna, or ten fillets of tilapia every day[1200] for weeks or months, overall, there was no benefit in terms of reducing key inflammatory markers.[1201]

The consumption of fish itself doesn't appear to affect markers of inflammation[1202] or lower inflammatory disease mortality—unlike plant-based omega-3 sources like nuts.[1203] Perhaps the benefits of the omega-3s are offset by the industrial toxins that now contaminate much of the aquatic food chain.[1204] That could also help explain the association found in the Harvard Nurses' Health Study between the consumption of non-dark-meat seafood (such as canned tuna, shrimp, scallops, and lobster) and higher inflammatory markers in the blood.[1205]

BERRY THE INFLAMMATION HATCHET

A study followed 10,000 Norwegian men for four decades and found that those eating berries more than fourteen times each month were significantly more likely to be alive at the end of the investigation.[1206] Higher intake of anthocyanins, berries' brightly colored pigments, has been associated with anti-inflammatory effects,[1207] but it takes interventional studies to prove cause and effect. I review dozens of such studies in my video see.nf/berryinflammation, showing that common berries like blueberries[1208] and strawberries[1209] can significantly reduce markers of inflammation.

This is not just an antioxidant effect. Free radicals can disfigure proteins in our body to the extent that they become so unrecognizable by our immune systems that our own body attacks them as foreign.[1210] We can help mitigate this inflammatory autoimmune response by saturating our body with sufficient antioxidants. High-antioxidant fruits and vegetables, such as berries and greens, have been found to douse systemic inflammation significantly better than the same number of servings of more common low-antioxidant fruits and veggies, like bananas and lettuce.[1211] However, no anti-inflammatory benefit was found for antioxidant vitamins and minerals like vitamins C and E, beta-carotene, or selenium,[1212] which takes us back to the bright red, blue, and purple anthocyanin plant pigments.

Dozens of randomized controlled trials on anthocyanin-rich supplements (mostly berry extracts) have demonstrated anti-inflammatory effects.[1213] This may be why red-fleshed plums beat out yellow-fleshed apricots in reducing CRP blood levels[1214] or why even super healthful fruits like mangos may be powerless against the inflammation caused by eating a meal of fatty meat,[1215] whereas a half dozen studies combined have shown that pomegranates, a fruit packed with ruby red anthocyanins, can bring down inflammation over time.[1216]

The anti-inflammatory effect of berries is so potent that you can actually feel it if you push yourself. The bioflavonoids in citrus can help with muscle fatigue during a tough workout[1217] (see.nf/citrus), but the anthocyanins in berries may help you deal with post-exercise inflammation. Muscle biopsies confirm eating berries can significantly reduce exercise-induced inflammation,[1218] which translates into faster recovery times.[1219] Watch see.nf/soreness for details. Antioxidant supplements, however, don't appear to help.[1220] In fact, men doing arm curls with added vitamin C ended up with *more* muscle damage and oxidative stress.[1221]

Optimizing recovery from a workout is considered to be the "holy grail of exercise science,"[1222] but what about discernible effects on inflammatory conditions of aging, such as arthritis? Tart cherries have been successfully used to treat gout.[1223] Delicious dietary treatments are more than welcome, as some gout drugs can cost $2,000 per dose,[1224] carry no clear-cut distinction among nontoxic, toxic, and even lethal doses,[1225] and can cause a rare side effect in which your skin detaches from your body.[1226] (Of course, the best way to deal with gout is to try to prevent it in the first place with lower alcohol consumption[1227] and a more plant-based diet.[1228]) As I detail in see.nf/berryinflammation, the most common inflammatory joint disorder, osteoarthritis of the knee, can also be mitigated with berry treatment.

How to Lose Count

Considering the anti-inflammatory effects of plant foods and their components, it's no surprise that a pooling of more than twenty studies shows that those eating more plant-based diets have lower CRP levels—especially among those eating purely plant-based.[1229] This has been confirmed with two dozen interventional studies that, overall, found that randomizing people to plant-based diets reduces systemic inflammation within a matter of months or even weeks.[1230] However, plant-based diets can be so effective at causing weight loss that some of the drop in inflammation may be indirect.[1231] Even when weight is taken into account, though, compared to those randomized to eat the American Heart Association's recommended diet, which includes more fruits and vegetables but also low-fat animal products like skinless chicken breast, skim milk, and egg whites, those randomized to an exclusively plant-based diet got a 33 percent drop in CRP within eight weeks.[1232]

In addition to lower CRP levels, those eating more plant-based also tend to have lower white blood cell counts, considered to be a "stable, well-standardized, widely available and inexpensive measure of systemic inflammation."[1233] As I explore in my video see.nf/whitecount, a higher white blood cell count may be an important predictor for cardiovascular disease incidence and mortality, decline in lung function, cancer mortality,[1234] diabetes,[1235] and premature death in general.[1236] Even within the normal range, every drop of just one point may be associated with a 20 percent drop in the risk of premature death.[1237]

How can we lower it? As I discuss in my follow-up video see.nf/idealcount, avoiding secondhand smoke can drop your white count by about half a point,[1238] losing about a quart of excess body fat can lower it by about one point,[1239] and exercising one to two hours a week for two months can drop it about a point and a half,[1240] as can eating a whole food, plant-based diet.[1241]

GO GREEN

The Low Inflammatory Foods Everyday (LIFE) Diet is based on Dr. Joel Fuhrman's high-nutrient-density principles, which includes a daily green smoothie and is packed with other fruits and vegetables.[1242] The LIFE Diet successfully lowered CRP, but participants were also encouraged to limit their consumption of all animal products. However, even looking only at those who drank the green smoothie each day without making any other changes to their usual diet saw an astounding 40 percent reduction in CRP within just one week, claimed to be the fastest diet-induced reduction in CRP ever reported in the medical literature. Here's Dr. Fuhrman's recipe if you want to try it yourself: half a pound of dark green leafy vegetables (such as baby kale), two and a quarter cups of blueberries, one banana, one tablespoon of unsweetened cocoa powder, one tablespoon of ground flaxseeds, half a cup of water, and half a cup of either plain or vanilla soymilk or unsweetened vanilla almond milk.[1243]

The secret to the green smoothie may lie in how it's made. High-speed liquification may enhance the liberation of nutrients. If you blenderize spinach, for example, the bioavailability of its beta-carotene is boosted by nearly 50 percent compared to mincing it, and you get closer to 90 percent more than if you ate the leaves whole.[1244] The same amount of food, but greater or lesser levels of nutrients make it into your bloodstream depending on how you prepare it. The chlorophyll itself may also play a role. It's been found to be anti-inflammatory in a petri dish[1245] and in animal studies,[1246] reducing "paw volume"—that is, how swollen their paws get when injected with some inflammatory irritant. However, the anti-inflammatory effects of chlorophyll have yet to be tested clinically.

Cruciferous vegetables, which encompass kale, collard greens, and others in the broccoli family, may be particularly anti-inflammatory,[1247] which could help explain why they are also more closely associated with living a longer life compared to other veggies.[1248] Special cruciferous compounds appear to inhibit NF-κB, which is a central mediator of inflammation that regulates a battery of pro-inflammatory genes, though it may take eating about two pounds a day to significantly drop IL-6 levels within two weeks.[1249] However, even just about an ounce of broccoli sprouts a day can significantly reduce CRP levels and cut IL-6 in half.[1250] They can easily be sprouted at home year-round in a mason jar for about twenty-five cents a cup.

Hot Tomato

Have any vegetables other than greens been shown to lower inflammation in people? Purple-fleshed potatoes,[1251] tomato juice[1252] and tomato paste[1253] (but not tomato extract supplements[1254]), and shiitake mushrooms.[1255] Details in see.nf/veggies.

GRAIN OF TRUTH

Consistent with recommendations from leading cancer[1256] and heart disease[1257] authorities, I suggest getting at least three daily servings of whole grains. A meta-analysis of eleven studies estimated that such intake would translate into a 17 percent lower overall risk for mortality.[1258] (Amusingly, the authors had a typo, writing instead about "risks for morality." Angel food cake versus devil's food cake?)

The findings aren't surprising, given that whole grain consumption has been associated with a lower risk of dying from cardiovascular disease, cancer, diabetes, and inflammatory diseases in general.[1259,1260] Put simply, millions of people around the world every year could potentially save their own lives by eating more whole grains.[1261] Interventional trials are required to establish cause and effect, though. I review the randomized controlled trials in see.nf/grains, which found that anti-inflammatory effects may be limited to certain subgroups.

THE FLAX OF LIFE

Like whole grains, nuts are linked to lower inflammation in population studies,[1262] as well as lower risks of death from inflammatory disease[1263] and all causes put together.[1264] The interventional trial data, however, are underwhelming. Only two of six of the inflammatory markers tracked in longer-term trials responded to nut consumption.[1265] Certain seeds hold more promise in this dimension.

Watch see.nf/sesame to learn what a quarter cup of sesame seeds a day can do for knee osteoarthritis pain[1266] and see.nf/oxylipins to see what happens when people are randomized to muffins with flaxseeds versus placebo muffins.[1267] Though flaxseeds also reduce conventional inflammatory markers,[1268] the mechanism by which ground flaxseeds reduce blood pressure appears to be through the reduction of oxylipins, pro-inflammatory compounds thought to be involved in inflammaging that rise with age.[1269] But middle-aged adults randomized to eat muffins containing ground flaxseed were able to drop their oxylipin levels down to what one would expect to see in a twenty-year-old within just four weeks.[1270]

THE SPICE OF LIFE

Spices have been used for centuries to treat inflammatory disorders.[1271] If you recall, turmeric is scored as the most anti-inflammatory food in the Dietary Inflammatory Index.[1272] In vitro, curcumin—the pigment in the spice responsible for its bright yellow color—has an anti-inflammatory profile that is stronger and broader than that of the powerful anti-inflammatory corticosteroid drug prednisolone.[1273] Many turmeric preparations have proven to be beneficial for inflammatory diseases of the joints,[1274] lungs,[1275] skin,[1276] and gut,[1277] including purified curcumin, turmeric extracts, and about a daily half teaspoon of the plain spice you can buy at your local market.[1278] Although curcumin from turmeric doesn't appear to blunt the acute pro-inflammatory effects of a milkshake,[1279] for example, when taken over time, randomized controlled trials clearly show a drop in a variety of inflammatory markers.[1280,1281]

Ginger and garlic follow turmeric as the most anti-inflammatory foods in the Dietary Inflammatory Index.[1282] A meta-analysis of more than a dozen randomized controlled studies lasting four to twelve weeks using a half teaspoon to one and three-quarters teaspoons of ground ginger found a significant reduction in inflammatory markers.[1283]

Ginger powder has been used to successfully treat rheumatoid arthritis[1284] and osteoarthritis.[1285] Its pain-reducing effects are on par with ibuprofen,[1286] and it is protective[1287] rather than damaging to the stomach lining.[1288] One-eighth of a teaspoon of powdered ginger, which can cost a single penny, can work as well as the migraine headache drug Imitrex without the medication's side effects.[1289] Taking a third of a teaspoon up to a full teaspoon each day for a few days before your period was shown to significantly lessen menstrual pain and dramatically stanch heavy bleeding.[1290] Dried ginger powder is expected to work better than fresh, since the most potent anti-inflammatory components are dehydration products formed during the drying process.[1291]

Garlic powder can also reduce inflammation blood markers.[1292] Compared to placebo, a third of a teaspoon a day was found to significantly improve pain intensity, tender joint count, fatigue, and disease activity among women with active rheumatoid arthritis.[1293] Any significant side effects? Just body odor and bad breath.[1294]

Anti-inflammatory effects have also been documented for cloves, rosemary,[1295] dill,[1296] cinnamon[1297] (choose Ceylon, not cassia[1298]), and cocoa (except when given with milk).[1299] Details in see.nf/spicy.

Chamomile Tea May Be *Too* Anti-Inflammatory During Late Pregnancy

The single most anti-inflammatory beverage in the Dietary Inflammatory Index is tea.[1300] Green tea is so anti-inflammatory it can be used for pain control as a mouthwash after wisdom tooth surgery.[1301] Chamomile tea is so anti-inflammatory that it may not be safe to drink regularly during late pregnancy, for fear it might prematurely constrict the fetal ductus arteriosus, a temporary blood vessel that the body keeps open with inflammatory compounds to allow the fetus to "breathe" in the womb.[1302] For details, see my video see.nf/thirdtrimester.

ANTI-INFLAMMATORY DRUGS

If inflammation plays a key role in the aging process, what about taking over-the-counter anti-inflammatory drugs like aspirin?

ASPIRIN

Aspirin has been shown to extend the lifespan of mice and other model organisms.[1303] It's been around in pill form for more than a century and is perhaps the most commonly used medication in the world.[1304] We've been using its active anti-inflammatory ingredient, salicylic acid, for thousands of years, though, in its natural form (as an extract of willow tree bark) to ease pain and fever.[1305] One reason it remains so popular despite the existence of even better anti-inflammatory painkillers today is that it's used on a daily basis by millions of people as a blood thinner to reduce the risk of a heart attack.

The benefits of taking a daily aspirin must be weighed against the risk of internal bleeding complications. My video see.nf/aspirin runs through all the numbers. In short, taking an aspirin a day is generally not recommended for those without a known history of heart disease or stroke,[1306] particularly among the elderly, as the risk of bleeding complications increases sharply in individuals over seventy years of age.[1307] How can we get the anti-inflammatory effects without the bleeding risk?

Aspirin is actually two drugs in one. It's technically acetylsalicylic acid. Within minutes of swallowing aspirin, enzymes in our gut split it apart into an acetyl group and salicylic acid.[1308] The acetyl group is what inactivates our platelets and thins our blood. If we could consume salicylic acid directly, we could combat inflammation without the risk of bleeding. That's exactly what we can do with diet.

Vitamin S

In my How Not to Die chapter on avoiding iatrogenic (doctor-induced) death, I note in the aspirin discussion that the willow tree isn't the only plant that contains salicylic acid precursors. They are widely found throughout the plant kingdom in many fruits and vegetables.[1309] In fact, the blood levels of people eating plant-based diets actually overlap with some of those taking low-dose aspirin,[1310] but they can end up with a significantly lower risk of ulcers[1311] due to gut-protective nutrients prepackaged in plants along with the salicylic acid.[1312]

Whole,[1313] organic,[1314] unpeeled[1315] plants have higher concentrations of these aspirin phytonutrients. Standouts include beets, green peas, avocados, dates, nuts, cocoa,[1316] lentils, and buckwheat, but herbs and spices contain the highest concentrations.[1317,1318] Dried basil,[1319] chili powder,[1320] coriander,[1321] dried oregano, paprika, and turmeric are rich in the compound, but cumin has the most per serving. A single teaspoon of ground cumin may have more salicylic acid than a baby aspirin.[1322,1323]

The spicier the better. A spicy vegetable vindaloo has been calculated to contain four times as much salicylic acid–type compounds as a milder Madras-style veggie dish. Approximately one in four vegetarians tested in rural India had blood levels above the lower end of those taking aspirin every day.[1324] This may help explain why India, with its traditionally spice-rich diets, has among the lowest worldwide rates of colorectal cancer[1325]—the cancer that appears most sensitive to aspirin's effects.[1326]

The benefits of salicylic acid are another reason you should strive to choose organic produce. Because a plant uses the compound as a defense hormone, its concentration may be increased when it is bitten by bugs. Pesticide-laden plants aren't nibbled as much, which may be why they appear to produce less salicylic acid. In one study, for example, soup made from organic vegetables was found to contain nearly six times more salicylic acid than soup prepared from conventional, nonorganically grown ingredients.[1327]

Given the strength of the aspirin evidence, some in the public health community talk of a widespread "salicylic acid deficiency" and have proposed that the compound be classified as an essential vitamin: "Vitamin S."[1328] Whether it's the salicylic acid or a combination of other phytonutrients that accounts for the benefits of whole plant foods, the solution is the same: Eat more of them.

Food for Thought

Aging can be thought of as an inflammatory disease.[1329] A single measurement of inflammatory markers, such as CRP or IL-6, can predict physical and cognitive performance, as well as remaining lifespan in elderly individuals. In a study of thousands of individuals followed over time, only about a third of those with age-related diseases starting out with a CRP above 10 mg/L were alive five years later, whereas, among those with a CRP of 3 mg/L or lower, only about a third were dead within the same time frame.[1330]

Thankfully, excess inflammation can be extinguished through changes in diet. Those eating lower on the Dietary Inflammatory Index in middle age are more likely to age successfully, which is defined as living independently with no major chronic diseases, no symptoms of depression, no function-limiting pain, and good overall self-perceived health—good social health, good physicality, and good mental function.[1331] The associated extension of both healthspan and lifespan suggests anti-inflammatory may be synonymous with anti-aging.[1332]

To help slow this aging pathway, on a daily basis, consider:
- reducing dietary and endogenous exposure to inflammatory AGEs (see the Glycation chapter)
- reducing senescent cell SASP inflammation (see the Cellular Senescence chapter)
- boosting autophagy to help clear out inflammatory cellular debris (see the Autophagy chapter)
- applying an emollient skin lotion
- avoiding pro-inflammatory food components, such as saturated fat, endotoxins, Neu5Gc, and sodium, by minimizing intake of meat, dairy, tropical oils, and salt (one lousy breakfast could double your

C-reactive protein levels within four hours before it's even lunch time[1333])

- eating foods shown to be anti-inflammatory, such as legumes, berries, greens, sodium-free tomato juice or tomato paste, oats, flaxseeds, turmeric, ginger, garlic, cinnamon, cocoa powder, dill, green and chamomile teas, and other fiber-, anthocyanin-, and salicylic acid–rich foods

mTOR

It sounds like science fiction. Bacteria in a vial of dirt taken from a mysterious island create a compound that prolongs life. Researchers called it rapamycin—named after the bacteria's home, the mystical Easter Island, known locally as Rapa Nui and famed for its rock-carved figures.[1334] Rapamycin inhibits an enzyme that came to be known as mTOR, or "mechanistic target of rapamycin." mTOR has since been characterized as a "master determinant of lifespan and aging."[1335]

OVER THE HILL AND PICKING UP SPEED

What does the enzyme actually do? mTOR is the major regulator of growth in animals,[1336] and its activation drives increases in both cell size and cell number.[1337] When we're young, mTOR is a life preserver, buoying our development, but when we're older, it can act like a block of cement chained to our ankles, pulling us under.

The action of mTOR has been described as the engine of a "speeding car without brakes." In this analogy, aging is a hurtling car that enters the low-speed zone of adulthood and wreaks havoc because it does not and cannot slow down. Living organisms don't have brakes because they've never needed them. In the wild, animals don't often live long enough to experience aging. Most die even before reaching adulthood, and the same used to be true for humans. Most Londoners, for example, apparently didn't even survive to age sixteen during the seventeenth century.[1338]

In the face of early-age mortality, living beings need to grow as fast as possible to be able to reproduce before dying from external causes. The best evolutionary strategy may be to run at full speed. However, once we pass the finish line, once we win the race to pass on our genes, we're still careening forward at an unsustainable pace, thanks in part to this enzyme. In our childhood, mTOR is an engine of growth, but, in adulthood, it can be thought of as the engine of aging. Nature simply selects for the brightest flame, which in turn casts the darkest shadow.

This is the so-called trade-off theory of aging, a concept technically known as *antagonistic pleiotropy*, in which a gene can have a positive effect when we're young and a negative one when we're old. That explains how genes with deleterious effects late in life can persist in a population.[1339] For example, the pro-inflammatory "Alzheimer's gene" appears to protect us against some childhood infections, major killers throughout most of human existence.[1340]

Unconstrained, mTOR plows full steam ahead, revving up construction pathways to churn out cellular building blocks for new growth and canceling any plans for renovation or demolition. To preserve growth at all costs, mTOR actively suppresses autophagy, countermanding cellular cleansing and rejuvenation.[1341] In the Autophagy chapter, I explained how this can lead to accelerated aging. Conversely, putting the brakes on mTOR and slowing things down appear to decelerate the aging process, extending life and health. Inhibiting mTOR is considered to be the best validated aging regulator.[1342]

The soil bacteria collected from Easter Island weren't making rapamycin to slow down aging but rather to slow down the growth of their natural enemy, soil fungi,[1343] just like fungi make penicillin to wipe out competing bacteria. Fungi, from yeast on up, have mTOR-equivalent genes, as do all plants and animals. mTOR is the universal growth regulator of advanced life-forms.[1344] So, while rapamycin originally drew attention as an antifungal drug, we soon learned it had many other effects.

UNIVERSAL ANTI-AGING DRUG

Dozens of published studies have demonstrated that, by slowing down mTOR, rapamycin extends both the average and maximum lifespans of laboratory mice.[1345] What if you aren't a rodent? Rapamycin appears to be a universal anti-aging drug that lengthens lifespan in all animals and other organisms tested to date,[1346] the only known drug to do so.[1347] It can even work when started in midlife.

The original experiment, conducted by the National Institute on Aging's Interventions Testing Program and published in 2009, was delayed because the researchers were having difficulty keeping rapamycin stable in food pellets for mice. (It can't just be dissolved in their drinking water because it's fat soluble.[1348]) By the time the experiment was up and running, the mice were six hundred days old, which is equivalent to sixty human years.[1349] Even though the mice started the drug so late in life, their lifespan was extended by about 12 percent, which could equate to more than seven additional years of human life.[1350]

Initially, it was debated whether rapamycin was a true anti-aging intervention or "merely" a potent anticancer agent, lengthening lifespans simply by preventing cancer formation.[1351] mTOR signaling is hyperactive in up to 80 percent of human cancers, where it plays a pivotal role in sustaining tumor growth.[1352] When rapamycin was used clinically to prevent the rejection of organ transplants (by suppressing the proliferation of immune cells that attack the new organ), a peculiar side effect was found:[1353] It made cancer disappear. In a set of fifteen patients who had biopsy-proven Kaposi sarcoma, a cancer that often affects the skin, all cutaneous sarcoma lesions disappeared in all subjects within three months after starting rapamycin therapy.[1354] As mTOR is the master regulator of cellular growth, the reduction in cancer incidence is unsurprising, but subsequent studies have shown that rapamycin can do so much more.

In animal models, it extends healthspan, too.[1355] Rapamycin has been shown to ameliorate age-related declines in cognitive and physical function,[1356] regenerate the periodontal bone that holds teeth in place,[1357] and prevent hearing loss,[1358] artery dysfunction,[1359] and tendon stiffening.[1360] It can even rejuvenate the hearts of aged mice.[1361] Remarkably, health and longevity benefits could be achieved with intermittent or transient dosing, such as receiving one dose every five days[1362] or just for a few months during middle age.[1363]

As a dog dad, I was excited to read about the Dog Aging Project, where paw-rents brought their middle-aged canine companions to be randomized to a low rapamycin, high rapamycin, or placebo group for ten weeks. As in the mouse studies, rapamycin appeared to at least partially reverse some age-related heart dysfunction in the dogs without any untoward side effects. Anecdotally, most of the owners of the dogs who covertly got the rapamycin reported their pets displayed increased activity and energy compared to only a minority of those whose pooches got slipped the placebos.[1364] It was time to try rapamycin in humans. I cover all the rapamycin trials to date in see.nf/rapamycin. Bottom line? It is not ready for prime time as an anti-aging drug. Is there any way to suppress mTOR without taking meds?

CALORIE RESTRICTION

For an organism to reach reproductive age as soon as possible, it certainly makes sense to plow full steam ahead, but there are times one has to slow down out of necessity. When we were evolving, we didn't have the luxury of Uber Eats and Instacart. Periodic famine was the norm. Those who didn't slow their roll (in terms of cellular growth) during times of scarcity might not live long enough to pass along their genes. That's why we evolved a braking mechanism triggered by caloric restriction.

Remember AMPK, our fuel gauge enzyme? When our tank is drained, AMPK switches us to energy conservation mode, in part by shutting down mTOR via two separate mechanisms to ensure we don't continue spending wildly while we have pennies in the bank. AMPK and mTOR can be thought of as the yin and yang of nutrient sensing and growth control.[1365] One goes up as the other goes down, based on nutrient availability.

Suppression of mTOR may be a central mediator of the lifespan-extending effects of dietary restriction.[1366] mTOR may explain why women hospitalized for anorexia were found to have half the risk for breast cancer.[1367] The severe caloric restriction caused by their disorder may have tamped down the very mTOR expression that has been noted in breast cancer tumors and associated with more aggressive disease progression, as well as a lower survival rate among breast cancer patients.[1368] Of course, as one of the deadliest psychiatric disorders,[1369] anorexia nervosa also carries tremendous risk, but serious long-term caloric restriction is no cakewalk either.

Caloric restriction has been heralded by some as a fountain of youth,[1370] but negative side effects may include dangerously low blood pressure, infertility, slower healing of wounds, menstrual irregularities, sensitivity to cold, and loss of strength, bone, and libido, as well as "psychological conditions such as depression, emotional deadening, and irritability." You're also walking around starving all the time. In the infamous Minnesota Starvation Study that used conscientious objectors as guinea pigs during World War II, many of the volunteers suffered a preoccupation with food, constant hunger, binge eating, and many emotional and psychological issues.[1371] Even researchers who study caloric restriction rarely practice it themselves.[1372] There's got to be a better way to suppress mTOR.

PROTEIN RESTRICTION

The breakthrough came when scientists discovered that the benefits of eating less may not be coming from restricting calories but, rather, from restricting protein. A comprehensive, comparative meta-analysis of dietary restriction in animal models found that the proportion of protein intake was more important for life extension than was the degree of caloric restriction.[1373] In fact, just reducing protein intake without any changes in caloric intake has sometimes been shown to have effects similar to restricting calories.[1374] Rats fed a diet of about 8 percent protein live almost 40 percent longer than rats fed a diet that's around 20 percent protein.[1375]

It makes sense that protein intake can drive mTOR activation. It's not enough to have energy (calories); construction crews need building materials. Yes, insufficient calories can shut down mTOR by cranking up AMPK, but calories aren't the primary inducer of mTOR activity—amino acids are, the building blocks of proteins.[1376] That's good news. Protein restriction is much easier and safer to maintain than dietary restriction, and it may be even more powerful because it suppresses mTOR *and* IGF-1, the two pathways thought responsible for the longevity and health benefits of caloric restriction.[1377]

A small handful of amino acids are particularly important: methionine and the three branched-chain amino acids (BCAA), isoleucine, leucine, and valine[1378] (so named since they happen to have fatty side-chains branching off from their central structure). Restriction of these specific amino acids recapitulates many of the beneficial effects of protein restriction, which itself is the fulcrum of caloric restriction, and restricting only methionine is sufficient to extend life in a lab.[1379] So, restricting all calories to boost lifespan via mTOR suppression is like fasting to manage a peanut allergy. It works, but it's unnecessary overkill.

Where are these mTOR-accelerating amino acids concentrated? In animal proteins. There is more mTOR-stimulating leucine in whey protein than in a comparable amount of wheat protein.[1380] Those eating strictly plant-based diets still tend to exceed overall protein requirements but end up taking in about 30 percent fewer BCAAs (including leucine) and 47 percent less methionine than omnivores. This translates into significantly lower levels in their blood, perhaps helping to explain the longer lives[1381,1382] and lower cancer rates among those eating more plant-based.[1383] (Tryptophan is the only other amino acid for which restriction alone can promote longevity, delay tumor onset, and increase average and maximum lifespans in rats.[1384] It is also found in lower levels in the diets and bloodstreams of those eating plant-based diets.[1385])

This may also help explain the longevity of long-living populations like that of Okinawa, Japan, who had about half the mortality rate of Americans from major age-related diseases. The traditional Okinawan diet is heavily plant-centric. Only about 10 percent is protein, and less than 1 percent is made up of animal products, the equivalent of one serving of meat a month and one egg every two months.[1386] Their longevity is surpassed only by those regularly eating no meat at all, the vegetarian Adventists in California,[1387] who have perhaps the highest life expectancy of any formally described population in history.[1388]

Individuals eating plant-based have the additional advantage of more easily avoiding palmitic acid, the saturated fat found mainly in meat and dairy that has also been shown to activate mTOR.[1389] A note of caution: Those following a plant-based diet who do not ensure a regular, reliable source of vitamin B_{12}, either through supplements or B_{12}-fortified foods, may have elevated levels of a methionine breakdown product called *homocysteine*.[1390] Homocysteine is also an mTOR activator,[1391] but it can be detoxified with adequate B vitamin intake.

LEUCINE RESTRICTION

To combat the diet-induced mTOR boost, some researchers have suggested that drugs could be developed to block some of the intestinal absorption of the offending amino acids.[1392] It makes more sense to me to just eat less of them in the first place. Leucine may be the most effective mTOR activator and is concentrated where it makes the most sense for growth promotion: in milk.[1393] Whey proteins contain the highest amount of leucine, 75 percent more than beef.[1394] A whey protein beverage can significantly boost mTOR activation within an hour of ingestion.[1395]

Bovine milk has more than three times the leucine of human milk,[1396] which is reasonable because calves grow about forty times faster than human babies.[1397] (Baby rats double their weight in five days, so it's understandable that rat milk has more than ten times the leucine compared to ours.[1398]) Different animals have different amounts of leucine in their milk, appropriate for the growth and development needs of their offspring. No animal—except humans—drinks milk after weaning.

Milk is not a simple beverage. It has a highly sophisticated hormone-signaling system designed to activate mTOR.[1399] When we drink the milk of a faster-growing species, especially later in our life, there is concern we may "over-stimulate" mTOR signaling.[1400] One early, visible manifestation of excessive mTOR stimulation may be acne.

Acne is considered a disease of Western civilization, as it was rare or even nonexistent in places like Okinawa.[1401] The acne-aggravating effects of milk drinking were first noted more than a century ago.[1402] Those who consume the most dairy have more than double the odds of developing acne as those who consume the least.[1403] Seventy-five to 90 percent of commercial dairy products in the marketplace comes from pregnant cows, so this may relate to the hormone content in milk, but mTOR alone appears to increase risk, in part by promoting the production of sebum, the oily sebaceous gland secretion.[1404]

Acne is considered the prototypical mTOR-driven skin disease.[1405] The fact that up to 85 percent of teens in Western countries exhibit acne implies overactivated mTOR signaling[1406] and offers an explanation why a history of acne has been associated with both breast[1407] and prostate cancer risk.[1408] mTOR is upregulated in nearly 100 percent of advanced human prostate cancers,[1409] which may help explain why milk consumption has been found to be a major dietary risk factor for both the development[1410] and spread of prostate cancer.[1411]

Milk drinkers also appear to live shorter lives, unless they drink fermented (soured) milk.[1412] In the fermentation process, the lactic acid bacteria break down some of the galactose, branched-chain amino acids, and bovine microRNAs[1413] (see page 528), which may explain why yogurt intake doesn't carry the same risk.[1414]

A CUP OF TEA AND BROCCOLI

Is there anything we can eat to dampen mTOR activity? Tomato powder decreases mTOR activation in aging rats[1415] and a tomato extract slowed mTOR in human breast cancer cells in a petri dish,[1416] but they have yet to be clinically evaluated. Broccoli compounds, however, have been put to the test.

There's a compound called DIM, which is formed when the cruciferous vegetable compound indole-3-carbinol hits our stomach acid,[1417] and it's been shown to suppress mTOR activation.[1418] Sulforaphane, another product of consuming vegetables in the broccoli family, also cools down mTOR,[1419] which may help explain why those who eat their greens live, on average, longer, more healthful lives.[1420]

Given that hyperactive mTOR signaling may play a role in autism,[1421] researchers from Johns Hopkins and Harvard conducted a double-blind, randomized, placebo-controlled trial with an amount of sulforaphane equivalent to a few cups of broccoli a day in young men with autism[1422] and showed benefits no drug has ever matched.[1423] (Details in see.nf/autism.)

Is there anything we can drink to dampen mTOR activity? Exposing yeast cells to the level of caffeine that would be found in your bloodstream after a cup of coffee led to an inhibition of TOR activity sufficient to extend life.[1424] In mice, both caffeinated and decaffeinated coffee consumption was able to downregulate mTOR to a similar extent, suggesting there's something other than caffeine in coffee that may be helping.[1425] Similarly, green tea contains the flavonoid EGCG that itself suppresses mTOR activity at physiologically relevant concentrations.[1426] This could help explain why a topical 2 percent green tea lotion can cut the number of pimples in half[1427] and why green tea consumption is associated with living a longer life.[1428]

WHAT ABOUT MUSCLE MAINTENANCE?

If dietary changes are so good at suppressing mTOR, might we be concerned about rapamycin-style side effects? The enzyme is part of two different protein complexes— mTOR complex 1 (mTORC1) and mTOR complex 2 (mTORC2). mTORC1 is the aging accelerator, whereas mTORC2 actually appears to be protective. Unfortunately, rapamycin inhibits both, and with mTORC2 disruption come many of its adverse effects. Protein restriction, however, targets only mTORC1, so you get the best of both worlds.[1429] Is there any downside to dietary mTOR suppression?

mTOR signaling is required for the bulking of muscle mass in response to resistance exercise,[1430] raising the possibility of, as one rehabilitation medicine journal editorial title put it, "The mTOR Conundrum: Essential for Muscle Function, but Dangerous for Survival."[1431] However, the suggestion that leucine restriction might accelerate the rate of muscle loss with aging does not seem to be supported. Higher mTOR activation in men may help explain why they tend to live shorter lives than women,[1432] yet men experience a higher rate of age-related muscle loss.[1433] And, giving months of leucine supplements with meals to elderly men did nothing to increase muscle mass or strength.[1434,1435]

In mice, blocking mTOR with rapamycin *protects* aging muscle. Mice genetically engineered to overstimulate mTOR suffer a catastrophic collapse of muscle mass, which is prevented by mTOR inhibition. This suggests that, if anything, mTOR may drive detrimental muscle aging.[1436]

Food for Thought

The enzyme mTOR is recognized as a major driver of aging,[1437] the "Grand ConducTOR" of aging, if you will.[1438] (mTOR seems to bring out the punny side of study authors: "TORwards a Victory over Aging"[1439] or, my favorite, "The Magic 'Hammer' of TOR."[1440]) Perhaps more so than any other single anti-aging strategy, mTOR inhibition disrupts a panoply of degenerative processes,[1441] explaining why the mTOR-blocking drug rapamycin is currently the most effective pharmacological approach ever devised for targeting aging.[1442] Nonpharmacological approaches to slowing this "pacemaker of aging"[1443] include the restriction of certain amino acids, such as methionine and leucine, protein restriction in general, or full dietary restriction.

To help slow this aging pathway, on a daily basis, consider:
- following all the steps to boost AMPK from pages 22–23
- striving to stick to the recommended daily intake of protein, 0.8 g per healthy kg of body weight (0.36 g per pound), which translates to about 45 g a day for the average-height woman and about 55 g a day for the average-height man
- choosing plant-based protein sources whenever possible

OXIDATION

Earl Stadtman, revered biochemist and recipient of the National Medal of Science, the highest honor for scientific achievement in the United States, once said, "Aging is a disease. The human lifespan simply reflects the level of free radical damage that accumulates in cells. When enough damage accumulates, cells can't survive properly anymore, and they just give up."[1444]

This concept, first proposed in 1972[1445] and known today as the mitochondrial theory of aging, suggests that, over time, free radical damage to our mitochondria leads to a loss of cellular function and energy. Our mitochondria are the power source for our cells. Think about charging your phone over and over; its capacity diminishes every time you recharge it. Similarly, as our power plant mitochondria accumulate free radical damage, they may also lose function over time.

HULK SMASH

For a refresher on what exactly free radicals are and how they are formed, see my comic-book characterization of the quantum biology of oxidative phosphorylation in the brain disease chapter in *How Not to Die*. Suffice it to say, free radicals tend to be unstable, violently reactive molecules with an unpaired electron.

Electrons, tiny building blocks of matter, like to travel in pairs. Free radicals try to pair their unmatched electrons by stealing electrons away from any molecule in their path.[1446] This can have varying effects, depending on what kind of molecule is mugged. When fat is attacked, cell membranes can be disrupted.[1447] When enzymes are targeted, they can become inactivated.[1448] When other proteins are damaged, they can unravel and create new structures that our very own immune system may attack as foreign, thus leading to a form of autoimmune inflammation.[1449] And, when free radicals rip electrons from our DNA, our genes can become mutated and our DNA strands literally broken.[1450] Thankfully, our body has an array of antioxidant defenses that can harmlessly donate spare electrons and thereby defuse free radicals.

An imbalance between excess free radicals and inadequate antioxidant defenses is known as oxidative stress. According to the theory, the resultant cellular damage essentially causes aging. So, aging and disease are conceptualized as the oxidation of our body. Those brown age spots on the back of your hands? Oxidized fat and protein under the skin. Oxidant stress is thought to be why we get wrinkles[1451] and become more forgetful,[1452] and why our organ systems break down as we get older. In sum, the theory goes, we're rusting.[1453] (Rust is the oxidation of metal.) That's the rationale for eating more antioxidants, but does that actually work? Despite 20,000 published reviews of more than a quarter million papers on antioxidants,[1454] it remains a controversial topic.[1455] First, let's examine if the theory about oxidation and aging is even true.

THE ONLY THEORY THAT EXPLAINS THE SPREAD

More than three hundred theories of aging have been proposed.[1456] Although none has achieved general acceptance,[1457] the mere fact that the mitochondrial theory has persisted for nearly half a century lends it a certain weight.[1458] Its origins can even be traced back decades earlier than Stadtman's proposal in the 1970s—back to when scientists noted a parallel between many of the manifestations of aging and the DNA-damaging effects of radiation exposure.[1459] This led to the free radical theory of aging of 1956, the proposal that aging was due to the accumulation of oxidative tissue damage.[1460] Then, with the realization that mitochondria were the major source of cellular free radical formation, it morphed into the mitochondrial theory.[1461]

Any successful theory of aging must be able to solve a fundamental mystery: *Why do the maximum lifespans of animals vary so widely?* There is a two hundredfold difference among mammals. Some shrews may only live for a year, while bowhead whales can reach two hundred years or more[1462]—and they're only the second-longest living animal.[1463] The ocean quahog, a clam in the North Atlantic, can live to be more than five hundred years old.[1464] That's *thousands* of times that of some other invertebrates that may only survive a few days. Just one theory of aging can account for the only known parameters that can explain this spread: the mitochondrial theory.[1465]

This theory proposes that the lower the rate of mitochondrial free radical production, the longer animals live. This is not a matter of metabolic rate. Bats and birds, for example, have high metabolisms yet relatively high longevity. The mitochondria of long-lived species simply appear to be more efficient. They often leak fewer electrons, which correlates with less oxidative damage to mitochondrial DNA.[1466] (Mitochondria have their own tiny loops of DNA commonly thought to code for just thirteen proteins,[1467] separate from the bulk of DNA coding of the more than 20,000 genes in the cellular nucleus.[1468]) Thankfully, mitochondrial efficiency is not some immutable characteristic. We may be able to reduce our mitochondrial free radical production rate through exercising,[1469] as well as by making a single dietary tweak—lowering our intake of the amino acid methionine.[1470]

HOW TO LOWER METHIONINE INTAKE

The methionine content of tissues is linked tightly to maximum lifespan among mammals. The lower the methionine, the longer the longevity. This makes sense within the mitochondrial theory, since methionine is the protein component most susceptible to oxidation.[1471] High methionine levels don't just make you vulnerable to oxidative stress, though—they actively cause it. This can even be demonstrated in a test tube. When methionine is dripped onto isolated mitochondria, they start churning out more free radicals.[1472] To see if diet can dial it down, researchers put it to the test.

In rodents, a dietary restriction of 40 percent less food decreases the rate of mitochondrial free radical generation and increases lifespan. This was found to be due to the drop in protein intake. Rather than restricting diet across the board, just cutting protein had the same effects, whereas fat or carbohydrate restriction alone affected neither free radical formation nor longevity. In turn, the beneficial effects of protein restriction on mitochondrial function were found to be due to the drop in the single amino acid methionine.[1473] Restricting all dietary amino acids except methionine had no effect on mitochondrial free radical flux or DNA damage, but restriction of just methionine did both.[1474] This led to the conclusion that the electron leakiness of mitochondria appeared to be controlled by the amount of methionine in the diet.[1475]

Within a period of seven weeks, restricting the intake of methionine in rats lessened electron leakage, free radical formation, and mitochondrial DNA damage.[1476] Consistent with the mitochondrial theory, this appeared to slow aging, as evidenced by a reduction in the incidence of a range of degenerative age-related ailments and an extension of lifespan.[1477] As discussed in chapters on other anti-aging pathways, such as autophagy (see page 23), there are many ways dietary restriction can prolong life, but methionine restriction alone is thought to account for about 50 percent of the lifespan extension attributed to full dietary restriction.[1478]

There are three ways to lower methionine intake. We can decrease our overall intake of food, but that can leave us hungry, and we can also lower methionine by just decreasing our overall intake of protein.[1479] Many Americans get more than twice as much protein as is needed,[1480] so it could be a matter of going from excessive intakes to the recommended intake.[1481] Doing so has been shown to offer a variety of metabolic payoffs within a matter of weeks, thought due to the concurrent drop in branched-chain amino acid intake.[1482] Speaking of bonus benefit, the third way to reduce our methionine intake is by swapping out animal protein for plant protein.[1483] (See the methionine sources graph on page 577.)

At one time, the comparably low methionine content in legumes (beans, split peas, chickpeas, and lentils) had been considered a nutritional disadvantage, but longevity researchers have concluded that the newly discovered multitude of benefits ascribed to methionine restriction "ironically converts such 'disadvantage' into a strong advantage."[1484] This is consistent with data showing legume consumption may be the most important dietary predictor of survival in older people around the world,[1485] a cornerstone of longevity Blue Zones diets.[1486] Plant-based diets are said to make methionine restriction "feasible as a life extension strategy."[1487]

WHAT ABOUT ANTIOXIDANT SUPPLEMENTS?

Antioxidant supplements are a multibillion-dollar industry[1488] and frequently touted as having anti-aging benefits, despite hundreds of studies failing to find clear evidence of such effects.[1489] Those taking antioxidant supplements don't appear to live any longer.[1490] What's more, when put to the test in randomized controlled trials, beta-carotene, vitamin A, and vitamin E supplements seem to *increase* mortality.[1491] In effect, supplement users may be paying to live a shorter life.

My video see.nf/antioxsupplements explains why. For example, supplements contain only a select few antioxidants, whereas our body relies on hundreds of them, all working together to create a network to help dispose of free radicals.[1492] High doses of a single antioxidant may upset this delicate balance.[1493] Rather than working in isolation, antioxidant compounds can act synergistically.[1494] In essence, the whole (food) may be greater than the sum of its parts.[1495]

As I explain in the video, the bottom line is that the close proximity or even physical contact between mitochondrial DNA and the source of free radical formation likely explains why antioxidants can't seem to slow the rate of aging,[1496] but that doesn't mean antioxidants can't prevent age-related diseases linked to oxidative damage to the 99.999995 percent[1497] of our DNA *outside* the mitochondria.

FREE RADICALS ACCELERATE AGING

Our nonmitochondrial DNA is compartmentalized inside the cell nucleus, out of the direct line of fire from the mitochondria, but it is still subject to constant assault from free radicals. Each day, our genome suffers an estimated 70,000 hits, manifesting largely as single-stranded breaks in the DNA double helix. Thankfully, we have an array of DNA repair mechanisms (the subject of a Nobel Prize in 2015) that may be able to fix a break before the cell divides and passes along the DNA lesion as a mutation.[1498] Unfortunately, our DNA repair capacity declines with age,[1499] which may explain the accumulation of DNA damage seen in older individuals[1500] (though centenarians tend to escape with relatively less oxidative damage).[1501] Why do we believe this is not just a consequence of aging but a cause of it? The most compelling evidence is that most of the rare genetic syndromes of premature aging are caused by mutations of DNA repair genes.[1502] Parallels have also been drawn with the long-term effects of cancer treatment.

Radiation therapy and genotoxic chemotherapy work by purposefully creating free radical–induced DNA damage to kill rapidly dividing cancer cells. All exposed cells are affected, though, not just cancerous ones. If DNA damage is a driver of aging, one would expect such cancer survivors to suffer prematurely from age-related disability, and that indeed appears to be the case, with survivors experiencing conditions such as arthritis decades earlier than expected. Twenty percent of survivors of childhood cancers have a heart attack or stroke by age fifty compared to only one percent of their siblings by that age. Ten percent of seniors aged sixty-five or older suffer from frailty, a disabling loss of endurance and strength. That's the same percentage of pediatric cancer survivors suffering from frailty in their thirties. Whether arising from congenital deficiencies in DNA repair or exposure to genotoxic agents, the consequence of excess DNA damage appears to be the same: accelerated aging.[1503]

Oxidative stress has been implicated in hair graying;[1504] the development of cataracts, arthritis, frailty, and neurodegenerative, cardiovascular, kidney, and pulmonary diseases;[1505] cognitive decline; age-related macular degeneration;[1506] and muscle loss.[1507] Lowering antioxidant defenses in mice results in accelerated hearing loss, cataract formation, and cardiac dysfunction, whereas increasing antioxidant capacity affects the reverse,[1508] delaying age-related disease.[1509] So, in this aging pathway, lifespan modulation may require quelling free radical formation, but healthspan enhancement may be achieved through bolstering our antioxidant defenses to help quash the resulting oxidant stress.

OUR ORIGINAL DIET

The paleo diet view of human nutrition posits that the agricultural revolution over the last 10,000 years is but an evolutionary eye blink and humans are adapted to Paleolithic diets heavy with lean meat.[1510] Why stop there? If our entire evolutionary timeline were scaled down to a year, the last 200,000 years of Stone Age humanity would be but a few days, representing just the last 1 percent of the roughly twenty million years we've been evolving since our common great ape ancestor.[1511]

During our truly formative years, perhaps the first 90 percent of our existence before we learned how to use tools, our nutritional requirements reflected an ancestral past in which we ate mostly leaves, flowers, and fruits,[1512] similar to that of our fellow great apes.[1513] This could explain why fruits and vegetables are not only good for us but are, in fact, vital to our survival.[1514]

Humans are one of the few mammals so adapted to a plant-based diet that if we don't eat enough produce, we could actually die from scurvy, a disease of vitamin C deficiency.[1515] Most other animals make their own vitamin C, but why would our body expend all that effort to do the same when we evolved hanging out in the trees and eating fruits and veggies all day long?[1516]

Presumably, it's not a coincidence that the few other mammals unable to synthesize their own vitamin C—such as guinea pigs, fruit bats, and some rabbits—are all strongly herbivorous, just like the great apes.[1517] Data from human fossilized feces deposited in the Stone Age tell us that we may have been getting up to ten times more vitamin C and ten times more dietary fiber than we do today.[1518,1519] Are these incredibly high-nutrient intakes simply an unavoidable by-product of eating whole plant foods all the time, or might they actually be serving some important function, like antioxidant defense?[1520]

Plants create an impressive array of antioxidants from scratch to defend their own structures against free radicals in the firestorm of photosynthesis.[1521] There is a reason plants can lounge about in the sun all day long without getting sunburned (which in us is an inflammatory reaction to the DNA damage created in part by UV ray–induced free radicals).[1522] The human body must defend itself against the same types of pro-oxidants, so we, too, have evolved an array of amazing antioxidant enzymes that are effective—but they aren't infallible. Indeed, free radicals can breach our defenses and cause cumulative DNA damage with age.[1523] This is where plants can come in.

Plants make antioxidants so we don't have to. Since antioxidant-rich foods traditionally formed such a major part of our ancestral diet, we didn't have to evolve that great of an antioxidant system. We could just let the plants in our diet pull some of the weight, like giving us vitamin C so we didn't have to be bothered to make it ourselves.[1524] Using plants as a crutch may well have relieved the pressure for further evolutionary development of our own defenses. So, we became dependent on getting massive quantities of plant foods in our diet, and, when we don't, we may suffer adverse health consequences.

At what point in our evolutionary history did we stop consuming enough antioxidant-rich plants? Even during the Stone Age, this may not have been a problem. Only recently did we start giving up on whole plant foods.[1525] Today, paleo and low-carb followers may actually be eating more vegetables than those on standard Western diets.[1526] Great! The problem isn't that people want to cut their carb intake by swapping out junk food in favor of vegetables. The concern is the shift toward animal-sourced foods. According to NYU nutrition professor emerita Marion Nestle, if there is one takeaway from anthropological studies of ancestral diets, it's that "diets based largely on plant foods promote health and longevity. . . ."[1527]

WHICH FOODS HAVE THE MOST ANTIOXIDANTS?

In many ways, our prehistoric ancestors consumed a larger amount of antioxidants than we do but had less need for them. In modern life, we are surrounded by new pro-oxidant stresses—from air pollution and cigarette smoke, to alcohol and junk food, and pesticides and industrial chemicals.[1528] This makes it even more important to buttress our inherent antioxidant defenses with antioxidant-rich foods. Today, we have the advantage of being able to get seasonal produce, such as frozen berries, from around the world at any time of the year, making it much easier to have a steady intake of antioxidants in our diet.

Given that the total antioxidant capacity of our diet correlates with a lower risk of getting[1529] and dying from cancer[1530] and all causes of death put together,[1531] scientists set out to find the most antioxidant-rich foods. Sixteen researchers from around the world published a database of the antioxidant power of more than 3,000 different foods, beverages, supplements, herbs, and spices. They tested everything from Cap'n Crunch cereal to the crushed dried leaves of the African baobab tree to see what has the most antioxidants. They even tested dozens of brands of beer. (Santa Claus beer from Eggenberg, Austria, tied for the most antioxidant-rich brew.)[1532] Beer actually represents Americans' fourth-largest source of dietary antioxidants.[1533] Check out the chart to find out where your favorite foods and beverages rank in see.nf/antioxidantlist.

There is no need to post the entire 138-page chart on your refrigerator. Just remember this simple rule: On average, plant foods contain sixty-four times more antioxidants than animal foods.[1534] As the researchers noted, "antioxidant-rich foods originate from the plant kingdom while meat, fish and other foods from the animal kingdom are low in antioxidants." Even iceberg lettuce, which is 96 percent water[1535] and the least healthy plant food I can think of, contains seventeen units (micromoles per decagram using a modified FRAP assay) of antioxidant power. To give you some perspective, some berries have more than one thousand units, making iceberg pale in comparison. But compare iceberg's seventeen units to some common animal products. Fresh salmon has only three units of antioxidant power, chicken as few as five units, and skim milk and a hard-boiled egg have just four units each. "Diets comprised mainly of animal-based foods are thus low in antioxidant content," concluded the research team, "while diets based mainly on a variety of plant-based foods are antioxidant rich, due to the thousands of bioactive antioxidant phytochemicals found in plants which are conserved in many foods and beverages."

Among plant foods, berries average about ten times the antioxidant power of other fruits and vegetables, and are beat out only by herbs and spices. Cherries may have up to 714 units, but there is no need to cherry-pick individual foods to boost your antioxidant intake. Simply strive to include a variety of fruits, vegetables, and salt-free seasonings at every meal. That way, you can continuously flood your body with antioxidants to help ward off age-related disease.

BOOSTING BLOOD ANTIOXIDANT CAPACITY

Just as you can measure the amounts of antioxidants in foods and beverages, you can measure the antioxidant level in the bloodstream. Compared to most foods in the produce aisle, the antioxidant level in our body is kind of pitiful. Like meat, we don't even make it up to iceberg lettuce level![1536] Then again, meat is what we're made of, so I guess it's not that surprising.

Rather than just measuring the antioxidant power of a food in a test tube, tracking the change in antioxidant capacity of our blood after eating provides confirmation that antioxidants are effectively being absorbed into our system. Antioxidant supplements may not be able to move the needle[1537] or decrease oxidative DNA damage,[1538,1539] but fruits and vegetables can do both.[1540,1541,1542] And the greater our blood antioxidant status, the longer we tend to live.[1543]

Bloodstream antioxidant capacity may just be a marker of healthier eating in general,[1544] but at least one study found that the mortality benefit persisted independent of fiber intake.[1545] This suggests that we aren't living longer just because we're eating more whole plant foods in general, though tea may be a confounder. Tea has no fiber and is the single leading contributor of antioxidants in the American diet.[1546] Tea consumption alone is associated with a longer lifespan,[1547] so it would be interesting to see if the protective antioxidant association with premature mortality would survive after controlling for tea intake.

ANTIOXIDANT-RICH FOODS AT EVERY MEAL

Every meal is an opportunity to tip the balance in a pro-oxidant or antioxidant direction. Eating a single meal deficient in antioxidant-rich foods can leave us in a pro-oxidant state for hours, coinciding with a drop in antioxidants in our blood as our body's stores are slowly used up.[1548] (Details in see.nf/antioxidantmeals.) We don't want to slide backward every day and end up with fewer antioxidants in our body than we woke up with. This is especially important in the context of increased oxidative stress due to illness, secondhand smoke, air pollution, or sleep deprivation.[1549]

There was a remarkable study published in the *Journal of Biomedical Optics* that detailed a novel experiment in which German researchers noninvasively tracked people's antioxidant levels using an argon laser to measure, in real time, the fluctuating antioxidant levels in their skin. Their most important finding was that antioxidant levels can plummet within two hours of a stressful event and may take up to three *days* to get back to normal.[1550] Hours to lose, but days to recover, so healthier eating is especially important when we anticipate we'll be stressed, sick, or tired. Ideally, we would be having antioxidant-rich foods at every meal and snack.

HOW TO REDUCE DNA DAMAGE

Sadly, most Americans eat a lot of pale foods—white bread, white potatoes, white pasta, and white rice—but colorful foods are often better for us because of their antioxidant pigments. Blueberries are one of the most vividly tinted foods, and the data don't disappoint. A half cup of blueberries is able to blunt the drop in antioxidant capacity of our blood in the hours after consuming a berry-free sugary breakfast cereal (though a quarter cup cannot).[1551] Over time, those randomized to twice-daily blueberry smoothies halved the levels of a potent free radical in their blood within six weeks, which could then translate into enhanced DNA protection.[1552]

Researchers drew blood from people before and after they ate two cups of defrosted frozen blueberries and exposed their white blood cells to free radicals in the form of hydrogen peroxide.[1553] The blueberries significantly reduced the ensuing DNA damage within an hour of consumption. However, the protective effect was transient. DNA vulnerability returned within two hours, so again, we should aim to eat supercharged antioxidant-rich foods multiple times a day.

In a test tube, lemons, persimmons, strawberries, broccoli, celery, and apples all conferred DNA protection to human cells, but that presumes that the active components would get absorbed into the bloodstream at the concentration found to be protective.[1554] There are, however, foods that have been demonstrated to reduce DNA damage when actually eaten:

- one daily ounce of mixed nuts (walnuts, almonds, and hazelnuts) can reduce damage within twelve weeks,[1555]
- five teaspoons a day of tomato paste within just two weeks,[1556]
- three-quarters of a cup of microwaved frozen spinach[1557] or one cup of other cooked green leafy vegetables a day within three weeks,[1558]

- about four daily teaspoons of spinach powder within two weeks,[1559]
- two cups a day of steamed brussels sprouts within six days,[1560]
- a single serving of watercress within two hours,[1561]
- about one and a half cups of green tea[1562] or tomato,[1563] orange,[1564] blood orange,[1565] or carrot juice[1566] within hours to weeks, and
- eight kiwifruit within four hours[1567] or one kiwifruit a day for three weeks (with no significant difference found between eating one, two, or three a day).[1568]

Kiwis,[1569] cooked carrots,[1570] and green tea[1571] have the additional distinction of being able to facilitate DNA repair, something previously presumed not to be readily affected by diet.[1572] Can we just take a pill? A supplement containing the same amounts of alpha- and beta-carotene as the carrots failed to achieve the same effect.[1573]

Whole-food extracts of apples,[1574] oranges,[1575] spinach,[1576] and blueberries[1577] have been shown to increase the lifespan of *C. elegans*, and there are individual phytonutrients, such as gallic acid, that can not only extend *C. elegans* lifespan[1578] but also reduce human DNA damage within days[1579]—and do so at the daily dose found in a half cup of strawberries, half a mango, or a few tablespoons of carob powder, though whole foods may work even better.[1580] Whole apple extract has been found to extend the average lifespan of *C. elegans* by 39 percent, which is twice that of individual apple fractions or single apple phytonutrients,[1581] such as quercetin, which only prolonged average lifespan by 15 percent.[1582] Lemon-infused water—not even the whole fruit—increased the lifespan and healthspan of mice compared to a lifetime of drinking regular water,[1583] and amla,[1584] cinnamon,[1585] cocoa,[1586] and turmeric[1587] have all been shown to extend the longevity of fruit flies. In humans, the daily dose of antioxidants associated with a 7 percent lower risk of premature death can be found in about one cup of cooked spinach or just two-thirds of a cup of blackberries.[1588]

SPICE IT UP

Spices are the most potent DNA protectors. Just one week of eating about two teaspoons of rosemary or sage a day, one and a half teaspoons of ground ginger or cumin, three-fourths of a teaspoon of paprika, or even just a tenth of a teaspoon of cooked turmeric can protect against breakage of our strands of DNA.[1589] A daily quarter teaspoon of amla—dried Indian gooseberry powder—was also found to decrease oxidative DNA damage.[1590] This is to be expected, as ounce for ounce, dried herbs and spices pack the greatest antioxidant punch.[1591]

Herbs and spices max out at ten times the antioxidant power of nuts and seeds, for example. Of course, it's easier to eat an ounce of nuts than it is to eat an ounce of nutmeg, but some herbs and spices are so off-the-charts that even just a small pinch can go a long way. For example, adding a single teaspoon of dried oregano to a bowl of whole-wheat spaghetti with marinara and steamed broccoli nearly doubles the antioxidant power of the dish. Even just two-thirds of a teaspoon of marjoram would offer the same boost. A half teaspoon of cinnamon more than quintuples the antioxidant content of a bowl of oatmeal,[1592] and we have verification of bioavailability. A dozen randomized controlled trials have shown that cinnamon—both the cassia and Ceylon varieties—can increase the antioxidant capacity of our bloodstream and reduce free radical damage at doses ranging from just half a teaspoon to one and a half teaspoons a day.[1593]

Don't forget fresh herbs. A tablespoon of fresh lemon balm leaves approximately doubles the antioxidant content of a salad of lettuce and tomato, as does half a tablespoon of oregano or mint or even three-fourths of a teaspoon of marjoram, thyme, or sage.[1594] When you're whipping up a dressing, keep in mind that dozens of randomized controlled trials have shown that small doses of ginger[1595] and garlic[1596] can increase the antioxidant capacity of your bloodstream and decrease free radical damage, so try to include one or both.

The leader of the pack? Cloves. One of my favorite ways to enjoy them only takes a few minutes to prepare. I simply microwave a sweet potato and then mash it up with some cinnamon and just a pinch of cloves, which gives it a delicious pumpkin pie profile. An inexpensive, simple, easy snack with more antioxidants than people on a standard American diet may get in a whole week.[1597]

What about cocoa? Consumption of cocoa has been found to decrease markers of oxidative stress[1598] as well as lower blood pressure.[1599] Dark chocolate can do the same for us, but not white chocolate[1600] or milk chocolate.[1601] Cocoa may, however, be able to neutralize the pro-oxidant effects of dairy milk,[1602] whereas soymilk can actually bring down free radical damage[1603] (though rice milk may make things worse).[1604]

Not Worth Your Salt

Sodium is a commonly neglected pro-oxidant dietary component. I cover this in depth in my video see.nf/salty, but basically, a single typically salted meal can significantly suppress artery function within thirty minutes[1605] by suppressing a powerhouse antioxidant enzyme in our body called *superoxide dismutase*,[1606] which can ordinarily detoxify a million free radicals per second.[1607]

DNA-PROTECTING BEVERAGES

Although eating whole fruits is best, randomized controlled trials have found a reduction in free radical damage after consumption of tart cherry,[1608] orange,[1609] pomegranate,[1610] tomato,[1611] wheat grass,[1612] and low-sugar cranberry juices.[1613] Grape juice can also improve the antioxidant capacity of the blood.[1614] What about wine?

Red wine can acutely improve blood antioxidant capacity[1615]—even to the extent of buffering (but not eliminating) the spike in oxidation caused by a Mediterranean meal including fried fish.[1616] However, chronic wine consumption doesn't seem to help. When smokers were randomized to drink about two glasses of red wine, white wine, or dealcoholized red wine every day for weeks, only those drinking the nonalcoholic wine experienced a drop in markers of oxidant stress.[1617] This was presumed to be due to the known pro-oxidant effects of alcohol ingestion.[1618]

Smokers who drink alcohol were found to suffer twice the chromosomal damage compared to teetotaling smokers, but, other factors being equal, smokers who drink green tea suffer about a third less. (Even better are those who don't smoke at all, who have ten times less damage.)[1619] Though neither coffee[1620] nor green tea[1621] can block the oxidant stress induced by a high-fat meal, both green and black teas can increase the total antioxidant capacity of the bloodstream within just thirty minutes of ingestion, which can last for at least two hours. (Green tea is about 50 percent better at boosting than black.)[1622] Although the data on the effects of adding milk to your tea are mixed, most studies have shown that taking your tea with dairy decreases or even completely inhibits tea's antioxidant properties.[1623]

Within just one hour, a single cup of green tea can significantly boost the activity of the initiating DNA repair enzyme that fixes oxidative DNA damage, and drinking two cups a day for a week boosts it even more.[1624] Within four weeks, drinking a mug (300 mL) of green tea every day improves DNA resistance to free radical damage in the first place.[1625] Tea is in fact so DNA-protective that it can be used to store fresh samples of sperm until they can be properly refrigerated.[1626]

HOW PRO-OXIDANTS CAN HAVE ANTIOXIDANT EFFECTS

Ironically, the rallying of antioxidant and DNA repair defenses appears to be a consequence of green tea's mild *pro*-oxidant qualities, a phenomenon paralleled to physical training.[1627] It's been called the "exercise-induced oxidative stress paradox."[1628] Ultramarathon runners may generate so many free radicals during a race that they can damage the DNA of a significant percentage of their own cells.[1629] Why would an apparently healthy act (exercise) lead to detrimental effects? Because exercise in and of itself is not necessarily the healthy act; it's the recovery period afterward.[1630] For example, exercise training has been shown to enhance antioxidant defenses by increasing the activities of our antioxidant enzymes. So, athletes may be taking hits to their DNA during a race, but, a week later, they don't just go back to the baseline level of DNA damage. Day-to-day DNA damage drops even lower, presumably because the prior exertion had revved up their antioxidant defenses.[1631]

In this way, the mild oxidative stress of green tea and exercise can be seen as beneficial, similar to vaccination. By challenging the body a little, we might induce a response that's favorable in the long run. The concept that low levels of a damaging entity can upregulate protective mechanisms—the whole "that which doesn't kill us makes us stronger" notion—is known as *hormesis*.[1632] (See page 507.)

Taking antioxidant pills, such as vitamin C and vitamin E supplements, can block that boost in antioxidant enzyme activity caused by physical activity and thereby blunt some of the ensuing health benefits, but eating antioxidant-rich foods may offer the best of both worlds.[1633] While vitamin C supplements seem to impair physical performance,[1634] fruits[1635] and vegetables[1636] can have ergogenic benefits, enhancing performance without undermining the protective adaptation response.[1637] In fact, fruits and veggies may even boost exercise benefits. Both black currants[1638] and lemon verbena,[1639] an antioxidant-rich herbal tea, were shown to protect against exercise-induced oxidative stress and, at the same time, improve some beneficial adaptations to exercise.

Given the hormetic benefits of certain mild pro-oxidant stresses, such as green tea and physical activity, the oversimplistic narrative of "antioxidants good, free radicals bad"[1640] must be revised.[1641] Perhaps nowhere is this more apparent than in the case of broccoli.

KALE FLIPS THE SWITCH

The dietary antioxidants we co-opt from plants represent only our second line of defense against free radicals.[1642] Our frontline defenders are our own antioxidant enzymes. The human body naturally produces 100,000,000,000,000,000,000,000 free radicals an hour.[1643] This is why we make enzymes like catalase, the fastest-reacting enzyme in our body, able to detoxify literally millions of molecules of hydrogen peroxide into water and oxygen each second.[1644] (You know that fizzing that occurs when you pour hydrogen peroxide on a wound? That's from the oxygen bubbles formed by the catalase enzyme.) Is there any way to boost this first line of antioxidant defense?

In the 1980s, scientists first began discovering a specific genetic sequence in the promoter regions of dozens[1645] and then hundreds of "cytoprotective" (cell-protecting) genes.[1646] It was found promoting genes that code for antioxidant enzymes that quench free radicals directly, like catalase,[1647] enzymes that make antioxidants like glutathione,[1648] and even genes for DNA repair enzymes[1649] and detoxification enzymes in our liver.[1650] Whatever bound to these so-called antioxidant response elements could activate our global antioxidant defense system all at once.

In the 1990s, this trigger was discovered—Nrf2, a protein floating in the cell's cytoplasm that is normally bound to a suppressor protein.[1651] But, when that suppressor protein gets oxidized, it releases Nrf2, which is then able to dive into the cell's nucleus to bind to the antioxidant response elements and activate the powerful battery of antioxidant protections.[1652] The entire process can be completed within fifteen minutes.[1653] Nrf2 is considered the "master regulator of the environmental stress response"[1654] and is expressed universally in all cells,[1655] just waiting to be freed to hit the panic button and rally cellular defenses.

Nrf2 is also called a "guardian of healthspan and gatekeeper of species longevity."[1656] Boosting Nrf2 signaling causes significant increases in longevity in *C. elegans*[1657] and fruit flies,[1658] and correlates with maximum lifespan potential across ten different species of rodents.[1659] For example, the Nrf2 gene is overexpressed sixfold in long-lived naked mole rats compared to mice,[1660] combined with lower suppressor protein expression.[1661] That may not only help explain why they live eight times longer[1662] but also why it takes up to a hundred times the concentration of toxins like heavy metals and chemotherapy drugs to kill the same percentage of skin cells taken from naked mole rats compared to mice.[1663] They are little nude detoxification machines.

Unfortunately, Nrf2 levels[1664] and signaling tend to decrease with age.[1665] Thirty minutes of cycling can boost them,[1666] for example, but the most potent natural Nrf2 inducer on the planet may be sulforaphane,[1667] the compound formed when we bite into cruciferous vegetables, such as broccoli, kale, collards, cabbage, and cauliflower. Sulforaphane, like the active components of green tea and turmeric, frees Nrf2 by oxidizing its suppressor protein, resulting in a rejuvenating effect on aged mice.[1668] Older mice fed sulforaphane actually had superior grip strength compared to younger mice and performed just as well on a treadmill.[1669] Nrf2 activation led to decreased DNA damage and muscle loss, and improved heart function and lifespan.

What about us? Sulforaphane can also restore Nrf2 activity in our aging tissues,[1670] which may explain why sulforaphane can delay the senescence of human stem cells.[1671] Just one stalk of broccoli a day can significantly reduce the DNA damage from cigarette smoke,[1672] and two daily cups of brussels sprouts can minimize the DNA damage from a type of cooked meat carcinogen (a heterocyclic amine).[1673] About a third of a cup a day of broccoli sprouts can help our body clear benzene from air pollution.[1674] One study found that sulforaphane could tamp down the inflammation from diesel exhaust that was squirted into subjects' noses at levels simulating hours of rush-hour exposure on a Los Angeles freeway.[1675]

Cruciferous vegetables so boost our detoxification pathways that heavy broccoli eaters might need to drink more coffee to get the same buzz, as the drug-metabolizing pathway that clears caffeine can get so revved up.[1676] The protection veggies from the cabbage family give us can even be demonstrated topically. Rubbing a broccoli extract on your skin before spending time in the sun can decrease the redness of a sunburn by 35 percent by reducing the tissue damage caused by UV rays through Nrf2 activation.[1677]

The discovery that sulforaphane can switch on Nrf2 arguably heralds a "new paradigm in nutrition science."[1678] No wonder cruciferous vegetable intake is associated with decreased risk of cardiovascular disease, cancer, and mortality from all causes put together.[1679] Even those who average just a single floret's worth of broccoli a day have lower mortality rates than those who eat little or none.[1680] However, the life-extending benefits of broccoli may extend even beyond sulforaphane. Animals fed 1 percent broccoli diets lived longer, but those given just the amount of sulforaphane found in that much broccoli (the compound without the broccoli itself) did not. Sulforaphane salads trump sulforaphane supplements.[1681]

Enhancing Sulforaphane Formation

Acidifying raw cruciferous vegetables can boost sulforaphane formation. Adding lemon juice to a shredded cabbage salad, for instance, may help a little, but adding vinegar is even better, presumably because of its higher acid content. However, the opposite may be true when cooking cabbage. Boiled red cabbage should be kept blue, not pink, indicating a more alkaline environment that helps keep the critical cruciferous components from degrading.[1682] (See see.nf/cabbageph.) The most critical factor when it comes to cooking, though, is pausing between chopping and heating, my "hack and hold" strategy detailed in my Cruciferous Vegetables chapter in *How Not to Die* and in my video see.nf/hackandhold.

FAT REACTOR

We know that some foods have antioxidant qualities, while others act, on balance, as pro-oxidants. Just as the Dietary Inflammatory Index was designed to weigh the balance of anti- and pro-inflammatory foods, more than twenty oxidative balance scoring systems have been developed. In general, the more the scale tips toward the pro-oxidant side, the higher the risk of heart disease, kidney disease, and getting and dying from cancer and all causes put together. Although all the different scoring systems have a different complement of components, they all agree that exercise, cruciferous vegetables, and certain constituents of whole plant foods, such as fiber and carotenoid phytonutrients, are net antioxidant, squelching free radicals, whereas meat, alcohol, fat, and activities like smoking are pro-oxidant, generating free radicals. Of all the dietary pro-oxidants, saturated fat is considered the worst.[1683]

Heterocyclic amines, the carcinogenic compounds formed when meat is cooked or tobacco is smoked,[1684] can induce free radical formation,[1685] but that's not the only reason meat and meat products contribute to oxidative stress.[1686] Our stomach acts as a "bioreactor"[1687] in which the heme proteins in blood and muscle oxidize the fat in the acid bath of our stomach. It turns out that during slaughter, chickens, for example, are bled of only about half their blood,[1688] and the remaining residual can be such a powerful promoter of fat oxidation that some within the industry are advocating for an additional decapitation step during the slaughter process.[1689]

When we consume the oxidized (rancid) fat, it can then make it into our LDL cholesterol particles that accelerate atherosclerosis, the hardening of arteries that, ultimately, is our leading cause of death.[1690] Oxidized fat levels in circulating LDL can double within four days of eating grilled turkey cutlets every day.[1691] (Damaging effects can be mediated by eating berries with meaty meals, though. See the Berries chapter.) This may help explain why vegetarians appear protected from cardiovascular disease,[1692] but oxidized fats are also created when vegetable oils are heated.[1693] It's no surprise then that the consumption of more ultraprocessed junk food is associated with higher rates of DNA damage compared to those eating less.[1694] However, the oxidation of animal fats may be even worse because of the "dreaded oxysterols."[1695]

Antioxidant Status of Vegetarians

Both systematic[1696] and nonsystematic[1697] reviews have concluded that plant-based diets protect against free radical damage, which "may explain why vegetarians live longer."[1698] Most studies show that vegetarians, for example, suffer lower levels of oxidative stress,[1699,1700,1701,1702,1703,1704,1705,1706] but some show no significant difference compared to meat eaters[1707,1708] or fish eaters,[1709] or even higher levels in the vegetarians.[1710,1711] As I detail in see.nf/antioxveg, the discrepant results may be due to vitamin B_{12} inadequacy among vegetarians and vegans who don't supplement their diet with B_{12} or B_{12}-fortified foods,[1712] as even subclinical (asymptomatic) B_{12} deficiency is associated with increased oxidative stress.[1713] A regular reliable source of vitamin B_{12} is critically important to take advantage of the full spectrum of benefits to plant-based eating.[1714]

DIRTY COPs

Too much cholesterol in the blood has long been considered to be a primary risk factor for developing Alzheimer's disease.[1715] Cholesterol cannot directly get across the blood-brain barrier,[1716] though, but cholesterol oxidation products (COPs) can. Also known as *oxysterols*, oxidized cholesterol present in the bloodstream accumulates in the brain,[1717] where it's considered to be a driving force behind the development of Alzheimer's disease.[1718] I present the chain of evidence in my video see .nf/copdementia.

COPs can be up to a hundred times more toxic than unoxidized cholesterol.[1719] They may contribute to a wide range of age-related diseases, including atherosclerosis,[1720] cataracts,[1721] kidney failure,[1722] osteoporosis,[1723] and cancer.[1724] This may explain why egg consumption[1725] and dietary cholesterol in general are associated with an increased risk of breast cancer.[1726] The main cholesterol oxidation byproduct in the blood, known as *27-hydroxycholesterol*,[1727] is estrogenic and increases the proliferation of most breast cancer cells[1728]—sometimes even in the context of estrogen-blocking drugs.[1729]

How can we cut down on the amount of oxidized cholesterol in our blood? Since oxidized cholesterol in the diet is a source of oxidized cholesterol in our bloodstream, one way is by not eating it.[1730] Levels of oxidized cholesterol rise in the blood within hours of consumption[1731] and circulate for more than six and even eight hours after a meal.[1732] Oxidized cholesterol is found in milk powders, meat and meat products (including fish), cheese, and eggs and egg products,[1733] such as powdered eggs, which are found in a lot of processed foods.[1734] Fresh, raw meat may start out with zero oxidized cholesterol, but cooking or storage can cause a dramatic increase in levels.[1735] All forms of cooking can do it, since maximum cholesterol oxidation can be achieved at only about 300°F (149°C), but some types of cooking are worse than others.[1736] See details in my video see.nf/stopcops.

In general, the cholesterol in white meat is more susceptible to oxidation than the cholesterol in red meat, due to white meat's higher polyunsaturated fat content. Fish tends to be the worst, followed by poultry, pork, then beef.[1737] Chicken has about twice the oxidized cholesterol of beef, even before it's irradiated.[1738] When chicken meat is irradiated to improve its food safety from an infectious disease standpoint, it may diminish food safety from a chronic disease standpoint, due to extra cholesterol oxidation.[1739]

Exposure to cholesterol oxidation products is said to be "unavoidable,"[1740] but let's take a step back. Only foods that start out with cholesterol can end up with *oxidized* cholesterol.[1741] So, the primary method to reduce dietary intake may be to reduce the total cholesterol content of the diet by centering one's diet around unprocessed plant foods, which don't have any cholesterol to get oxidized in the first place.

Clarifying a Mystery

Until relatively recently, our understanding of dietary oxidized cholesterol has been limited by the lack of testing methods and procedures to accurately analyze the amount in various foods.[1742] Though oxidized cholesterol products have been found throughout animal products, the levels in canned tuna are surprisingly high, fifteen times higher than in beef or pork chops, for example, but ghee takes the cake.[1743]

Ghee, clarified butter, is commonly used in Indian cooking.[1744] Boiling, the method of preparation, appears to multiply oxidized cholesterol levels tenfold. This dietary exposure to oxidized cholesterol may help explain why the subcontinent of India is ravaged by heart disease even though a significant proportion of the population eschews meat and eggs.[1745] A number of Indian dairy-based desserts are also made in a similar way.[1746]

SUPPLEMENTS

I had known antioxidant supplements had grown into a multibillion-dollar business, but I was surprised to learn that Big Pharma had turned it into "the biggest, most elaborate, longest lasting, and most harmful of the international cartels discovered by the U.S. Department of Justice (DOJ) [in] the 1990s," according to a textbook on global price fixing. Before being busted with dozens of criminal convictions and record-setting fines, drug companies had conspired in a complex, illegal, monopolistic price-fixing scheme to overcharge for vitamin supplements by the billions.[1747] To make matters even more egregious, people were cheated for nothing—or worse. No antioxidant supplement has ever been shown to reduce mortality, and supplemental beta-carotene, vitamin E, and higher doses of vitamin A may even cut people's lives short.[1748] This parallels many animal studies that found either no effect at all or significant lifespan shortening.[1749]

There are countless antioxidant supplements on the market, many of which make "strongly exaggerated and . . . flawed" claims.[1750] Here's a short rundown of some of the lesser-known ones.

ALPHA-LIPOIC ACID

Alpha-lipoic acid is an antioxidant our body manufactures internally.[1751] Is there any advantage to taking extra in supplement form? I discuss the pros and cons in see.nf/lipoic. Bottom line? I would exercise caution until we have a better idea of its dosing safety window.

COENZYME Q_{10}

Coenzyme Q_{10}, more commonly known as CoQ_{10}, is the only fat-soluble antioxidant produced by the human body.[1752] Because we synthesize it from scratch, there's no need to consume any,[1753] yet it's one of the most popular dietary supplements.[1754] Centenarians have low levels compared to seventy-six-year-old controls,[1755] but this fact can be used to argue two diametrically opposed positions: Some posit that CoQ_{10} levels decrease with age so we should supplement to regain youthful levels, while others maintain that low levels may be beneficial to achieving such remarkable longevity.

Animal studies echo this ambiguity. Indeed, both added CoQ_{10}[1756] and subtracted CoQ_{10} (by repressing synthesis) have been found to extend lifespan in *C. elegans*[1757] but mostly have no effect on rats and mice.[1758] In people, CoQ_{10} supplementation reduces markers of inflammation[1759] and oxidative stress[1760] and may benefit patients with heart failure[1761] and migraines, reducing headache frequency and duration but not severity.[1762] Those who choose to take it need to keep it in a cool, dark, airtight container since it's sensitive to heat, light, and oxidation.[1763] I prefer to regenerate it naturally using the technique I described in my Greens chapter in *How Not to Die*. It involves eating a chlorophyll-rich diet,[1764] which may be especially important for those on cholesterol-lowering statin drugs, as these medications can interfere with CoQ_{10} production.[1765]

GINSENG

Ginseng root is a popular herbal medicine.[1766] Like the word "panacea," ginseng's Latin name, *Panax*, is derived from the Greek roots *pan* and *akos* for "cure-all." However, although there have been more than a hundred clinical trials on various ginseng formulations,[1767] to date, the results for even one of its most promising usages (blood sugar regulation)[1768] have been less than impressive.[1769]

From an oxidative stress standpoint, American (*Panax quinquefolius*),[1770] Chinese (*Panax notoginseng*),[1771] and Korean (*Panax ginseng*) ginseng[1772] have all been shown to acutely protect against free radical–induced DNA damage within hours of consumption, but one longer-term trial raised red flags. Although four weeks of consuming Korean ginseng reduced levels of oxidative stress,[1773] four months of consuming American ginseng caused an uptick in DNA damage from less than a quarter teaspoon a day of whole root powder.[1774] Until it can be shown that the chronic intake of other ginsengs isn't also DNA-damaging, I'd recommend steering clear.

N-ACETYLCYSTEINE

N-acetylcysteine (NAc) increases the lifespan of male mice, but not female mice, and only because it apparently led to reduced food and water consumption.[1775] In *C. elegans*[1776] and fruit flies, lifespan was extended at one dose but, at a higher dose, was dramatically cut short by up to 70 percent, raising a "serious concern" for taking NAc supplements.[1777] More details in see.nf/nacse.

SELENIUM

Selenium, a critical component of key antioxidant enzymes, is considered an essential trace mineral,[1778] though, given its narrow safety margin, it's also been termed an "essential poison."[1779] Indeed, the consumption of just a single high-selenium Brazil nut a day was found to have pro-inflammatory effects.[1780] I also cover selenium in see.nf/nacse, but basically, both low[1781] and high[1782] blood levels are associated with dying prematurely, and certain doses of selenium supplements may shorten your life,[1783] as well as worsen blood sugar control in diabetics[1784] and increase the risk of developing diabetes in the first place.[1785]

What About Vitamin C?

Vitamin C is likely the most abundant antioxidant in the body,[1786] but levels decline with age. Vitamin C levels in the blood cells of those aged eighty-five and older may be only half that compared to those at age sixty.[1787] Vitamin C levels in the brain seem to drop about 40 percent (comparing those sixty and older to those fifty-nine and younger).[1788] Might restoring youthful levels be beneficial? It's been tried and flopped. Vitamin C supplements fail to extend life, improve quality of life or cognitive performance, or prevent eye diseases, infections, cardiovascular diseases, or cancer.[1789]

There is insufficient evidence to even claim vitamin C supplements are effective in preventing DNA oxidation[1790] and, at higher doses (about 900 mg plus NAc), may actually cause *more* oxidative damage.[1791] This Janus-faced nature of vitamin C has similarly been demonstrated in animal models: an antioxidant at lower doses but a pro-oxidant at higher doses.[1792] This may help explain why animal studies have shown that vitamin C treatments are all over the map, resulting in increased, decreased, and neutral effects on longevity.[1793]

Although high-dose vitamin C supplementation may result in oxidative DNA damage, so can slipping below the recommended dietary allowance (RDA). Over the last twenty years, vitamin C consumption has declined in the United States by more than 20 percent, due largely to the decrease in fruit juice consumption without a compensatory increase in whole fruit intake. It's gotten to the point that nearly half of all Americans now fall below the estimated average requirement.[1794] What's the optimal intake? See see.nf/vitaminc for details, but the magic number appears to be about 200 mg a day. Since a single serving of fruits and vegetables may have about 50 mg of vitamin C, just four or five servings of fruits and veggies a day should get you up to ideal blood levels.

Another reason to avoid megadoses of vitamin C is the risk of kidney stones, at least in men.[1795] Those taking 1,000 mg or so of vitamin C a day may as much as double their risk, from having a one-in-six-hundred chance of getting a kidney stone every year to a one-in-three-hundred chance.[1796] We don't yet know if women are similarly at risk.

Food for Thought

The mitochondrial theory of aging explains why animals with the lowest rate of free radical production live the longest. We can slow this rate through exercise training and methionine restriction, which can be achieved with a predominantly whole food, plant-based diet.[1797] Such an eating pattern would also cut down on pro-oxidant foods rich in cholesterol, salt, saturated fat, and sugar, while boosting the intake of plant foods that have the dual benefit of enhancing our primary oxidant defense via Nrf2 activation and our second line of radical resistance, the symphony of natural antioxidant compounds that can work in concert in a way in which antioxidant supplements have failed.

To help slow this aging pathway, on a daily basis, consider:

- exercising
- restricting methionine intake by choosing plant-based protein sources and reducing overall protein intake to recommended levels
- activating Nrf2 defenses by eating green (cruciferous vegetables) and drinking green (tea)

(continued)

- eating berries and other naturally vibrantly colored foods
- using herbs and spices, such as cinnamon, cloves, garlic, ginger, and marjoram
- avoiding added salt, sugar, and saturated fat– and cholesterol-rich foods

SIRTUINS

Each of us contains tens of billions of miles of DNA—enough for 100,000 trips to the moon and back if each strand were uncoiled and placed end to end.[1798] How does our body prevent these precious ribbons of information from getting all twisted and tangled? Enzymes known as *sirtuins* keep our DNA neatly and nicely wrapped around spool-like proteins and, by doing so, silence whatever genes are in that stretch of DNA. The name *SIR*tuins stands for Silencing Information Regulator.[1799]

THE GUARDIANS OF HEALTHSPAN

Since this seminal discovery, myriad other functions of sirtuins have been discovered, including their ability to activate or deactivate more than fifty other proteins.[1800] What most excited the scientific community about these regulatory enzymes is that boosting their activity could extend yeast lifespans by as much as 70 percent.[1801,1802] Boosting sirtuins also boosts the lifespans of other model organisms—worms and flies—leading to great hopes that it could do the same in mammals.[1803]

In a few mouse models, sirtuin upregulation was found to extend life,[1804,1805] but most mice studies just showed healthier lives, rather than longer ones,[1806] thereby earning sirtuins the title of "guardians of mammalian healthspan."[1807] In addition to preserving DNA integrity,[1808] sirtuin activation improves DNA repair,[1809] downregulates inflammation,[1810] and contributes to telomere maintenance,[1811] which I discuss in the next chapter. This translates into better blood sugars and bone mass, and less DNA damage and cancer.[1812] So, in the few cases in which lifespan was extended, it may have been more a matter of suppressing age-related diseases than slowing the rate of aging per se.[1813] Regardless, these effects were found in mice and have yet to be confirmed in humans. We do know, however, that there doesn't seem to be an association between exceptional longevity in people bearing any of the different variants of at least one of the sirtuin genes.[1814] As one reviewer mused, sirtuins may have lost their "Methuselah" image but may still be a helpful metabolic "Samaritan."[1815]

As you'll recall, the fuel gauge enzyme that I discussed in the AMPK chapter boosts sirtuin activity.[1816] So, activating AMPK via metformin,[1817] caloric restriction,[1818] or exercise[1819] can lead to sirtuin activation. However, since the sirtuin boost is an indirect effect caused by AMPK, chugging sugar water before a sprint, for example, a sports or energy drink, blunts the sirtuin response to exercise.[1820] While mild caloric restriction—by about 15 percent, roughly 350 calories a day—had no effect on sirtuin activity,[1821] a 30 percent reduction in calories for eight weeks did,[1822] but not for just five days.[1823] However, Buchinger fasting (consuming only a limited selection of juices and vegetable broth) can boost sirtuin activity within five days,[1824] as can alternate-day fasting for three weeks,[1825] dropping down to 1,000 calories a day for a month,[1826] or six months of 25 percent calorie restriction.[1827]

The way AMPK enhances sirtuin activity is by increasing levels of cellular nicotinamide adenine dinucleotide (NAD^+).[1828] NAD^+ is a critical cofactor necessary for sirtuin activity. Alternate means of boosting NAD^+ levels include taking a variety of NAD^+ precursors,[1829] as I'll discuss in the Anti-Aging Eight section. Raising NAD^+ levels is one of two basic approaches to sirtuin stimulation.[1830] The other is via STACs, sirtuin-activating compounds, the most widely known of which is resveratrol,[1831] a natural compound concentrated in the skin of grapes.

RESVERATROL

Resveratrol, the "red wine molecule,"[1832] became a household word[1833] in 1991 when a scientist from Bordeaux University[1834] appeared on the popular TV show *60 Minutes* and attributed the so-called French Paradox to the French habit of drinking red wine.[1835] As you can see in see.nf/resveratrol, the "paradox" was effectively debunked,[1836] but not before resveratrol research had already taken root, culminating in more than 15,000 scientific publications to date.[1837,1838]

As I show in the video, animal data are mixed. For example, resveratrol extends the lives of worms[1839] and bees,[1840] but not flies[1841] or fleas.[1842] Unfortunately, most studies on mammals (mostly mice) failed to show a lifespan benefit.[1843] Even its purported sirtuin activity has been called into question.[1844] Commentaries with titles like "Is Resveratrol an Imposter?"[1845] and "Promising Therapeutic or Hopeless Illusion?"[1846] were published, suggesting that seeming sirtuin activity was probably the result of experimental artifact.[1847] It didn't help matters when a leading resveratrol researcher was found guilty of 145 counts of fabrication and falsification of data, throwing the whole field into turmoil.[1848]

In a 2014 medical journal editorial titled "The Resveratrol Fiasco," the editor in chief summarized the state of the science: "The conclusions are quite clear-cut: after more than 20 years of well-funded research, resveratrol has no proven human activity."[1849] However, since that publication, more than 150 human clinical trials have been published.[1850] I present the update in see.nf/resveratrolhealth. No impact on inflammation, cancer, cardiovascular disease, long-term frailty,[1851] or death[1852] has been found epidemiologically for dietary resveratrol exposure, and meta-analyses of randomized controlled trials of resveratrol supplements failed to find clinically[1853] or even statistically[1854] significant effects on systemic markers of oxidative stress, helping to explain the lack of apparent DNA protection.[1855]

For almost all outcomes measured in randomized controlled trials of type 2 diabetes, metabolic syndrome, or nonalcoholic fatty liver disease, the effects of resveratrol were trivial at best,[1856] but a meta-analysis found that doses ranging from 5 to 500 mg twice a day resulted in an average twenty-point drop in fasting blood sugars.[1857] There was also a significant benefit for longer-term (HbA1c) blood sugar control, though this only appeared to be the case in shorter-term studies.[1858] What's the point of better longer-term control if resveratrol only works in studies lasting less than three months? Well, there was a study suggesting accelerated healing of diabetic foot ulcers,[1859] a leading cause of lower-limb amputations.[1860]

In see.nf/resveratrolclinical, I run through what else resveratrol supplementation might be able to do clinically. In rats[1861] and mice,[1862] resveratrol can help ameliorate the effects of experimentally induced periodontitis, the inflammatory gum disease. It appeared to have no effect, however, on the progression of chronic periodontitis in human sufferers.[1863] Resveratrol may help with the inflammatory bowel disease ulcerative colitis[1864,1865] and knee osteoarthritis,[1866] though.

Resveratrol has some estrogenic activity,[1867] and, although it doesn't appear to help with hormonal migraines,[1868] it does appear to help with a few symptoms of polycystic ovary syndrome (PCOS)[1869] and menopause.[1870] Unfortunately, a meta-analysis of studies on resveratrol supplementation to improve bone quality found no significant effect on bone health markers or bone mineral density of the spine, hip, or overall skeleton.[1871] The same was true for cognitive effects, leading one systematic review to suggest resveratrol may be a "cognitive enhancer for mice only."[1872] The largest trial of resveratrol for Alzheimer's disease even found a tripling of brain shrinkage in those randomized to the resveratrol group compared to placebo.[1873]

Negative or null findings are often marginalized by the resveratrol research community.[1874] As I review in see.nf/resveratrolsafety, there are no long-term safety data,[1875] but even supplementation purported to be "safe"[1876] (150 mg to 250 mg a day) found that resveratrol may blunt some of the positive effects of exercise training, undercutting physical fitness in both the young[1877] and the old.[1878]

A recent review overreacted to these data by suggesting that "foods containing resveratrol should not be consumed during exercise,"[1879] but to reach even the lower dose of 150 mg, you'd have to eat more than a hundred pounds of grapes.[1880] The exercise impairment with supplemental resveratrol does make sense, though, given its purported mechanism. Sirtuin activation by resveratrol is thought to occur via the activation of the body's fuel gauge AMPK by impairing energy production in our cells' mitochondria.[1881] Mouse cells react by increasing mitochondria to compensate,[1882] but human cells apparently do not,[1883] so the energy-dimming effect of resveratrol may explain why the effects of exercise are impaired.

The hype surrounding resveratrol, concluded one review, may "turn out to be nothing more than a slight-of-hand [sic] marketing device using peer-reviewed, published, non-human research as a cover."[1884] The fitness-blunting exercise study of older adults was supported in part by a manufacturer of resveratrol supplements. To their credit, however, the researchers responded to an angry letter by a supplement company consultant that "it is our opinion that we, as scientists, have a responsibility to report what we find, and not to twist our findings to fit the commercial interests."[1885]

HOW ABOUT THEM APPLES?

Resveratrol may be the most familiar STAC, but thousands of others have been discovered.[1886] In vitro, apple extracts have been shown to activate sirtuins, as well as AMPK and autophagy, while suppressing mTOR signaling.[1887] It's perhaps unsurprising, then, that a meta-analysis of population studies found that those who ate more apples had a 15 percent lower risk of premature death.[1888] How many apples is "more"? The "high" category of apple consumption averaged only about a quarter of an apple a day. The one study that looked at the greatest apple intake— half an apple a day compared to less than one apple in an entire month—found a 35 percent lower risk of dying early.[1889] Over a lifetime, that could translate into around four more years of life.[1890] Forget just the doctor. An apple a day may keep the mortician away, too.

A single apple phytonutrient, *phloridzin*, was found to boost sirtuin expression and extend the lifespan of yeast, though it also increases levels of the antioxidant enzyme superoxide dismutase, so it's not clear what role the sirtuin played.[1891] In fruit flies, at least, the increase in average lifespan from an apple extract requires intact antioxidant enzymes, suggesting it may be more of an antioxidant effect.[1892]

Even just straight apple fiber (pectin) had a lifespan-extending effect, and this wasn't solely due to caloric dilution (dietary restriction achieved through bulking the diet with fiber). The pectin group actually ate more food yet lived longer.[1893] The whole apple, however, may be better than the sum of its parts.

Adding the flesh of an apple to a prematurely aging mutant yeast that normally only lives about ten days bumped up its lifespan to eleven days, whereas adding the skin of an apple extended its life up to fourteen days. Seems like most of the good stuff is in the peel, right? What do you predict would happen if you add both the flesh and the skin? I would have guessed the whole apple would extend the lifespan somewhere between eleven and fourteen days since the components of the peel would get diluted, but I would have been wrong. The *whole* apple more than *doubled* lifespan, taking it to twenty-one days.[1894]

Similarly in *C. elegans*, whole apple extracts increased average lifespan up to 39 percent, which is more than three times the 12 percent achieved with a subfraction of purified apple compounds (though the studies also used different apples, Red Delicious[1895] and Fuji, respectively). In *C. elegans*, at least, sirtuin dependency of the longevity benefit was confirmed.[1896]

If the components of apple peel and pulp can synergize, providing benefits greater than the sum of the parts, what about combining apples and blueberries? In *C. elegans*, both apple and blueberry extracts extend life, but using half of each extended life significantly more than either could alone.[1897] Results like these buttress the commonsense notion that, whenever possible, we should strive to acquire our nutrition from combinations of whole foods rather than isolated components in pill form.

THE QUEEN OF SPICES

Are there any other "sirtfoods," foods with sirtuin-activating properties?[1898] Numerous food components boost sirtuin activity in cells in a petri dish, but very few have been put to the test in people.[1899] Two hundred daily micrograms of selenium for ten weeks can upregulate sirtuin expression,[1900] but, as I note in see .nf/nacse, that dose used long-term has been shown to increase diabetes risk.[1901] Curcumin, the pigment that makes turmeric yellow, works in vitro[1902] and in an animal model[1903] but flops when it comes to significantly changing sirtuin gene expression in humans, even after taking the equivalent of about a quarter cup of turmeric every day for months.[1904] One spice that might work, though, is cardamom.

A member of the ginger family, green cardamom (*Elettaria cardamomum*) is known as "the queen of spices."[1905] In a trial of patients with fatty liver disease, those randomized to a half teaspoon of cardamom three times a day with meals for three months not only had improvements in liver function and markers of systemic inflammation but they also saw a significant increase in sirtuin levels in their bloodstream.[1906] Now, we aren't exactly sure about the origin or implication of sirtuins in the blood. It's not like a hormone. Each cell appears to make and use its own sirtuins internally. However, blood levels do decline with age,[1907] and accelerated decline in sirtuins is associated with age-related impairments such as frailty,[1908] cognitive decline, and Alzheimer's disease,[1909] suggesting it may be a biomarker of aging.[1910]

As a bonus, the same cardamom dose over two to three months can significantly improve markers of inflammation and oxidative stress,[1911] and be a safe, cheap, convenient way to decrease the level of triglycerides in the blood by about twenty points (mg/dL).[1912] I enjoy it in my chai tea and like adding it to cocoa powder any time I'm chocolating anything up. No significant adverse side effects have been reported from taking such doses, though there are no long-term data available at this time.[1913]

AGEs SUPPRESS SIRTUINS

Is there anything we need to avoid to preserve sirtuin function? Smokers have diminished sirtuin levels in their lungs,[1914] and in vitro, cigarette smoke extracts actively decrease sirtuin levels and activity in lung cells, helping to establish cause and effect.[1915] The advanced glycation end products (AGEs) in smoke may be contributing, since AGEs alone suppress sirtuin expression in vitro and feeding AGEs to mice causes a sirtuin brain deficiency, along with an impairment of learning and memory.[1916] Unfortunately, as we learned in the Glycation chapter, people are also exposed to dietary AGEs.

Increasingly, sirtuin activity is being seen as playing a significant role in protecting against Alzheimer's dementia.[1917] The fact that dietary AGE intake is linked to lower sirtuin expression may help explain why high blood, brain, and dietary AGE exposure is associated with cognitive decline in elderly adults. Researchers have concluded that human sirtuin deficiency is "both preventable and reversible by AGE reduction," suggesting that avoiding high-AGE foods may offer a new strategy to combat the Alzheimer's epidemic.[1918] However, dietary AGEs are unlikely to pose a central role in sirtuin regulation, as no differences have been found in sirtuin expression or activity in a cross-sectional comparison of healthy omnivores, vegetarians, and vegans.[1919]

Food for Thought

Sirtuins are a class of protein regulators that appear to play a key role in protecting us against a variety of age-related diseases, though their role in longevity is questionable.[1920] Dependent on a molecule called NAD^+, sirtuins can be up-regulated by anything that increases NAD^+ levels, including AMPK activation. Certain foods and supplements may also be able to activate sirtuins in other ways, but research on resveratrol has been largely disappointing and raised certain safety concerns.

To help boost this anti-aging pathway, on a daily basis, consider:
- elevating cellular NAD^+ levels (see the NAD^+ chapter)
- following the recommendations on AMPK activation (see the AMPK chapter)
- snacking on apples and experimenting with adding cardamom to meals
- not smoking
- avoiding foods high in AGEs (see the Glycation chapter)

TELOMERES

In each of our cells, we have forty-six strands of DNA coiled into chromosomes. At the tip of each chromosome is a protective cap called a *telomere*, which keeps our DNA from fraying or fusing with other chromosomes,[1921] analogous to how the plastic tips on the ends of our shoelaces keep them from unraveling. ("Telomere" comes from the Greek words *telos* for "end" and *meros* for "part."[1922]) Each time our cells divide, however, a bit of that cap is lost. When telomeres become critically short, the exposed ends of our chromosomes appear like double-stranded DNA breaks, an emergency signal that sends the damaged cells into senescence, or death.[1923] Our body does this on purpose, it is thought, to protect us from cancer.[1924]

ON A SHORT FUSE

Remember the "Hayflick limit" from the Cellular Senescence chapter? Telomere shortening is the mechanism by which many cells are restricted from dividing more than about fifty times.[1925] This cap on cellular immortality may limit our lifespan potential, but it may also protect us from tumor formation. This may explain, for example, why those of European ancestry tend to have shorter telomeres than those from sub-Saharan Africa.[1926] The Europeans' lighter skin tones made them more susceptible to melanoma skin cancer, so their cells were presumably forced to adapt. This may be another example of antagonistic pleiotropy.[1927] What may have been helpful in letting us reach reproductive age so we could pass along our genes (not dying from a childhood cancer) may not bode well for successful aging and longevity (the littering of our tissues of zombified senescent cells from critical telomere shortening).[1928]

At birth, our telomeres start out at maximum length, but then they tend to get progressively eroded year after year as we age.[1929] That's why telomeres are often thought of as a "life clock."[1930] Based on how much the length of your telomeres changes every year, you can approximate the rate of biological aging. Two people can have the same chronological age but suffer more, or less, effective cellular aging. If you smoke a pack of cigarettes a day for a decade, your cells may age about three years faster, for example, and drinking just 8 oz of sugar-sweetened soda every day is associated with nearly two years of additional aging.[1931]

Our telomeres can start shortening as soon as we are born, and when they're gone, we are, too. Though a gross oversimplification, they're kind of like life's fuse. Accelerated telomere shortening has been identified as a key biomarker for accelerated aging, disease, and diminished longevity,[1932] and shortened telomeres have been associated with arthritis, diabetes, heart disease, kidney failure, liver failure, lung disease, osteoporosis, stroke, and vision loss.[1933] Telomere length is also tied to a reduction of muscle mass and performance (measured in grip strength),[1934] as well as reduced immune function. When the common cold virus is dripped into people's noses, those with shorter telomeres in key immune cells are significantly more likely to get sick.[1935] Alzheimer's disease, though not necessarily cognitive decline in general,[1936] is one of the age-related diseases most strongly linked to short telomeres.[1937] Shorter ends may also lead to a faster end.

LOOKS CAN BE PERCEPTIVE

Large-scale studies have found that research subjects with the shortest telomeres had a 17 to 66 percent increase in mortality risk when compared to subjects with the longest ones.[1938] In other words, longer telomeres may mean a longer life. Studies of hundreds of twins, for example, found that the twin with shorter telomeres was more likely to die at an earlier age.[1939] And, not only did the twin with the longer telomeres live longer, but they looked younger, too.[1940]

Looking "old for your age" is actually an indicator of poor health and a strong predictor of mortality, independent of physical and mental functioning. When geriatric nurses were given high-quality photographs of hundreds of pairs of twins, they were able to pick out who was more likely to die first—just based on which twin looked older. Perceived age is linked to telomere length, too.[1941] Even those born with a genetic predisposition to longer telomeres grow up to experience less facial aging, suggesting the relationship is cause and effect[1942] rather than due to some third variable, like smoking, that may concurrently age your appearance and snip away at your telomeres.[1943]

As one might expect, women tend to have longer telomeres than men and a presumed slower telomere erosion rate, consistent with the fact that women typically live longer.[1944] The telomere shortening rate is a powerful predictor of lifespan across species,[1945] as well as within them. For example, telomere length is a strong predictor of average lifespan among fifteen different breeds of dogs, who sadly lose their telomeres at approximately ten times the rate of humans and have about tenfold shorter lives.[1946]

ON THE CLOCK

Is telomere length a cause of aging or merely a consequence? Mice manipulated to start out with longer telomeres at birth do live longer and healthier lives.[1947] The case for causation in humans is buttressed by rare genetic disorders of telomere maintenance that manifest as accelerated aging, from premature hair graying and skin pigmentation to untimely heart attacks.[1948] Telomere shortening is thought to actively drive aging through cellular senescence and the ensuing constellation of SASP inflammation.[1949] (See the Cellular Senescence chapter.)

The concept of telomeres as a constantly ticking biological clock is not quite accurate.[1950] By taking DNA from a blood stain, forensic scientists may be able to roughly estimate a person's age simply based on the length of the blood cell's telomeres,[1951] but the shortening rate and baseline length vary widely between individuals.[1952] The fuse burns faster in some people than in others. On average, across an adult population, there appears to be a constant, inexorable yearly loss in length, but the individual data are scattered such that it's not uncommon to run across an eighty-year-old whose telomeres are as long as those of a thirty-year-old.[1953]

In addition to this, there is variability within the same person—and also within the same cell within the same person. Each cell has ninety-two telomeres capping off either end of our forty-six chromosomes.[1954] All it takes is a single critically short telomere to send the entire cell into a spiral of senescence or death.[1955] Most studies track the average telomere length of individuals, usually from their blood cells for convenience's sake; however, the length of our *shortest* telomeres may provide a better predictor of remaining healthy years of life.[1956] Thankfully, there's a way not only to slow down the rate of telomere attrition but to build back up our shortest telomeres.

BUILD BACK BETTER

The answer lies in an enzyme found in Methuselah. That's the name given to a bristlecone pine tree growing in California's White Mountains. When it was named, the tree was the oldest recorded living being. Today, it's nearing its 4,800th birthday. For context, Methuselah had already been alive for centuries before construction of the Egyptian pyramids had even begun. An enzyme found in the roots of bristlecone pines appears to peak a few thousand years into the trees' lifespan and actually rebuilds telomeres.[1957] Scientists named the enzyme *telomerase*. Once they knew what to look for, they found that the enzyme is present in our cells, too.

It makes sense that such an enzyme exists. If we didn't have a telomere-maintaining mechanism in our testicles and ovaries so our sperm and eggs could start out with fully intact telomeres, every generation would begin with at least a puberty's worth of telomere loss.[1958] And, how could we explain cancer? The vast majority of cancer cells crank up telomerase activity to obtain effective immortality.[1959] In most cells, though, telomerase becomes relatively inactive after birth, so our telomeres usually lose ground year after year[1960]—but not every year and not in everyone.

Longitudinal studies that tracked telomere length in the same people over time unexpectedly found that 1.5 to 25 percent of individuals experienced an elongation in their telomeres.[1961] In the Bogalusa Heart Study, for example, 16 percent of all participants showed telomere lengthening over a period of seven years, but, by year twelve, that figure decreased to 1.5 percent.[1962] So, eventually, time may win out, but from one year to the next, we may be able to keep telomere shrinkage at bay, thanks to telomerase activation.

Your trajectory of telomere length over time may have serious health consequences. In the MacArthur Study of Successful Aging, for example, elderly men whose telomeres shortened over a two-and-a-half-year period had a threefold higher chance of death from cardiovascular disease over the subsequent decade compared with participants whose telomere length was lengthened or even just maintained.[1963] Centenarians appear to be particularly good at maintaining their telomeres,[1964] especially those who successfully escape the major age-related diseases.[1965] So, is telomerase the "fountain of youth," as it's been described?[1966] An "anti-aging molecular switch"?[1967]

Mice engineered to be deficient in telomerase suffer critical telomere shortening and experience premature aging and death, which can be prevented by reinstating telomerase.[1968] Conversely, when mice were engineered to express even more of the enzyme, there was a striking 40 percent extension of average mouse lifespans.[1969] Further demonstrating its anti-aging activity, telomerase activation in various mouse models has also been shown to lead to a reduction in age-related osteoporosis[1970] and improvements in heart,[1971] liver,[1972] and kidney function,[1973] as well as coordination, balance,[1974] and movement.[1975] Telomerase may even have additional beneficial "non-canonical" activities, such as DNA repair.[1976]

What About Cancer?

Since telomerase can be hijacked by cancer cells, should we be concerned that boosting its activity would increase our cancer risk? Drug companies have been trying to come up with anti-telomerase chemotherapy in an effort to stop cancer, but they haven't been successful. Not only are there toxic effects on stem cells that rely on telomerase, but cancer can't be stopped in time. Even if telomerase were completely blocked and cancer cell telomeres began getting ratcheted down, we could be dead long before the Hayflick limit was reached. (The amount of cancer produced during fifty doublings is more than enough to kill us.[1977])

Ramping up telomerase activity does not, however, seem to be a problem. Telomerase is a permissive, but not sufficient, cause of cancer, meaning the enzyme can be used by cancer cells but does not itself cause it.[1978] Skin cells (taken from circumcised foreskins) in a petri dish "immortalized"[1979] with telomerase activation, for example, were not transformed into skin cancer cells.[1980] Similarly, in mice, telomerase activation delays aging and increases lifespan without increasing cancer risk.[1981] Since we're left with apparently all upsides, we should try to boost activity of the age-defying enzyme.

DIETARY TELOMERE PROTECTION

Approximately 30 percent of the difference in telomere-shortening rates between people is genetically determined, but the majority of influence over whether our telomeres lengthen or shorten and at what rate is determined by external factors, such as environment, lifestyle, and diet.[1982] This helps explain the correlation of telomere length shared by spouses,[1983] for example, but it doesn't necessarily mean we have control over that full 70 percent of our telomeric destiny. For instance, we can suffer telomere loss before we're even born due to prenatal exposure to alcohol,[1984] smoking,[1985] or air pollution.[1986] But, the choices we make every day—or three times a day—can make a difference.

The main drivers of accelerated telomere loss may be oxidative stress and inflammation.[1987] (For an explanation why, watch see.nf/ttaggg.) No surprise, then, that a systematic review on the role of nutrition concluded that longer telomeres were associated with the intake of vegetables, fruits, legumes, nuts, and other foods high in fiber and antioxidants. In contrast, the consumption of processed meats, alcohol, soda, and other foods and beverages rich in saturated fat and sugar was linked to shorter telomeres.[1988] So, a whole food, plant-based diet was put to the test.

HOW TO WIND BACK THE CLOCK

Research pioneer Dean Ornish was the first to show, in a randomized controlled trial, that a whole food, plant-based lifestyle could reverse the progression of heart disease.[1989] He then showed that the same dietary changes could also help reverse the trajectory of early-stage prostate cancer,[1990] and he is currently pitting plants against dementia in an attempt to reverse the course of early-stage Alzheimer's disease.[1991] In a study partially funded by the U.S. Department of Defense to see what a healthy diet and lifestyle could do for cellular aging, Ornish teamed up with Dr. Elizabeth Blackburn, who was awarded the Nobel Prize in medicine for her role in the very discovery of telomerase.[1992]

Thirty men aged forty-nine to eighty were encouraged to eat a low-fat diet centered around whole plant foods—fruits, vegetables, whole grains, and beans—as well as walk for exercise and practice stress management. Within three months, their telomerase activity jumped by nearly 30 percent. This was the first ever intervention that showed significant boosting of the telomerase enzyme. The study was published in one of the world's leading medical journals,[1993] and the accompanying editorial concluded that the landmark findings "should encourage people to adopt a healthy lifestyle in order to avoid or combat cancer and age-related diseases."[1994]

In the five-year follow-up study, the researchers measured the lengths of the subjects' telomeres to determine if the telomerase boost actually translated into a slowing of telomere loss. For similarly aged men in the control group who maintained their regular diets, their telomeres predictably shrank with age. In the healthy-living group, however, the subjects' telomeres didn't just shrink less or hold steady—they *grew*. Five years after that first intervention, their telomeres were even longer on average than when they had started participating in the study, suggesting for the first time ever that a healthy plant-based diet and lifestyle can boost telomerase enzyme activity and effectively reverse cellular aging.[1995] But, was it the diet, the exercise, or the stress management?

CAN WE DE-STRESS OUR TELOMERES?

In the Hollywood blockbuster *The Holiday*, Cameron Diaz's character announces, "Severe stress . . . causes the DNA in our cells to shrink until they can no longer replicate."[1996] Did Tinseltown get that right? As I review in see.nf/destress, the data on stress and telomeres are conflicting, finding, for example, decreased telomerase activity among one set of dementia caregivers[1997] and increased telomerase activity among another.[1998] In the video, you'll see the data are also mixed on the role of meditation.[1999] Regardless, there appears to be more to the remarkable Ornish results than just the stress reduction component. What about the exercise and weight loss?

TELOMERE LENGTH IN THE LONG RUN

We can't always change our station in life, but we can always go out for a walk. A study of thousands of twins found that those who exercised more appeared to pump up their telomeres along with their muscles.[2000] Although some findings suggest that walking as little as 150 minutes a week is associated with longer telomeres[2001] and, on average, those who exercise tend to have longer telomeres than those who don't,[2002] the majority of studies on physical activity and telomere length actually came up short, finding no significant association.[2003] "[I]t is not clear," concluded one review, "whether P[hysical]A[ctivity] is protective for the shortening of telomere DNA."

The data are more consistent with elite athletes. Those taking part in national or international competitions[2004] and master athletes competing in professional sports tend to have longer telomeres than age-matched non-athletes.[2005] Ultramarathoners,[2006] marathoners, and triathletes running fifty miles a week for thirty-five years[2007] may have longer telomeres, but what about those of us who haven't run the equivalent of three times around the Earth's equator?

Of the five randomized controlled trials that have actually put exercise to the test, only one found a significant difference in changes in telomere length.[2008,2009,2010,2011] Six months of aerobic endurance training (running) or high-intensity interval training (HIIT) increased telomerase activity and telomere length, whereas resistance training for the same period did not.[2012] But none of the other interventional trials found any significant effect regardless of the regimen, calling any telomere effects of exercise into question, at least in the short term.[2013]

WAS IT THE MENU OR THE MOVEMENT?

To tease out the critical Ornish study question—*Was it the plant-based nature of the diet, the exercise, or the weight loss?*—ideally a study would randomize people into at least three groups: a control group who did nothing (sedentary on a typical diet), a group who just exercised, and a group who lost weight eating pretty much the same diet but in smaller portions. And just such a study was published by a team of American and Canadian researchers.[2014]

About four hundred postmenopausal women were randomized into one of four groups for a year: a control group, an exercise group, a portion-controlled diet group, and an exercise *and* portion-controlled diet group. As expected, after twelve months of doing nothing, there was little change in the control group. What about after a year of exercise? They did no better, and this study's exercise group did more than just walk for half an hour like those in the Ornish study; they were tasked with forty-five minutes of moderate-to-vigorous exercise, like jogging. And the portion-controlled diet group? The weight loss had no effect, nor was there a significant change in telomere length in the combined exercise and weight-loss group. This is on par with inconsistent findings across the board with weight-loss interventions attempting to restore telomere integrity.[2015]

So, as long as we're eating the same diet, it may not matter how small our portions are, how much weight we lose, or how much we exercise; after a year, the subjects saw no benefit. In contrast, the individuals in the Ornish study on a whole food, plant-based diet who exercised only half as much and enjoyed the same amount of weight loss after just three months[2016] appeared to acquire significant telomere protection.[2017] In other words, neither the weight loss nor the exercise reversed cell aging by rebuilding telomeres. It was the food—and not just any diet. A similar study across a similar time frame—four and a half years of more moderate nutritional advice, such as choosing low-fat dairy and skinless chicken breast, along with more fruits, vegetables, and whole grains[2018]—failed to significantly affect telomere length.[2019]

FOODS TO AVOID

Not all plant foods are good for you. For example, eating french fries is associated with shorter telomeres.[2020] Yes, vegetable intake goes hand in hand with longer telomeres, but that may be trumped by a deep fryer.[2021] Refined carbs, like cookies and crackers, may also snip at your telomeres.[2022] So, part of the benefit of centering one's diet around *whole* plant foods may be from cutting out junk. Those eating the most ultraprocessed foods have nearly twice the odds of having shorter telomeres,[2023] not to mention a higher risk of obesity,[2024] depression, heart disease, stroke, and premature death in general.[2025]

Alcohol is another processed plant product. Researchers followed a cohort of Helsinki businessmen for nearly thirty years and found that those who drank the most ended up with an extra decade of telomere aging. Although they also found that even minor alcohol consumption during middle age might result in shortened telomeres,[2026] a systematic review of evidence published in 2021 concluded that any negative effects of alcohol on telomeres appeared to be limited to heavier drinkers with alcohol dependence.[2027]

In addition to eschewing alcohol, the Ornish study participants were asked to cut out processed meat. Consumption of foods like bacon, ham, hot dogs, lunch meat, and sausage has been associated with both cancer[2028] and shorter telomeres, although unprocessed red meat—a steak, for example—does not appear to be similarly associated with telomere length.[2029] There have been studies implicating meat, including wild game, poultry,[2030] and fish,[2031] but, more broadly, it appears to be more of an issue with processed meat.[2032]

Long-chain omega-3 fats in fish and fish oil were presumed to benefit telomeres because they score as anti-inflammatory in the Dietary Inflammatory Index.[2033] A 2010 population study correlated higher baseline blood levels of omega-3 fatty acids with less telomere shortening over a five-year period, which launched a series of randomized controlled trials.[2034] Though a secondary analysis of a clinical trial on schizophrenics found an increase in telomerase activity,[2035] unfortunately, not a single one of the randomized controlled trials putting fish oil supplementation to the test could demonstrate a significant effect on telomere length.[2036,2037,2038,2039]

The most pro-inflammatory food component is saturated fat.[2040] Figuring it's never too early to start eating more healthfully, researchers randomized more than a thousand infants to a diet low in saturated fat or a control group for their first twenty years of life. This remarkable Finnish study found that, compared to those growing up in the healthier diet group, subjects in the control group suffered twice the annual rate of telomere loss. However, this may be more than an effect of saturated fat reduction. Although that was the main focus of the study, those in the intervention group were also encouraged to reduce their salt intake and eat more fruits, vegetables, and whole grains, making it impossible to pinpoint the decisive factor.[2041]

On the other end of the research spectrum is a series of randomized controlled dietary trials that only lasted four weeks but had an innovative study design. Cells from umbilical cords (a convenient source of human tissue) were cultured in the blood of elderly subjects after a month of eating a diet high in butter versus a similar diet high in olive oil. A greater percentage of cells bathed in the buttery blood had shortened telomeres.[2042] A Mediterranean-style diet, which is typically higher in olive oil and lower in dairy, may be insufficient, though. Although cross-sectional studies have found that higher adherence to a more Mediterranean diet correlated with longer telomeres, the only longitudinal and controlled trials found telomere lengths to be the same or even shorter.[2043]

The adverse effects of saturated butterfat may help explain the association between increased biological aging and the consumption of high-fat milk in a national survey of thousands of Americans. Even increasing milk fat by just 1 percent—for example, going from 1% low-fat milk to 2% reduced-fat milk—correlated with the equivalent of more than four years of telomere loss, presumed to be due to the inflammatory response and oxidative stress triggered by the saturated fat.[2044]

TELOMERE-FRIENDLY FOODS

The most anti-inflammatory food component is fiber.[2045] The same representative sampling of thousands of U.S. adults found that the more fiber people consumed, the longer their telomeres tended to be. Since there appeared to be a straight-line increase, researchers could do the math. It seems that just a 10 g increase in fiber per 1,000 calories equates to four fewer years of telomere aging.[2046] That's comparable in magnitude to the additional years of aging associated with consumption of processed meat (4.0 extra aging years),[2047] drinking 20 oz of soda a day (4.6 more years),[2048] or smoking (also 4.6 extra aging years).[2049]

Fiber intake may just be a marker for the consumption of plant foods, since, by definition, they are the only place fiber is found.[2050] So, the apparent link between fiber consumption and telomere length may have nothing at all to do with fiber; it could be related to some other protective component or components of plant foods. It's like the studies showing longer telomeres in people with higher dietary intakes[2051] or blood levels[2052] of carotenoids, plant pigments like beta-carotene. Again, that could just be a proxy for the intake of plants. Also associated with longer telomeres is consumption of coffee,[2053] and that has neither fiber nor carotenoids. Interestingly, while coffee intake is linked to longer telomeres, *caffeine* intake seems to be coupled with shorter telomeres,[2054] presumably because so much caffeine intake these days is from sodas and sugary energy drinks.[2055]

Green tea consumption has been associated with longer telomeres in elderly men[2056] and shown to protect telomeres in rats,[2057] but it wasn't put to the test clinically in an interventional trial until 2016. It's hard to make a convincing placebo tea, so researchers used green tea extract capsules. In my video see.nf/nutsandtea, I show how those randomized to the equivalent of about four cups[2058] of green tea a day for five months experienced a significant boost in telomere length in the green tea group over placebo.[2059] (It is unclear if nuts help our telomeres or not.)

Green tea is essentially a green leafy vegetable dipped in hot water. What about *eating* green leafy veggies? In the video, I profile a dietary intervention that showed that eating the equivalent of one and a quarter daily cups of kale—cooked, not raw—boosted telomerase activity in as little as five days. The study provided, for the first time, evidence that telomerase activity can respond in a matter of days to a food intervention. Not just any food, though, but the healthiest food out there—cruciferous, dark green leafy vegetables. Within sixteen days of stopping the kale, however, telomerase activity was back to baseline.[2060] So, as I recommend in my Daily Dozen, try to fit cruciferous veggies into your regular dietary routine.

SUPPLEMENTS

One of the reasons I don't recommend taking green tea extract supplements is the risk of liver toxicity. We used to think such reactions were rare, on the order of one in a hundred thousand.[2061] But, now that there are large studies like the Minnesota Green Tea Trial, we realize it may be more like one in twenty.[2062] (In contrast, not a single liver problem has been reported in any of the trials that used green tea in regular beverage form.[2063]) Are there any other supplements that aren't as risky yet may protect our telomeres?

VITAMIN D

Nearly every supplement study to date has failed to find benefits for our telomeres. None of the fish oil trials successfully delayed telomere shortening,[2064,2065,2066,2067] nor did extra-virgin olive oil,[2068] B vitamins,[2069] or zinc supplements.[2070] Of the ten studies on vitamin D and telomeres, only two were double-blind, randomized, placebo-controlled trials,[2071] but they both showed benefits (at 60,000 IU once a month[2072] and 800 IU once a day[2073]). Details in see.nf/dtelomeres.

ASTRAGALUS

Astragalus root is one of the most popular herbs in traditional Chinese medicine,[2074] widely marketed for millennia as a "life-prolonging" tonic.[2075] A compound in the root called *cycloastragenol* (branded as "TA-65") appeared to moderately enhance telomerase activation in vitro,[2076] but the only study suggesting clinical benefit was funded by the company that sells it[2077] for $600 a bottle online. It grossed more than $50 million before being charged with false and deceptive claims and practices by the Federal Trade Commission.[2078] For those interested in learning more, I explore the pros and cons in see.nf/astragalus.

GOTU KOLA

In 2019, the most powerful telomerase activator to date was discovered in *Centella asiatica*, also known as *gotu kola*. It was found to cause a nearly ninefold increase in telomerase activity, four times that of TA-65.[2079] Widely used in both Ayurvedic and traditional Chinese medicines,[2080] gotu kola is a green leafy vegetable, commonly eaten fresh in salads or cooked in soups in Malaysia and Indonesia or juiced or brewed as tea in India and Thailand. In India, it is primarily considered a "brain food"[2081] and has been found to enhance cognitive function in mice,[2082] but a meta-analysis of the handful of studies done to date with people found no significant effect on human cognition.[2083] Should clinical benefits be discovered, gotu kola tea can be purchased online for only about a nickel per cup.

Food for Thought

Telomeres are one of the aging pathways that have crept into the public consciousness. Increasing telomere length to slow or even prevent aging is a popular idea, though, as I've addressed, the science is controversial.[2084] Telomere elongation is possible through activation of the telomerase enzyme, but there is a constant battle between the forces hacking away at our telomeres, such as aging, oxidative stress, and inflammation, and the lifestyle decisions that can help build them back up.[2085]

Some people have expressed concern that boosting telomerase activity could theoretically increase cancer risk,[2086] since tumors have been known to hijack the telomerase enzyme and use it to ensure their own immortality,[2087] but the same lifestyle changes that Dr. Ornish used to protect telomeres appeared to slow, stop, or even *reverse* tumor progression of cancer in a randomized controlled diet and lifestyle program of early-stage prostate cancer.[2088]

In response to Ornish's work showing that telomerase may be boosted and telomeres elongated with a plant-based diet and lifestyle, an accompanying editorial suggested that such studies might uncover mechanisms that can be exploited by Big Pharma since "adopting a healthy lifestyle is not always possible in today's world. . . ."[2089] Hopefully, if you're reading this book, you're motivated to take at least a step or two toward living more healthfully, which, in the case of telomere protection, may involve quitting smoking[2090] and reducing your intake of refined grains,[2091] soda,[2092] processed meat,[2093] and dairy,[2094] while increasing consumption of fruits,[2095] vegetables,[2096] and other antioxidant-rich foods.[2097]

(continued)

To help boost this anti-aging pathway, on a daily basis, consider:

- following the recommendations in the Inflammation and Oxidation chapters
- eating a high-fiber diet centered around whole plant foods
- choosing to drink tea or coffee over soda or milk
- eating cruciferous vegetables
- supplementing with 800 to 2,000 IU of vitamin D_3 a day if your vitamin D blood level is under 20 ng/mL (50 nmol/L)

CONCLUSION

Most of the major advances made in our understanding of these aging pathways have occurred in the last twenty years, after I had already graduated from medical school; hence, much of the research I uncovered while working on this book has been eye-opening to me, too. The more we learn about them, the more we discover their interconnectedness. Rather than existing as distinct entities, the aging pathways are intertwined in a complex circuitry: A boost in AMPK downregulates mTOR while upregulating autophagy and NAD^+ levels, which in turn raise the sirtuin activity that then lowers IGF-1 and feeds back on AMPK.[2098] It is therefore no surprise that they share many common triggers.

Here is a chart of interventions that may help slow aging by hacking each of the eleven aging pathways:

Interventions to Regulate the Eleven Aging Pathways

	Exercise	Smoking Cessation	Caloric Restriction	Protein Restriction	Decrease in Certain Animal Foods	Decrease in Certain Processed Foods	Increase in Certain Plant Foods
AMPK	✓		✓	✓	✓	✓	✓
Autophagy	✓		✓	✓	✓	✓	✓
Cellular Senescence	✓	✓	✓	✓		✓	✓
Epigenetics	✓	✓	✓	✓	✓		✓
Glycation	✓	✓	✓	✓	✓	✓	✓
IGF-1				✓	✓		
Inflammation	✓	✓	✓	✓	✓	✓	✓
mTOR		✓	✓	✓	✓		✓
Oxidation	✓	✓	✓	✓	✓	✓	✓
Sirtuins	✓	✓	✓	✓	✓	✓	✓
Telomeres	✓	✓		✓	✓	✓	✓

It is remarkable that, just since the turn of the century, research has uncovered a half dozen single compounds that can significantly extend the lifespan of mammals. Though there is elaborate cross-talk between many of the aging pathways, the drugs or supplements that extend life primarily target only one or another. Metformin, for example, can extend the lifespan of mice by boosting AMPK, and rapamycin by suppressing mTOR.[2099] When they're taken together, they appear to work synergistically—not only better than each taken alone but better than just adding together each of their independent effects.[2100] This may be a major advantage of diet and lifestyle approaches, as they can target multiple aging pathways at the same time.

II. The Optimal
Anti-Aging Regimen

DIET

Worldwide each year, physical inactivity has potentially accounted for more than ten million years of healthy life lost, but what we eat may account for nearly twenty times that amount.[2101] According to the Global Burden of Disease Study, the most comprehensive and systematic analysis ever undertaken of the causes of death,[2102] the number one killer in the United States[2103] and on planet Earth is a bad diet.[2104] Unhealthy diets shave hundreds of millions of disability-free years off people's lives annually.[2105] That is why I've dedicated my life to the study of nutrition.

THE BEST FOODS

Funded by the Bill & Melinda Gates Foundation, the Global Burden of Disease Study pulled together nearly five hundred researchers from more than three hundred institutions in fifty countries and examined almost 100,000 data sources.[2106] Among the findings, they determined that the number one killer of Americans is the American diet, bumping tobacco down to number two. Smoking now only kills an estimated half million Americans every year, whereas our diet appears to kill many more.[2107]

Diet is considered to be the most important modifiable lifestyle factor when it comes to aging, healthspan, and lifespan.[2108] When studies find that "optimal nutrition," "healthy dietary patterns," or "higher diet quality" are associated with increased life expectancy, lower risk of all types of chronic disease,[2109] a higher quality of life,[2110] or more successful aging, what do they mean by *healthy diet?*[2111]

Tallying higher on each of the four major dietary quality scoring systems has been associated with an extended lifespan and lowering of heart disease and cancer mortality,[2112] and they share only four fundamental elements: more fruits, more vegetables, more whole grains, and more nuts and beans.[2113] They are all built on a common core of a plant-rich diet, whereas food patterns that are rich in refined and animal foods and poor in plant foods, referred to as the Western diet or westernized diets, are associated with higher risks.[2114]

In the Global Burden of Disease Study, four of the top five dietary risk factors for death were foods of which we're not eating enough. Eating more vegetables could potentially save about one and a half million lives around the world every year. Eating more nuts and seeds? Two million lives. More fruits? Close to two and a half million lives. And inadequate intake of whole grains may be responsible for the loss of three million lives annually. Salvation for millions may lie not in some new medicine or vaccine but in eating more whole, healthy plant foods.[2115] (Note that pickled vegetables, with added salt, and canned fruit, with added sugar, may do more harm than good.[2116])

THE WORST FOODS

When making critical life-or-death decisions, like what is best to feed ourselves and our families, how should we evaluate our choices? "Best available balance of evidence" is a phrase I often use, but what does it mean? What a single study says matters less than what the totality of peer-reviewed science has to say.

Individual studies can lead to headlines like this one from *Forbes*: "Study Finds No Link Between Secondhand Smoke and Cancer."[2117] To know if there's *really* no link between secondhand smoke and lung cancer, it would be better to look at a review or meta-analysis that compiles multiple studies together. The problem is that even these collated findings can sometimes contradict each other. For instance, some reviews say that breathing secondhand tobacco smoke is a cause of lung cancer,[2118] while others not only say that the effects are insignificant, and such talk may "foster irrational fears," but claim that you can even *directly* smoke four to five cigarettes a day and not worry about it.[2119] (You can imagine who funded that one.)

Why do review articles on the health effects of passive smoking reach different conclusions? It may not surprise you that about 90 percent of reviews written by researchers affiliated with the tobacco industry said it was not harmful, while about 90 percent of independent reviews concluded that it was. In fact, reviews written by industry-affiliated authors had eighty-eight times the odds of concluding that secondhand smoke was harmless.[2120] It was all part of a deliberate corporate strategy to discredit the science by, in the words of the US Tobacco Institute's market research advisers, "developing and widely publicising . . . medical evidence that passive smoke is not harmful to the nonsmoker's health."[2121]

In that case, can't we just stick to independent reviews? If only we could figure out which are truly impartial. Industry-funded researchers have all sorts of sneaky ways of getting out of declaring conflicts of interest, so it's hard to follow the money. Regardless, even without knowing who funded what, the majority of reviews still concluded that secondhand smoke is harmful. So, just as a single study may not be as helpful as a compilation of studies, a single review may not be as useful as a compilation of reviews. Looking at a review of reviews can provide a better sense of where the best available balance of evidence may lie. For second-hand smoke, with 63 percent of reviews concluding that it is deleterious for your health, 37 percent concluding it's neutral, and none suggesting protective benefits, it's probably best not to inhale.[2122]

If only there were a review of reviews for different foods. There is! An exhaustive review of meta-analyses and systematic reviews on the associations between food and beverage groups and major diet-related chronic diseases was finally published. To offer the broadest takeaway, the researchers first split the food groups into plant-based and animal-based. The vast majority (94 percent) of reviews on whole plant foods show either protective or, at the very least, neutral effects, whereas most (77 percent) reviews of animal-based foods identified deleterious health effects or, at best, neutral ones.[2123] (Note that due to rounding of percentages, not all totals equal 100.)

Percentages of Pooled / Meta-Analysis or Systematic Reviews Reporting Protective, Neutral, or Deleterious Effects on Major Diet-Related Chronic Diseases

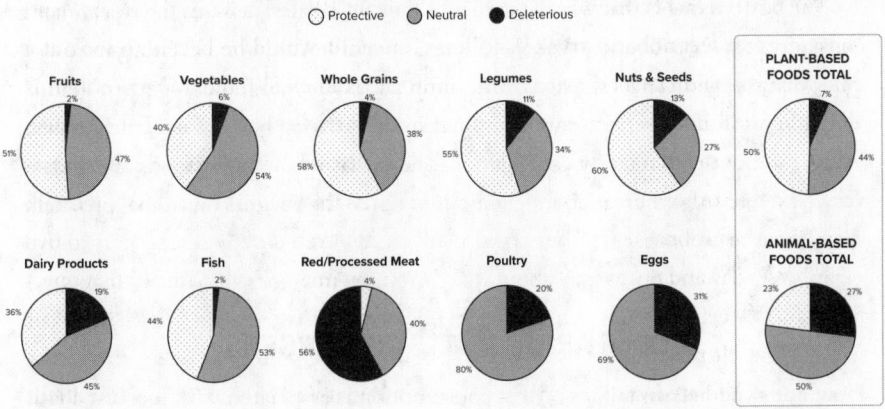

The plant-based category was broken up into five groups—fruits, vegetables, whole grains, legumes, and nuts and seeds—and each consistently rated well, between 87 and 98 percent protective or at least neutral. The five groups of animal foods, however, varied considerably. As you can see in the figure, if it weren't for dairy and fish, the animal foods total would be rated almost entirely (98.7 percent) neutral or negative.[2124]

In the Beverages chapter, I'll talk in detail about the impacts of dairy industry funding, as well as substitution effects. For example, those who drink milk may be less likely to drink soda, a beverage even more universally condemned, so any protective benefits may be relative, arising not necessarily from what is consumed but rather from what is avoided. This may help explain the fish findings, too. After all, the prototypical choice is between chicken and fish, not chicken and chickpeas. Not a single review found a single protective effect of poultry consumption. As you will see in the figure on page 164, even the soda industry received 14 percent protective effects, but chicken and eggs got big fat goose eggs—and that's even in spite of all the funding supplied by the National Chicken Council and the American Egg Board. Like the secondhand smoke reviews, perhaps a whitewash is sometimes all the best money can buy.

Like the calcium in dairy, there are some healthy components of fish, namely the long-chain omega-3 fatty acids EPA and DHA. Not necessarily for heart health, though. In the most extensive systematic assessment to date of effects of omega-3 fats on cardiovascular health, increasing intake of the fish oil fats has little or no effect on cardiovascular health. In fact, if anything, only the *plant*-based omega-3s found in flaxseeds and walnuts might be protective.[2125] The long-chain omega-3s are important for brain health, though. Thankfully, just like there are best-of-both-worlds nondairy sources of calcium,[2126] there are pollutant-free (algae-based) sources of EPA and DHA.[2127]

The bottom line is that when it comes to the diet-related diseases the researchers considered, such as obesity, type 2 diabetes, mental health, bone health, cardiovascular disease, and cancers, even if you lump all the animal foods together, ignore any industry-funding effects, and simply take the existing body of evidence at face value, nine out of ten study compilations show that whole plant foods are, in the very least, *not bad*, whereas about eight out of ten of the reviews on animal products show them to be *not good*.[2128]

COMPARING BUTTS TO BURGERS

How not good are we talking? Meat consumption is associated with increased risk of more than twenty different diseases, but by how much?[2129] To compare different chronic risks to one another, researchers came up with the concept of a "microlife," defined as thirty minutes of your life expectancy. Someone in their twenties may have about fifty-seven years left of life on average. That's about 20,000 days, a half-million hours, or one million half hours. A microlife is one of the million half hours we may have left. Smoking two cigarettes or drinking two pints of beer, on average, would cost a thirty-year-old man one microlife, as would each day he is eleven pounds overweight.[2130] See how helpful this can be in terms of comparing risks? Drinking a pint of strong beer, for example, cuts your life expectancy as much as smoking one cigarette does. If it's unthinkable for you to have so little respect for your own health that you'd light up twice a day, then it should be just as unthinkable to be eleven pounds overweight.

Alternately, you can compare life-extending behaviors. For instance, eating at least five daily servings of fruits and veggies may add an average of four years onto your lifespan. That's about twice as beneficial as the estimate for exercising every day. But, even exercising for twenty minutes may add an hour (two microlives) to your life. So, for everyone who says they don't have time to work out, exercising potentially gives a three-to-one return on investment. Give twenty minutes of your life to theoretically get sixty minutes of life. Beyond that, there's a bit of diminishing returns, but exercise an hour a day and you still may get back more time than you put in.[2131]

What about meat? A single burger is associated with losing a microlife. Is eating a burger worth thirty minutes of your life?[2132] So, in terms of lifespan, one burger appears to equal two cigarettes. If you wouldn't light up before and after lunch, maybe you should consider a bean burrito instead.

An egg salad sandwich wouldn't be a great choice either. In 2021, the largest prospective study ever done on eggs and mortality was published, the NIH-AARP Diet and Health Study, sponsored by the National Institutes of Health and the American Association of Retired Persons, which followed more than half a million people for an average of sixteen years. Each half-an-egg-a-day was associated with a 7 percent increase in all-cause mortality,[2133] which would make one egg on par with one burger for reducing lifespan.[2134]

BACON CAUSES CANCER

Processed meat is even worse. Imagine two people who are identical in every way, except one consumes around 50 g of processed meat a day—about one large sausage or hot dog, or a few strips of bacon—and the other doesn't have any. Eating just that single daily serving of processed meat is expected to take off around two years of life.[2135]

Alternately, you can frame it as a daily loss. Eating a sandwich with just two slices of deli meat like baloney or ham is expected to take off around one hour of your life.[2136] Do you ever feel like there are never enough hours in the day? Well, you may have effectively one less hour depending on what you pack for lunch.

Processed meat—bacon, deli meats, hot dogs, and the like—causes cancer. In 2015, the most prestigious cancer research institution in the world classified processed meat as a group 1 carcinogen—a substance known to cause cancer.[2137] Critics questioned putting processed meat in the same carcinogenic classification as asbestos, tobacco,[2138] and mustard gas,[2139] but the classifications relate to the strength of evidence that the agent causes cancer or not, not how *much* cancer.[2140] All substances with group 1 classification are not equally dangerous.[2141] Even though they are both group 1 carcinogens, it's safer to eat a sandwich filled with pastrami than plutonium.

Just how dangerous is processed meat? The elevated risk of colorectal cancer is 18 percent for every 50 g of processed meat consumed a day, so if you have a sandwich with two small slices of baloney every day for lunch, you would increase your colorectal cancer risk by 18 percent. A half-pound pastrami on rye could bump it up by more like 80 percent.[2142] How does "18% increased cancer risk" compare to other risky behavior? When I testified before the 2020–2025 U.S. Dietary Guidelines Scientific Committee, I said, "We try not to smoke around our kids, so why would we send them to school with a baloney sandwich?" That may sound like a hyperbolic metaphor, but it isn't an exaggeration. According to the surgeon general, living with a smoker increases your risk of lung cancer by 15 percent.[2143] So, breathing in secondhand smoke day in and day out increases your risk of lung cancer almost to the same extent that eating a single daily serving of processed meat increases your risk of colorectal cancer.

Colorectal cancer is the second leading cause of cancer death, after lung cancer.[2144] So, if you don't smoke, colon and rectal cancer may be your greatest cancer nemesis. But, you can drop that risk by nearly a fifth just by cutting a serving of processed meat out of your daily diet.

BACK TO NATURE

Given that the healthiest foods tend to come from plants, it should come as no surprise that healthy plant-based diets are associated with a lower risk of premature death in the general population[2145] and, specifically, among older adults.[2146] For healthy aging,[2147] longevity,[2148] and delaying age-related diseases,[2149] recommended diets center around whole plant foods. Such a diet may cut the risk of Alzheimer's disease by more than half, for instance, and could save billions in healthcare costs.[2150] Just one additional serving of fruits or vegetables a day could potentially slash $5 billion off U.S. medical expenditures each year.[2151]

The benefits of plant-based eating likely derive from the dual action of increasing protective dietary factors like fiber while decreasing intake of pathogenic (disease-causing) dietary factors like saturated fat.[2152] For eighteen years, the Baltimore Longitudinal Study of Aging followed individuals who had started out at an average age of around sixty. Researchers found that more fruits and vegetables, as well as less saturated fat, were associated with a lower likelihood of dying from heart disease within that period, but only the *combination* of elevated produce consumption and decreased saturated fat intake significantly reduced the risk of dying from all causes put together.[2153] This kind of diet is in line with what's natural based on our ancestral history.

For the millions of years before we began to mill grains, sharpen spears, or boil sugarcane, our entire physiology is presumed to have evolved in the context of eating what our great ape cousins did—leaves, stems, and shoots (that is, vegetables), seeds, nuts, and fruits.[2154] We started using tools during the Paleolithic period, which only goes back about two million years, but we and other great apes have been evolving since the Miocene era, which goes back about *twenty* million years.[2155] So, our body evolved on mostly plants for the first 90 percent of our hominoid existence.[2156] We were built to have nutrition from wild plant foods—especially fruits[2157]—continuously flowing throughout our system,[2158] with extremely low intake of cholesterol and saturated fat.[2159] Perhaps it's no wonder that our body thrives best on the diet we were designed to eat. Maybe we should get back to our (edible) roots.

NOT WORTH YOUR SALT

The skyrocketing intake of salt has been one of our most dramatic dietary changes. For most of human existence, we only got the pinch of salt that's naturally found in whole foods.[2160] Today, due primarily to processed foods, we're exposed to ten times more than our body was meant to handle,[2161] and it's having devastating health consequences.[2162]

I've mentioned four of the five deadliest dietary traps defined in the Global Burden of Disease Study—not eating enough whole grains, fruits, nuts and seeds, and vegetables—but the most fatal flaw about humanity's diet is not what we're getting too little of but what we're getting too much of. Excess sodium appears to be humanity's number one dietary risk factor for death.[2163]

Please see my High Blood Pressure chapter in *How Not to Die* for an in-depth review. The evidence that sodium raises blood pressure is clear, including double-blind, randomized trials dating back decades.[2164] Even just a single meal can do it. When subjects with normal blood pressure were given a bowl of soup containing the amount of salt typically found in an average American meal,[2165] their blood pressure climbed up over the next three hours compared to those who ate the same soup without any added salt.[2166] Having a "normal" salt intake can lead to a "normal" blood pressure, which can contribute to us dying from "normal" causes like heart attacks and strokes.

In the United States, most adults aged forty-five and older have high blood pressure, including nearly nine out of ten after age seventy-four,[2167] whereas there is no rise in blood pressure with age in no-salt cultures like the Amazon Yanomami, who eat a normal-for-the-human-species sodium intake. Not a single case of high blood pressure was found. Their average pressures start out about where all human infants do,[2168] at about 100 over 60, and stay that way throughout life.[2169]

A number of simple strategies can help you shake your salt habit.[2170] Don't cook with salt or add it to food. The food may taste a little bland when you first start skipping the salt, but, within just two to four weeks, the salt-taste receptors in your mouth become much more sensitive so the flavor of your food improves. After two weeks, you may actually *prefer* the taste of less salty food.[2171] Play around with pepper, lime, onions, basil, garlic, tomatoes, thyme, sweet peppers, parsley, celery, chili powder, lemon, rosemary, smoked paprika, curry, and coriander to find new, deeper flavors to enjoy.[2172] An editorial in the prestigious *New England Journal of Medicine* argued that "the individual approach is probably impractical" since 75 percent or so of salt exposure comes from manufactured foods,[2173] but that perversely presumes that processed foods are somehow preordained. We have control over the foods we buy, though some high-sodium foods may come as a surprise.

For example, the greatest contributor of sodium to the diet of twenty- to fifty-year-olds is chicken.[2174] The poultry industry routinely injects chicken carcasses with salt water to artificially inflate their weight, yet they can still be labeled as "100 percent natural." *Consumer Reports* found some chickens in grocery stores so pumped full of salt that they had a whopping 840 mg of sodium per serving. That could be more than a full day's worth of sodium in just a single chicken breast.[2175]

The now defunct Salt Institute reliably railed against public health recommendations to reduce sodium intake. In testimony before a congressional dietary guidelines committee, the presumption that healthier diets would cut healthcare costs was challenged. "Indeed," one processed food industry defender testified, "healthcare expenditures *increase* if the lifespan is prolonged." If people live longer because they eat more healthfully, it could be *more* expensive, it was argued, noting that "[i]f tobacco were banned the increase in the expected lifespan would simultaneously increase the cost of care of old people. . . . ."[2176]

Tongue Scraping

As we age, our sense of taste may decline. As a consequence, older adults often oversalt their foods.[2177] An innovative way to counter this loss in salt sensitivity is cleaning the whitish-gray coating off your tongue that can block your taste

pores.[2178] Check out my video see.nf/tonguecleaning on how tongue brushing or scraping has been shown to improve the ability to taste saltiness in both
younger[2179] and older adults,[2180] effectively decreasing your taste for death.[2181]

POTASSIUM-BASED SALT SUBSTITUTES

Hypertension, or high blood pressure, is called the "silent and invisible killer" because it rarely causes symptoms but is one of the most powerful independent predictors of some of our leading causes of death.[2182] The American Heart Association's
recommended limit is 1,500 mg of sodium a day.[2183] Care to guess what percentage
of Americans exceed that? An incredible 99.4 percent.[2184] The overwhelmingly vast
majority of U.S. adults consume too much sodium and, at the same time, too little
potassium, a mineral that lowers blood pressure. (Less than 2 percent of U.S. adults
consume the recommended daily minimum intake of potassium.)[2185] This is even
more striking when we compare our current intake with that of our ancestors, who
consumed huge amounts of dietary potassium.[2186] We likely evolved getting more
than 10,000 mg a day.[2187] The recommended daily minimum is to only get about
half of that, yet most of us don't come anywhere close.

Put the two guidelines together, and sodium and potassium goals are currently
met by less than 0.015 percent of the U.S. population.[2188] Close to 99.99 percent
noncompliance, with only one in about seven thousand Americans meeting even
the minimal recommendations. What about using potassium-based salt substitutes? Instead of flavoring our food with sodium chloride (salt), why not shake on
some *potassium* chloride? A naturally occurring mineral salt, potassium chloride
is obtained in the same way as regular sodium salt.[2189] Randomized controlled
trials have found that simply swapping in some potassium chloride for regular salt
can not only lead to significant reductions in blood pressure[2190] but can prevent
hypertension in the first place and, most important, save lives. Even just switching
to half potassium salt appeared to effectively make people more than a decade
younger when it came to the risk of death.[2191] I review the studies in my video
see.nf/ksalt.

It seems a little too good to be true. Why haven't more people embraced this
salt substitute if it works so well and can taste just as good?[2192] Potassium chloride
is "generally regarded as safe" by the Food and Drug Administration (FDA).[2193] The
reason healthy people don't have to worry about getting too much potassium is
that our kidneys just pee out the excess.[2194] However, people with known kidney
disease, diabetes (since diabetes can lead to kidney damage), severe heart failure,
or adrenal insufficiency, and those on medications that impair potassium excretion

need to be careful.[2195] Older adults should ask their doctor to get their kidney function tested before starting salt substitutes. For more details on this, go to see .nf/ksaltsafety.

The only downside for healthy individuals is the taste. If you go 100 percent sodium-free and use straight potassium chloride, you may find that it has a bit of a bitter or metallic taste.[2196] Personally, I've found it depends on what I'm putting it on. Potassium chloride works perfectly on some foods, but, for me, makes others inedible. When I learned about the sodium science and threw out my salt shakers for good, my palate totally changed within a few weeks and everything tasted fine without salt—except pesto. For some reason, pesto without any salt just never tasted like it used to, so I tried the potassium chloride salt substitute and it worked fabulously. I couldn't tell the difference at all, so I got the best of both worlds. Enthused, I decided to re-create a childhood favorite. I used to put a tiny sprinkle of salt on watermelon to make it even sweeter, a traditional southern culinary trick, but when I tried it with the potassium salt, I almost gagged!

WE ARE WHAT WE EAT

Not only is the American diet the leading killer of Americans, but, thanks in part to the obesity epidemic, our diet is also the leading cause of disability in the United States.[2197] So, what we eat is the number one determinant of how long we live and what most determines whether we will become disabled or not.

If our diet is the number one cause of death and disability,[2198] and if most deaths are preventable and related to nutrition,[2199] then, obviously, nutrition is the number one subject taught in medical school, right? It's the number one thing your doctor discusses with you at every single visit, right?

How can there be such a disconnect between the science and the practice of medicine?

Unfortunately, doctors suffer from a severe nutrition deficiency—in education. Most medical students are never taught about the impact that healthy nutrition can have on the course of illness, so they graduate without this powerful arsenal of knowledge.[2200] There are also institutional barriers, such as time constraints and lack of reimbursement. In general, doctors aren't paid for counseling their patients on how to better care for themselves.[2201] Of course, the drug companies also play a role in influencing medical education and practice. The director of the Institute for the Medical Humanities concluded an ethics journal article on Big Pharma's influence on medical education with these words: "I am not sure which is the more severe condemnation of our professionalism—our willingness to be bought; or our willingness to rationalize and deny, to make it seem as if we are not being bought."[2202] Ask your physician when they were last wined and dined by Big Broccoli.

It's like smoking in the 1950s. Even then, we already had decades of science linking cigarettes with cancer, but it was largely ignored in part because smoking was *normal*.[2203] The average per capita cigarette consumption was 4,000 cigarettes a year[2204]—meaning the average American smoked half a pack a day. Back then, the American Medical Association reassured everyone that "smoking in moderation" was just fine.[2205] After all, most doctors themselves smoked cigarettes.[2206] There was the same disconnect between the science and medical practice: overwhelming evidence versus the inertia of personal habit.

It took more than twenty-five years,[2207] 7,000 studies, and the deaths of countless smokers before the first surgeon general's report against smoking was published in the 1960s.[2208] You'd think maybe after the first *6,000* studies they could have given people a little heads-up or something, but no. Big Tobacco was a powerful industry, and today's alcohol, meat, sugar, dairy, salt, egg, and processed food industries are using the same tobacco industry tactics to try to twist the science and confuse the public.[2209]

Big Food is a trillion-dollar industry with thousands of trade associations spending hundreds of millions of dollars on lobbying our legislative leaders. After the processed food sector, which is led by PepsiCo, the next top three food lobbies are sugar, meat, and dairy.[2210] (Dairy is the only food trade group with a budget exceeding $100 million.[2211]) This tells us a lot about the American diet. *Cui bono?* Follow the money.

Today, only 1 to 2 percent of doctors smoke,[2212,2213] but most continue to eat foods that are contributing to our epidemics of dietary disease.[2214] Until the system changes, we have to take personal responsibility for our own health and our family's. We can't wait until society catches up to the science again, because it's a matter of life and death.

Master of Your Own Destiny

Longevity experts consider nutrition likely "the most important intervention for the promotion of health and the prevention of the great majority of age-associated chronic diseases."[2215] Changing from a typical diet to a more optimized one starting at age twenty would be expected to increase the lifespan of women by about eleven years and men by thirteen. The largest lifespan gains would be made by eating more legumes, then whole grains and nuts, and cutting down on meat, then sugary beverages like soda. And it's never too late. At age sixty, starting to

(continued)

at more healthfully could mean eight or nine more years of life. Even starting as late as age eighty could add years to your life.[2216] Changing your health destiny can start with your very next meal.

BEVERAGES

You may have heard that the human body is 70 percent water. That's true of newborn babies, but as Aristotle said, "Old age is dry and cold." Older individuals may only be about 50 percent water.[2217] With smaller fluid reserves, a diminished sensation of thirst,[2218] and waning ability of the kidneys to concentrate urine, the elderly are particularly susceptible to dehydration,[2219] especially when taking laxatives or diuretic drugs.[2220] What's the best way to remain hydrated?

CONSENSUS PANEL RECOMMENDATIONS

There are scads of dietary guidelines for what we should eat, but what about for what we should drink? A Beverage Guidance Panel was assembled to bring together leading health experts like Dr. Walter Willett, then chair of the Harvard University School of Public Health's nutrition department. The panel's task was to provide recommendations on the nutritional risks and benefits, as well as the relative healthfulness, of different beverage categories, ranked on a six-tier scale from best to worst.

Unsurprisingly, soda came in last. Beer and whole milk were grouped together as two other beverages to be avoided. They cited concerns about the association between milk and prostate cancer and aggressive ovarian cancer, arising from well-documented effects on circulating levels of insulin-like growth factor 1, which I covered in the IGF-1 chapter. Tied as the second *healthiest* beverages were tea and coffee, preferably without sweetener or creamer. And the top-ranked drink? Water.[2221]

HELL OR HIGH WATER?

In the *How Not to Die* beverages chapter, I trace the origins and bust the myth of the "drink at least eight glasses of water a day" recommendation, as well as discuss the difficulty of establishing cause and effect in the multitude of studies correlating low water intake with a wide range of diseases.[2222] I review all the studies on water consumption and mortality in see.nf/h2olongevity. Basically, three studies showed a mortality benefit,[2223,2224,2225] whereas four did not,[2226,2227,2228,2229] so the connection remains murky.

SO HOW MUCH WATER SHOULD YOU DRINK?

Based on snapshot-in-time blood sampling, between 20 to 30 percent of older adults are dehydrated at any one time.[2230] Such individuals are at increased risk for heart attacks, pneumonia, and blood clots, which results in a doubling of the odds of becoming disabled over the subsequent four years.[2231] How do you know if you're dehydrated? Younger folks can just check the color of their urine. The gold standard for hydration—or rather, the *pale* gold standard—is the color of straw, a light yellow. A darker yellow, amber, or brownish coloring has been validated as a way to detect dehydration in athletes,[2232] pregnant and lactating women,[2233] and the broader general population,[2234] but it does not appear to work in older adults.[2235] Not one of sixty-seven different assessments for dehydration—including urine color or volume, or having a dry mouth or feeling thirsty—appeared consistently useful in determining hydration status for adults older than sixty-five. Only the combination of experiencing fatigue and missing some drinks between meals appeared predictive for impending dehydration in older men and women.[2236]

Based on the best evidence to date, authorities from the World Health Organization and the U.S. Institute of Medicine recommend eight to eleven cups of water a day for women and ten to fifteen daily cups for men.[2237] This includes water from all sources, though, not only beverages. We get about four cups of water from the food we eat and what our body produces on its own[2238] (for example, when our body burns fat), so the guidelines translate roughly into a daily recommendation for drinking four to seven cups of water for women and six to eleven cups for men, assuming moderate physical activity at moderate ambient temperatures.[2239] The kidney capacity of older individuals tends to be limited to approximately three to four cups per hour, though, so under normal circumstances, avoid exceeding that limit.[2240] Drinking more than the recommended amount could critically dilute the electrolytes in your brain.[2241]

What Kind of Water Should We Drink?

Many are distrustful of the safety of tap water,[2242] but bottled water may not be any cleaner than water right out of the faucet.[2243] How much is that saying, though? Drinking water safety isn't only about preventing waterborne diseases.

(continued)

In fact, our fight against microbial contaminants introduced a new kind of contamination in our water—in the form of disinfection by-products caused by the chlorination of drinking water. In my video see.nf/water, I quantify the potential bladder cancer risks and review the efficacy of two fridge filters (Whirlpool and GE) and three pour-through pitchers (Brita, PUR, and ZeroWater) to remove contaminants.

BEVERAGES RANKED FROM BEST TO WORST

Other than water, what are the best beverages? Below is another graphic from the exhaustive study that encompassed hundreds of pooled meta-analyses and systematic reviews cataloging protective, neutral, or deleterious associations with diet-related chronic diseases.[2244]

Percentages of Pooled / Meta-Analysis or Systematic Reviews Reporting Protective, Neutral, or Deleterious Effects on Major Diet-Related Chronic Diseases

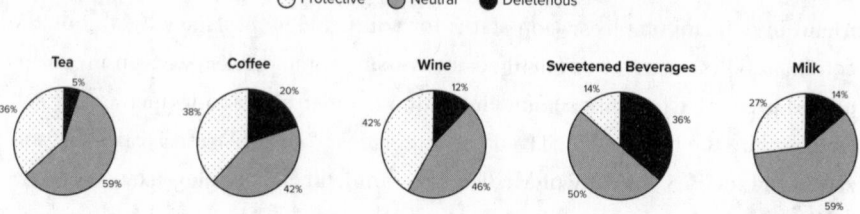

As expected, sweetened drinks like soda ranked most deleterious, but 14 percent of reviews reported *protective* effects of soft drinks. How is that possible? Most were references to cross-sectional studies like one that found that eighth-grade girls who drank more soda were skinnier than girls who drank less.[2245] That was just a snapshot in time, though. What do you think is more likely? Heavier girls weighed more because they drank less soda, or they drank less sugary soda because they were heavier? Soda abstention may be a *consequence* of obesity rather than a cause, yet it gets marked down as protective because less of the beverage was associated with less of the disease.

Study design flaws may also account for findings about wine. The review of reviews was published in 2014, before the revolution in our understanding that the purported health benefits from "moderate" alcohol intake may have just been a mirage.[2246] (See page 169 for a discussion of the systematic error of misclassifying former drinkers as if they had been lifelong abstainers.[2247]) Sometimes, however, there are unexplainable associations. For instance, one of the soft drink studies found that increased soda consumption was associated with *lower* risk of certain types of esophageal cancers. Let me guess. Was the review funded by Coca-Cola? Yes, the review was funded by Coca-Cola.[2248] Do similar conflicts of interest help explain the "protective" milk studies? Were those funded by the National Dairy Council? In fact, even *more* conflicts of interest have been found among milk studies than soda studies, and exclusively industry-funded studies of all such beverages are four to eight times more likely to be favorable to the financial interests of the sponsor.[2249]

Funding bias aside, though, there could be legitimate reasons for the protective effects associated with dairy milk consumption. After all, those who drink more milk may drink less soda, which is an even more deleterious beverage, so the milk drinkers may come out ahead. But it may be more than just relative benefits. Even something as universally condemned as tobacco isn't universally bad. More than forty studies have consistently found a protective association with Parkinson's, thanks to the effects of nicotine on the brain.[2250] Even secondhand smoke may be protective.[2251] Of course, you'd still want to avoid it. Tobacco may decrease the risk of Parkinson's, but its use increases the risk of stroke, an even deadlier brain disease, not to mention lung cancer and heart disease, which have killed millions of Americans since the first surgeon general's report against smoking was released.[2252]

Thankfully, by eating certain nicotine-containing vegetables, we may be able to get some of the benefits without the risks[2253] (see.nf/nightshades), and the same concept may be true of dairy. The consumption of milk is associated with increased risk of prostate cancer,[2254] which has led to recommendations suggesting that men may want to cut down or minimize their intake,[2255] but dairy consumption is also associated with *decreased* colorectal cancer risk.[2256] This protection appears to be a calcium effect.[2257] Thankfully, we may be able to get the best of both worlds by eating high-calcium plant foods, such as greens and beans.[2258]

I explored dairy in greater detail (see page 106) and covered the benefits of coffee (see page 25). However, based on the bird's-eye view provided in the figure on page 164, every cup of coffee may be a lost opportunity to drink something even healthier, like a cup of tea.

The Healthiest Type of Milk

There is a constellation of new choices in the dairy case these days, with milks made from everything from almonds to oats,[2259] so much so that major dairy corporations are going out of business.[2260] Of all the options, soymilk is probably the healthiest. See page 27 and watch my video see.nf/milks. All plant-based milks lack lactose, which is a benefit worthy of emphasis.[2261]

(continued)

The majority of adult humans are lactose intolerant, meaning they have trouble digesting dairy milk. Throughout childhood, the enzyme we have that breaks down the milk sugar lactose begins to decline in most of us around the world, which makes sense since milk is for babies.[2262] Why would we need to be able to digest it after we've weaned from the breast? So, when drinking milk, most people on the planet can experience symptoms like bloating, abdominal pain, intestinal gas, and watery stool, or even nausea and vomiting.[2263]

The estimated global prevalence of lactose malabsorption is more than two out of three people. In the United States, it's more like one out of three,[2264] but 95 percent of Asians, 60 to 80 percent of African Americans and Ashkenazi Jews, 80 to 100 percent of American Indians, and 50 to 80 percent of Hispanics have trouble digesting milk. It's those of northern European origin who are more likely able to handle it throughout adulthood.[2265] So, saying that everyone should drink milk seems like an example of racial bias in federal nutrition policy.[2266] Spoiler alert: Not everyone in the United States is of northern European descent.

For reasons like these, Canada removed dairy as a separate food group in its national dietary guidance. After a thorough review, the Canadian dietary guidelines and food guide were updated and rereleased in 2019. Emphasis was placed on the importance of consuming more plant-based foods.[2267] The reduced emphasis on dairy products and the increased focus on plant-based foods were based in part on the removal of industry-funded studies from consideration by the Canadian experts.[2268] What a concept! Many leading medical journals already refuse to accept papers funded by Big Tobacco.[2269] It's time to consider extending this to all commercial entities intent on skewing the science to place profits over public health.

GREEN AND BLACK TEAS

Around the world, we consume literally billions of cups of tea every day.[2270] Even just the purified green tea compound EGCG (epigallocatechin gallate), purported to be the main active ingredient, can extend the lifespan of *C. elegans* under stressful conditions,[2271] as well as delay the deaths of rats by eight to twelve weeks (extending average lifespan by about 14 percent).[2272] Although we are still waiting for long-term randomized controlled clinical trials, an umbrella review of ninety-six meta-analyses of observational studies found that increasing tea consumption by three cups a day may decrease the risk of premature death from all causes put together by 24 percent,[2273] which is the equivalent of adding about two years onto your lifespan.[2274] This applies to both green tea and black tea, though green tea may have a slight edge.[2275] (Details in see.nf/greenblack, where I also review some rather disappointing data on the use of matcha to treat Alzheimer's disease.)

Don't Add Milk

The apparent mortality benefit of tea is thought to derive largely from cardiovascular protection, as both green and black tea consumption can significantly improve arterial function within hours of ingestion.[2276] This may only work, however, if you skip the milk. In 2007, we first learned that the addition of dairy milk "completely blunted the effects of tea" when it came to improving artery function.[2277] In 2018, we then learned it was even worse than that. Men and women were randomized to a month of drinking their black tea black, a month of drinking black tea with milk, or a month just drinking plain hot water. The straight black tea group experienced a significant improvement in artery function, as expected. The tea-with-milk group, however, not only did worse than the plain tea group but they had significantly impaired artery function compared to the plain hot water group. So, the milk didn't just neutralize the beneficial effects; drinking tea with milk was worse than not drinking any tea at all.[2278] Milk also appears to undercut the benefits of berries,[2279] chocolate,[2280] and coffee.[2281] (See page 390.)

RED TEA

Black, green, and white teas all come from the same evergreen plant (*Camellia sinensis*), whereas herbal tea involves pouring water over any plant other than the tea plant. I covered hibiscus tea in the AMPK chapter and chamomile in the Glycation and Inflammation chapters. Rooibos, also known as red tea or redbush tea, is another notable herbal tea that may have anti-aging properties. It has been shown to increase the lifespan of *C. elegans* by as much as 23 percent under conditions of oxidative stress, presumed to be due to its antioxidant properties.[2282] In a head-to-head comparison of fifteen herbal teas, rooibos came in second (after dandelion) in a measure of in vitro antioxidant power.[2283]

I review optimal tea brewing techniques in see.nf/red. Red tea should ideally be simmered[2284] for at least five minutes.[2285] Brew black tea for four minutes,[2286] green tea for three minutes at 85°C (185°F),[2287] and white tea for seven minutes at

98°C (208°F).[2288] Surprisingly, bags are better than bulk, because the leaves in tea bags are much more finely chopped, allowing for greater extraction.[2289]

SODA

Now that we've covered some of the best beverages, what about some of the worst?

A typical can of soda contains about nine spoonsful of sugar. Given that sugar-sweetened beverages are the single largest source of added sugar in the American diet,[2290] it should come as no surprise that their consumption is associated with dying prematurely. Each additional daily can of soda's worth of sugar appears to increase all-cause mortality by about 8 percent,[2291] likely due to associated increased risks of heart disease[2292] and diabetes.[2293]

Diet soda is still associated with increased mortality risk, but at an 8 percent elevated risk from *two* servings a day, it's only half as bad as regular soda.[2294] Now, those who drink a lot of artificially sweetened soda also tend to be more likely to be overweight or obese. Rather than diet soda leading to health problems, maybe health problems led people to drink diet drinks—so-called reverse causation. However, all the analyses took weight into account and the mortality risk remained significant. This was the case even when studies didn't count the first few years of follow-up in order to eliminate those who may have switched to diet soda to address health problems right before their deaths. An editorial accompanying a Women's Health Initiative study linking diet soda and stroke risk summed it up in its title: "Artificial Sweeteners, Real Risks."[2295] Read my Not Sweet Nothings section in *How Not to Die* for details on how artificial sweeteners may mess with our microbiomes and metabolism.

ALCOHOL

When I sat down to research this section, I was surprised to find a paper titled "Tequila . . . Extends Life Span in *Drosophila melanogaster*"—fruit flies.[2296] I imagined hordes of buzzed little flies buzzing around, but, alas, no. "Tequila" is just the name a creative fly geneticist gave to some fruit fly gene.[2297] So, tequila (the spirit) may not help fruit flies live longer, but what about us?

Alcohol use appears to be the seventh leading risk factor for death globally, leading to millions of people dying annually[2298] and resulting in three times more healthy years of life lost than all illicit drug use combined.[2299] About half of all alcohol-related deaths may be due to sudden causes, such as vehicular accidents; the other half are slower, with alcoholic liver disease the leading cause.[2300] Over the last twenty or so years in the United States, there has been about a 50 percent increase in alcoholism rates, annual alcohol-related emergency room visits,[2301] and alcohol-related death rates.[2302]

There is agreement that binge drinking, drinking during pregnancy, and heavy drinking are bad for you, but what about "moderate" drinking? In terms of aging pathways, even one to two drinks' worth of alcohol[2303] can decrease NAD$^+$ levels and sirtuin activity in human brain cells in vitro.[2304] On the other hand, alcohol is detoxified in our body into acetic acid,[2305] which activates AMPK.[2306] Unfortunately, before alcohol is fully converted into acetic acid, a toxic intermediate, *acetaldehyde*, is formed, and it's a known carcinogen. This may be the reason alcohol is believed to increase the risk of several different cancers,[2307] including breast and colorectal—even among light drinkers who only have up to one alcoholic beverage a day.[2308]

Yes, alcohol may be an addictive, intoxicating carcinogen that can cause birth defects,[2309] but what role might it play when it comes to our heart? Could it help reduce heart disease risk, particularly since alcohol consumption has clearly been shown to raise HDL, the supposed "good" cholesterol?[2310] Sadly, HDL is no longer considered to be protective, based in part on Mendelian randomization studies that found that having a high HDL throughout your entire life doesn't appear to help lower heart disease risk[2311] (whereas a lifelong reduction of bad LDL cholesterol, thanks to nothing more than luck-of-the-draw genetics, does indeed decrease risk).[2312]

So, the boost alcohol gives our HDL may not matter, and if you look at early signs of atherosclerosis, like the thickening of the wall of the carotid arteries in your neck, those who completely abstain from alcohol seem to be at the lowest risk.[2313] We see the same with coronary calcium scores, where, in general, the lower the alcohol consumption, the lower the risk.[2314] Alcohol bumps up our blood pressure a bit, too, which would be expected to raise, not lower, our cardiac risk.[2315] So, where did we get this idea that moderate alcohol consumption was good for us? From the famous *J curve*.[2316]

WHAT HAPPENED TO THE J CURVE?

In large populations followed over time, in general, the more people drink, the higher their risk of dying prematurely. However, those with the lowest risk, those who tend to live the longest, are not the abstainers who drink zero alcohol but those who imbibe a few drinks a week.[2317] The mortality-versus-drinking curve, therefore, resembles the letter *J* rather than being a straight diagonal line up like a slash.

I describe our evolution in understanding in my video see.nf/jcurve, but, long story short, this appears to be an artifact of the "sick quitter effect" arising from the systematic misclassification of former drinkers as lifelong abstainers.[2318] It's the same reason studies can find higher mortality rates among those who quit smoking compared to those who continue to smoke. It's not that abstention led to poor health but rather that poor health led to abstention.[2319]

When researchers went back and controlled for the error of misclassifying former drinkers as if they were lifelong abstainers, the J-shaped curve disappeared. In other words, the death-versus-alcohol relationship became more consistent with a linear dose response, meaning more alcohol, more death, with no protection at low levels of consumption.[2320]

MENDELIAN RANDOMIZATION

Confusing nondrinkers with those who quit drinking alcohol in response to ill health raises the issue of reverse causation. We've also seen this with studies that purport to show that those who tend to sit around and watch more TV have worse health. Is more TV leading to illness, or is illness leading to more TV?[2321] That's one of the reasons why, if you look at the "hierarchy of evidence," interventional trials with control groups tend to offer better evidence than observational studies of populations, which can suffer from both reverse causation[2322] and confounding factors. For example, as a group, light drinkers may be more likely to sip their glass of wine with a salad than a cheeseburger, so maybe that's why the wine appeared protective.[2323] Moderate alcohol intake is also strongly linked to higher socioeconomic status, which itself is a predictor of a longer life.[2324] But sometimes it's hard to do randomized controlled trials. It would be impractical—not to mention unethical—to randomize people to smoke a pack a day for a few decades, for instance, so you sometimes have to base public health decisions on observational data.[2325] We now have an extra tool, though: "nature's clinical trial," Mendelian randomization.[2326,2327]

In cases where randomized controlled trials are not feasible or practical, Mendelian randomization can provide reliable cause-and-effect evidence.[2328] As I mentioned, the unraveling of HDL as a protective factor was based in part on Mendelian randomization studies, where people who were randomly assigned higher lifelong HDL levels genetically from birth didn't go on to suffer less heart disease.[2329] Instead of researchers doing it, the randomization was accomplished through chance meeting of that exact sperm and egg. Is there any way to study people who were randomly assigned since conception to not drink as much? Remarkably, yes.[2330]

Alcohol is detoxified in the liver to carbon dioxide and water by two enzymes, but, in the process, acetaldehyde is produced, the toxic intermediate metabolite I mentioned earlier, which can cause unpleasant nausea and flushing sensations. So, if you are born with either a slow variant of acetaldehyde-removing enzyme or a superfast variant of the acetaldehyde-forming enzyme, acetaldehyde can build up, making drinking alcohol a relatively unpleasant experience throughout your life. In this way, some people are born less likely to drink. Do they have an *increased* risk of heart disease like the original J-curve observational studies would suggest? No, they have a *reduced* risk of heart disease. This suggests that even light to moderate drinkers may benefit from reducing their consumption.[2331]

ACTUAL RANDOMIZATION

Some observational studies continue to find a J-shaped curve even after controlling for confounding factors and reverse causation,[2332] and it's possible that the genetic variants related to reduced alcohol intake have independent protective effects, which would undermine the strength of the Mendelian randomization data.[2333] We are left with a raging, bitter controversy in the medical literature,[2334] with some scientists continuing to push the J-shaped curve narrative[2335] (particularly those who've received industry funding[2336]) and others dismissing any purported benefits as outdated wishful thinking[2337] or alcohol industry spin-doctoring.[2338] What we need, concluded the National Institutes of Health (NIH), is a randomized controlled trial to put the question to rest once and for all. Enter the Moderate Alcohol and Cardiovascular Health Trial.[2339]

Thousands of volunteers aged fifty and older at high risk for cardiovascular disease were to be recruited. Half would be randomized to abstain from alcohol for the next six years, and the other half told to drink one serving of alcohol every day. Which group would suffer more heart attacks, strokes, diabetes, or death?[2340] There was a problem, though. NIH researchers, in violation of federal policy,[2341] solicited the likes of Anheuser-Busch and Heineken to pick up most of the $100 million tab for the study. The lead investigator and NIH officials swore that the industry funders would play no role in influencing the study design, but, predictably, we learned otherwise from an exposé published in *The New York Times* based in part on emails obtained through the Freedom of Information Act.[2342] Critics questioned, for example, why study endpoints didn't include cancer and heart failure, known alcohol-associated harms.[2343] The trial was summarily canceled after an internal investigation revealed, in the words of the then NIH director, that "[s]o many lines have been crossed that people were frankly shocked."[2344] The Moderate Alcohol and Cardiovascular Health Trial was no more.

Even if unbiased funders could be found, at this point it may not be ethical to randomize people to drink alcohol.[2345] Soon after the original trial was conceived, the Global Burden of Disease Study published the most comprehensive estimate on the overall effect of alcohol use,[2346] summarizing evidence from nearly seven hundred data sources.[2347] The conclusion, echoed by the World Health Organization[2348] and the World Heart Federation,[2349] was clear and unambiguous: "The safest level of drinking is none."[2350]

WINE

Even wine? A twenty-year study of older adults found that any apparent mortality benefit of moderate wine drinking seemed to disappear when variables such as sociodemographic differences were taken into account.[2351] I cover the not-so-paradoxical French Paradox in see.nf/resveratrol. The grape polyphenols in red wine have antioxidant properties when tested in isolation,[2352] but alcohol acts as a pro-oxidant, increasing markers of oxidative damage within hours of consumption.[2353] So, which wins out when you drink them together in wine? In the short term, the antioxidant power of red wine is enough to counteract the LDL oxidation of a bacon cheeseburger from McDonald's,[2354] but, over a period of weeks, consumption of wine, whether white or red, does not reduce markers of oxidative damage—unless the alcohol is removed.[2355] Even when sugar is added to the de-alcoholized wine to make the calorie count similar to regular red wine, a month of red wine consumption results in significantly more oxidative damage compared to consumption of the same wine with the alcohol removed.[2356] A comparable benefit-blunting effect was found with blood pressure: Nonalcoholic red wine lowers blood pressure, but regular red wine does not.[2357] So, might de-alcoholized wine offer the best of both worlds?

If you eat cheese and crackers with red wine, you can end up with five times more triglycerides (fat) in your blood six hours later than if you had drunk water with them instead. We know it's the alcohol, because the same wine with the alcohol removed doesn't cause the same spilling of fat into the bloodstream.[2358] Red wine and white wine also cause inflammation—a 56 percent (red) or 62 percent (white) rise in IL-6 levels over the six hours after consumption, which is significantly higher than drinking a sugary beverage (11 percent).[2359] Although the effects of wine on artery function are mixed,[2360,2361,2362,2363] the fatty, inflammatory reaction could explain the results of the largest such study that showed that de-alcoholized wine improved artery function, while regular red wine made things worse.[2364]

FRUIT JUICE

What about just drinking grape juice? Rats given access to Concord (purple) grape juice improved their cognitive performance compared to sugar water[2365] and white grape juice,[2366] but what about people? For a review of the available data, see my video see.nf/grapejuice. The bottom line is that the evidence is underwhelming, despite the spin Welch's-funded researchers tried to put on it.[2367]

My first instinct was to unreservedly recommend whole fruit over juice, given that fruit consumption is associated with living longer while fruit *juice* consumption is not,[2368] but the Kame Project study I profile in see.nf/juicybrain inspired me to dig a little deeper. It was a cohort study in which those drinking fruit or vegetable juice three or more times a week seemed significantly less likely to develop Alzheimer's disease compared to less than once a week.[2369] It's possible that the high-pressure extraction methods used to make commercial juices draw out more brain-protecting polyphenols from the pulp, peel, or seeds,[2370] but as I document in the video, the interventional studies to assess at least short-term cognitive effects are largely disappointing.

In see.nf/juicyarteries, I review studies on fruit juice and cardiometabolic health. The bottom line: If you are going to drink juice, cloudy apple juice is preferable to clear,[2371] red (blood) orange juice is preferable to regular,[2372] and drink juice with meals rather than between them.[2373] Pomegranate juice got its own video for its disappointing data (see.nf/pomjuice). Salt-free tomato may be the healthiest juice. Tomato juice can lower LDL cholesterol[2374] and improve artery function,[2375] helping to explain why higher tomato product intake has been associated with a significantly lower risk of premature death, even after controlling for other diet and lifestyle factors.[2376]

Fruit juice can carry a similar load of sugar to soft drinks but, unlike soda, is not associated with a shortened lifespan.[2377] This is presumed to be because of the presence of polyphenols,[2378] natural compounds in fruit thought to account for many of the benefits associated with fruit consumption. Fruit juice may be better than soda, but it is not as good as whole fruit for living to a ripe old age. Consumption of whole fruit is associated with significantly lower risk of premature death—11 percent lower risk with just a single serving a day compared to none.[2379]

WHAT DO CENTENARIANS EAT?

To study the lifestyle habits of our eldest elders, you first have to establish how old people really are. Centenarian science has long been plagued by rampant age exaggeration.[2380] According to an editor of *The Guinness Book of World Records*, "No single subject is more obscured by vanity, deceit, falsehood and deliberate fraud than the extremes of human longevity."[2381] It's a tale as old as time, dating back at least to biblical times with boasts of patriarch Methuselah living to 969.[2382]

One of the most famous blows to the credibility of studies of long-lived individuals was a 1973 cover story in *National Geographic*. It fascinated readers with its description of extraordinary rates of centenarians in the Caucasus region of the former Soviet Union, the Hunza Valley in Pakistan, and the village of Vilcabamba in Ecuador. Upon closer inspection, however, not only had none of the "centenarians" actually reached a hundred years of age, but none of the "nonagenarians" had even made it to ninety. Given the age exaggeration, whether for social status or to promote local tourism, the average "100-year-old" turned out to be eighty-four.[2383] The debacle was eventually recognized and acknowledged by the physician-author,[2384] but not before casting a shadow over the entire field.[2385]

Despite this inauspicious start, there are now more than a dozen major ongoing studies of actual centenarians that can offer insight into their exceptional longevity.[2386]

BLUE ZONES FOOD GUIDELINES

Careful checks have systematically invalidated nearly all claims of allegedly long-living populations as being inflated or undocumented, so we're left with five authenticated "blue zones"[2387]—longevity hot spots named for the color a demographer used in a global "heat map" of mortality.[2388] The five generally accepted blue zones are the Nicoya Peninsula in Costa Rica, the island of Sardinia in Italy, Ikaria in Greece, Okinawa in Japan, and Loma Linda, California, in the United States.[2389] These are the regions with high concentrations (up to ten times the U.S. average) of centenarians[2390] and other seniors who have reached old age in good health and remain active members of the community.[2391]

They share a number of lifestyle characteristics, including low smoking rates, daily moderate physical activity, and social engagement, and, nutrition-wise, they all center their diets around whole plant foods.[2392] Dan Buettner, the founder of the Blue Zones organization, along with a team of researchers, distilled findings from more than 150 dietary surveys from the world's longest-living people to create a set of ten food guidelines. The foundation of the Blue Zones Food Guidelines is "See that your diet is 95%–100% plant-based." Vegetables are emphasized (especially leafy greens), along with fruits, whole grains, and legumes. The list ends with "Retreat from meat," noting that blue zones centenarians only eat about 2 oz or less of meat about five times per month.[2393] Traditionally, people of the blue zones eat at least 90 percent plant-based.[2394] And the population with perhaps the highest life expectancy in the world, the Loma Linda Adventist vegetarians, don't eat any meat at all.[2395]

The Blue Zones Food Guidelines

To follow in the footsteps of people with the longest lifespans and healthspans, consider following the official Blue Zones Food Guidelines[2396]:

1. "95–100% plant-based"
2. "Go wholly whole" (reduce intake of processed foods)
3. "Daily dose of beans" (one to two servings of beans, chickpeas, lentils, or split peas)
4. "Drink mostly water"
5. "Snack on nuts"
6. "Go easy on fish"
7. "Eliminate eggs"
8. "Slash sugar"
9. "Reduce dairy"
10. "Retreat from meat"

LEGUME LONGEVITY

The emphasis on minimally processed plant foods is consistent with studies on long-lived persons that date back more than a century,[2397] including ones on modern-day centenarians.[2398,2399,2400,2401] Of all plants, beans appear most often as the dietary cornerstones for centenarians, as well as for individuals throughout each of the blue zones.[2402,2403]

A paper titled "Legumes: The Most Important Dietary Predictor of Survival in Older People of Different Ethnicities" detailed a study in which researchers looked at five cohorts in Australia, Greece, Japan, and Sweden. Of the food factors investigated, the only one found to have a consistent and significant association with a longer lifespan across the board was intake of legumes, whether it was Swedes eating their brown beans and peas, Japanese eating their soy, or Greeks eating their lentils, chickpeas, and white beans. The researchers identified an 8 percent reduction in risk of death for every 20 g increase in legumes consumed each day,[2404] which is just about two tablespoons' worth.[2405] This is consistent with data from the Global Burden of Disease Study that found that of all foods considered, the largest lifespan gains would be expected from eating more legumes.[2406]

In the United States, for more than a decade now, the federal government has aimed to encourage Americans to build healthy meals with its MyPlate campaign using the visual guide of a dinner plate. Vegetables and whole grains should fill most of it, and fruits and proteins should take up the remaining space. Legumes are given special treatment, straddling both the protein and vegetable groups.[2407]

Legumes are loaded with protein, zinc, and iron, as you'd expect from other protein sources like meat, while being naturally low in sodium and saturated fat, and they have zero cholesterol. But they are also chock-full of nutrients concentrated in the vegetable kingdom, like fiber, potassium, and folate, making beans among the best bargains for nutrition density per dollar.[2408]

In Costa Rica, researchers found that those who ate beans every day had a 38 percent lower risk of heart attack compared to non-bean-eaters, and this was after controlling for saturated fat and cholesterol, so it apparently wasn't just because they were eating beans instead of beef.[2409] Randomized controlled trials dating back as far as sixty years[2410] have proven that cardiovascular risk factors, such as cholesterol levels, blood pressure, and markers of inflammation, can be lowered simply by eating legumes, typically about a cup a day for four to eight weeks.[2411] One study found that two daily servings of beans, chickpeas, lentils, and split peas cut cholesterol levels so much that many participants, aged fifty and older, fell out of the range that typically results in the prescribing of cholesterol-lowering statin drugs.[2412] Dozens of randomized controlled trials have found that soy can lower cholesterol[2413] and blood pressure,[2414] but compilations of more than sixty randomized controlled trials have found that other beans also lower cholesterol,[2415] as well as benefit blood sugars and lower insulin levels.[2416] Despite this overwhelming evidence, surveys suggest that most American consumers are unaware of these benefits.[2417] They don't know beans!

In some of the studies, beans replaced meat, which makes it impossible to tease out the effects of boosting beans versus moderating meat.[2418,2419] Nevertheless, even interventional studies that pit beans, chickpeas, or lentils head-to-head against other healthy foods, like whole grains, show benefits in terms of cholesterol, blood pressure, and weight loss.[2420] One particularly instructive study added chickpeas to the diet for five months, which resulted in average total cholesterol dropping from levels typical in the Western world (around 206 mg/dL) down to about 160,[2421] which is close to the target of under 150.[2422] Interestingly, the study was performed in northern India, so the participants' cholesterol levels actually started out at an average of 123. Only after packing their diets with saturated fat were they able to *raise* their cholesterol to typical American levels in order to test out the effects of chickpeas. So, while it would be better to just eat healthier in the first place, why not eat healthier with hummus—a diet low in saturated fat with lots of legumes?

REVERSING ARTERIAL DISEASE WITH BEANS

Legumes are not interchangeable, though. A Venn diagram of the phytochemicals found in lentils, beans, soybeans, and chickpeas shared only a 7 percent overlap, so we should strive for variety.[2423] That's easier than ever before given the variety of ways to enjoy them. Have you had pasta made from legumes? Substituting just 40 percent of the semolina flour in pasta for sprouted chickpea flour can significantly improve artery function within hours of consumption, compared to regular pasta.[2424]

Are the improvements we get from eating legumes enough to actually reverse arterial disease? Researchers looked at legumes and peripheral artery disease, which results from the buildup of atherosclerotic plaque that causes decreased blood flow down to the legs. The way the disease is diagnosed and monitored is with the ankle-brachial index—the ratio of blood pressure at the ankle compared to the arm. If the index falls below 0.9, it indicates a clog in the flow of blood to your lower body. Researchers had twenty-six individuals with peripheral artery disease eat a half serving of beans, split peas, chickpeas, and lentils every day for a week, followed by one full daily serving for the next seven weeks. After just two months of eating beans, the ankle-brachial index of four participants jumped up into the normal range. The researchers concluded that "a legume-rich diet can elicit major improvements in arterial function."[2425] The study didn't have a control group, but peripheral artery disease patients tend to get worse, not better.

If you know my personal story, you may remember that my grandmother suffered from this disease. It was one of the reasons she was confined in a wheelchair waiting to die—until her life was saved by evidence-based nutrition. That's what inspired me to dedicate my life to do for everyone's family what Nathan Pritikin did for mine.

SLOW YOUR BEATING HEART

In chemistry and physics, there are constants—physical quantities thought to be both universal and unchanging. Biology, though, was considered too complex and too messy to be governed by simple, natural laws. In 1997, however, a theoretical high-energy physicist from Los Alamos joined two biologists to describe universal scaling laws that appear to apply across the board.[2426] For example, the number of heartbeats per lifetime is remarkably similar whether you're a hamster or a whale. Mice, who typically live for less than two years, have a heart rate of about five hundred to six hundred beats a minute—up to ten beats a second. In contrast, the heart of a Galápagos tortoise beats a hundred times more slowly, but they live about a hundred times longer.[2427]

There's such a remarkable consistency in the number of heartbeats mammals get in their lifetimes that a group of researchers started to ask a provocative question: *Can human life be extended by reducing the average heart rate?* For further exploration, see my video see.nf/pulse, but the bottom line does seem to be that a faster heart rate may lead to a faster death rate.[2428] We should shoot for an average resting heart rate of no more than sixty-five beats per minute, so a goal of about one heartbeat per second to beat the clock.[2429] Every ten-beats-per-minute increase in resting heart rate above about sixty-five beats per minute is associated with a 10 to 20 percent increase in the risk of premature death.[2430] Men with no apparent evidence of heart disease who have a pulse of ninety beats per minute had five times higher risk of sudden cardiac death compared to those in the apparent safety zone of less than sixty beats per minute.[2431] Resting heart rates around ninety beats per minute increase heart disease risk at a level similar to smoking.[2432] Thankfully, as I explore in my follow-up video see.nf/heartrate, we can slow our pulse with pulses.

Diabetics randomized to eat around a cup of beans, chickpeas, or lentils each day for three months not only experienced a significant improvement in blood sugar control but a drop of three beats per minute in average resting heart rate[2433]—as much as a twelve-week aerobic conditioning program of cycling, stair-climbing, and running on a treadmill.[2434]

All these short-term bean benefits appear to translate out in population studies to a decreased risk of heart disease, high blood pressure, obesity,[2435] and, most important, premature death.[2436] A single daily serving of beans, chickpeas, or lentils may be associated with a 10 percent decrease in all-cause mortality risk.[2437] The fact that the lowered risk was found even in studies that controlled for meat consumption suggests it's not just a substitution effect.[2438]

Beans, Beans, They're Good for Your Heart

Sadly, only one in twenty-five Americans approaches even a single serving of legumes a day.[2439] Why aren't more people clamoring for beans? For some, it's fear of flatulence.[2440] Beans have been christened the musical fruit, but could that just be a lot of hot air? A randomized controlled crossover study put it to the test, and the researchers concluded that "[p]eople's concerns about excessive flatulence from eating beans may be exaggerated."[2441]

Study participants were randomized in separate trials to eat pinto beans, black-eyed peas, or vegetarian baked (navy) beans. During the first week, 35 percent reported increased flatulence, but that fell to 15 percent by week three, 5 percent by week five, and only 3 percent by week eight.[2442] It turns out that much of beans' bad rap may have grown out of short-term studies in the 1960s that did not account for our body's ability to adapt.[2443]

In the long term, most people bulking up on high-fiber foods do not appear to have significantly increased problems with gas.[2444] When we first start incorporating more beans and foods higher in fiber in our diet, though, "[a] little bit of extra flatulence," reads the *Harvard Health Letter*, "could be an indication that you're eating the way you should!"[2445] The indigestible sugars in beans that make it down to our colon may even function as prebiotics to feed our good bacteria and make for a healthier colon.[2446]

Some of it may also just be in our heads. Preconceived notions about beans may be so strong that just the *expectation* of flatulence from eating them may influence our perceptions of having gas.[2447] Studies show that when we eat a product that's labeled as having an ingredient that may cause intestinal distress, it causes more intestinal distress—whether or not it actually contains that ingredient.[2448] In other words, the mere belief that we're eating something that causes us to pass more gas can cause us to perceive that we're passing more gas. Don't let the fartcebo effect prevent you from eating more healthfully.

THE HISPANIC PARADOX

The benefits of beans may help explain the so-called Hispanic Paradox. Hispanic Americans—despite socioeconomic patterns that generally lead to worse health outcomes like disparities in education and healthcare, as well as higher rates of poverty[2449]—tend to live longer than other ethnic groups in the United States.[2450] With lower risks of nine out of the top fifteen causes of death, notably including less heart disease and cancer, Hispanics have a 24 percent lower risk of premature death.[2451] For more on this topic, check out my video see.nf/hispanic.

In a study of Mexican Americans, researchers found that, compared with other groups, they not only eat more beans but also more fruits and vegetables,[2452] including tomatoes and corn.[2453] (These healthy dietary patterns extend down to Central America, too. After rice and beans, corn tortillas are the most commonly eaten food in the Costa Rican blue zone.[2454]) They also eat more chili peppers.[2455] Can chilies spice up longevity?

PEPPER UPPER

The spicy compound in hot chilis can extend the lifespan of fruit flies,[2456] but what about us? See my twin videos see.nf/spicy and see.nf/peppers for details, but basically, four out of four studies on spicy food and mortality found a significant decrease in death risk from any cause in people who ate more spicy chilis.[2457,2458,2459,2460] I wrote an entire section on chili peppers in my Fat Burners chapter in *How Not to Diet*, detailing how cayenne pepper can counteract the metabolic slowing that accompanies weight loss and, as a bonus, accelerate fat burning,[2461] but the apparent longevity benefits of chili pepper consumption remain after controlling for body mass index.[2462]

There are at least a half dozen no-salt-added hot sauces on the market. Even Tabasco is pretty low in sodium, though only the original flavor. (Spin-off flavors have up to five times more salt.) You can also add straight powdered chilis. I have different ones in shaker bottles for every occasion, including powdered adobo chilis, chipotle peppers, and crushed Thai bird's eye chilis for when I really want to kick up the heat.

THE MEDITERRANEAN DIET

Two of the world's blue zones, Ikaria and Sardinia, are located in the Mediterranean, home to the Mediterranean diet, about which the "father of preventive cardiology,"[2463] Jeremiah Stamler, once wrote, "Uncritical laudatory coverage is the common parlance."[2464] Does it live up to the hype?

CLUB MED

More than a dozen countries border the Mediterranean Sea. The Mediterranean diet refers to what was being eaten on the Greek isle of Crete more than a half century ago. After World War II, the government of Greece asked the Rockefeller Foundation to come in and assess postwar conditions.[2465] Impressed by the low rates of heart disease in the region, nutrition scientist Ancel Keys—after whom "K" rations, the prepackaged daily rations for American soldiers, were named— initiated his famous Seven Countries Study, the longitudinal study of diet and cardiovascular disease in men in seven regions of the world. The researchers, led by Keys, found that the rate of fatal heart disease in men on Crete was twenty times lower than in the United States and they also had the lowest cancer rates and fewest deaths overall.[2466] What were they eating? Their diets were more than 90 percent plant-based, which may explain why coronary heart disease was such a rarity there.[2467] A rarity, that is, except in a small class of wealthy residents whose diet differed from that of the general population—they ate meat every day instead of once every week or two.[2468]

The main characteristic of the Mediterranean diet is that it is mainly plant-based,[2469] low in the meat and dairy Dr. Keys considered to be the "major villains in the diet" due to their saturated fat content. Unfortunately, few really eat the traditional Mediterranean diet anymore, even in the Mediterranean. The prevalence of coronary heart disease skyrocketed by an order of magnitude within a few decades in Crete, blamed on the increased consumption of meat and cheese at the expense of plant foods.[2470]

So, even though many talk about the Mediterranean diet, few actually follow it.[2471] People often think of pizza or spaghetti with meatballs when they think of Italian food. While "Italian restaurants brag about the healthy Mediterranean diet," Dr. Keys wrote, "they serve a travesty of it."[2472] If no one's really eating this way anymore, how do you study it?

Researchers came up with a variety of scoring systems to assess adherence to the Mediterranean diet to see if people who are eating more Mediterranean-ish do better. You get higher points the more plant foods you eat, and, effectively, points are deducted with just a single daily serving of meat or dairy. So, it's no surprise those with relatively higher scores on the scale have a lower risk of heart disease, cancer, and death overall.[2473] The Mediterranean diet is protective compared to the standard American diet—no question—but any diet rich in whole plant foods and low in animal-fat consumption could be expected to confer protection against many of our leading killers.[2474]

Based on dozens of prospective cohort studies, the more adherent people are to a Mediterranean-style diet, the lower their risk of premature death.[2475] The difference in average age at death between those eating the least and the most Mediterranean may be on the order of two years.[2476] Mediterranean diet adherence is also associated with healthier aging[2477] and a lower risk of frailty.[2478] What about the diet is particularly protective?

A meta-analysis of studies on the most protective components of the Mediterranean diet found that, food-wise, the mortality benefit appeared to be derived from greater fruit and vegetable intake and reduced meat consumption. In contrast, eating fish, the only animal-based food promoted in the Mediterranean diet, did not seem to matter.[2479]

Criticism of Dr. Keys has become sort of a cottage industry as of late[2480] by "bloggers, commercial book writers or journalists in quest of sensationalism or financial gain," but the scientific record is clear that such invective constitutes "either investigative incompetence or plain dishonesty at the edge of scientific fraud."[2481] Ever the consummate scientist, Dr. Keys, when asked on his hundredth birthday whether he thought his diet contributed to his long life, answered, "Very likely, but no proof."[2482]

Dr. Stamler said as much about the Mediterranean diet on the occasion of *his* hundredth birthday.[2483] The centenarian remained committed to his pioneering research[2484] even after turning one hundred. We lost him on January 26, 2022, at the age of 102.[2485]

OLIVE OIL

Olive oil is commonly used in the Mediterranean to dress vegetables and salads, beans and other legumes, so its consumption can be an indicator of a more traditional, healthier diet.[2486] To better tease out the effects of the olive oil itself, then, it would be more instructive to study olive oil consumption in a non-Mediterranean country. Harvard researchers took up the mantle and dug through decades of data from nearly 100,000 women and men in the Nurses' Health Study and the Health Professionals Follow-Up Study. They found that replacing about a teaspoon of butter, mayonnaise, margarine, or dairy fat with about a teaspoon of olive oil every day would be expected to lower heart disease risk by 5 to 7 percent. So, olive oil is better than butterfat, but no significant difference was found between olive oil and other oils.[2487]

What about the study often cited by advocates of low-fat eating that implicated not only saturated fat but also monounsaturated and polyunsaturated fats in the appearance of new atherosclerotic lesions in coronary arteries?[2488] I discuss the critical flaw in their reasoning in my video see.nf/mediterranean. The fact is that olive oil is better for us than butter when it comes to LDL cholesterol level[2489] or artery function,[2490] though olive oil[2491]—even extra-virgin olive oil—can still acutely impair our arterial function,[2492] even to an extent similar to fast food and cheesecake.[2493]

Palm oil, soybean oil,[2494] and sunflower oil[2495] can also impede our arteries' ability to relax and dilate normally, which does not occur after we eat Green Light sources of fat, like nuts[2496] or avocados.[2497] (In *How Not to Die*, I defined Green Light fare as foods of plant origin to which nothing bad has been added and from which nothing good has been taken away.) Whole plant foods may even be able to mediate oil's ill effects. Consuming that extra-virgin olive oil with a salad, for example, as part of a balsamic vinaigrette, was shown to neutralize the artery-impairing effects of the oil. Unfortunately, because of the typical brining process, the whole-food source of olive oil—olives—is too high in sodium for regular consumption. Just twelve jumbo olives could take up nearly half of your recommended sodium limit for a whole day.[2498]

How might we see if major sources of plant fats, like olive oil or nuts, help or hurt in terms of hard endpoints, such as diagnosed disease? Ideally, we would run a multiyear, randomized study with thousands of participants and have one-third eat more nuts, another third eat more olive oil, and the final third essentially do nothing, then see who does better. And that's exactly what researchers ended up doing.

PREDIMED

In the PREDIMED study, from the Spanish *PREvención con DIeta MEDiterránea*, an impressive 7,447 people at high risk for heart attack were randomized into three groups.[2499] For all the nitty-gritty, watch my video see.nf/predimed, but basically, though it wasn't the researchers' original intention, it turned out that the participants were effectively randomized for about four years to either (1) switch from consuming about three tablespoons of half-virgin olive oil a day to four tablespoons of all-virgin olive oil, (2) go from eating about half an ounce of nuts a day to a whole ounce, or (3) pretty much continue their regular diet.[2500] The results were published in *The New England Journal of Medicine*.[2501]

Wasn't PREDIMED Retracted?

The PREDIMED trial is one of the most influential randomized dietary studies ever performed,[2502] yet, in 2018, the original paper was withdrawn due to irregularities in randomization procedures at two of the eleven sites where the study had been run.[2503] Household members were invited to participate and were allocated to the same diet. This makes sense to avoid assigning different diets to people in the same household, but the whole point of *randomized* controlled trials is to assign diets *randomly*. Thankfully, this only applied to about 6 percent of study participants. And, when the data were corrected, reanalyzed, and republished, the original results and conclusions remained the same.[2504,2505]

What happened to the amount of plaque in the arteries of the PREDIMED subjects over time? There was significant worsening of carotid artery thickening and plaque in the essentially-no-dietary-changes control group, and no significant changes in the olive oil group, but those in the added-nuts group showed a significant reversal in thickening and an arrest in plaque progression. The researchers concluded that nuts may not only be a preferable source of fat compared to olive oil but they may "delay the progression of atherosclerosis, the harbinger of future cardiovascular events," such as having a stroke.[2506] And that's exactly what seemed to happen. Those who switched to extra-virgin olive oil had about one-third fewer strokes, and those who added more nuts to their daily regimen cut their stroke risk nearly in half, dropping their ten-year risk of stroke from about 6 percent down to 3 percent.[2507] If nuts worked as well in the general population, that would mean the potential for preventing more than 85,000 strokes a year in the United States alone.[2508] Imagine that: About ten strokes an hour around the clock potentially prevented simply by adding about five almonds, walnuts, and hazelnuts to one's daily diet.

With no significant differences in meat and dairy intake across the study groups, there were no significant differences in saturated fat or cholesterol intake, so no surprise that there were no significant differences in their blood cholesterol levels or the number of subsequent heart attacks.[2509] In the five or so years the study ran, there were thirty-seven heart attacks in the olive oil group, thirty-one in the nut group, and thirty-eight in the essentially-no-dietary-changes control group. Similarly, there weren't significant differences among the three groups in the number of subjects dying from a heart attack, stroke, or from any cause. Those in the olive oil group and especially the nut group, however, did have significantly fewer strokes.

Regardless of which group the PREDIMED participants were in, those consuming a greater amount of nuts each day had a significantly lower overall risk of dying prematurely.[2510] Those consuming more olive oil or extra-virgin olive oil, what I consider Red and Yellow Light sources of fat, respectively, failed to get any survival benefit.[2511] This is consistent with Ancel Keys's take on olive oil. The so-called father of the Mediterranean diet considered its benefit to be more as a means of replacing animal fats like lard and butter.[2512]

VIRGIN TERRITORY

PREDIMED's bottom line for olive oil is that if you are going to use it, use extra-virgin. Extra-virgin olive oil is produced by simply pressing the oil out of olive paste, whereas "pure," "regular," and "light" olive oils are further refined, which results in a greater loss of the original olive phytonutrients. Those randomized to swap out their refined olive oil for extra-virgin not only had fewer strokes but they ended up with better global cognition[2513] and significantly less atrial fibrillation,[2514] peripheral artery disease,[2515] diabetes,[2516] diabetic vision loss,[2517] mild cognitive impairment,[2518] and breast cancer.[2519] This may be because extra-virgin olive oil doesn't appear to induce the same spike in inflammatory markers that regular (refined) olive oil does[2520] and may also be better at reducing oxidative stress,[2521] presumably due to the greater extraction of anti-inflammatory and antioxidant olive compounds.[2522] There are also potentially toxic chemical contaminants formed when refined oils are deodorized, such as 3-MCPD (3-monochloropropane-1,2-diol).[2523]

Regular olive oil has up to twenty-five times the 3-MCPD levels as extra-virgin olive oil.[2524] In fact, that's how you can discriminate among the various processing grades of olive oil. If a bottle of oil is labeled as "extra-virgin olive oil" but it contains a lot of 3-MCPD, then it must have been diluted with some refined olive oil. The ease of adulteration, the difficulty of detection, the economic drivers, and the lack of control measures all contribute to the susceptibility of extra-virgin olive oil to fraud.[2525] How widespread is the problem?

Of eighty-eight bottles of olive oil purchased in California that were *labeled* as extra-virgin, only thirty-three were found to be authentic when tested.[2526] Does it make a difference if you stick to the top-selling imported brands, such as Colavita, Star, Bertolli, Filippo Berio, and Pompeian? No. A whopping 73 percent of those extra-virgin olive oil samples failed. Only about one in four appeared to be entirely genuine, and not a single top-selling brand had even half of their samples pass the test.[2527] So, even if you want to switch to extra-virgin olive oil, it may not be so easy.

THE LYON DIET HEART STUDY

Our understanding of the Mediterranean diet, in general, is limited by the quantity and quality of the existing body of scientific research. Ironically, there may be more meta-analyses or systematic reviews of Mediterranean diet studies for cardiovascular health than there are actual original studies.[2528] And, most such reviews have been found to be faulty, using inappropriate statistical methods to combine study findings.[2529]

It also doesn't help that different studies used up to thirty-four different Mediterranean diet scoring systems.[2530] For example, some gave points for eating potatoes or subtracted them for consuming eggs, while others did neither.[2531] Most scored olive oil and nuts as characteristic components of a Mediterranean diet, which led to accusations that the research was in some way a conspiracy of vested Big Fat commercial interests; however, the vast majority of studies on the Mediterranean diet have been publicly, not privately, funded.[2532] That doesn't prevent questionable work from being published, of course. Consider the "Indo-Mediterranean Trial," which has been largely discredited as being, at the very least, "severely flawed"[2533] due to evidence that the researcher had "either fabricated or falsified data."[2534] When challenged to produce the original research records, he declined, responding they had been "eaten by termites."[2535]

One famous Mediterranean diet trial that has stood the test of time is the Lyon Diet Heart Study.[2536] About six hundred individuals who had each already had a heart attack were randomized into two groups. The control group received no dietary advice, apart from whatever their doctors had told them, while the experimental group was instructed to eat more of a Mediterranean-type diet, supplemented with a canola oil–based spread that would give them the plant-based omega-3s they would have normally gotten from foods like walnuts if they had actually lived on a Greek isle in the 1950s.[2537] Canola oil also lowers LDL cholesterol better than olive oil does,[2538] and, unlike olive oil, canola has been shown not to acutely impair artery function.[2539]

The Mediterranean group did end up taking some of the dietary advice to heart. They ate more breads and fruits, and less butter, cream, processed meat, and meat in general. Other than that, though, no significant changes in diet were reported in terms of wine, olive oil, or fish consumption. So, they ate less saturated fat and cholesterol and increased their intake of plant-based omega-3s, but otherwise didn't make any other great changes.[2540] Even so, at the end of about four years, forty-four individuals from the control group had a second heart attack, some fatal, but only fourteen suffered another attack in the group that had changed their diet.[2541] The Mediterranean diet group went from having a 4 percent chance of having a heart attack each year down to just 1 percent.

A cynic might say that while there was less death and disease, the Mediterranean diet continued to feed their heart disease, so much so that fourteen of them suffered new heart attacks while on the diet. There was a remarkable drop in heart attack rates, but, yes, ideally we would want a diet that could stop or even reverse heart disease.

Dr. Caldwell Esselstyn and his colleagues at the Cleveland Clinic published a case series of 198 consecutive patients with serious cardiovascular disease who had been counseled to switch to a diet composed entirely of whole plant foods.[2542] Of the 198 participants, 177 stuck to the diet, whereas the other 21 fell off the wagon. This set up a natural experiment. What happened to the noncompliant 21? In about the next four years, more than half suffered a fatal heart attack or needed angioplasty or a heart transplant. In contrast, of the 177 participants who stuck to the plant-based diet over the same time period, just a single patient had a major event as a result of worsening cardiovascular disease—0.6 percent versus 62 percent in the noncompliant group, an apparent hundredfold drop in risk.

Dr. Esselstyn's was not a randomized trial, so it can't be directly compared to the Lyon study. It also included very determined patients. Not everyone is willing to dramatically change their diets, even if it may literally be a matter of life and death. In that case, rather than doing nothing, eating a more Mediterranean-type diet may cut the risk of subsequent heart attacks by about two-thirds. Cutting 99 percent of risk would be better if Esselstyn's results were replicated in a controlled trial, but even a 70 percent drop in risk could save countless lives every year. "Although the results may seem simply too good to be true," wrote the director of the Harvard Program in Cardiovascular Epidemiology, "given the 20-fold or more differences in coronary rates across countries, such results for dietary change are entirely plausible."[2543]

THE OKINAWAN DIET

The U.S. Dietary Guidelines recommend that we choose meals or snacks that are high in nutrients but lower in calories to reduce the risk of chronic disease.[2544] By this measure, the healthiest foods on the planet—that is, the most nutrient dense— are vegetables, which contain the most nutrient bang for our caloric buck. What would happen if a population centered their entire diet around vegetables, like the Okinawa Japanese did traditionally? They would end up having among the longest lives in the world.[2545] (And yes, a validation study did confirm true centenarian prevalence.[2546])

The traditional Okinawan diet revolved around steamed sweet potatoes, simmered or steamed leafy greens and other vegetables, and soy, mostly in the form of tofu and miso soup.[2547] There's a common misconception that their traditional diet included a substantial contribution from fish or other meat,[2548] but if you look at their actual dietary intake, that doesn't seem to be the case. The United States occupied the island of Okinawa from 1945 until 1972, when it was returned to Japan's control, so we have data on what Okinawans were eating in the U.S. National Archives.[2549]

How did the traditional diets of more than 2,000 Okinawans break down? Only 1 percent of their diet was fish, less than 1 percent was other meats, and less than 1 percent was dairy and eggs, so it was more than 96 percent plants, with few processed foods.[2550]

A greater than 90 percent whole food, plant-based diet would be highly anti-inflammatory and highly antioxidant.[2551] When the level of oxidized fat was measured within centenarian Okinawans' systems, there was compelling evidence of less free radical damage,[2552] despite similar antioxidant enzyme activity.[2553] What may be making the difference are all the extra antioxidants they were getting from their mostly vegetable diet. Okinawa has had six to twelve times fewer heart disease deaths per capita than the United States, two to three times fewer colon cancer deaths, seven times fewer prostate cancer deaths, and five and a half times lower risk of dying from breast cancer.[2554]

Their traditional cuisine was not only whole food, plant-based and not only centered around vegetables, but one vegetable in particular, purple and orange sweet potatoes.[2555]

SWEET SPOT

Sweet potatoes have formed the bulk of the traditional Okinawan diet since the 1600s, accounting for 69 percent of daily caloric intake.[2556] This may be one of the secrets to Okinawan longevity. A study in China of 14,000 men and women followed for an average of fourteen years found that those who ate sweet potatoes had a significantly lower chance of dying prematurely (by 18 percent), even after controlling for a wide range of dietary, lifestyle, and socioeconomic factors.[2557] And no wonder. The Center for Science in the Public Interest ranked sweet potatoes as one of the healthiest foods on the planet[2558]—and, one day, perhaps even off the planet, as NASA has chosen the sweet potato for space missions.[2559]

Sweet potatoes are also a nutritional bang-for-your-buck bargain. A study of dozens of different vegetables found that some of the healthiest foods, like dark green leafy vegetables, may also be the most affordable, with the single highest nutrient-rich food score per dollar going to sweet potatoes.[2560] And purple sweet potatoes may be the best of the best.

Anthocyanins are a class of natural purple, red, and blue pigments in such plants as berries, grapes, plums, red cabbage, and red onions. The anthocyanins in red rice, black rice, and purple wheat have been shown to have anti-aging and/or life-extending properties in model organisms such as yeast, worms,[2561,2562] flies,[2563] and mice.[2564] Of all the plant pigments tested in a head-to-head comparison, the purple in purple sweet potato beat out the pigments in grape skins, elderberry, red cabbage, and purple corn for antioxidant activity.[2565]

Even regular sweet potatoes have been shown to exert both acute and chronic anti-inflammatory effects in rats,[2566] but the purple sweet potato pigment goes above and beyond with its ability to reverse or repair the damage resulting from inflammatory[2567] or oxidative[2568] insults to the brain in mice. From an anti-aging perspective, the color compounds in purple sweet potatoes also reduce inflammation, amplify autophagy, and delay senescence in human blood vessel cells in a petri dish,[2569] as well as activate sirtuin activity by boosting levels of NAD$^+$ in mice.[2570]

The autophagy activation is thought to underlie the 15 percent life extension in fruit flies fed a purple sweet potato extract, which is accompanied by a decrease in age-related gut leakiness, suggesting a healthspan benefit as well. Researchers fed fruit flies blue food coloring, which stains the digestive tract of young flies but seeps out of the leaky intestines in older flies, turning their entire bodies blue. It's called—no joke—the "Smurf assay." The number of "Smurf flies" was significantly lower in the purple sweet potato extract group.[2571]

Have any of these benefits been validated in clinical studies? Purple sweet potato anthocyanins have been shown to have prebiotic effects in human fecal culture studies, enhancing the proliferation of the good bacteria *Bifidobacterium* and *Lactobacillus*, along with a boost in protective short-chain fatty acids.[2572] That may help explain the anti-inflammatory effects found in the only double-blind placebo-controlled study I could locate. Men with inflamed livers were randomized to drink a cup a day of a purple sweet potato smoothie and experienced a significant improvement in their liver function tests within eight weeks, compared to those given a placebo beverage with a similar look and taste.[2573]

SOY SALUBRITY

The primary source of concentrated protein in the traditional Okinawan diet is soy. Eating an average of 3 oz of soy products a day—as mentioned, mostly in the form of tofu and miso—they had among the highest soy intake in the world.[2574] Might this also play a role in their longevity? How well does the science support the old Chinese saying "vegetables and tofu keep you healthy"?[2575]

For more than two decades, soy's ability to protect against heart disease has been recognized as one of the rare "FDA-approved" food-label health claims. Randomized controlled trials have shown that soy consumption can result in small decreases in cardiovascular risk factors, such as blood pressure[2576] and cholesterol.[2577] A billion-dollar industry, Big Soy has a lot of money to fund research touting the benefits of its bean. But, is soy really the top bean or are other legumes just as powerful? It turns out that *non*-soy beans, including lentils, lima beans, navy beans, and pinto beans, can drop bad cholesterol levels as effectively as soy protein—an eight-point drop in LDL cholesterol,[2578] compared to five (mg/dL) for soy.[2579] But, if you separate out the studies, natural soy products, such as soymilk and soybeans, really do seem to pull ahead, leading to an average eleven-point drop in LDL versus three points for highly processed soy extracts.[2580]

This appears to translate into reduced risk of heart disease and stroke,[2581] along with lower risk of death from both cancer and cardiovascular diseases. However, a significant reduction in all-cause mortality was only apparent in higher-quality studies, such as those with at least 10,000 participants. Compared to the lowest category of intake, the highest intake of isoflavones (the natural phytoestrogens in soy) was associated with a lower risk of premature death across the board. "Our findings," conclude the meta-analysis researchers, "may support the current recommendations to increase intake of soy for greater longevity."[2582]

What About the Sodium in Miso?

The process of producing miso involves adding a lot of salt, so it was always something I avoided—until I actually looked into it. Read my Beans chapter in *How Not to Die* for the details, but it turns out miso is not associated with the stomach cancer risk attributed to the salt in other fermented foods, like kimchi,[2583] nor the risk of developing high blood pressure.[2584] But what if you are already hypertensive?

Men and women with stage 1 or 2 hypertension (blood pressures ranging from 130 to 159 over 85 to 99) were randomized to eat either two bowls a day of miso soup, which alone exceeded the recommended daily sodium limit, or soybeans with no added salt for two months. Surprisingly, the miso group ended up with *lower* nighttime blood pressures than the soybean control group. The mechanism is unclear.[2585] Given a slight drop in body weight in the miso group, the miso may have a diuretic effect by increasing sodium excretion through the kidneys, a phenomenon that has been demonstrated in rats.[2586,2587] Regardless, miso is now a staple of my kitchen and cookbooks.

WAKAME THIS WAY

Sea vegetables are another important component of the Okinawan diet.[2588] Sea veggies have been associated with significantly lower all-cause mortality among those in Japan eating seaweed five or more times a week compared to fewer than three times.[2589] In addition to being an excellent source of trace minerals, sea vegetables have multiple unique components, including the olive-brown carotenoid *fucoxanthin*[2590] and a type of fiber called *porphyran* found to have lifespan-extending effects in model organisms.[2591]

One way seaweed could contribute to longevity is by lowering high blood pressure. With seaweed consumption associated with better blood pressure control in both children[2592] and adults,[2593] researchers decided to put it to the test and found significantly lower blood pressures from 6 (but not 4) g a day for a month of dried wakame (the sea vegetable in seaweed salad). A nice thing about whole food, plant-based interventions is that you sometimes get *good* side effects. In this study, one participant who had been suffering from gastritis saw their stomach inflammation resolved, and another's chronic headaches disappeared.[2594] Seaweed salad may also boost immune function, as I note in the Preserving Your Immune System chapter.

The Healthiest Source of Iodine

One advantage of cow milk over plant milk is iodine,[2595] a mineral essential for thyroid function. Dairy milk supplies about a quarter to one half of the daily iodine requirement in the United States, though, ironically, milk itself has little native iodine. The iodine residues in dairy appear to originate mainly from the contamination of the surface of the cow's udders from iodine-containing teat disinfectants that leach into their milk.[2596]

For a comparison of the healthiest iodine sources, see my video see.nf/iodine. In short, I recommend the dark-green leafies of the sea. The recommended daily intake can be had in about two sheets of nori,[2597] the seaweed used for sushi. I just nibble on them as snacks. A teaspoon of mild seaweed, like dulse or arame, or a tablespoon of seaweed salad would also fulfill your iodine needs for the day. You can sprinkle dulse, sold as pretty purple flakes, onto just about anything, and arame is one of my favorite ingredients to add to soups. Given that iodine is extensively stored in the thyroid, it can safely be consumed intermittently, meaning you don't have to get it every day.[2598] For more on safe sources, see my Supplements chapter at the end of *How Not to Die*.

ERGOTHIONEINE: THE "LONGEVITY VITAMIN"

Another component that may contribute to successful aging in Okinawa is mushroom consumption.[2599] Fruit flies fed a diet of 1 percent oyster mushrooms showed a slight but significant survival advantage,[2600] perhaps because oyster mushrooms are one of the most concentrated sources of ergothioneine.[2601]

To describe nutrients that may not necessarily be essential for life but may be required for long-term health,[2602] famed biochemist Professor Emeritus Bruce Ames coined the term "longevity vitamin" and identified ergothioneine as a likely candidate.[2603] Of more than a hundred compounds measured in the bloodstreams of thousands of individuals, the one most associated with the lowest rates of disease and death was ergothioneine,[2604] thought to function as a potent intramitochondrial antioxidant.[2605] I review what it can do and the best way to get it in see.nf/ergo.

In short, mushrooms and tempeh—a fungi-fermented soybean cake—are the only concentrated dietary sources.[2606] Porcinis lead the pack, with about three times more ergothioneine than oyster and shiitake mushrooms, which in turn have about three times more than the typical white, cremini, or portobello varieties.[2607] Ergothioneine may explain why mushroom consumption is associated with a lower risk of dying prematurely from all causes put together.[2608]

Interestingly, blood ergothioneine levels in the brain appear to decline after age sixty and this reduction is tied to both cognitive decline[2609] and frailty,[2610] and does not appear to be due to decreasing mushroom intake.[2611] Perhaps the function of the ergothioneine transporter at the blood-brain barrier declines with age, potentially making mushroom intake all the more beneficial as we grow older.

Mushroom Monition

Morel,[2612] shiitake,[2613] and *Agaricus* mushrooms, like white, cremini, and portobello, should be cooked before eaten. Oyster mushrooms can be safely consumed raw.[2614] For the reasons why and other potential provisos, go to see.nf/caveats.

THE "MUSHROOM OF IMMORTALITY"

Can mushrooms be medicinal? Mushroom-based products make up a sizable chunk of the $50 billion supplement market. As a senior editor of the journal *Fungal Biology* wrote, "This profitable industry provides a powerful incentive for companies to test the credulity of their customers and unsupported assertions have come to define the medicinal mushroom business," recalling the quackery of patented "medicines" with names like the very real "Dr. Bonker's Celebrated Egyptian Oil."[2615]

Now, it wouldn't be surprising if mushrooms had some potent properties. After all, a lot of drugs have been developed from fungi, not the least of which is penicillin, but also the cholesterol-lowering statin lovastatin and the powerful immunosuppressant drug cyclosporin.[2616] Still don't think a humble little mushroom can have pharmacological effects? Don't forget that they can also produce some of our most powerful poisons.[2617] Some look the part, like the polka-dotted fly agaric toadstool popularized by *Super Mario Bros.*, but others have a much more innocent look,[2618] like the mushroom actually named the "destroying angel." As little as one teaspoon of it can cause "a painful, lingering death."[2619]

I discuss the immune-boosting properties of mushrooms in the Preserving Your Immune System chapter. One of the most popular so-called medicinal mushrooms is called *reishi* in Japan (*lingzhi* in China), and it's revered as "the mushroom of immortality."[2620] It's a white-rot fungus that grows off decaying wood.[2621] It isn't edible in the culinary sense, as it's corky and bitter, but it's traditionally been revered in some Asian countries as an herbal concoction for longevity.[2622] Is it worthy of such reverence? Well, it works for wee worms, significantly prolonging the lifespan of *C. elegans*,[2623] and a related mushroom species has been shown to have anti-aging properties when injected into the abdomens of mice.[2624] Unfortunately, nearly every human clinical trial of reishi mushrooms over the last few decades for a variety of conditions has failed.[2625] The area where it may hold the most promise is cancer. For details, check out my video see.nf/reishi.

Of course, to be effective, a reishi mushroom supplement presumably needs to actually contain reishi mushrooms. No thanks to the 1994 Dietary Supplement Health and Education Act, the supplement manufacturers themselves—as opposed to the FDA—are responsible for the safety and integrity of their own products.[2626] You can imagine how well that has gone. Out of nineteen reishi supplements tested, none contained actual reishi.[2627]

GARLIC FOR ARTERY HEALTH

I've covered sweet potatoes, soy, sea vegetables, and mushrooms. What about the foods that have spiced up the traditional Okinawan diet—garlic, ginger, and turmeric?

In ancient Greece, the art of medicine was divided into three areas: cures through diet, cures through drugs, and cures through surgery. Garlic, Hippocrates wrote, was one such medicinal food—but it was used to treat a nonexistent entity called displacement of the womb, so ancient wisdom only goes so far.[2628]

Over a thirteen-year period, about 9,500 octogenarians, 9,500 nonagenarians, and 8,500 centenarians were recruited from twenty-three provinces in China to study the effect of garlic consumption on the eldest elderly. Compared to those who rarely ate garlic, those who ate garlic at least five times a week had about a 10 percent lower mortality rate, which translated into them living about a year longer.[2629] The investigators suspect that a reduction in cardiovascular disease may have played a role. Those who eat the equivalent of at least one large clove of garlic a day do seem to have better artery function than those who eat less,[2630] but you don't know if it's cause and effect until you put it to the test.

Check out see.nf/garlic for a remarkable series of interventional trials showing that, compared to placebo, a quarter teaspoon of garlic powder can dramatically improve artery function[2631] and slow the progression of atherosclerosis.[2632] Garlic can also significantly lower cholesterol[2633] and blood pressure.[2634] If plain old garlic powder can do that, what about those fancy Kyolic aged garlic extract supplements? They're up to thirty times more expensive and don't seem to work at all.[2635]

As I explored in *How Not to Diet*, a quarter teaspoon of garlic powder can also cause overweight men and women to lose nearly six pounds of straight body fat in fifteen weeks, compared to placebo.[2636] In the Preserving Your Immune System chapter, I'll talk about its immune-boosting effects. A systematic review concluded that plant-based medicine can provide beneficial effects, with little or no side effects, and "compared to other medicine are relatively cost effective."[2637] I'd say so, at as little as one or two pennies a day.

> ## Garlic for Those Who Vant to Suck Your Blood
>
> No data yet on its efficacy against vampires, but eating garlic can protect against other bloodsuckers. Check out <u>see.nf/repellent</u>, but basically, eating garlic has been shown to be useless against mosquitoes[2638] but to successfully reduce tick bites[2639] (though not as much as permethrin clothing treatments[2640]).

GINGER

For thousands of years, ginger has been used to treat disease in China and India.[2641] In India, in fact, it's known as *maha-aushadhi*, "the great medicine." Of course, Indian and Chinese systems of medicine have both also prescribed mercury,[2642] so there are limits to what we can glean from "traditional use." That's why we have science.

More than a hundred randomized controlled trials of ginger have been published.[2643] The most well established use of ginger is the alleviation of nausea and vomiting. It was first shown to beat out Dramamine in a head-to-head test forty years ago in which volunteers were blindfolded and spun around and around in a tilted, rotating chair.[2644,2645] Today, ginger is considered to be a nontoxic, broad-spectrum antiemetic (antivomiting) agent, effective in countering nausea induced by motion sickness, nausea during pregnancy, nausea after chemotherapy and radiation, and nausea after surgery.[2646] Even just inhaling ginger essence has been shown to help.[2647]

Randomized, double-blind, placebo-controlled trials have also found ginger to be effective for treating osteoarthritis,[2648] premenstrual syndrome,[2649] and menstrual pain;[2650] preventing[2651] and treating migraine headaches;[2652] and reducing cholesterol, triglycerides,[2653] blood sugars,[2654] blood pressure,[2655] excess body weight,[2656] and signs of oxidative stress[2657] and inflammation[2658]—typically for just pennies a day using the type of ground ginger you'd find at any grocery store. When ginger is dried, fresh ginger's main pungent compound *6-gingerol* is converted into *6-shogaol*[2659] (from the Japanese word for ginger), which may be even more potent.[2660]

Okinawans have traditionally eaten shell ginger, which is a species in the same family but separate from common ginger.[2661] Extracts of shell ginger leaves have been shown to increase the lifespan of *C. elegans*, but who eats ginger leaves?[2662]

We technically don't eat the root either, but rather the ginger rhizome, which is an underground part of the stem.[2663] Thankfully, 6-shogaol, the dehydration product found in common ground ginger, can on its own further increase the average lifespan of *C. elegans* by up to more than 25 percent.[2664]

The lifespan enhancement may be due to DNA protection. If a tissue sample is taken from a random person, about 7 percent of their cells may show evidence of DNA damage, actual breaks in the strands of their DNA. If we then blast those cells with free radicals, we can cause even more damage, taking that number up to about 11 percent. But, if the person had been eating one and a half teaspoons of ginger powder a day for a week, oxidative stress–induced DNA damage drops about 25 percent, down to 8 percent of cells, which is similar to what's been found in those fed the same amount of rosemary. Researchers also tested cumin, paprika, sage, and turmeric. The first three don't seem to help in this regard, but turmeric worked best.[2665]

TURMERIC

Turmeric is another common component of traditional Okinawan cuisine that has been shown to prolong the longevity of model organisms, including yeast,[2666] invertebrates, and mammals. Turmeric compounds resulted in a 39 percent increase in the average lifespan of *C. elegans*,[2667] a 20 percent increase for fruit flies,[2668] and a 12 percent increase for mice,[2669,2670] along with anti-aging effects demonstrated in the brains of aged rats.[2671]

In the DNA damage experiment where people ate different culinary doses of spices for a week before having their cells blasted with free radicals, turmeric led the pack. When people were fed just a pinch of turmeric a day, DNA damage rates were cut by 55 percent. This was not some proprietary turmeric extract either; study participants consumed about an eighth of a teaspoon each day of the plain spice you can buy at any grocery store. And this was not mixing turmeric with cells in some petri dish. This was just comparing what happens to the cells of those randomized to eat a modest amount of the spice each week and merely counting the DNA fracture rates.[2672]

Without the free radical blast, counting the DNA breaks in people's cells before and after a week of eating spices revealed no significant intrinsic protection in the ginger or rosemary groups. However, the turmeric still appeared to reduce DNA damage by about 40 percent.[2673] This may be because turmeric can boost the activity of our body's own antioxidant enzymes. Catalase is one of the most active enzymes in our body. Each one of these enzymes can detoxify millions of free radicals every second. If we consume the equivalent of about three-quarters of a teaspoon of turmeric a day for a month, the activity of the catalase enzyme in our bloodstream may get boosted by more than 50 percent.[2674] Taking a daily half teaspoon of a 50:1 ratio of turmeric to powdered black pepper for five days before radiation therapy reduced a measure of oxidative damage by about 50 percent compared to control.[2675]

For a review of clinical effects and doubts surrounding turmeric, both founded and unfounded, see my video see.nf/turmericskeptic. My Daily Dozen recommends a quarter teaspoon of turmeric every day.

Okinawa-Inspired Smoothie

I've been experimenting with a recipe for a delectable bright-purple smoothie that tastes like you are drinking a pumpkin pie. The sweet potato gives it an especially silky-smooth texture. There are a lot more recipes to come in my forthcoming *The How Not to Age Cookbook*, but to whet your appetite:

½ cooked then frozen purple sweet potato
¼-inch piece of turmeric root
¾ teaspoon matcha
1 cup unsweetened soymilk
1 ½ teaspoons ground flaxseed
1 ½ teaspoons wheat germ
¼ cup frozen cranberries
½ cup frozen strawberries
3 pitted dates
¼ teaspoon pumpkin pie spice
Dash of cardamom

Scrub one purple sweet potato under running water, then pierce it a few times with a fork. Microwave on high until it is fork-tender. When it is cool enough to be handled, cut it in half and freeze both halves. (You'll use half for this recipe and the other half next time you're craving this smoothie.) Place all the ingredients in a blender, and blend until smooth.

Tips: To preserve my turmeric root, I cut it into quarter-inch pieces, then freeze. Also, since learning about spermidine (see page 29), I've been cutting my ground flaxseed with wheat germ, half and half, so I just scoop in one full tablespoon of my flax–wheat germ mixture. Also, please note that the amount of matcha (2 g) used in this smoothie can carry more caffeine than a shot of espresso, so you may not want to drink this late in the day.

SPREAD THIN

Based on the best available studies with the longest follow-up, including an "unusually slim cohort" from the Oxford Vegetarian Study,[2676] the ideal body mass index (BMI) for the longest life appears to be 20 to 22 (kg/m^2).[2677] Okinawans traditionally fell smack dab in the middle at a stable BMI of 21. Although there was a cultural norm not to stuff oneself, the fact that they only averaged about 1,800 calories a day is probably more a function of the quality rather than quantity of the foods they were eating.[2678] The Okinawans were actually eating a greater amount of food, but whole plant foods are so calorically dilute that they were effectively practicing an 11 percent calorie restriction.[2679]

This mild, long-term restriction in calories consumed may have contributed to their exceptional survival, though the plant-based nature of the diet may trump caloric restriction. The one population who lives even longer than the Okinawa Japanese doesn't eat only a 98 percent meat-free diet, but rather 100 percent meat-free.[2680]

The Adventist vegetarians in California have "perhaps the highest life expectancy of any formally described population."[2681] Adventist vegetarian men and women live to be about eighty-three and eighty-six, respectively, which is comparable to Okinawan women, but longer-lived than Okinawan men.[2682] The best of the best were Adventist vegetarians who also practice such healthy lifestyle habits as exercising and not smoking. They live to the ages of eighty-seven and eighty-nine, on average. That's ten to fourteen years longer than the general population.[2683]

THE RED, WHITE, AND BLUE ZONE

Sadly, Okinawan longevity is a thing of the past. Okinawa is now home to more than a dozen KFC restaurants,[2684] and Okinawans' saturated fat intake levels have tripled in the years since World War II. They went from eating essentially no cholesterol on a daily basis to a few Big Macs' worth.[2685] They tripled their sodium intake and are now as potassium-deficient as Americans, getting less than half the recommended minimum daily intake of 4,700 mg. In just two generations, Okinawans have gone from the leanest Japanese to the fattest.[2686] As a consequence, there has been a resurgence of interest from public health professionals in getting Okinawans to eat the Okinawan diet, too.

The same can be said of nearly all the other blue zones, like those in the Mediterranean: They are artifacts of history.[2687] Only one blue zone survives and thrives to this day in the modern era: the Seventh-day Adventists in Loma Linda, California. Another aspect that sets it apart is that it is nondistinctly situated, surrounded by the rest of society. All the other blue zones were geographically isolated from their respective mainlands, as mostly islands, which allowed for the maintenance of divergent diets and lifestyles.[2688]

The diets of other blue zones were also economically constrained; people were in effect "forced" to eat healthier. For example, the average Okinawan wasn't eating much meat, sugar, salt, cooking oil, and polished white rice because they simply couldn't afford it.[2689] Okinawa was Japan's poorest prefecture.[2690] After World War II, their reliance on sweet potatoes went from forming the bulk of their diet to constituting less than 5 percent as imported white rice and bread started to crowd out healthier foods.[2691] In contrast, the United States is one of the richest countries in the world, with an average per capita GDP exceeding $65,000 a year,[2692] yet ranks as low as forty-fifth in life expectancy.[2693] What can we learn from the Adventists in Loma Linda, the one remaining active blue zone community right here in the United States that seems to exceed all others in terms of life expectancy?[2694] How have they been able to retain their healthy eating habits surrounded by the excesses of the modern world?

Adventists have a health philosophy built around a biblical notion that the human body should be treated as a temple.[2695] As such, they've been promoting vegetarian eating for more than 140 years. Adventists are unique in that the majority have adopted a meat-free or low-meat diet.[2696] In the Adventist Health Study-2, for example, which has been following nearly 100,000 North American Adventists for more than a decade, approximately 50 percent are vegetarian or vegan and the other half only eat meat about three times a week on average.[2697]

LIVING RELIGIOUSLY

Seventh-day Adventists are a Protestant Christian denomination. Might religiosity play a role? A poll of one thousand U.S. adults reported that 79 percent of respondents believed that spiritual faith can help people recover from disease.[2698] Might there be some truth to that? A meta-analysis of more than seventy studies on the topic found that measures of religiosity or spirituality were associated with reduced mortality rates in healthy populations, but not sick ones, and also identified evidence of publication bias, implying that some studies non-flattering to spirituality may have been quietly shelved.[2699]

Even if the association were robust, there are important confounding factors. For example, mainline (non-evangelical) Protestants and Jews have the lowest mortality rates among major religious groups in the United States, but they are also likely to be disproportionally white, wealthy, and well educated, and each factor on its own is linked to longevity.[2700] There is also the specter of reverse causation. In these studies, a common measure of faith is attendance of religious services, and you can imagine how developing a disease may prevent you from attending.[2701]

Religious involvement has also been associated with longer telomeres,[2702] though, unexpectedly, the longest telomeres were found in the least religious—for example, people reporting never praying or studying holy books like the Bible. But, among those who were at least somewhat religious, more spiritual involvement was associated with longer telomere length.[2703]

Religiosity could certainly be related directly to health outcomes through lifestyle choices, such as electing not to smoke or drink in excess, which tend to be characteristic of religious people or, in the case of the Adventists, a healthier diet.[2704] Might a predilection to stricter adherence to codes of conduct enable religious people to better stick to healthy lifestyle advice?[2705] Many of the Adventist plant-based diet and lifestyle tips have been put into action in the Complete Health Improvement Program (CHIP, though recently rebranded as Pivio), the most extensively published community-based lifestyle intervention in the medical literature.[2706] (Read all about it in my Optimal Weight-Loss Diet section in *How Not to Diet*.) The influence of religious affiliation on responsiveness to the program was tested in a group of 7,000 participants.

Even though Adventists make up less than 1 percent of the U.S. population, about one in five CHIP participants were in the church. How did they do compared to the nonbelievers? Substantial reductions in cardiovascular risk factors were achieved for both Adventists and non-Adventists, and some of the reductions were actually greater among the non-Adventists. The researchers concluded that this indicates that Seventh-day Adventists "do not have a monopoly on good health. . . ."[2707]

Fertility vs. Longevity?

Adventist vegetarians may be longest living, but might that come at a cost? A semen analysis in a Loma Linda fertility clinic raised questions about their sperm quality. Though still within the normal range,[2708] vegetarians had about a 25 percent lower

(continued)

sperm count.[2709] The few vegans tested also had a lower sperm concentration, though not significantly so, and this was made up for by their 30 percent greater ejaculate volume. The vegans did have significantly fewer activated sperm, however, which is a sign of decreased fertility. The researchers suggested soy consumption as a possible mechanism based on the potential for hormonal effects. Californian Adventist vegetarians average about a half serving a day of plant-based meats, many of which contain soy. But, when soy phytoestrogens were put to the test, months of consuming up to the equivalent of nearly twenty servings of soy a day resulted in no adverse effects on sperm parameters.[2710]

There were only five vegans in the study, so the sperm quality findings could just be a fluke, but, if verified, it could reflect an evolutionary trade-off between fertility and lifespan that was first proposed nearly a century ago.[2711] Using a finely tuned laser, it's possible to selectively destroy individual cells as *C. elegans* develops,[2712] and terminating the cells that give rise to the sperm and eggs significantly extends lifespan.[2713] The same phenomenon can be demonstrated in fruit flies, potentially shifting the body's priorities from reproduction to survival.[2714]

The fertility versus longevity trade-off may be one reason why spaying and neutering our pets can extend their lives. Based on a study of millions of dogs and cats,[2715] sterilized male and female dogs live about 20 percent longer than "intact" dogs, spayed female cats live about 40 percent longer, and neutered male cats a remarkable 60 percent longer.[2716]

What about men who have been castrated? Eunuchs seem to live 25 percent longer than uncastrated men.[2717] In the United States, people who were deemed "feebleminded" were involuntarily sterilized by the government by the tens of thousands until the 1950s,[2718] a practice upheld by none other than famed Supreme Court justice Oliver Wendell Holmes. Writing for the eight-to-one majority in *Buck v. Bell*, the decision upholding the eugenics practice, he penned: "The principle that sustains compulsory vaccination is broad enough to cover cutting the Fallopian tubes."[2719] The heinous practice of compulsory sterilization did allow for a natural experiment, though, and one mental institution found that castrated men lived an average of fourteen years longer than intact men in the same hospital.[2720]

A genealogy database of nearly 200,000 men and women across three centuries in sixteen countries found that those who had fewer children seemed to live longer.[2721] Centenarians, for example, were found to have fewer children and had them at later ages.[2722] This is not to suggest that having fewer children will make you live longer but rather that constitutional factors that enhance human lifespan may come at the expense of reduced reproductive potential, another example of the antagonistic pleiotropy theory. (See pages 102 and 137.) For instance, selection for lifespan extension in model organisms can lead to longer-lived animals but with reduced fertility.[2723] It makes intuitive sense when you consider the context of food scarcity.

In lean times, it is reasonable to put off reproduction until more favorable conditions return to ensure long-term survival.[2724] Caloric restriction can extend the lives of animals but can also cause a reduction in the number of their progeny. A similar pattern may be seen in humans. In the Minnesota Starvation Study, the subjects rapidly lost their libidos after their calorie intake was cut in half.[2725] Remember the nutrient-sensing aging pathways—AMPK, IGF-1, and mTOR? There can be a seesaw between tissue acceleration and reproduction on one side and tissue preservation and rejuvenation on the other.[2726] Thankfully, we can shift the weight to a more optimal balance with diet.

The later girls start their periods, the longer they tend to live. Each year later is associated with significantly lower risk of dying from heart disease,[2727] cancer,[2728] and stroke, plateauing with the lowest overall mortality among those who don't start menstruating until age fifteen.[2729] Earlier breast development (before age ten versus twelve or thirteen) is associated with as much as 23 percent greater breast cancer risk later in life,[2730] and each year earlier a girl starts to menstruate is linked to significantly higher risk of cancers of the bladder, breast, colon, liver, lung, skin, and uterus.[2731]

A century ago, the age of first menstruation averaged as late as nearly seventeen,[2732] but now the average age is under twelve.[2733] Similarly, around the world, the age breast development begins has dropped an average of about three months per decade over the last half century, down to just nine or ten years old in the United States, necessitating a change in textbook definitions of "premature" puberty.[2734] But it's something over which we have a degree of control.

Higher levels of IGF-1 are associated with earlier sexual maturity,[2735] so it's no surprise that kids eating more animal protein experience puberty significantly earlier; this effect is not seen with plant protein.[2736] A meta-analysis of sixteen studies on diet and development found that, for each additional 1 g of daily animal protein intake in childhood, one's first period appears to move up by two months.[2737] So, for example, seven-year-old girls consuming more than twelve servings of meat a week had 75 percent greater odds of beginning menstruation within the next five years or so compared to seven-year-olds who ate less than four servings a week,[2738] a relationship found for consumption of both red meat and poultry.[2739] IGF-1 and other aging pathways may not fully explain these findings, however, as persistent pollutants that build up in meat, like DDT,[2740] have also been linked to precocious puberty.[2741]

PLANT-BASED EATING

The principal component considered to be responsible for the extraordinary lon-gevity of the Adventist blue zone in California is its plant-based diet.[2742] Vegetarian Adventists not only live longer than nonvegetarian Adventists who eat relatively little meat but they also have a lower incidence of all cancers combined and less high blood pressure and diabetes.[2743] Overall, a comprehensive meta-analysis and systematic review of the major observational studies examining plant-based eating and chronic diseases found that a vegetarian diet had a significant protective effect on getting or dying from heart disease and on the incidence of total cancer, with a vegan diet conferring about twice the reduced cancer risk.[2744]

What about those who decided to stop eating vegetarian and start eating meat? The Adventist Health Study found that, compared to those who stayed vegetarian, individuals who began eating meat suffered about a 230 percent increased risk of gaining weight, a 170 percent increased risk of developing diabetes, and a 150 percent increased risk of having a stroke or being diagnosed with heart disease.[2745] And, if they continued eating meat, they appeared to cut their lifespan by 3.6 years. A comparable flip-side survival advantage was found for long-term vegetar-ians. Those who avoided meat for seventeen or more years had an estimated life expectancy of 86.5 years, while those who were vegetarian for fewer than seven-teen years had an estimated life expectancy of 82.9.[2746] Compared to longtime vegetarians, those who ate any meat, including poultry and fish, were found to be three times as likely to develop dementia.[2747]

Without guaranteed mental and physical health, most people don't want to live extended lives.[2748] Beyond the longevity advantage, vegetarian Adventists also appear to be in better health as evidenced by taking fewer medications and logging fewer X-ray exams, surgical procedures, and overnight hospital stays. Vegetarians also enjoy the improved quality of life that just comes with suffering fewer chronic diseases.[2749] A study of 15,000 American vegetarians found that they have signifi-cantly less coronary artery disease, fewer strokes, less high blood pressure, less diabetes, less diverticulosis, fewer allergies, and significantly fewer diseases overall, after controlling for nondietary factors like smoking. The researchers also noted that the nonvegetarians were more likely to have had surgeries for conditions as varied as varicose veins and hemorrhoids to even more hysterectomies, as well as be on a slew of different drugs. Those eating meat had about twice the odds of being on aspirin, sleeping pills, tranquilizers, antacids, painkillers, blood pressure medications, laxatives, and insulin.

This all translates into significantly fewer medical costs. Compared to non-vegetarians who similarly didn't smoke or drink, vegetarians were found to have significantly lower inpatient, outpatient, and total medical care expenditures, including a nearly 50 percent drop in depression-related medical expenses.[2750] One reason there has been such good compliance with plant-based dietary intervention studies is that participants not only tend to get measurably better but also tend to feel much better. Those randomized to plant-based diets report a significantly better quality of life and significantly higher mood scores than their counterparts assigned to conventional diets, which presumably encourages them to sustain this eating pattern over the long run.[2751]

Success breeds success. After just a few days or weeks following the shift, patients may experience palpable benefits of plant-based eating, beyond just improvements in measurements like blood sugar levels and weight, reinforcing the positive impacts of their new eating habits and providing further motivation to continue.[2752] In fact, sometimes, plant-based diets can work a little too well. In studies where people are switched on and off plant-based nutrition, they sometimes feel so much better eating healthier that they violate study protocol and refuse to go back to their original baseline diets.[2753]

Which do you think is more effective? Asking patients to make large dietary changes or smaller ones? Paradoxically, diet studies have shown that recommending greater changes leads to greater changes, leading researchers to conclude: "It may help to replace the common advice, 'all things in moderation' with 'big changes beget big results.'"[2754] But, it needn't be all or nothing.

SWAP MEAT

In the United States, the number one risk factor for dying is the American diet. Associated with the most deaths, primarily from cardiovascular disease, about half a million mothers, fathers, sisters, brothers, and friends die every year simply because of what they eat.[2755] In stark contrast, plant-based diets are associated with a lower risk of developing cardiovascular disease to begin with, a lower risk of dying from cardiovascular disease, and, in fact, a lower risk of dying from all causes put together. Progressively increasing our intake of plant foods by reducing how many animal foods we consume may enable us to live longer, healthier lives[2756]—and it doesn't take much.[2757]

As I mentioned, the largest cohort study of diet and health in history, the NIH-AARP study, found that replacing just 3 percent of daily calorie intake from animal protein with plant protein was associated with a 10 percent lower overall mortality in both men and women.[2758] Meat consumption alone was associated with greater risks of dying from heart disease, cancer, and prematurely in general.[2759] This led to an accompanying editorial titled "Reducing Meat Consumption Has Multiple Benefits for the World's Health," published in the *Archives of Internal Medicine*, the journal of the American Medical Association, calling for a "major reduction in total meat intake."[2760]

Of all the animal protein sources, eggs were found to be the worst. Swapping in 3 percent of daily calories with plant protein instead of egg protein (found mostly in the egg whites) was associated with twice the benefit of swapping out meat protein, exceeding 20 percent lower mortality in men and women. So, eggs appeared to be worse than red meat. The researchers concluded that the finding that plant protein was preferable provides evidence for "dietary modifications in choice of protein sources that may promote health and longevity."[2761]

What about the effects of dietary intake of animal versus plant protein on aging? Healthy aging is defined as "the process of developing and maintaining the functional ability that enables wellbeing in older age." A higher intake of plant protein has been associated with less accumulation of deficits, based on functional impairments, self-reported health and vitality, mental health, diseases, and the use of health services.[2762]

Swapping in just 1 percent of calories from plant protein in place of animal protein led to significantly less deficit accumulation. Now, you may be thinking that animal protein and animal fat travel alongside each other in the same foods, so the benefits of this swap may have just been a saturated fat effect. But even after accounting for fat, there still seems to be something about the animal versus plant protein sources.[2763] It's still not clear, however, if the beneficial health effects are due to an avoidance of deleterious effects associated with animal foods or the addition of beneficial effects of plants, though it may be a little of both.[2764]

EATING PLANTISH

Since the benefits of the Mediterranean diet appear primarily due to the added plant foods,[2765] PREDIMED researchers created what they called a "provegetarian" scoring system to test the effects of one's dietary plant-to-animal ratio. They knew "pure" vegetarians lived longer but figured recommendations to just eat "more plant-based foods, less animal-based foods" might be easier to swallow. Would simply moving along the spectrum toward more plants actually enable people to live longer? Check out see.nf/flexitarian for details, but indeed, this appeared to translate into a 40 percent lower risk of premature death, evidence that "the simple advice to increase the consumption of plant-derived foods with compensatory reductions in the consumption of foods from animal sources confers a survival advantage."[2766]

Though there are vested interests that fight hard to maintain the status quo, such as the processed food and pharmaceutical industries, one corporate sector actually benefits from keeping people healthy: the insurance industry. In a nutritional update published about ten years ago in its official medical journal, Kaiser Permanente, the largest managed-care entity in the United States, urged its nearly 15,000 physicians that healthy eating may be "best achieved with a plant-based diet." The update read:

> Too often, physicians ignore the potential benefits of good nutrition and quickly prescribe medications instead of giving patients a chance to correct their disease through healthy eating and active living. . . . Physicians should consider recommending a plant-based diet to all of their patients, especially those with high blood pressure, diabetes, cardiovascular disease, or obesity.[2767]

In other words, doctors should give their patients the chance to first correct their diseases themselves. The major downside that Kaiser Permanente's nutritional update identified is that a plant-based diet may work a little too well. If individuals adopt the diet while still taking medications, their blood sugar or blood pressure could drop so low that they may need their physicians to adjust their meds or take them off them completely. Ironically, the "side effect" of the diet may be not having to take drugs anymore.

As with many articles, this one ends with a familiar refrain: "Further research is needed. . . ." In this case, though, the call was not for more studies on efficacy but rather: "Further research is needed to find ways to make plant-based diets the new normal. . . ."[2768]

In Kaiser Permanente's guide "The Plant-Based Diet: A Healthier Way to Eat," a plant-based diet is defined as completely excluding animal products, but it expressly points out: "If you find you cannot do plant-based eating 100% of the time, that's OK. Any movement toward more plants and fewer animal products, processed foods, and sweets can improve your health!"[2769]

Vegetarian vs. Mediterranean

The Mediterranean diet is primarily, but not exclusively, plant-based,[2770] so much so that vegetarians have three times the odds of having their diets rated as highly adherent in the classic Mediterranean diet scoring system and vegans have more than thirty times the odds.[2771] After all, the traditional Mediterranean diet itself can be considered to be a "near-vegetarian diet."[2772] What happened when the two diets were pitted head-to-head?

(continued)

Researchers randomized overweight individuals to either a low-calorie Mediterranean diet plan or a low-calorie vegetarian one. With the same enforced caloric restriction, both groups lost the same amount of weight, but the vegetarian group edged out an advantage with a significant drop in LDL cholesterol.[2773] What if there were no specific calorie or portion restrictions? That's the tack a different study took, and obese subjects randomized to advice to eat a Mediterranean diet lost no weight at all over four months compared to thirteen pounds lost by those advised to eat a strictly plant-based diet with no added fats.[2774]

VEGAN JUNK FOOD IS STILL JUNK FOOD

Is a plant-based diet just another way of saying *vegan*? No. Although it's often confused with vegan or vegetarian diets, it can have very different health implications. Vegan diets are free of any animal-derived ingredients, and vegetarian ones are meat-free but can include dairy and eggs. Both may exclude animal products for religious or ideological reasons, but neither is necessarily focused on healthy choices. A plant-based diet, on the other hand, has been defined as a way of eating that minimizes consumption of meat, dairy, eggs, and processed junk, while maximizing intake of whole plant foods, such as vegetables, fruits, whole grains, legumes (beans, split peas, chickpeas, and lentils), mushrooms, nuts and seeds, herbs and spices—basically real food that grows out of the ground.[2775]

These days, "junk" is the predominant food group.[2776] Corporations willfully engineer products to maximize eating for profit, and the industry will happily make all the vegan junk we're willing to buy.[2777] In fact, one study found that when the consumption of ultraprocessed junk, like ramen noodles, potato chips, and cookies, was compared across different eating patterns, vegetarians and vegans ate the most.[2778] Oreos are vegan, and there are vegan Doritos, Pop-Tarts, and Krispy Kreme pies. Vegan does not necessarily mean health-promoting.

From a health perspective, this may help explain why vegans in the United States tend to do better than vegans in the United Kingdom.[2779] The number one reason Americans choose to eat plant-based is for their health,[2780] so they tend to eat more plants (as evidenced by higher fiber and vitamin C intakes,[2781] which are only found concentrated in whole plant foods). On the other side of the Atlantic, however, the top reason for veganism is ethical concerns,[2782] so British vegans may be more likely to just switch to vegan crumpets.[2783] Similarly, U.S. vegetarians have been found to eat fewer refined grains and sweets than veg Brits.[2784]

In order to distinguish between healthful and unhealthful vegan diets, Cornell professor emeritus in nutritional biochemistry Dr. T. Colin Campbell introduced the term *whole food, plant-based diet*.[2785] If you look at India, for example, you see a decrease in the whole plant food content of their diet, along with increasing risk of obesity and noncommunicable chronic diseases. There's been a shift from brown rice to the more processed white rice and the substitution of other refined carbohydrates, packaged snacks, and fast food in place of India's traditional staples of vegetables, lentils, fruits, nuts, whole grains, and seeds. This may help explain why disease rates are on the rise even in a country with a large vegetarian contingent.[2786]

Professor Campbell's physician son and daughter-in-law tried putting a group of vegetarians and vegans on a whole food, plant-based diet for eight weeks. On average, the study participants lost ten pounds and dropped their LDL cholesterol by sixteen points.[2787] In other words, vegans may benefit from eating more plant-based, too.

SETTLING THE SCORE

In the medical literature, when "anti-aging diets" are discussed, the conversation isn't only about eating more whole plant foods and cutting down on meat, but also cutting down on junk. Here are some examples: "A diet portfolio rich in fruits and vegetables, legumes and whole grains, but reduced in animal products and accompanying saturated fat, salt, sweets, and refined carbohydrates."[2788] "Such a diet would include wholegrain cereals, legumes, fruits and vegetables, with a low intake of saturated fat and trans fatty acids,"[2789] and "anti-aging" eating involves "minimizing meat, salt, added sugar, and heavily processed foods while emphasizing phytochemical-rich foods."[2790]

If people just concentrate on decreasing their intake of animal foods, they may end up increasing their consumption of highly processed junk, like Coke and Wonder Bread.[2791] It's worth repeating that you can't assume that simply avoiding animal foods will necessarily produce a healthy diet.[2792] In recognition of the fact that all plant foods are not created equal, "healthful" plant-based diet indexes were created that, like the "provegetarian" system, positively score healthy plant foods, but negatively score both animal foods *and* processed junk.[2793]

Using these more sophisticated plant-based scoring systems, we learned that simply giving points for any plant foods (junk or not) and docking points for any animal foods (meat, dairy, or eggs) results in scores that are associated with a significantly lower risk of premature death.[2794,2795,2796,2797] However, just replacing animal products with highly processed junk doesn't do your body any favors. Plant-based junk diets are associated with neutral[2798] or even increased mortality risk.[2799] Over time, as assessed in 75,000 health professionals over a dozen years in the Harvard cohorts, those who made the greatest improvements in minimizing all animal foods and increasing any plant foods, particularly healthy ones, had a lower risk of dying, but those who kept animal products to a minimum but piled on the most junk, like sodas and sweets, increased their risk of dying overall.[2800]

These studies suggest we shouldn't lump together all plant-origin foods. Kidney beans are different from jelly beans. All the animal foods were still being treated the same, though, so researchers tried making an animal food–based quality index as well. They put processed meats, red meat, and eggs in an "unhealthy animal foods" category but treated fish, other seafood, dairy, and poultry as "healthy animal foods." They found that the higher the quality of plant foods, the lower the all-cause mortality, but no independent association was found for the quality of animal foods, meaning they all seemed to be roughly just as bad in terms of cancer mortality, heart disease mortality, and all-cause mortality.[2801]

The Simplest Dietary Quality Index

In general, the dividing line between foods that promote health and those that promote disease may be less plant versus animal and more whole plant foods versus everything else. This has been encapsulated by a dietary quality index that reflects the percentage of calories gotten from nutrient-rich, unprocessed plant foods on a scale of zero to one hundred. So, if half of your food calories are from unprocessed plants, you'd score a fifty. A strictly whole food, plant-based diet, meaning a vegan diet that excludes refined grains, white potatoes, alcohol, and added sugars and oils, could achieve a perfect score of a hundred.[2802] Sadly, most Americans hardly make it above a score of ten.[2803]

The standard American diet only rates an eleven out of one hundred. According to U.S. Department of Agriculture (USDA) estimates, 57 percent of our calories come from processed plant foods, 32 percent from animal products, and only 11 percent from whole grains, fruits, beans, nuts, and vegetables.[2804] In other words, on a scale of one to ten, the American diet only rates about a one.

Why do we care? Because those with higher scores appear to lose more body fat over time and have a lower risk of abdominal obesity,[2805] high blood pressure,[2806] high blood sugars,[2807] metabolic syndrome,[2808] high cholesterol, and high triglycerides,[2809] as well as depression, anxiety, and psychological distress.[2810] A higher score also correlates with 70 percent lower odds of benign breast diseases like fibrocystic lumps.[2811] What about malignant disease?

When researchers compared the diets of 100 women with breast cancer to 175 healthy women, they concluded that scoring higher on the whole plant food diet index (eating just twice the proportion of plants compared to the standard American diet) may reduce the odds of breast cancer by more than 90 percent.[2812]

PRODUCE LONGEVITY

Probably the least controversial advice in all of nutrition is to eat more fruits and vegetables, which is to say: Eat more plants. After all, the term *vegetable* basically means all parts of the plant that aren't fruit. How much longer might we get to live if we eat more produce? Compared to those getting five servings of fruits and veggies a day, those only eating two daily servings may live seven fewer months. Having only one serving a day may equate to living about a year and a half less. With just a half serving a day, we may live two fewer years. And, if we don't eat any servings of fruits and vegetables a day, we could lose three years of our lives.[2813] So, for someone eating sufficiently unhealthfully, eating just a single serving of fruit each day, like one apple, could potentially mean a nineteen-month difference between life and death. One daily salad might mean years more time on this planet.

In contrast, the potential lifelong damage of any pesticides on those fruits and vegetables has been estimated to only cut a few *minutes* off the average person's life.[2814] So, while there are many reasons people choose organic produce over conventional, concerns over pesticide residues should not discourage us from stuffing our faces with as many fruits and vegetables as possible.

The fruit and vegetable dose-response longevity study mostly looked at people in their fifties and sixties.[2815] Is it too late to make a difference by the time we're in our seventies? Apparently not. Women in their seventies with the most carotenoid phytonutrients in their bloodstream were twice as likely to survive five years as those with the least, potentially doubling their likelihood of survival merely by eating more fruits and vegetables.[2816] In a study out of Taiwan, spending just fifty cents a day on fruits or vegetables appeared to buy participants about a 10 percent drop in mortality.[2817] That's quite a bargain. Imagine if there were a drug that could lower the risk of death by 10 percent——with only good side effects. How much do you think drug companies would charge? Probably more than fifty cents.

Eating Low on the Food Chain

Eating from the lowest rung of the food chain gives plant-based eaters another advantage in the modern world: suffering less exposure to the industrial pollutants that bioaccumulate up the ladder.[2818] I explore the role of contaminants in aging and disease, such as PCBs, dioxins, and long-banned pesticides like DDT, in see.nf/eatlow. Studies of the pollutants in the breast milk of vegetarians dating back more than forty years found the average levels of some pollutants were fifty to one hundred times lower in the vegetarians compared to the national average. In fact, for six out of seven pollutants researchers investigated, there was no

(continued)

overlap in the range of scores: The highest vegetarian value was lower than the lowest value obtained in the general population.[2819] Lower pollutant levels may help explain why those on a plant-based diet appear to be less likely to develop all forms of cancer combined.[2820]

Based solely on levels of dioxin contamination, the USDA determined that American children who consume meat could be ingesting more than the daily safety limit.[2821] Surprisingly, as I explore in see.nf/organicmeat, the differences in pollutant contamination between organically and conventionally produced meats were minimal.[2822] Indeed, even just eating half of the average U.S. per capita meat intake[2823] could exceed the maximum tolerable limits, whether organic or not.[2824]

What, then, can we do to reduce our exposure? We can eat high-fiber foods, as fiber can bind to some of the contaminants and potentially flush them out of the body.[2825] We can exercise, as blood levels of persistent pollutants have been found to be lower among physically active individuals,[2826] perhaps due to sweating,[2827] boosting detoxing enzymes,[2828] or increasing clearance through the bile.[2829] We also can trim fat when preparing meat and further trim and thoroughly drain fat after cooking,[2830] though given current contamination levels, a recent review concluded that "meat consumption in general . . . should be significantly modified downward, as much and as soon as possible."[2831]

THE VEGETARIANS' ACHILLES' HEEL

The largest association of nutrition professionals in the world, the Academy of Nutrition and Dietetics, is clear in its latest position paper on the subject: Plant-based diets are not only "appropriate for all stages of the life cycle" but may "provide health benefits in the prevention and treatment of certain diseases." (I'm honored to report that the academy directed readers to NutritionFacts.org as a trusted resource.)[2832] As the emeritus dean of the School of Public Health at Loma Linda University once said at a nutrition conference, "Attitudes toward vegetarian diets have progressed from ridicule and skepticism to condescending tolerance, to gradual and sometimes grudging acceptance, and finally to acclaim."[2833]

A comparison of the dietary quality of different popular diets scored Ornish's plant-based plan the highest and Atkins's low-carb plan the lowest.[2834] Using a number of nutritional quality indexes, researchers found that individuals' diet scores generally ranked healthier the more plant-based they ate.[2835] Despite plant-based eaters eschewing entire categories of foods, they ironically tend to get more nutrition. One study found that those eating more plant-based got more of nearly every nutrient—more fiber, more vitamins A, C, and E, more of the B vitamins thiamin, riboflavin, and folate, and more of the minerals calcium, magnesium, and iron.[2836] This shouldn't be surprising. Responded the *Journal of the American Dietetic Association* editor in chief, "What could be more nutrient dense than a vegetarian diet?"[2837]

Nowadays, the most widely published cases of classic nutrient-deficiency syndromes are people following extreme diets, like the American service member who was hospitalized for a muscle tear due to scurvy. He reported eating only skinless chicken and candy bars.[2838] Ironically, one of the healthiest eating patterns, an exclusively plant-based diet, is perhaps the most life-threateningly incomplete, lacking vitamin B_{12}.

Vitamin B_{12} isn't made by plants. It isn't made by animals either, but rather by microbes that blanket the earth.[2839] However, B_{12} produced by bacteria in the guts of animals can suffuse through their tissues to provide a human source. Unfortunately, the B_{12} made in our colons is too far down to be absorbed.[2840] We all presumably used to get B_{12} by drinking out of a mountain stream or sipping well water,[2841] but today we chlorinate the water supply to kill off any bacteria. We don't get a lot of B_{12} in our water anymore, but we don't get a lot of cholera either!

Vegetarians living in developing world slums appear to have fewer B_{12}-deficiency problems,[2842] but the more hygienic our meals, the less B_{12} we may get.[2843] Our fellow great apes, like gorillas, get all the B_{12} they need by eating their own feces.[2844] I prefer supplements.

In our modern, sanitized world, vitamin B_{12} can be found reliably only in supplements, animal products, and B_{12}-fortified foods. Vegans and vegetarians should take supplements containing at least 50 mcg of cyanocobalamin (the most stable form[2845]) each day or at least 2,000 mcg once a week,[2846] as should all individuals between fifty and sixty-five, regardless of their diets (since we lose some of the ability to absorb B_{12} from food as we age).[2847] After that, however, the recommendations change.

After age sixty-five, a single dose of 50 mcg a day—even 100 daily mcg—may not be enough.[2848] Researchers set out to find an adequate dose for this age bracket, and it seems most need at least 650 mcg to 1,030 mcg a day, so I recommend 1,000 mcg of cyanocobalamin a day for *everyone* after age sixty-five, ideally as a chewable, sublingual, or liquid supplement.[2849] Absorption is boosted when B_{12} mixes with saliva, because we secrete a B_{12}-binding protein from our salivary glands that helps transport the vitamin safely through our digestive tract.[2850] Chewing a B_{12} tablet can cause our levels to go up ten times more than had we simply swallowed the exact same vitamin.[2851]

Vitamin B_{12} deficiency is serious business, with the potential to cause a wide range of disorders of the blood, gut, brain, and nervous system.[2852] With the ever-increasing demand for cleanliness in our food chain, it is of special importance that we secure a regular, reliable source of B_{12}, and supplements are probably the easiest, safest, and cheapest.[2853]

What About Vitamin K_2?

For a deep dive, check out my video see.nf/vitamink, but in short, purported benefits for the bones, heart, and brain have failed to materialize (taking into account that some of the major trials were found plagued with admissions of data fabrication).[2854] Even if such evidence arose, we can get all the vitamin K we need from the vitamin K_1 in greens since there's no requirement for the vitamin K_2 found in certain animal products and fermented foods.[2855] And, even if some evidence arose that there was some unique benefit to K_2, our microbiome makes K_2 from the K_1 in greens, which we then absorb into our system. But what about the one type of K_2 made only by mammals? We're mammals! So even if we had some problem with our microbiome, our own cells can make K_2 from K_1 just like other animals.[2856]

Of all the dietary components correlating with all-cause mortality, the best evidence appears to support the intake of green leafy vegetables and salads to maximize our time on Earth.[2857] So it's no surprise that lower circulating levels of vitamin K_1 in the bloodstream—a marker of inadequate greens intake—are associated with dying prematurely.[2858] Eat. Your. Greens.

LIFESTYLE

In the thirteenth century, the renowned scholar Roger Bacon recommended a good diet, proper rest, exercise, moderation in lifestyle, and good hygiene for lifestyle prolongation, as well as, all too conveniently, the "breath of a virgin."[2859] But he was right about the first few!

"Diet" derives from the ancient Greek word *diaita*, which means "way of living," not just dietary needs.[2860] In 1903, Thomas Edison predicted that "[t]he doctor of the future will give no medicine, but will instruct his patient in the care of human frame in diet and in the cause and prevention of disease."[2861] A hundred and one years later, the American College of Lifestyle Medicine (ACLM), of which I am a proud founding member, was born.[2862]

As physicians, we still prescribe medicines when necessary, but we understand that lifestyle behaviors are most often the root causes of what ails us and, as such, place an emphasis on what we put into our mouths. Food and cigarettes are our leading causes of disability and death.[2863] More broadly, a recent research summit described lifestyle medicine as "the use of a whole food, plant-predominant diet, regular physical activity, restorative sleep, stress management, avoidance of risky substances and positive emotions/social connection as a primary therapeutic modality for treatment and reversal of chronic disease."[2864]

Based on seventy-four studies that enrolled millions of participants, those with the healthiest lifestyles had less than half the risk of dying compared to those checking all the unhealthy boxes during the average study's more-than-decade-long duration.[2865] We have all heard stories of cigar-chomping, gin-guzzling hundred-year-olds that capture the public's imagination, but the truth about lifestyle and longevity is more prosaic.[2866] Adhering to just four simple healthy lifestyle factors can have a strong impact on the prevention of some of our deadliest diseases: not smoking, not being obese, getting thirty minutes of exercise a day, and eating more healthfully, which is defined as consuming less meat and more fruits, vegetables, and whole grains.

Those four factors alone appear to account for 78 percent of our chronic disease risk. If you start from scratch and manage to tick off all four, you may eliminate more than 90 percent of your risk of developing diabetes and more than 80 percent of your risk of suffering a heart attack, halve your risk of having a stroke, and reduce by more than a third your overall cancer risk.[2867] For some cancers, like our number two cancer killer, colon cancer, up to 71 percent of cases appear to be preventable through simple diet and lifestyle changes.[2868] Think of what that means in terms of the numbers. As it stands now, each year, a million Americans will suffer their first heart attack or stroke, a million will get diabetes, and a million will be diagnosed with cancer.[2869] It's time we stop blaming genetics and focus on the 80 percent or so of risk that appears to be directly under our control.[2870]

What does that mean for mortality? A similar batch of healthy behaviors predicted a fourfold difference in total mortality, with an estimated impact equivalent to fourteen years in chronological age. Put another way, those taking better care of themselves were dying at such a slow rate that it was as if they were fourteen years younger.[2871] Imagine turning back the clock fourteen years—not with a drug or a DeLorean but just by eating and living more healthfully.

What if you already decided to go the drug route and are treating your risk factors like high blood pressure and cholesterol with medications? Adherence to basic healthy lifestyle behaviors appeared to effect the same mortality advantage for users and nonusers of preventive medications alike.[2872] What's more, it's never too late to turn back the clock. A midlife switch to even the basics—eating at least five daily servings of fruits and vegetables, walking just about twenty minutes a day, maintaining a healthy weight, and not smoking, for instance—results in a substantial reduction in mortality even in the immediate short-term future. We're talking about a 40 percent lower risk of dying in the subsequent four years. The researchers concluded that "making the necessary changes to adhere to a healthy lifestyle is extremely worthwhile, and that middle-age"—in this case, ages forty-five through sixty-four—"is not too late to act."[2873]

Healthier lifestyles can also delay the emergence of chronic disease by about a decade.[2874] Most seventy-two-year-olds who don't smoke or have diabetes, obesity, hypertension, or a sedentary lifestyle make it to age ninety, but among those plagued with those risk factors, the probability dropped to less than 5 percent.[2875] Even over the age of seventy-five, basic behaviors—not smoking, walking at least a half hour a day, and eating at least three daily servings of fruits and vegetables—may delay death and disability by about eighteen months.[2876]

No, Sitting Is Not the New Smoking

A media analysis found hundreds of news articles claiming that prolonged sitting each day is comparable to smoking cigarettes. This is decidedly not the case. Smoking is expected to cause a billion deaths in this century.[2877] Tobacco use is responsible for up to ten times or more greater mortality risk:[2878] twenty excess deaths per thousand people each year for the heaviest smokers, compared to less than two such deaths for the heaviest sitters. Even light smoking of a few cigarettes a day is associated with a higher risk.[2879] The good news is that quitting cigarettes even as late as age sixty-five may add years onto our lifespan.[2880]

Plummeting tobacco use is one of our great public health victories. The share of adults who smoke declined from 42 percent in 1965[2881] to just 14 percent today.[2882] Cigarettes now kill only about a half million Americans a year, whereas our diets kill many thousands more.[2883] To be victorious in the dietary realm, plant-based diets have been proposed to be "the nutritional equivalent of quitting smoking."[2884]

EXERCISE

When people retire, they don't appear to improve their diets, but they do tend to become more active.[2885] For many, leaving the workforce allows for more time for activities like playing sports, gardening, or entertaining friends and family. What role may physical activity play in longevity? In terms of combating the hallmarks of aging (see page 13), aerobic exercise can induce autophagy, lower inflammation, decrease DNA damage, and facilitate DNA repair,[2886] though, after controlling for weight reduction, it may not actually affect the rate of aging.[2887] There is, however, a strong body of evidence supporting its role in preserving higher functioning as we age.[2888] A meta-analysis of cohort studies of middle-aged and older individuals with follow-ups lasting as long as twenty years found that adults who exercised were more likely to age successfully than those who were sedentary,[2889] though less than 3 percent of those sixty and older may meet the recommended physical activity guidelines.[2890]

EXERCISE IS MEDICINE

Population studies have found a correlation between regular aerobic exercise and decreased risk of at least thirty-five different diseases,[2891] but what have interventional trials proven in terms of cause and effect? Randomized controlled experiments of older adults have demonstrated that physical activity can improve muscle mass, strength, balance,[2892] and mobility,[2893] as well as decrease the risk of falls[2894] and, potentially, fractures, while helping to minimize bone loss.[2895,2896] Exercise has also been shown to improve cognition,[2897] enhance mood,[2898] successfully treat depression as well as the prescription antidepressant drug Zoloft,[2899] improve erectile function in men,[2900] and generally improve quality of life.[2901] The evidence supporting the overall health benefits of physical activity is overwhelming.[2902] More on aging benefits in see.nf/perks.

Who Should Check with Their Doctor First?

If you are a man over the age of forty-five or a woman over fifty-five, have diabetes, or experience symptoms such as chest pain, dizziness, or shortness of breath, I would recommend checking with your health professional before starting a new exercise regimen.[2903]

SURVIVAL OF THE FITTEST?

Researchers who accept grants from the Coca-Cola Company[2904] call physical inactivity "the biggest public health problem of the 21st century."[2905] Not true. Exercise is fantastic, but in terms of risk factors for death and disability in the United States, physical inactivity ranks down at number ten and eleven, respectively.[2906] Globally, inactivity doesn't even scratch the top twenty when it comes to years of healthy life lost.[2907] A poor diet, as I've discussed, is by far our greatest killer, followed by smoking cigarettes.[2908]

Exercise has been described as the "only intervention that has shown a remarkable efficacy for . . . increasing mean and maximum lifespan in humans."[2909] View see.nf/lifelongexercise for an extensive review. But whether physical inactivity is said to be related to 6 percent of premature mortality,[2910] 9 percent,[2911] or even 15 percent,[2912] these estimates are all derived from observational studies and predicated on the presumption of cause and effect. I was surprised by how much controversy appears in the medical literature over whether the apparent longevity benefits of exercise are even real. You can imagine the confounding factors and potential for reverse causality. I review some of the critical studies in see.nf/fitnesslongevity.

For example, researchers have compared the effects of leisure-time physical activity to occupational physical activity. If the link between exercise and longevity were truly causal, then the context in which you exert yourself shouldn't matter.[2913] As you can probably guess, manual labor is associated with a shorter, not longer, life, again suggesting the primacy of confounders like socioeconomic factors.[2914]

CAN WE EXERCISE POWER OVER OUR LIFESPAN?

Is it possible a genetic predisposition to physical fitness is what accounts for the exercise-longevity link, rather than the physical activity itself? This question was raised by experiments comparing two strains of rats, one bred to have a high intrinsic running capacity and another bred to have a low one. Even without exercising, the rats with high fitness ability lived longer than those with the low fitness ability. But unexpectedly, when the rats were provided with running wheels, longevity dropped for both the high and low fitness strains. Voluntary exercise cut their lives short.[2915]

Using twin studies, we can show there are also genetic predispositions to exercise in humans. When identical twins leave home to start their separate lives, their exercise habits are much more likely to be "concordant" than those of fraternal twins, meaning if one twin vigorously exercises, the other twin is more likely to do the same if the two share 100 percent of their DNA instead of just 50 percent, like typical brothers and sisters. By looking at the rare cases of identical twins whose exercise habits diverge, we can tell if it's this genetic predisposition to exercise or actual exercise that accounts for athletic longevity. With the same DNA, would intense physical activity make a difference? Apparently not. The same mortality rates were found in identical twins whether they exercised vigorously or not.[2916]

So, does working out make you live longer or not? A critical analysis concluded that "the undisputed health-related benefits of exercise have yet to translate into any proven causal relationship with longevity." More details in see.nf/exerciselongevity.

HOW MUCH IS TOO MUCH?

Centuries ago, Hippocrates said, "Everything in excess is opposed to nature." Is it possible to exercise too much?[2917] Details in see.nf/toomuch, but basically, like any powerful medicine, there may be a safe range of dosing.[2918] It may be prudent to limit chronic, vigorous exercise to no more than an hour a day and no more than five hours a week, with at least a day or two off.[2919] For runners, the recommended upper limit for potential longevity benefits is thirty miles a week.[2920] Only about half of U.S. adults even reach the recommended minimum exercise level, though,[2921] so public health advocates tend to focus on the "even a little is great" message[2922] rather than worry about the 2 to 3 percent of Americans who may be overdoing it.[2923]

RUNNING THE RISK

What's the best diet to support our physical fitness? I was shocked to learn that endurance athletes, compared with sedentary individuals, have been found to have *worse* atherosclerosis.[2924] See see.nf/athletes for a review of that research. It's not that they seem to be overstressing their heart with movement but rather with meals.[2925] Endurance athletes can eat five, six, or even seven thousand calories a day. So, if they're eating twice the saturated fat and cholesterol, no wonder their hearts are getting hammered.

What do you think happened when researchers put people on a paleo diet, along with a CrossFit-based, high-intensity circuit training exercise program? Normally, if you lose enough weight by any means—whether by working out, getting your stomach stapled, or developing tuberculosis for that matter—you can temporarily lower your cholesterol levels no matter what you eat. However, after ten weeks of intensive workouts and weight loss on the paleo diet, the participants' LDL cholesterol levels actually went *up*. Counterbalancing changes in LDL cholesterol size or HDL cholesterol are not considered sufficient to offset this risk.[2926] And, those who started out the healthiest experienced the worst increase. The subjects who began the study with optimal LDL levels (under 70) experienced a 20 percent increase in this leading risk factor for our number one killer, heart disease.[2927] Exercise is supposed to make things better, not worse.

On the other hand, people placed on a plant-based diet and a modest, mostly walking-based exercise regimen, can drop their bad cholesterol by 20 percent within three weeks,[2928] whereas the paleo diet appeared to have "negated the positive effects of exercise."[2929] That is why all athletes should eat more plant-based. It doesn't matter how shred if you're dead.

PLANT POWERED

There has been a surging interest in plant-based eating among athletes,[2930] thanks in part to documentaries like *The Game Changers*. (I was honored to play a small role in that film as a scientific adviser.) There is a desire not only to score long-term health benefits but to improve performance and accelerate recovery.[2931] The artery-dilating, antioxidant, and anti-inflammatory properties of plant-based nutrition can certainly lead to improved blood flow and reduced oxidative stress and inflammation, and indeed, plant-based athletes have been found to have superior cardio-respiratory fitness[2932] and an endurance advantage,[2933] perhaps due to superior heart function.[2934] (Check out see.nf/fitness for a run-through of all the studies.) The more important question from a public health standpoint, though, is what about dietary effects on fitness for exercise training programs in *non*athletes?

Type 2 diabetics were randomized to a vegetarian versus conventional calorie-controlled diet and exercise program. All meals were provided to enhance compliance, and the exercise was closely monitored. Despite the same allotment of exercise in each group, VO_2 max (a measure of aerobic fitness) increased by 12 percent and maximal performance increased by 21 percent in the vegetarian group, both significantly better than the nonvegetarian group, who didn't significantly improve at all in either dimension. In other words, the results indicated that a more plant-based diet more effectively leads to improvements in physical fitness—in terms of better aerobic capacity and power output—than a less plant-based diet after the same aerobic exercise program.[2935]

The meat-free group also experienced reduced feelings of depression[2936] and a greater improvement in quality of life and mood.[2937] This is consistent with randomized crossover trials that show that covertly increasing saturated fat intake can reversibly induce negative changes in brain function, inflammation, mood, and resting metabolic rate, and perhaps even undercut exercise motivation.[2938,2939] Study participants became 12 to 15 percent less physically active when they were on diets high in saturated fat compared to low.[2940]

Compared to the conventional calorie-controlled diet group, the vegetarian group also experienced superior effects on body weight, blood sugar control, cholesterol, insulin sensitivity, and oxidative stress. Both diets contained the same number of calories, yet simply eating meat-free led to about six pounds more weight loss, as well as more *waist* loss (a significantly slimmer waist); less superficial fat, meaning the external jiggly fat; and, most important, significantly greater loss of visceral fat, the most metabolically dangerous deep belly fat.[2941] This is all in addition to leading more effectively to improvements in physical fitness.

WEIGHT CONTROL

Over the last forty years, obesity rates have tripled among older adults.[2942] Forty-three percent of Americans over the age of sixty are not just overweight but obese.[2943] This can't just be ascribed to a slower metabolism. Resting metabolic rate (the calories we burn just to keep us alive) remains stable from the time we're twenty through sixty, after which it only declines by about ten calories a day per year.[2944] So, don't blame your metabolism. As I documented in detail in my book *How Not to Diet*, blame the food.

Obesity is associated with accelerated cellular aging, as measured by telomere shortening or advanced epigenetic age,[2945] presumably due to the oxidative stress[2946] and systemic inflammation that accompany excess body fat.[2947] Obesity is associated with declining physical function in terms of mobility limitations, as well as declining cognitive function.[2948] MRI scans of hundreds of individuals across the age spectrum found that the brain shrinkage of white matter in overweight and obese individuals corresponded to having a brain that was up to ten years older.[2949] A meta-analysis of nineteen studies following more than a half million people for up to forty-two years found that midlife obesity was associated with a 33 percent increased risk of developing dementia,[2950] and each one-point increase above a body mass index (BMI) of 20 at age fifty appears to move up the onset of Alzheimer's disease by about seven months.[2951] What about obesity and mortality?

VISCERAL REACTION

Thanks in part to the obesity epidemic, we may now be raising the first American generation to live shorter lives than their parents.[2952] This downward trend in lifespan is expected to accelerate as the current younger generation, who started out even heavier, earlier, ages into adulthood.[2953] Some predict that, in the coming decades, we may lose two to five years of life expectancy in the United States, or even more. To put that into perspective, a miracle cure for *all* forms of cancer would only add three and a half years to the average American lifespan.[2954] In other words, reversing the obesity epidemic might save more lives than curing cancer.

Even a moderate midlife weight gain of approximately ten to twenty pounds may significantly reduce the odds of healthy survival later in life.[2955] In a study of more than six hundred centenarians, less than 2 percent of the women and not one of the men were obese.[2956] After the age of forty, obesity may reduce life expectancy by as much as six or seven years.[2957]

As we age, the fat on our body also tends to redistribute from the superficial jiggly flab under our skin (subcutaneous fat) to deep stores that wrap around our internal organs and bulge out our abdomens (visceral fat), especially in women.[2958] Between twenty-five and sixty-five, women lose approximately thirteen pounds of bone and muscle, while quadrupling stores of visceral fat. (Men's visceral fat stores typically only double.[2959]) So, even if the bathroom scale doesn't indicate any weight gain, a woman may be gaining the worst kind of fat. Even at the same overall body fat or BMI, the greater one's waistline, the shorter one's lifeline.[2960]

Visceral fat is the killer fat. In contrast, superficial fat is relatively benign. *The New England Journal of Medicine* published a study of fifteen obese women, assessed before and after having about twenty pounds of superficial fat sucked from their bodies, which resulted in an almost 20 percent decrease in their total body fat.[2961] Significant improvements in blood sugars, inflammation, blood pressure, cholesterol, and triglycerides are typically seen with just a 5 to 10 percent loss of body weight in fat,[2962] but, after the massive liposuction, none of those benefits materialized.[2963] This suggests that the subcutaneous fat under our skin is not the problem, but, rather, the visceral fat is what's responsible for the metabolic insults of obesity. The good news is the riskiest fat is the easiest to lose. Our body appears to preferentially shed the villainous visceral fat first.[2964] And lifestyle interventions appear to have a similar weight-loss efficacy in older compared with younger people.[2965]

The life-shortening effects of visceral fat have been proven in rats. Surgical removal resulted in a significant extension in average and maximum lifespans.[2966] What about in people? Those who get bariatric weight-loss surgery do go on to live significantly longer than weight-matched controls who don't[2967] (details in see .nf/bariatric), but there haven't been any randomized trials to confirm it. There are, however, randomized weight-loss trials using diet and lifestyle interventions.

ALL FAT CALORIES AREN'T THE SAME

A meta-analysis of fifteen studies that randomized men and women to weight-loss regimens for up to twelve years found that losing weight doesn't only decrease inflammation, blood pressure, blood sugars, and disability, but it extends life, decreasing the risk of premature death by about 15 percent.[2968] So, what's the best weight-loss diet?

A whole food, plant-based diet was found to result in the greatest weight loss ever reported in the medical literature at six and twelve months compared to any other diet in randomized control studies that similarly didn't limit calories or mandate exercise.[2969] One of the reasons may be its lower fat intake. When people were randomized to eat a low-fat plant-based diet, they naturally ate about 600 fewer calories a day compared to those randomized to a high-fat ketogenic diet. This led to a significant loss of body fat and a preservation of lean body mass, the opposite of what was found with the ketogenic dieters, who saw no significant loss in body fat but did experience a reduction of lean body mass as their bodies appeared to cannibalize their own body protein (even though they were eating more protein).[2970]

All fat is not equal, though.

In *How Not to Diet*, I bust the myth that "a calorie is a calorie." A calorie from one source isn't always as fattening as a calorie from any other. If you eat about the same number of calories and the same amount of fat, for instance, but replace meat and butterfat with nuts, avocados, and olive oil, you could lose nearly six more pounds of fat in just one month.[2971] Saturated fat can also cause twice the accumulation of visceral fat compared to the same amount of other fats.[2972] Why? One reason saturated fats may be more fattening is that they appear more likely to be stored immediately rather than burned. For instance, oleic acid, the primary monounsaturated fat in nuts, avocados, and olives, is promptly burned about 20 percent more readily than palmitic acid,[2973] which is sourced mainly from meat and dairy and is the predominant saturated fat in the American diet.[2974] In fact, you can drip palmitic acid on muscle cells in a petri dish and openly demonstrate the suppression of fat utilization.[2975]

For other reasons why healthier eating can be so effective at weight loss, check out *How Not to Diet* from your local library.

Going to BAT Against Fat

At birth, we emerge, all wet and slimy, from the balmy 98.6°F (37°C) of our mothers' wombs directly into room temperature. To maintain warmth, we developed an adaptive mechanism around 150 million years ago—the appearance of a unique organ called *brown adipose tissue*, or *BAT* for short, which enables us warm-blooded mammals to maintain our high body temperatures.[2976] BAT generates heat by consuming fat calories in response to exposure to the cold. The white fat in our belly stores fat, but the *brown* fat that is found high in our chest *burns* fat. BAT activation is not only a potential means to blunt the age-related decline in metabolic rate but it may also play a role in longevity.[2977]

BAT activity appears to be higher in long-lived animals and diminished in

(*continued*)

short-lived ones,[2978] and a gene that increases longevity in mice was found to boost BAT activity.[2979] Experiments surgically removing and transplanting brown fat between animals confirmed the role of BAT in healthy aging, at least in mice.[2980] If the same is true for humans, that could possibly help explain why women live longer than men, as females have greater BAT deposits throughout life.[2981] BAT activation enhances secretion of the fasting and longevity hormone FGF21 (see the Protein Restriction chapter), but, unfortunately, BAT activity decreases with age.[2982] Cold-stimulated BAT activity can be as high as 100 percent in those younger than forty, but that may drop down to less than 10 percent in older individuals.[2983]

You don't have to be left out in the cold, though. As I describe in *How Not to Diet*, there are dietary components that can boost BAT activation. Chili pepper compounds, for example, can do it and have been tested up through age sixty-four.[2984] The dosing works out to a whole raw jalapeño pepper or a half teaspoon of red pepper powder a day.[2985] To help beat the heat, finely chop or very thinly slice the jalapeño to reduce its kick, or mix the red pepper into soup or the whole-food vegetable "V8" smoothie I feature in one of my cooking videos on NutritionFacts.org. Alternately, there's ground ginger. It increases weight loss (potentially through BAT activation[2986]) at a teaspoon a day,[2987] which you can just stir into hot water to make ginger tea.

WHAT'S THE IDEAL WEIGHT FOR LONGEVITY?

We seem to have become inured to the mortal threat of obesity. If you go back a half century or so in the medical literature, when obesity wasn't run of the mill, the descriptions are much more grim: "Obesity is always tragic, and its hazards are terrifying."[2988] But it's not just obesity. Of the four million deaths attributed to excess body fat each year, nearly 40 percent of the victims are merely overweight, not obese.[2989]

But what about the so-called obesity paradox, evidence suggesting overweight individuals live longer? The Global BMI Mortality Collaboration busted this myth using data from more than ten million people from hundreds of studies conducted in dozens of countries around the world.[2990] (Go to see.nf/paradox for details.) So, what's the optimal BMI?

The largest studies in the United States[2991] and around the world found that having a normal body mass index between 20 and 25 is associated with the longest lifespan.[2992] When you put together all the best available studies with the longest follow-up, that ideal range can be narrowed down even further to a BMI of 20 to 22,[2993] which is about 124 to 136 pounds for someone who stands five feet six inches tall.[2994] You can use this unisex chart to see what your optimal weight might be based on your height:

Optimal Weight Based on Height

Height	Ideal Weight		Height	Ideal Weight		Height	Ideal Weight		Height	Ideal Weight
4'9"	92–102		5'2"	109–120		5'7"	128–140		6'	147–162
4'10"	96–105		5'3"	113–124		5'8"	132–145		6'1"	152–167
4'11"	99–109		5'4"	117–128		5'9"	135–149		6'2"	156–171
5'	102–113		5'5"	120–132		5'10"	139–153		6'3"	160–176
5'1"	106–116		5'6"	124–136		5'11"	143–158		6'4"	164–181

SLEEP

I'm wondering if calling this section "Do as I Say, Not as I Do" would have been more accurate. (I find I'm just not as productive when I'm unconscious!) In fact, in the wee hours this morning, I thought, *I've got to get up and write the sleep chapter!* It's something I'm working on.

There is a perception that time spent sleeping is time wasted,[2995] but inadequate sleep is associated with multiple acute and chronic conditions and may result in increased risk of death and disease.[2996] Force people to go one week with six hours of sleep a night, and you change the expression of more than seven hundred genes.[2997] The most dire effect may be endothelial dysfunction.[2998] The endothelium is the thin layer of cells that covers the internal surface of blood vessels and is responsible for allowing our arteries to properly relax and dilate open.[2999] Randomize people for about a week to get five rather than seven hours of sleep, though, and just that difference of two hours a night results in a significant impairment in artery function.[3000] But how significant?

Sleep deprivation is no joke. The magnitude of impairment from a week of five-hour nights is similar to that reported in people who smoke, have diabetes, or have coronary artery disease. Yet, more than a quarter of the population may routinely get six or fewer hours a night.[3001] Sufficiently long, restful sleep sessions each night are considered an "indisputable cornerstone of good health."[3002] However, whether or not the link between sleep and mortality is cause and effect remains controversial.

In Living Color

In my research for this chapter on the potential for light therapy to help with insomnia, I ran across some supremely weird research findings—for example, a paper titled "Green Light Extends *Drosophila* Longevity" from the journal *Experimental Gerontology*. Researchers found they could "dramatically" increase by 24 percent the lifespan of fruit flies by raising them under green light.[3003] Conversely, they could dramatically reduce their lifespans by exposing them to blue light, and this was true even in mutants that had no eyes! Even when the flies couldn't detect the color of the light at all, their lifespans were significantly altered. How?

A clue was unearthed when the researchers found that the longevity-boosting effect of green light was greatly reduced when the flies were fed an antibiotic, suggesting that their gut flora may somehow be involved.[3004]

In humans, skin exposure to ultraviolet light can alter the intestinal microbiome, but this is assumed to be an effect of vitamin D.[3005] It makes some sense that flies might somehow be nourished by green, a predominant color in their natural environment.[3006] I have videos on NutritionFacts.org about the beneficial effects of "forest bathing" for humans, though they appear to be due to the aromatic compounds, like pinene, which are given off by the trees,[3007] rather than the colors of the woods.

Lest you be tempted to order some green bulbs, note that in rats, green light (but not red or blue) induces glucose intolerance, which means higher blood sugars.[3008]

THE BIG SLEEP

There have been dozens of prospective studies on sleep duration and mortality. The most consistent finding is that there is no association at all. The second most common finding is a link between premature death and sleeping *longer*, typically more than nine hours a night. A quarter of the findings support a U-shaped effect, where those who don't get much sleep (typically less than six or seven hours) or get too much (more than nine) died at higher rates than those in the sweet spot, getting around seven to eight hours. Less than 5 percent of findings found a higher mortality risk only for those not getting enough sleep.[3009] Given these results, it's not surprising that a 2020 meta-analysis concluded that the only sleep category associated with higher risk for both older men and women was those sleeping the most at eight or more hours a night.[3010]

Seven hours of sleep a night may not sound like enough, but it may actually be what's natural for our species. Scientists studied three preindustrial societies, isolated from one another across two continents, and found surprising uniformity. Despite the absence of electric lighting or electronic gizmos, they usually stayed up until three or so hours after sunset and then arose before dawn, getting a solid six and a half hours of sleep out of about seven and a half hours in "bed."[3011] Even the studies showing risk at both ends of the sleep-duration spectrum tended to find a greater risk on the longer side.[3012]

A mechanism by which excess sleep might be harmful remains elusive, so a cause-and-effect relationship between sleeping eight or more hours a night and increased risk of death and disease has been dismissed by some as implausible.[3013] Could it be reverse causation, like sickness leading to more time in bed instead of vice versa? Maybe it's due to confounding factors, such as employment status?[3014] After all, who may be more apt to sleep in? Those without a job. Long sleepers (those sleeping at least nine hours a night) are more likely to be sedentary, obese, depressed, unmarried, and diabetic, and have a host of diseases that could confound the link between mortality and sleeping late.[3015] Studies have taken socioeconomic status and health conditions into account, but it's hard to control for everything.[3016] The bottom line? For adults sixty-five and older, the National Sleep Foundation recommends seven to eight hours of sleep a night,[3017] which correlates with about the sleep duration associated with the lowest risk of frailty[3018] and age-related muscle loss.[3019]

How to Get a Good Night's Sleep

Those who have sleep apnea, a common consequence of obesity that interferes with sleep, can benefit from the use of CPAP machines while they're losing the weight to treat the underlying cause.[3020] But what if that's not your problem and you still have difficulty falling or staying asleep? Check out my four rules of sleep conditioning and hygiene in see.nf/sleeprules, which involves cognitive behavioral therapy techniques,[3021] along with regulating the dose and timing of exercise, caffeine, nicotine, and alcohol, as well as establishing the best bedtime routines and sleep environment.

RISK WITHOUT REWARD

There is a common misconception that older individuals need less sleep.[3022] The reality is sleep may just be harder to get as we age. Insomnia symptoms increase with advancing age, with prevalence rates approaching 50 percent in adults sixty-five and older, and remission rates as high as 50 percent over three years.[3023] Thankfully, insomnia symptoms do not appear to correlate with mortality risk, though this may be partly because most people diagnosed with insomnia may actually end up getting more than six hours a night when their sleep is measured by objective means.[3024] Based on twin studies, insomnia has a heritability of 40 percent, meaning our genes account for less than half of insomnia risk.[3025] What can we do to flex the bulk we may have control over?

Sleeping pills are a nonstarter. Hypnotics are the class of sleeping pills that includes Ambien, the one most commonly prescribed.[3026] People who are prescribed even just half a dose or more a year appear to have more than three times the risk of dying prematurely compared to those receiving none.[3027] Up to 10 percent of the adult population are prescribed these drugs,[3028] so if these pills are truly killing people, that means they could be responsible for a six-figure death toll each year.[3029] Not surprisingly, the manufacturer of Ambien questioned the study,[3030] but it wasn't a one-off. It was one of two dozen studies that found a significant association between sleeping pills and premature death.[3031] In response to criticism for "reporting alarmingly high death risks from commonly used medications,"[3032] the principal investigator at the Scripps Clinic Sleep Center replied: "We cannot hide risks, even if they might frighten patients out of taking hypnotics. Patients have a right to know."[3033]

We also have a right to know that they may not even work. The most authoritative meta-analysis concluded that Ambien and Ambien-type drugs do not significantly increase total sleep time.[3034] How can that be? My patients used to tell me how much better it made them sleep. As it turns out, people only *think* they sleep better. Despite reporting that hypnotics gave them an extra half hour of sleep, objective measurements tell us they weren't getting significantly more sleep at all.[3035] The subjective sense that you sleep better after popping a pill appears to be a result of the drug's amnesic properties, meaning the hypnotics can erase your memories of just how badly you slept.[3036] The American Academy of Sleep Medicine recommends against the use of these drugs as a primary treatment for chronic insomnia.[3037]

Dip Your Toes In

Eating late at night not only exacerbates weight gain, as I cover in *How Not to Diet*, but may hinder our ability to fall asleep. Normally, around bedtime, there is a drop in our core body temperature,[3038] which seems to be one of our cues that it's time to sleep, but late-night munchies may interfere with that. In that case, wouldn't taking a hot shower be counterproductive? No. The moment you step out of the bath, the rapid decline in your skin temperature can enhance that natural nighttime drop and actually improve your sleep.[3039] Just soaking your feet in a warm bath may help you fall asleep about fifteen minutes faster.[3040]

Footbaths have been called a "safe, simple, and non-pharmacological method to improve sleep quality."[3041] A meta-analysis of trials found that enjoying a warm shower, footbath, or full-body bath for just ten minutes one to two hours before bedtime can help people fall asleep more quickly and sleep better.[3042]

Special blood vessels that connect the arteries and veins in the palms of our hands and the soles of our feet are dilated by the warm water, enhancing the transfer of heat from our core to our hands and feet, where it can be dissipated more efficiently to achieve that sleep-inducing drop in core temperature.[3043] Older adults have a blunted temperature response—perhaps helping to explain some of the age-related sleep difficulties—and that potentially makes measures to increase circulation in our hands and feet even more important.[3044]

Is there any way to accomplish this without getting wet? A hot water bottle by our feet might do it.[3045] Can we just wear warm socks? A study in which young men wore socks starting an hour before bedtime didn't subjectively improve sleep quality. Objectively, however, they slept about a half hour more than when sockless, thanks to falling asleep more quickly and waking up fewer times throughout the night.[3046]

MELATONIN AND LONGEVITY

Some experts recommend melatonin, a hormone secreted by the "third-eye" pineal gland in the middle of our head, as a first-line agent to treat insomnia in older adults.[3047] The World Sleep Society disagrees, due to its low efficacy.[3048] Subjectively, people report better sleep on melatonin,[3049] though, objectively, a meta-analysis of studies found that melatonin only helped people get to sleep four minutes faster and extended overall sleep duration by thirteen or so minutes.[3050] Concerning contaminants have also been found[3051] (see.nf/melatoninsupplements), though there are also natural sources in the diet (see.nf/melatoninfoods). I was more intrigued by its purported anti-aging benefits, but, as I document in see.nf/melatoninaging, the data are all over the place.[3052] In rats, for example, melatonin significantly improved survival, but so did a drug that *blocks* melatonin![3053]

Herbal Sleep Aids?

Valerian root is one of the most frequently studied herbs for sleep.[3054] However, most studies, including all the latest, most methodologically sound ones, found no significant benefit over placebo.[3055] Randomized controlled trials found that lemon verbena could help insomnia patients, at least subjectively,[3056] but chamomile could not.[3057] Chamomile may improve subjective sleep quality in noninsomniacs, though, based on a meta-analysis of five trials.[3058]

DON'T SLEEP WITH THE FISHES

In terms of food, low fiber intake, as well as high saturated fat and sugar intake, is associated with lighter, less restorative sleep.[3059] Meat consumption is associated with napping, which has been suggested as a proxy for sleepiness.[3060] This may be one of the reasons insomnia has been reported as a side effect of low-carb, ketogenic diets.[3061] Even after controlling for obesity, higher meat consumption appears to double the odds of snoring, with each daily serving of meat associated with 60 percent higher odds of diminished sleep quality and quantity in older adults. Both red meat and poultry were implicated,[3062] and no significant difference in objective sleep measures has been found for fish compared to chicken, pork, and beef.[3063]

Researchers have suggested that the amino acids like methionine in meat compete with tryptophan, which is the precursor to both melatonin and the "happiness hormone" serotonin, for transport to the brain.[3064,3065] This may help explain why randomizing people to restrict fish, poultry, and red meat has been shown to improve mood within two weeks.[3066] Plant proteins, on the other hand, tend to be relatively lower in methionine, which may help explain why a study of thousands of people put through the plant-based Adventist CHIP program reported a greater than 50 percent drop in reported insomnia and restless sleeping, not to mention declines in easy emotional upset and feelings of fearfulness or depression within four weeks.[3067,3068]

Salad Nights

Any vegetables that might help? *Lactuca sativa* is a plant that has traditionally been used in the treatment of insomnia.[3069] What is this exotic-sounding vegetable? Lettuce![3070] Lettuce extracts have evidently been used from the time of the Roman

Empire for sedation and sleep induction. Lettuce has a hypnotic substance in it called *lactucin*, which is what makes lettuce taste a little bitter. Sleep in both mice and rats is enhanced by romaine lettuce,[3071] which tends to have a higher lactucin content compared to other lettuces,[3072] but what about in people? I go through all the studies in see.nf/lettuce. The bottom line: A quarter teaspoon of ground lettuce seeds beat out placebo in a double-blind trial for improving sleep quality.[3073]

STRESS MANAGEMENT

According to the director of the largest and most comprehensive study of centenarians in the world,[3074] the average life expectancy with optimal health behaviors—meaning no tobacco or alcohol use, regular exercise, vegetarianism, and the effective management of stress—should reach into the late eighties. "[T]he vast majority of why one lives to their sixties or seventies versus these later octogenarian years," he and a colleague wrote, "would be explained by health habit choices."[3075] I've discussed diet and exercise. How important is stress management?

The American Psychological Association conducted national surveys and found that the majority of Americans report moderate to high levels of stress.[3076] Even though the prevalence of anxiety disorders has not experienced much change over the last few decades, the level of general psychological stress seems to be worsening.[3077] What implications does this have for life expectancy?

When stressed, the majority of people not only eat more[3078] but they tend to gravitate toward foods high in calories, fat, and sugar.[3079] When study participants were randomized to solvable and unsolvable word puzzles, for example, those in the more stressful situation chose less healthy snacks, M&M's rather than grapes.[3080] It's called *comfort food* for a reason. Overeating may be a sign that something is eating us.

Similar experimental studies have shown that acute stress tests can also induce cigarette cravings,[3081] increase alcohol intake,[3082] and contribute to relapses in illicit drug use.[3083] So, when studies show stressful life events, like the death of a child or a spouse, are associated with a shortened lifespan,[3084] what's really to blame? Might it just be these concomitant unhealthy behaviors?

Once you control for these secondary mediators, the significant link between stress and mortality does appear to disappear.[3085]

Keeping Occupied

Among the most poignant illustrations of the subordinate role of stress to lifestyle behaviors are the natural experiments set up by wartime deprivations. After all, what could be more stressful than living under Nazi occupation? Heart attack rates must have skyrocketed, right? No, studies in Nazi-occupied Norway,[3086] Finland, and blockaded Sweden showed the rates plummeting, dropping down to as little as only about one-fourth the preceding rate.[3087] Check out see.nf /worldwars to see what happens when meat, eggs, and butter are rationed,[3088] and food shortages result in diets dominated by garden produce.[3089] In reference to the Nazi occupation of Norway, an editorial in the *Journal of the American Medical Association* noted, "[S]tress has little or no effect if the diet is poor in animal fat."[3090]

SOCIAL TIES

Social connectivity is a blue zone attribute scrutinized for its potential role in supporting longevity.[3091] People who are married, for example, appear to have lower mortality rates than those who are single.[3092] The loss of a spouse or partner appears to increase mortality risk for both widowers and widows. However, "death from a broken heart"[3093] may be due in part to bereavement's association with increased use of cigarettes and alcohol.[3094] Higher mortality rates haunt those who lose a spouse not only through death but also through divorce. The never-married also seem to be at higher risk. Most of the studies documented no difference by gender, but, of the minority that did, most found that the risk of premature dying was greater for single men than single women.[3095]

The marriage advantage may be a consequence of selection bias or confounding factors. For example, healthier individuals are more likely to marry or stay married, and higher socioeconomic status and better health behaviors are found among married individuals. Nevertheless, studies that have tried to control for such factors continue to find a betrothal benefit.[3096]

Single or not, social isolation—an objective measure of social disconnectedness[3097]—and the subjective feeling of loneliness[3098] are both associated with an increased risk of premature death. But the effect is diminished when controlling for confounding factors,[3099] such as tobacco use or problems with alcohol associated with feelings of loneliness.[3100] There is also the nagging chicken-or-the-egg possibility of reverse causation, where, instead of social isolation leading to impaired health, the correlation may be due to ill health leading to the isolation.[3101]

Who Is Rescuing Whom?

Does slobbery social contact count? More than two-thirds of U.S. households, including mine, include a pet.[3102] In an "awww"-inspiring paper published in the prestigious journal *Science* titled "Oxytocin-Gaze Positive Loop and the Coevolution of Human-Dog Bonds," researchers found that petting or looking into the eyes of a canine companion leads to oxytocin release in the brains of both the humans and the dogs—the same "love hormone" that bonds breastfeeding mothers to their infants.[3103]

I was reading about the potential mechanisms by which our animal companions might improve our survival after a heart attack when I ran across a passage about a "profound" cardiovascular response when petting dogs or horses. "This response usually takes the form of a significant reduction in the heart rate and blood pressure." I could totally see that. But then the next sentence made me do a double take: "Unfortunately, we have no information about the physiological responses of the person doing the petting."[3104] The researchers were talking about the heart rate and blood pressure of the animals!

To my surprise, studies of the effects of companion animals on human health have, as one review put it, produced a "mishmash of conflicting results."[3105] For all the details, check out my video see.nf/pets. As you can imagine, the observational studies are rife with the potential for confounders[3106] and reverse causation,[3107] and the one interventional study that actually put animal companionship to the test involved "pet insects."[3108] Still, it can't hurt to heed this advice from a medical journal article published in 1925: "The best prescription to be written for a walk is to take a dog, a cane and a friend."[3109]

III. Preserving Function

PRESERVING YOUR BONES

Literally meaning *porous bone*, osteoporosis is characterized by reduced bone formation, excessive bone loss, or a combination of both, which leads to bone fragility[3110] and contributes to millions of fractures a year.[3111] Overall, the disease is estimated to affect two hundred million people worldwide.[3112]

Bone mineral density is used as a robust and consistent predictor of osteoporotic fracture.[3113] Although the bone density cutoff for an osteoporosis diagnosis is arbitrary,[3114] using the current definition, the disease may affect about one in ten women at age sixty, two in ten by age seventy, four in ten by age eighty, and six or seven out of ten by age ninety. Osteoporosis is typically thought of as affecting mostly women, but one-third of hip fractures occur in men.[3115] For fifty-year-old white women and men, for example, the lifetime risks for osteoporotic fractures are 40 percent and 13 percent, respectively.[3116]

The good news is that osteoporosis need not occur. Based on a study of the largest twin registry in the world, less than 30 percent of osteoporotic fracture risk is heritable. Researchers concluded that "fracture-prevention efforts at older ages should be focused on lifestyle habits."[3117] This is consistent with the enormous variation in hip fracture rates around the world, with the incidence of hip fracture varying tenfold, or even a hundredfold, between countries, suggesting that excessive bone loss is not an inevitable consequence of aging.[3118]

The U.S. Preventive Services Task Force (USPSTF), an independent scientific panel that sets evidence-based clinical prevention guidelines, recommends osteoporosis screening (such as the DXA scan of bone mineral density, also called DEXA) for all women from age sixty-five and potentially even earlier for postmenopausal women at increased risk, such as having a history of parental hip fracture, smoking, excessive alcohol consumption, or low body weight.[3119] What should you do if you're diagnosed? More important, what should you do to never *get* diagnosed? Before we explore the drugs on offering to treat osteoporosis, let's look at the drugs that may cause the disease.

ACID BLOCKERS MAY BE BAD TO THE BONE

Stomach acid–blocking "proton pump inhibitor" (PPI) drugs with brand names like Prilosec, Prevacid, Nexium, Protonix, and AcipHex are among the most popular medications in the world, raking in billions of dollars a year,[3120] but they come with a cost. As I document in see.nf/ppi, dozens of studies totaling more than two million people show higher hip fracture rates among both long- and short-term users at all dose levels.[3121] This class of drugs has been linked to increased risk of other possible adverse effects, such as pneumonia,[3122,3123] intestinal infections, kidney failure,[3124,3125] stomach cancer,[3126] cardiovascular disease,[3127] and premature death.[3128] What's more, once you start them, it can be hard to stop due to withdrawal symptoms.[3129] And, as I document in the video, the irony is that most people taking these drugs shouldn't even be on them in the first place.[3130]

To deal with acid reflux without drugs, recommendations include weight loss,[3131] smoking cessation,[3132] avoiding fatty meals,[3133] not eating within two to three hours of reclining,[3134] increased fiber consumption,[3135] and an overall more plant-based diet.[3136]

> ## Bones and Joints
>
> For decades, we've recognized that cigarette smoking can have a major effect on bone health, increasing the lifetime risk of hip fracture by about half.[3137] It also appears to impair bone healing,[3138] so much so that surgeons ask if they should discriminate against smokers because wound and bone healing complication rates are so high.[3139] Instead of cigarettes, what about smoking cannabis?[3140] I cover that in see.nf/joints. The bottom line: Heavy cannabis use does appear to be an independent predictor of weaker bones.[3141]

HOW EFFECTIVE ARE OSTEOPOROSIS DRUGS?

Drug therapy for osteoporosis is recommended for postmenopausal women or men aged fifty and older with a history of past hip or vertebral (spine) fractures, those with hip or spine "T-scores" ≤ -2.5, or those who don't make that cutoff but have an estimated 20 percent or greater risk of a major osteoporotic fracture over the subsequent decade or, specifically, an estimated 3 percent or higher risk of hip fracture.[3142]

T-score? That's a measure of how dense your bones are compared to the average thirty-year-old white woman. (Seriously.) Since we tend to lose bone as we get older, we can be labeled as having osteoporosis even if we have completely normal bone density for our age. However, just because our bone density may be normal doesn't mean it's necessarily optimal. That's one reason why the National Osteoporosis Foundation set out guidelines for drug treatment. Another reason, perhaps, is that it gets substantial funding from the pharmaceutical companies that rake in literally billions of dollars in profits from osteoporosis drugs.[3143] What does the science say? I run the numbers in see.nf/drugefficacy. Basically, surveys show that most people wouldn't take these osteoporosis drugs if they knew the truth,[3144] but it's for you to decide.

HOW SAFE ARE OSTEOPOROSIS DRUGS?

Most people prescribed these drugs stop taking them within a year, and it's not just because of the lack of perceived efficacy.[3145] Osteonecrosis of the jaw and atypical femur fractures are two rare but serious side effects. When they came to light, they contributed to more than a 50 percent drop in the use of these drugs.[3146] A *New York Times* article noting the decline began: "Reports of the drugs' causing jawbones to rot and thighbones to snap in two have shaken many osteoporosis patients so much that they say they would rather take their chances with the disease."[3147] In see.nf/drugsafety, I review just how likely these are and what can be done to reduce the risk.

HOW SAFE AND EFFECTIVE ARE CALCIUM SUPPLEMENTS?

Are there any supplements that might help reduce the risk of osteoporosis? In the Preserving Your Muscles chapter, I discuss how creatine can benefit muscle health in older adults, which could potentially translate into lower risk of falls, but it failed to do so when put to the test.[3148] The vast majority of studies show no benefit from creatine for bone health.[3149] What about supplementing calcium and vitamin D?

In just a dozen years, expert panels shifted from suggesting widespread calcium supplementation to prevent osteoporosis[3150] to telling patients "do not supplement,"[3151] the suggestion still in effect for most people today.[3152] I detail what happened in my video see.nf/calciumsafety. In short, calcium supplements appear to raise the risk of heart attacks and strokes[3153] by leading to unnaturally large, rapid, and sustained calcium levels in the blood[3154] that increase the risks of abnormal clotting.[3155]

Having a heart attack or stroke can be devastating, but so can fracturing your hip. How effective are calcium supplements in preventing hip fractures? Calcium intake in general does not seem to be related to hip fracture risk at all.[3156] If anything, randomized controlled trials suggest a 64 percent *greater* risk of hip fractures with calcium supplementation compared to placebo. In my video see .nf/calciumeffectiveness, I explore how we even got the idea that taking calcium supplements might help our bones. Basically, evidence suggests that dietary calcium intake is not something most people need to worry about,[3157] given our body's ability to absorb more and excrete less at lower intakes.[3158] Don't push it too far, though. Once you get down to just a few hundred milligrams per day, you can suffer significantly more bone loss.[3159]

THE BEST VITAMIN D DOSING TO PREVENT FALLS

Too much vitamin D can be harmful, too. In my video see.nf/vitamindfalls, I run through the studies showing that periodic megadoses, like a single dose of 500,000 units once a year, can increase fall risk compared to placebo.[3160] Increased falls were also seen after giving 100,000[3161] or 60,000 units once a month.[3162] On a daily basis, a yearlong randomized, double-blind, placebo-controlled trial of seven different doses of vitamin D found that elderly women randomized to the medium doses (1,600, 2,400, or 3,200 units a day) were significantly less likely to fall than those given either the lower doses (400 or 800 units a day) or the higher doses (4,000 or 4,800 units a day).[3163] Additionally, taking 4,000 or 10,000 units a day for three years *decreased* bone mineral density,[3164] especially in women,[3165] so you don't want to overdo it.

DOES MILK REALLY DO A BODY GOOD?

Which foods might help our bones? Milk comes to mind, but it appears that's just an empty marketing ploy. There haven't been any randomized controlled trials,[3166] but most meta-analyses of dairy milk consumption and hip fracture population studies have shown no overall protection.[3167] In fact, Dr. Walter Willett, past chair of Harvard's nutrition department, went so far as to suggest that it might even contribute to the high incidence of hip fractures in countries with the greatest milk consumption.[3168] It was that enigma that inspired a Swedish research team to perform a set of studies involving 100,000 men and women followed for up to twenty years.[3169] They found that milk intake appeared to *increase* bone and hip fracture rates, as well as shorten people's lives.[3170]

As I explore in my video see.nf/milkbones, the culprit appears to be the galactose, a breakdown product of the milk sugar lactose. Galactose is actually used by scientists to induce premature aging in lab animals. In one such study, after being given galactose, the "life-shortened animals showed neurodegeneration, mental retardation and cognitive dysfunction . . . diminished immune responses and reduction of reproductive ability."[3171] It doesn't take much, either—just the human equivalent of one to two glasses' worth of milk a day.[3172] But humans aren't lab animals. We've known for nearly a century, for instance, that you can cause cataracts in rats by feeding them a lot of lactose or galactose.[3173] The epidemiological data, however, are mixed as to whether dairy does the same in people.[3174]

With the then largest-ever study on milk intake and mortality showing such adverse effects, Harvard researchers stepped in with three of their cohorts to form a study twice as big to see whether the Swedish findings were just a fluke. After following more than 200,000 men and women for up to three decades, they confirmed the bad news in 2019. Those who consumed more dairy lived significantly shorter lives.[3175] Every additional half serving of regular milk a day was associated with a 9 percent increased risk of dying from cardiovascular disease, an 11 percent increased risk of dying from cancer, and an 11 percent increased risk of dying from all causes put together. More details in see.nf/milkupdate.

Highly influential advocacy organizations, such as the U.S. National Osteoporosis Foundation and the European-based International Osteoporosis Foundation, continue to push dairy, drugs, and calcium supplements. Perhaps their objectivity is compromised by the influence of their commercial sponsors, which include companies that market (you guessed it) dairy, drugs, and supplements.[3176] Conflict of interest is a legitimate concern. Most recent reviews on dairy and osteoporosis in the English-language medical literature were found to be written by those with ties to the dairy industry.[3177] A primary justification for inclusion of dairy in federal nutrition recommendations is based on purported bone benefits that are not supported by the available scientific evidence.[3178]

What if dietary guidelines were drafted without commercial influence? As I've mentioned, Canada recently decided to exclude industry reports and stick to the science in the formation of its new dietary guidelines. Major changes included a new emphasis on plant-based food intake, along with the removal of the dairy food group.[3179]

ACID/BASE BALANCE AND BONE

For most of the last century, a prevailing theory within the field of nutrition was that eating acid-forming foods such as meat was, in essence, putting us at risk of peeing our bones down the toilet.[3180] But as I describe in my video see.nf/acidbone, we've come to learn that most of the extra calcium people lose in their urine after a protein-rich meal comes from increased calcium absorption, not their bones.[3181] So, if our body isn't using our bones to primarily buffer the acid formed from our diet, how is it neutralizing the acid? As I explore on page 412 in Caught Off Base, the answer may lie with our muscles. (Our kidneys can buffer acid with a base they make from the muscle breakdown product *glutamine*.[3182])

At high enough acid loads, though, bone may be affected, too. Sadly, bone fractures are a side effect that disproportionately plagues kids with intractable epilepsy who are placed on ketogenic diets.[3183] Even a few weeks on a keto diet may have negative effects on bone remodeling markers.[3184] Such diets appear to cause a steady rate of bone loss as measured in the spine,[3185] thought due to the fact that ketones themselves are acidic[3186] and can result in a mild metabolic acidosis.[3187] It could also be all the saturated fat. The predominant saturated fat, palmitic acid, is toxic to bone-building cells in a petri dish.[3188] In general, the intake of saturated fat is significantly associated with increased hip fracture risk.[3189]

As we grow older, the pH of our blood falls to the lower (more acidic) end of the spectrum, perhaps due in part to the declining ability of our kidneys to excrete acid with age.[3190] In vitro studies suggest that this drop in pH may lead to activation of the cells that break down bone, as well as an inhibition of bone-building cells.[3191] This may explain why, when researchers removed alkaline-forming foods (fruits and vegetables) from people's diets, a marker of bone formation (bone-specific alkaline phosphatase) significantly dropped and a bone resorption marker (carboxy-terminal cross-linking telopeptide) shot up, and vice versa when they then added six cups of fruits and vegetables to the participants' daily diets.[3192]

In individuals sixty-five or older, the greater the estimated ratio between acid-forming foods and alkaline-forming foods, the greater the risk of hip fracture.[3193] (To see which foods are which, see the figure on page 413.) To prove cause and effect, two-year randomized, double-blind, placebo-controlled trials were performed in which three added servings of fruits and vegetables[3194] or the equivalent of six failed to have an effect, but nine daily servings of fruits' and vegetables' worth[3195] of an alkaline-forming compound (potassium citrate) was able to successfully increase bone volume and density.[3196] This shows that buffering the dietary acid load of a typical Western diet with enough fruits and vegetables may help prevent bone loss.

PRUNING YOUR SKELETON

Inflammation and oxidative stress may also play a role in osteoporosis. The intake of pro-inflammatory foods[3197] and an elevation of inflammatory markers in the blood, such as C-reactive protein, are both associated with osteoporotic fractures,[3198] and postmenopausal women with osteoporosis tend to harbor greater signs of oxidative damage and fewer antioxidants in their blood.[3199] These are two more reasons why a higher intake of fruits and vegetables is associated with lower fracture risk.[3200] Vitamin C is a third. The consumption of vitamin C–rich foods is associated with lower risk of bone loss, osteoporosis, and hip fracture[3201]—a 5 percent lower hip fracture risk for every 50 mg of vitamin C a day, which is about the amount in one orange.[3202] Are there any fruits and vegetables that are particularly good?

After feeding rats more than fifty different foods, the fruit found to preserve their bones the best was the prune and the leading vegetable was the onion.[3203] What about in people? I review the available evidence in see.nf/prunes. The bottom line is that five or six prunes a day may help preserve bone density.[3204]

CRY YOUR WAY TO THE BANK

What was that about onions? I review both the preclinical and clinical data in see.nf/onionstomatoes. Basically, onions can lead to an improvement in a marker of bone loss in people,[3205] but the study didn't last long enough to see if this translated into tangible bone benefits. However, a clinical trial on the other vegetable put to the test did.

HITTING THE SAUCE

In the same video (see.nf/onionstomatoes), I review all the tomato juice[3206] and sauce[3207] studies, as well as the Scarborough Fair Diet (which includes prunes, onions, tomatoes, and presumptive bone-protecting herbs parsley, sage, rosemary, and thyme, from the song popularized by Simon and Garfunkel).[3208] The bottom line is that we can probably just focus on stuffing our faces with fruits and vegetables of any stripe.

TEA AND TEETOTALING

What about beverages? A meta-analysis on the effect of alcohol on osteoporosis found that, compared to abstainers, people who sipped one to two drinks a day had a 34 percent increased risk of developing osteoporosis.[3209] Having more than two a day bumped up that elevated risk to 63 percent, which appears to translate into an increase in hip fracture risk.[3210] This may be partially from alcohol's negative effect on bone health and also because of fall risk due to impaired coordination.[3211]

One way sugary soda appears to cause negative effects on bone is the same way[3212] sodium does: by increasing calcium loss through the urine.[3213] It doesn't appear to be the caffeine, though: Drinking three or more cups of coffee daily is associated with a doubling of hip fracture risk, but habitual tea consumption is associated with significantly *lower* risk.[3214] Hope was raised that the tea link was cause and effect when a randomized trial found an improvement in bone turnover markers in women[3215] and higher actual bone mass in tea-fed rats.[3216] But, in the Minnesota Green Tea Trial, the largest and longest clinical trial on the effects of green tea extracts on postmenopausal women, no significant benefit on bone mineral density was found.[3217]

NUTS AND BONES

Researchers in the world-famous lab of Dr. David Jenkins exposed human osteoclasts, the bone-eating cells, to blood obtained before, as well as four hours after, eating a handful of almonds. Details in see.nf/bonenuts, but basically, almonds may be able to help prevent bone loss but not build bones,[3218] whereas the opposite was found for prunes—so a combo prune-and-almond trail mix may be in order.

ESTROGENS VS. PHYTOESTROGENS

When the Women's Health Initiative study found that menopausal women taking hormone replacement therapy suffered "higher rates of breast cancer, cardiovascular disease, and overall harm," a call was made for safer alternatives.[3219] Yes, the Women's Health Initiative found that supplemental estrogen does have positive effects, such as reducing menopausal symptoms, improving bone health, and reducing hip fracture risk, but negative effects include increased risk of blood clots to the heart, brain, and lungs, as well as breast cancer.[3220]

Ideally, to get the best of both worlds, we'd need what's called a selective estrogen receptor modulator—something with pro-estrogenic effects in tissues like bone but, at the same time, *anti*-estrogenic effects in other tissues like the breast.[3221] Drug companies are trying to make these, but the phytoestrogens in soybeans like genistein, which is structurally similar to estrogen, appear to function as natural selective estrogen receptor modulators. How could something that looks like estrogen act as an *anti*-estrogen?

In my video see.nf/phytoestrogens, I explain how soy can have it both ways, thanks to the discovery of two different types of estrogen receptors in the body—bone-strengthening effects without this risk of clots[3222] and cancer.[3223] A 2020 meta-analysis of more than five dozen randomized controlled trials of soy phytoestrogens with postmenopausal women found significantly improved bone mineral density compared to control in the hip, spine, and wrist.[3224] When tested head-to-head, it was even comparable to hormone replacement therapy.[3225] In a two-year study, for example, soymilk was compared to a transdermal progesterone cream and a placebo control group. The control group lost significant bone mineral density in their spine over the two years, whereas the progesterone group lost significantly less. However, the group drinking two glasses of soymilk a day ended up with *more* bone than when they started.[3226]

Soymilk also appears to have the additional benefits of reducing risk of breast[3227] and prostate[3228] cancers, improving gut health,[3229] and decreasing inflammation[3230] and free radical DNA damage compared to rice milk or dairy milk.[3231] It can also improve insulin resistance[3232] and help with stroke rehabilitation, improving walking speed, exercise endurance, grip strength, and muscle functionality,[3233] as well as lower blood pressure better than dairy milk.[3234] Soymilk can even lower your LDL cholesterol as much as 25 percent after just twenty-one days.[3235] Nutritionally, soymilk is considered the best choice for replacing dairy milk in the human diet.[3236]

The reason we care about bone mass is that we want to prevent fractures. Dairy products can also increase bone density,[3237] but this fails to translate into decreased hip fracture risk.[3238] Soy foods, however, have consistently been significantly associated with 20 to 50 percent lower risk of fracture in women,[3239] starting with as little as a single serving of soy a day—the equivalent of just 5 to 7 g of soy protein or 20 to 30 mg of phytoestrogens,[3240] which is about a cup of soymilk or, even better, a single serving of a whole soy food like tempeh, edamame, or the mature beans themselves.[3241] We have no fracture data on soy supplements, but it's better to stick to whole foods anyway rather than taking pills or powders, especially since "huge differences" have been found in isoflavone content when identically labeled commercial soy isoflavone supplements have been tested.[3242]

WHAT ABOUT THE "ANTI-NUTRIENTS" IN BEANS?

So-called anti-nutrients are plant compounds that purportedly reduce the absorption of nutrients. But recently, the whole concept of "anti-nutrients" has been called into question, and some of them may in fact be beneficial.[3243] Details in see.nf/milks.

Plant-Based Bones

With studies showing that an increased consumption of plant foods is associated with increased bone mineral density,[3244] while a more animal-sourced nutrient pattern is associated with a higher risk of fractures, one would expect less osteoporosis in those eating plant-based diets. The data, however, are mixed.[3245] In see.nf/vegbone, I review the last half century of available evidence.

Vegetarians and vegans tend to have lower bone mineral density compared to meat eaters,[3246] but most of the difference effectively disappeared once body size was taken into account. Thus, it's not so much the composition of the diets of vegetarians and vegans as much as it's the fact that they are typically so much slimmer.[3247]

Hip fracture risk goes down as weight goes up. Nearly half of under-weight women have osteoporosis, for example, but less than 1 percent of obese women, which makes total sense.[3248] Being obese forces your body to make your bones stronger to carry around extra pounds. That's why weight-bearing exercise is important; it constantly puts stress on your skeleton. And vegetarians—especially vegans—have such low rates of obesity that it's no won-der they would have lower bone density on average. Does this translate into elevated fracture risk?

I review all the fracture data in my video see.nf/vegfractures, but, in short, the answer is yes[3249]—and not only because vegans are generally more slen-der[3250] but because of the potential for inadequate vitamin D status and calcium intake.[3251] I recommend 2,000 IU of supplemental vitamin D a day for those getting inadequate sun exposure[3252] and at least 600 mg of calcium daily[3253] via calcium-rich plant foods—preferably low-oxalate dark green leafy vegeta-bles, which include all greens except spinach, chard, and beet greens. (All very healthy foods, but just stingy with their calcium.)

EXERCISE EARLY AND OFTEN

When it comes to bone health, it's use it or lose it. That's why astronauts can lose 1 percent of their bone mass *every month* they're not on planet Earth.[3254] Their bodies aren't stupid. Why waste all that energy making a strong skeleton if you're just floating around and not putting any weight on it? Physical activity is consid-ered a "widely accessible, low cost, and highly modifiable contributor to bone health."[3255] However, some exercises are more effective than others, as I detail in see .nf/weightbearing.

Not by Any Stretch

Lower-impact activities like yoga are generally not considered to be bone-building,[3256] despite misleading studies[3257] purporting otherwise. (Details in see .nf/yogabones.) In fact, yoga may even result in vertebral compression fractures. Safer poses include those with mild spine extension and leg stretching, like the warrior pose; poses to be avoided include extreme spinal flexion or extension (like the forward fold or the camel), neck strain (like the plow), or low back/hip strain (like the one-legged pigeon), which may cause fractures even in people with normal or near-normal bone mass density.[3258]

Based on a systematic review involving more than 9,000 yoga practitioners, the risk of yoga-associated injuries is lower than from higher-impact activities[3259] such as running,[3260] with the exception of meniscus damage in the knee, presumed to be due to yoga postures like the lotus position.[3261] Hot (Bikram) yoga carries its own risk.[3262] Watch see.nf/yogarisk for a list of recommendations to stay safe.

THE SINGLE MOST IMPORTANT THING TO DO TO PREVENT OSTEOPOROTIC FRACTURES

Bone mineral density screening is a billion-dollar industry,[3263] so it shouldn't be that surprising that's the focus of osteoporosis and treatment. But among women sixty-five and older, only 15 percent of low-trauma fractures (meaning from a fall from no more than standing height) are due to osteoporosis.[3264] Between the ages of sixty and eighty, hip fracture risk increases thirteenfold in men and women, whereas the age-related decline in bone mineral density accounted only for a twofold increased risk.[3265] So, 85 percent of the age-related rise in hip fracture risk has nothing to do with the measured density of your bones.

Without a fall, even fragile hips don't fracture. The primary cause of fractures—including vertebral fractures—are falls.[3266] The disparity between men and women in hip fracture rates seems primarily not because men have stronger bones but because women fall more often.[3267] Doctors simply asking the question *"Do you have impaired balance?"* can predict about 40 percent of all hip fractures,[3268] which is more than a bone scan diagnosis of osteoporosis can.[3269] Even a weak osteoporotic bone is strong enough to survive normal life activities without the excessive loading that comes from the impact of a fall or, in the case of the spine, bending with your back rather than your knees to lift something.[3270]

The primacy of falls in fracture risk explains a number of apparent osteoporosis paradoxes. For example, despite the fact that about 70 percent of bone mass is determined by your genes,[3271] the heritability of hip fractures appears negligible[3272] because the propensity to fall is much less inherited.[3273] It also explains the poor predictive value of DXA scanning for fractures. Adding bone mineral density measures to a hip risk score based just on age, sex, height, weight, the use of a walking aid, and cigarette smoking status did little to improve its predictive power.[3274] A provocative editorial published in the *Journal of Internal Medicine* titled "Osteoporosis: The Emperor Has No Clothes" suggested it would therefore be safer and more effective to focus on fall prevention rather than pharmaceutical intervention.[3275]

Though only about 5 percent of falls result in a fracture, falls are very common among the aged.[3276] Due in part to age-related muscle weakness and loss of balance,[3277] more than a third of those sixty-five and older fall each year.[3278] After a hip fracture, less than 50 percent may regain their pre-fracture function in terms of walking ability and independence.[3279] What can we do to prevent injurious falls? Exercise.[3280] Based on dozens of randomized controlled trials, exercise is the single intervention most strongly associated with a reduction in falls rate.[3281]

HOW TO PREVENT FALLS

Based on eighty-one trials, compared to control groups, those randomized to exercise reduced the rate of falls by 23 percent and lowered the number of people who end up falling by 15 percent. So, if you followed 1,000 people around age seventy-five for a year and 480 of them fell a total of 850 times without exercise, adding exercise would be expected to result in 72 fewer people falling and 195 fewer falls. Tai Chi appears to reduce falls by 19 percent, balance and functional exercises (like sit to stand) may reduce falls by 24 percent, and multiple exercises—typically balance and functional exercise plus strength training—may reduce falls by 34 percent.[3282]

The reduced-falls rate translates into fewer fractures. A recent meta-analysis found that exercise interventions—ones mostly using a combination of resistance exercise to improve lower limb muscle strength training and balance training—cut fracture rates nearly in half.[3283] One yearlong trial combining strength training with step and jumping aerobics that focused on balance and agility[3284] resulted in 74 percent fewer fractures over the five-year period after the study ended.[3285] More than 70 percent of the women in the exercise group did not have a single injurious fall during those five years, compared to more than half in the control group who did.

Trials on hip protectors, which use plastic shields or foam pads sewn into special underwear to cushion a sideways fall on the hip, are often plagued with poor compliance due primarily to discomfort, particularly in bed.[3286] Studies have not found them to be useful for reducing hip fracture rates among those living at home, but trials in nursing homes and residential care facilities do show a small reduction in risk, translating into about eleven fewer people out of a thousand suffering hip fractures due to wearing hip protection.[3287]

There are also commonsense measures we can employ. Quality improvement trials involving interventions like patient education have shown a 10 percent reduction in falls rates.[3288] We can, for example, keep things within reach so we don't need to use step stools, use nonslip mats in the bath and shower,[3289] add grab bars in the bathroom, keep floors clutter-free, remove small throw rugs or use double-sided tape to keep them from slipping, and make sure all staircases have handrails and adequate lighting.[3290] We could also avoid walks during inclement weather and, for those of us who walk leashed dogs, consider adopting smaller breeds or ensuring proper training to prevent them from lunging.[3291]

Otherwise, the main ways to prevent fractures may not have changed much over the last thirty years since the classic paper titled "Strategies for Prevention of Osteoporosis and Hip Fracture"[3292] exhorted us to "stop smoking, be active and eat well."[3293]

PRESERVING YOUR BOWEL AND BLADDER FUNCTION

Lasting for more than 3,000 years, ancient Egypt was one of the greatest early civilizations. They had a vastly underestimated knowledge of medicine, which even included medical subspecialties. The pharaohs, for example, had access to dedicated physicians to serve as "guardian[s] of the royal bowel movement,"[3294] a title alternatively translated from the hieroglyphs to mean *Shepherd of the Anus*.[3295] How's that for a résumé builder?

Today, the primacy of the bowel movement's importance continues. Some have called for bowel habits, along with heart rate, blood pressure, and breathing rate, to be considered a vital sign of how the body is functioning.[3296] Optimal frequency, as derived in see.nf/bms, is probably two or three bowel movements a day. However, the most important criterion for establishing a constipation diagnosis is not frequency[3297] but, rather, consideration of the most prevalent symptom: straining.[3298] Ideally, bowel movements should be effortless.

CONSTIPATION

Constipation is considered the most common gastrointestinal complaint in the United States,[3299] leading to millions of doctors' appointments each year[3300] and 800,000 emergency room visits.[3301] Older adults are at increased risk, perhaps due to decreased dietary fiber, fluids, and physical activity.[3302] Constipation affects up to 30 percent of those sixty-five and older, up to 50 percent of individuals older than eighty-five,[3303] and as many as two-thirds of those living in geriatric-care facilities.[3304] Other than straining at hard stool and infrequent bowel movements, symptoms of constipation can include abdominal discomfort and pain, bloating, nausea, and rectal bleeding during defecation.[3305] Though it can often be benign, any sign of blood from bathrooming should always be something you get checked out by a medical professional. Other red-flag symptoms include unintentional weight loss of more than 10 percent over three months, a family history of inflammatory bowel disease or colorectal cancer, jaundice, new-onset symptoms starting after age fifty, and rectal tenesmus, which is the sensation of being unable to empty your bowels even though there's nothing in there.

DON'T STRAIN YOURSELF

A systematic review of the impact of constipation on people's lives found that the decrease in quality of life was comparable to that experienced by persons suffering from conditions such as osteoarthritis, rheumatoid arthritis, chronic allergies, and diabetes.[3306] Despite the shadow cast over everyday life, surveys show that many U.S. adults suffering from chronic constipation have never discussed their symptoms with a healthcare provider. The taboo appears to go both ways, as health professionals seldom pay sufficient attention to bowel function,[3307] which has been recognized as a "serious oversight" of the medical profession by a consensus panel of experts.[3308]

Even people who don't think they are may very well be clinically constipated.[3309] In one study in Ohio, for example, a quarter of the so-called healthy subjects reported experiencing incomplete emptying and almost half indicated increased straining when defecating[3310]—so much so, in fact, that more than half had found blood on their toilet paper within the past year.

Straining when trying to pass small, firm stools can certainly cause discomfort, but, beyond the pain, firm stools may contribute to a variety of health problems. For example, more than one in five Americans suffer from hiatal hernias,[3311] a condition where part of the stomach is pushed up and through the diaphragm into the chest. Hiatal hernias are uncommon among populations eating plant-based diets, who have rates closer to one in a thousand.[3312] Why such a great discrepancy?

Plant-based eaters tend to smoothly pass large, soft stools. If you routinely strain during bowel movements, over time, the increased pressure to push out stool can actually push part of the stomach up and out of the abdomen, which allows acid to reflux up toward the throat and cause symptoms like heartburn.[3313] This same pressure exerted on the toilet week after week can also cause other issues, including hemorrhoids and varicose veins,[3314] as well as anal fissure and other painful conditions.[3315]

Have you ever squeezed a stress ball? If you have, then you know how tightening your hand around it causes balloon-like bubbles to bulge out. Similarly, the pressure from straining on the toilet may cause pockets to pop out from the wall of the colon, a condition known as diverticulosis. The increased abdominal pressure may also back up blood flow in the veins around the anus, causing hemorrhoids, and even push blood flow back into the legs, resulting in varicose veins.[3316] But, a fiber-rich diet can relieve the pressure—in both directions. Those who eat diets that revolve around whole plant foods tend to pass unforced bowel movements,[3317] which results in more than twenty-five times lower rates of "pressure diseases," such as diverticulitis, hemorrhoids, varicose veins, and hiatal hernias.[3318]

(As a TMI side note—don't say I didn't warn you!—once when I was showering, to my chagrin, I detected a . . . well . . . "posterior" lump. How could I, of all people, have a hemorrhoid? I even named one of my guinea pigs after "fiber man" Denis Burkitt! After a few more seconds of inspection, I realized that I *wished* I just had a hemorrhoid. The lump had legs. Thus concludes the story of how I discovered a huge, bloated anal tick.)

Protracted straining can also cause heart rhythm disturbances and a reduction in blood flow to the heart and brain, which may result in defecation-related fainting and even, under certain circumstances, death.[3319] Just fifteen seconds of straining can temporarily cut blood flow to the brain by 21 percent[3320] and to the heart by nearly 50 percent, thereby providing a mechanism for "bedpan death" syndrome.[3321] If you think you have to strain a lot while sitting, try having a bowel movement while you're flat on your back. Bearing down for just a few seconds while supine can send up our blood pressure to nearly 170 over 110, which may help account for the notorious frequency of sudden and unexpected deaths of patients while using bedpans in hospitals.[3322]

When treated inadequately, constipation can also lead to fecal impaction, which could require emergency hospitalization.[3323] Older individuals facing a "half in, half out" crisis[3324] may try manual self-disimpaction—removing stool by hand—a procedure that can be painful, distressing, and potentially harmful.[3325] The optimal remedy is to prevent constipation in the first place.

Best Pooping Position for Constipation

What about the influence of body position on defecation? While squatting remains the traditional position in some parts of Asia and Africa, Westerners have become accustomed to sitting on toilet seats. When you sit upright, however, your "anorectal angle" doesn't straighten enough. That kink at the end of the rectum helps keep us from pooping our pants. In a sitting toilet posture, your poop must make a nearly ninety-degree turn, defeating the purpose of this brilliant design.[3326] Trying to poop while seated is like trying to drive a car without releasing the parking brake.[3327] Check out see.nf/positioning for all the research, but basically, we can manipulate the anorectal angle through squatting or leaning to more easily pass unnaturally firm stools, but why not just treat the cause and eat enough fiber-containing whole plant foods to create stools so large and soft that you could pass them effortlessly at any angle?[3328]

LAX LAXATIVE EFFICACY

The desperation to treat constipation is embodied by medical gadgets that range from automated abdominal massage devices that strap around your midsection[3329] to vibrating capsules you swallow to buzz you from the inside out.[3330] More ominously, colectomies for chronic constipation are on the rise.[3331] Complications of colon resection occur in approximately 1 in 4 operations, and 1 in 250 procedures result in death.[3332] The most common treatments, though, are over-the-counter remedies, such as laxatives, that cash out in excess of a billion dollars in sales every year.[3333]

Despite more than a hundred randomized clinical trials on various constipation treatments,[3334] we still lack high-quality evidence on the safety and effectiveness of laxatives in older adults.[3335] The stool softener docusate, for example, which is sold as Colace, doesn't appear to effectively relieve constipation despite its frequent use as one of the most common over-the-counter agents.[3336] Stimulant laxatives, such as senna or bisacodyl (Dulcolax), are only approved for short-term usage of fewer than four weeks, but, unfortunately, long-term use for months or even years is widespread.[3337] Biopsies taken from long-term stimulant laxative users show that the nerves innervating their colon can be "severely damaged."[3338]

The over-the-counter laxative with the best safety[3339] and efficacy[3340] record is probably polyethylene glycol, which is sold as MiraLAX or Glycolax—not to be confused with *ethylene* glycol, or antifreeze, which can be fatal if ingested.[3341]

The majority of drugs currently available for the treatment of constipation are generally safe when used as directed, but their effectiveness leaves much to be desired.[3342] In a survey of more than one thousand men and women suffering from chronic constipation, the majority taking over-the-counter medications reported little or no satisfaction at all with the drugs' effect on their constipation (62 percent) or constipation-related abdominal symptoms (78 percent).[3343] There has got to be a better way.

SMOOTH MOVES

There are many lifestyle approaches to treating constipation, such as eating breakfast with a hot beverage to help kick off the gastrocolic reflex,[3344] but the holy trinity that doctors preach about most often is dietary fiber, fluids, and exercise.[3345] In terms of exercise, population studies don't seem to show a clear association between constipation and physical activity after other factors, like fiber consumption, are taken into account, but you can't know for sure until you put it to the test.[3346]

Inactivity does seem to slow things down. When active older individuals became sedentary, dropping their daily step counts from about 13,000 down to 4,000, they nearly doubled their colonic transit time within two weeks.[3347] (The time it takes food to get from mouth to anus can be measured by using the "blue poo" test with food coloring or just eating some beets.[3348]) Conversely, even mild physical activity has been shown to reduce symptoms of abdominal distention and bloating, but what about constipation?

To date, there have been nine randomized controlled trials in adults of exercise for constipation. Even moderate aerobic exercise, such as walking twenty minutes a day, was shown to be able to improve mild constipation symptoms,[3349] though this has not been tested for severe constipation.[3350] What about fluids?

I review all the interventional studies on increasing fluid intake and constipation in see.nf/mineralwater, including the risks and benefits of using Epsom salts (magnesium sulfate) and minerals introduced in the opposite direction via sodium phosphate enemas (sold as Fleet). I conclude that the best remedy for constipation may be to *treat the cause* by ensuring an adequate intake of fiber, considered the first-line treatment for the management of constipation.[3351]

A FIBER DEFICIENCY DISEASE

Constipation can be considered a disease of nutrient deficiency—and that nutrient is fiber.[3352] Not even 3 percent of Americans meet the recommended minimum daily intake of fiber, meaning Americans are not eating enough whole plant foods, the only place fiber is found in abundance.[3353] No wonder those eating strictly plant-based diets are three times more likely to have daily bowel movements.[3354] If just half of the adult U.S. population ate an additional 3 g of fiber a day—a quarter cup of beans or a bowl of oatmeal—we could potentially save billions in medical costs for constipation alone, based on an estimate that, on a population scale, a daily increase of just 1 g of dietary fiber would lead to about a 2 percent reduction in constipation prevalence.[3355] It's hard to create a shredded wheat placebo, but you can prove cause and effect with randomized, double-blind, placebo-controlled trials using fiber supplements.

FIBER SUPPLEMENTS

By far the most commonly used treatment for constipation,[3356] fiber supplements are recommended as first-line management by American, European, and global guidelines.[3357] Soluble nonfermentable fibers, such as psyllium (also known as is-paghula and sold as Metamucil), are touted as the most appropriate first choice.[3358] Psyllium traps water in the intestine, increasing stool water content and bulk to ease defecation, but it's for this very reason that it's important to take it as directed—with sufficient fluid intake.[3359] Otherwise, psyllium itself can cause its own intestinal obstruction.[3360] Check out see.nf/fibersupplements for details on efficacy and potential ancillary benefits.

FIBER FROM FOODS, NOT FILLERS

The best way to get fiber is not from the supplement aisle but from the produce aisle and, even more so, from the bulk bean and whole grain section. In addition to bowel regularity, high dietary fiber intake is associated with a reduced risk of heart disease,[3361,3362] cancer,[3363] obesity,[3364] diabetes,[3365] depression,[3366] and premature death in general.[3367] Every 7 g of daily fiber intake correlates to a 9 percent reduced risk in heart disease, our number one killer.[3368] So, would 77 g a day drop our risk by 99 percent? That's about how much fiber they used to eat in Uganda,[3369] a country in which coronary heart disease was almost nonexistent.[3370]

Heart disease was so rare among those eating traditional plant-based diets in Uganda that papers were published with such titles as "A Case of Coronary Heart Disease in an African."[3371] After twenty-six years of medical practice in East Africa, doctors finally recorded their first case of coronary heart disease. (The patient was a judge who consumed a "partially Westernized diet," in which fiber-free foods, such as meat, dairy, and eggs, displaced some of the plant foods in his traditional diet.) Of course, since eating habits have been westernized across the continent, cardiovascular disease is now the noncommunicable disease killing the most people there as well—going from virtually nonexistent to an epidemic.[3372]

The early rarity of typical Western diseases in rural regions of sub-Saharan Africa led to the *dietary fiber hypothesis*, which suggested that diets centered around whole plant foods are so protective against chronic disease because of their fiber content.[3373] Predictably, a multibillion-dollar fiber supplement market arose.[3374] There's a problem, though. They don't work.[3375]

Fiber supplements can be helpful with constipation, but they don't seem to provide any of the other chronic disease benefits. Indeed, studies associating lower risk of disease and death with high fiber intake relate exclusively to fiber from *food*— *not* from fiber isolates or supplements.[3376] This may be because fiber is a marker of healthy, whole plant food intake, or because of its role as a smuggler.[3377]

The primary role of dietary fiber may be to encapsulate nutrients to deliver them to our gut microbiome. Fiber is the brick that builds the cell walls of plants, and those cell walls act as indigestible physical barriers. So, when you eat structurally intact plant foods, some of the nutrition remains trapped. You can chew all you want, but you'll still end up with nutrients like starch completely surrounded by fiber, delivering sustenance to your friendly flora. Your good gut flora then get to eat not only the fiber but all the food it's wrapped around, too. Fiber supplements like psyllium, however, fail to carry any bounty to our bacteria and aren't even fermentable themselves, so we may miss out on all the auxiliary benefits high-fiber diets give your microbiome.[3378]

Flax and Rye

Ground flaxseeds are an excellent whole-food source of fiber.[3379] For twelve weeks, constipated diabetics were randomized to cookies containing about a tablespoon a day of milled flaxseeds or flax-free placebo cookies. Not only did the flax improve constipation symptoms, such as defecation pain, straining, and hard stools, but, compared to placebo, its consumption resulted in an eight-pound weight loss, twenty-five-point lower fasting blood sugars, an astounding 1.8 percent lower HbA1c, and a seventeen-point lower LDL cholesterol.[3380] For a head-to-head test between flaxseed and psyllium, a second cookie group was added containing 10 g of psyllium. The flaxseed still won, beating out the psyllium for constipation relief, weight loss, blood sugars, and cholesterol.[3381] (Flax can also be about four times cheaper than even generic psyllium.) Flaxseeds have also been compared directly to—and beat—the laxative lactulose, increasing bowel movement frequency from two per week to seven per week, as opposed to six per week for lactulose.[3382]

High-fiber rye bread with 5 g of fiber per slice has also been tested, with study participants randomized to eight slices a day. Compared to white bread with only 1 g per slice, the fiber-rich rye "clearly relieved constipation," increasing bowel movement frequency, comfort, stool softness, and intestinal transit time. The rye group experienced increased flatulence and bloating, however, especially in the first week, but, as the gut flora adapted and a balance of gas-producing and gas-utilizing bacteria was established, those symptoms diminished.[3383] (As an aside, the term "old farts" may not only be derogatory but a misnomer. Based on a survey of 16,000 Americans, older individuals tend to wind less often than younger age groups.[3384])

Prunes and Mangos

Decades ago, a paper was published in the journal *Geriatric Nursing* titled "A Special Recipe to Banish Constipation," anecdotally documenting the efficacy of an ounce a day of a specific concoction. The basic recipe was two cups applesauce, two cups unprocessed wheat bran, and one cup of 100 percent prune juice, doled out in little medicine cups for nursing home residents.[3385] Such a regimen might only cost about half that of psyllium (calculated at $77 a year versus $147 for the psyllium).[3386] But how good is the science on prunes?

I review the evidence in see.nf/prune. Basically, ten prunes a day beat out psyllium in a head-to-head test in terms of stool frequency and consistency, increasing regularity from two bowel movements a week to four in the prune group versus three in the Metamucil group.[3387] (For context, those eating plant-based diets average about eleven bowel movements a week.[3388]) With the acknowledged caveat that their study was funded by the California Dried Plum Board, the researchers proposed that prunes should be "considered as a first line therapy for chronic constipation."[3389]

Figs failed,[3390] but a Mango Board–funded study found that fresh mangos were also able to beat out psyllium. Men and women with chronic constipation were randomized to eat either a mango a day or the equivalent amount of added fiber in the form of psyllium, which was one daily teaspoon. At the end of one month, not only did the mangos work better in terms of constipation relief but the fruit had a significant anti-inflammatory effect, dropping blood IL-6 levels by more than 20 percent.[3391] This was assumed to be due to the prebiotic effect of mango pulp based on mice microbiome studies,[3392] which was confirmed in humans in 2020 when a mango a day for eight weeks was found to significantly increase the abundance of *Lactobacillus*, the good bacteria in our gut.[3393]

COLORECTAL CANCER

Colorectal (colon and rectal) cancer takes 50,000 lives annually in the United States and is one of the most commonly diagnosed of all cancers. Over the course of their lifetime, the average person has about a one-in-twenty chance of developing it.[3394] Fortunately, it is one of the most treatable cancers if caught early enough, and routine screening has enabled physicians to detect and remove it before it metastasizes. In the United States alone, there are more than one million colorectal cancer survivors, and, for those who are diagnosed before the cancer has spread beyond the colon, the five-year survival rate is about 90 percent.[3395] In its early stages, however, colorectal cancer rarely causes symptoms. If left uncaught until a later stage, treatment is less effective and more difficult. In *How Not to Die*, I recommend getting screened for colorectal cancer starting at age fifty,[3396] but forty-five may be the new fifty.

In 2018, the American Cancer Society became the first major organization to suggest that individuals at average risk for colorectal cancer begin screening from age forty-five instead of fifty.[3397] The American College of Physicians, however, reaffirmed starting at fifty, while the U.S. Preventive Services Task Force, the most prestigious U.S. guidelines organization I mentioned earlier, debated the pros and cons. Given the recent increase in late-stage tumors among those in their forties,[3398] the USPSTF agreed in 2021 that the starting age for colorectal cancer screening should probably be moved up to forty-five.[3399]

"Early-onset" colorectal cancer, defined as diagnosis before age fifty, still accounts for only about 10 percent of cases, but that number has increased by 50 percent since the mid-1990s.[3400] The current incidence rate among forty-five-year-olds is comparable to the rate among fifty-year-olds back in the nineties that led to the original recommendations to begin screening at fifty.[3401] This rise has been blamed partly on the growing prevalence of obesity,[3402] though the increased overuse of antibiotics in children may have also played a role.[3403] African American men are at particular risk,[3404] as illustrated by the tragic death of actor Chadwick Boseman from colorectal cancer at age forty-three. Compared to white Americans, Black Americans have a 40 percent greater risk of dying from colorectal cancer,[3405] yet, when surveyed, most mistakenly thought they were at lower risk for the disease.[3406] The American College of Physicians has recommended that African Americans begin screening at age forty.[3407]

SCOPING OUT COLONOSCOPIES

According to the USPSTF, there are six acceptable colon-cancer screening strategies. From age forty-five, everyone should do one of the following screening procedures: get a colonoscopy once a decade; have their stool tested for hidden blood every year; have their stool tested for DNA markers every one to three years (by Cologuard, for example); get a "virtual" colonoscopy using CT scan X-rays; or have a flexible sigmoidoscopy either every five years or every ten years with annual DNA marker testing.[3408]

Why do nearly all U.S. doctors recommend colonoscopies[3409] when noninvasive stool testing appears to be the preferred screening method in most of the rest of the world?[3410] Perhaps it's because most doctors practicing in the rest of the world do not get paid by procedure.[3411] As one U.S. gastroenterologist framed it,

"Colonoscopy . . . is the goose that has laid the golden egg."[3412] See my extensive coverage of colonoscopy risks versus benefits in *How Not to Die* to help you make your decision. In the end, the best method of screening is the one that you will actually do.[3413]

COLORECTAL CANCER PREVENTION

Ironically, one downside of screening is what's been called the "health certificate effect," in which those who pass their screenings perceive themselves to be certified as healthy and have a reduced incentive to adopt healthy lifestyles.[3414] Indeed, those randomized to colorectal cancer screening ended up lowering their intake of fruits and vegetables,[3415] which could potentially end up outweighing the beneficial effect of screening.[3416] The answer may be to introduce lifestyle counseling as part of the screening visit.[3417]

While regular screenings to detect colorectal cancer are certainly sensible, preventing the cancer in the first place is even better. The fraction of colorectal cancer cases that might be prevented by colonoscopies and sigmoidoscopies has been estimated at about 30 percent,[3418] but up to 71 percent of cases appear to be preventable through a simple portfolio of diet and lifestyle changes, such as decreasing meat intake.[3419] To home in on the most consequential lifestyle elements, researchers looked to where colon cancer rates are lowest.

While colon cancer remains the second leading cancer killer in the United States, rural Africa has ten times lower incidence. Migrant studies show that the differences in global rates aren't genetic, since it may only take a single generation for immigrants to assume the colon cancer incidence of their new home country. Changes in diet are considered most likely to be responsible, but there are all sorts of changes when you move from one culture to another—from smoking rates to different exposures to chemicals, infections, and antibiotics.[3420] You don't know if it's the diet until you put it to the test.

Watch my video see.nf/switchdiets to find out what happens inside the colons of African Americans switched to a traditional, high-fiber African-style diet and the colons of native Africans given the SAD standard American diet.[3421] In short, as the lead investigator put it, "change your diet, change your cancer risk!"[3422]

Based on studies of more than three million individuals, plant-based diets are associated with significantly lower rates of tumors of the digestive tract, including cancers of the colon and rectum.[3423] Given the "stunningly positive impact" a diet centered around whole plant foods can have on cancer risk, one commentator concluded: "While it would be unrealistic to expect rapid and profound lifestyle changes in the general population, it is gratifying to have sound, effective advice to offer to those who are willing to take the steps needed to optimize their healthful longevity."[3424]

URINARY INCONTINENCE

We've covered the ins and outs of preserving our bowel function. What about our bladder? Urinary incontinence is defined as any involuntary leakage of urine.[3425] There are two types: urgency incontinence, defined as an involuntary loss of urine associated with a sudden strong desire to urinate, and stress incontinence, where an activity such as sneezing triggers an involuntary accident.[3426] Women are affected at two to three times the rate of men, especially as they age.[3427] The number of voluntary muscle fibers in the female urethral sphincter decreases as they mature.[3428] This is combined with a decline in the ability of aging kidneys to concentrate urine and a bladder with reduced capacity, which can also become more irritable and less likely to empty completely. All this may be complicated by delays in sensations of bladder fullness.[3429]

About a third of people surveyed in the United States believe the myth that incontinence is an inevitable part of aging, but it certainly does become more common as we get older.[3430] Over the age of seventy, 40 percent of women may be affected,[3431] and over eighty, that number may rise to 55 percent.[3432] At whatever age, urinary incontinence is associated with a poorer quality of life.[3433] What can we do to prevent and treat it?

PISS OFF WITH DIET

One of the reasons women tend to be more affected than men is a history of childbirth. Compared to cesarean section, vaginal birth can triple the future prevalence of urinary incontinence,[3434] thought due to the stretching of muscles and nerves during the birthing process.[3435] This especially appears to be the case when having children later in life.[3436]

Obese women are at three times the odds of severe incontinence compared to healthy-weight women.[3437] This may be due to increased intra-abdominal pressure bearing down on the bladder.[3438] Beyond observational data, interventional studies show that even modest weight loss may help.[3439] For example, the Program to Reduce Incontinence by Diet and Exercise (PRIDE) trial randomized hundreds of overweight and obese women to a weight-loss program or a control group that just got general educational health sessions. The weight-loss program participants lost an average of about fourteen pounds more than the control group and experienced significantly fewer episodes of incontinence. At the end of six months, the frequency of incontinence was cut by more than half in 61 percent of women in the weight-loss group compared to only 34 percent in the control group.[3440]

With or without incontinence, overactive bladder is defined as urinary urgency, often accompanied by increased urinary frequency. More than one in three women experience an overactive bladder in their lifetime, with an increasing prevalence with advancing age.[3441] However, a randomized, double-blind, placebo-controlled trial showed that relief may just be ½ g of dried cranberry powder away. Bladder-relaxing drugs to control symptoms, like tolterodine (Detrol), are a multibillion-dollar industry,[3442] yet may only reduce average monthly urinations by sixteen, about one less pee every other day.[3443] But, less than a quarter teaspoon of cranberry powder worked nearly four times better, resulting in almost two fewer trips to the bathroom a day. And, that's without suffering from the drug's side effects, which may include dry mouth, constipation, sedation, impaired cognitive function, rapid heartbeat, urinary retention, and visual disturbances that lead almost two-thirds of users to discontinue taking it.[3444]

In the popular press, sufferers are counseled to reduce their consumption of "bladder irritants," such as spicy, salty, and acidic foods. There doesn't appear to be any published evidence to support this recommendation, but the beauty of safe, simple dietary tweaks is that there isn't any harm in giving them a try and seeing if you feel better.[3445] The only two dietary components found to be significantly associated with stress incontinence in a longitudinal study of more than 5,000 women were saturated fat and cholesterol,[3446] though they may just be proxies for unhealthier diets and/or lifestyles. There doesn't appear to be any association between phytoestrogen intake (such as soy or flaxseeds) and urinary symptoms.[3447] What about cutting down on coffee?

U.S.[3448] and European[3449] guidelines both suggest reducing caffeine intake. This makes sense. Caffeine is a mild diuretic, especially at doses found in more than two or three cups of coffee, though daily consumers may habituate to the effect.[3450] Surprisingly, though, a meta-analysis of observational studies did not uncover any link between urinary incontinence and coffee intake, or caffeine more generally.[3451] Two of four interventional studies of caffeine reduction found a reduction in urinary frequency (and the other two found no notable effects), but only two of seven such studies measuring episodes of incontinence found a significant benefit. Again, though, what's the harm of giving it a try?

Fluid restriction in general may be counterproductive, as more concentrated urine may irritate the bladder lining and, paradoxically, worsen symptoms of frequency and urgency.[3452] I would, however, suggest trying to cut out diet drinks. A head-to-head comparison found that Diet Coke increased urinary frequency and urgency more than regular Coke. The researchers blamed the artificial sweeteners based on in vitro studies on rat bladders showing increased muscle contraction.[3453]

JACKED IN THE BOX

Drugs that inhibit the bladder muscle from contracting can be prescribed for urge incontinence.[3454] The average cure rate is nearly 50 percent, but they have the list of common side effects I describe above.[3455] This may help explain why only 14 to 35 percent of people prescribed these drugs are still on them one year later.[3456] There are no FDA-approved drugs for stress incontinence,[3457] but surgical interventions have a cure rate exceeding 80 percent.[3458]

Surprisingly, there is considerable evidence that systemic (oral) estrogen therapy may actually worsen incontinence.[3459] For example, in the Women's Health Initiative, continent women receiving estrogen were approximately twice as likely to develop stress incontinence within the first year, compared to placebo.[3460] Topical (vaginal) estrogens do seem to help, though, reducing one or two accidents a day.[3461] However, first-line management for urinary incontinence is nonpharmacological and nonsurgical.[3462] Working five times better than local estrogens in a head-to-head test: pelvic floor (Kegel) exercises.

In 1948, Dr. Arnold H. Kegel published a paper describing a successful therapy for urinary incontinence that involved exercising the hammock of muscles extending from the pubic bone in the front, down and around to the tailbone in the back.[3463] To find the right muscles, stop urination midstream. The Mayo Clinic suggests you imagine sitting on a marble and trying to lift it up with your vaginal muscles.[3464] Contractions held for ten seconds and followed by at least ten seconds of relaxation are recommended thirty to a hundred times day for at least a month to start seeing results.[3465] For added motivation to stick with it, improved orgasms and sexual satisfaction are a happy side effect of a toned pelvic musculature.[3466]

Once your pelvic muscles are in shape, you can use the "freeze and squeeze" technique to suppress the need to pee when urgency strikes or before you sneeze.[3467] For urge incontinence, this can be combined with bladder training, which consists of an hourly pee schedule while you're awake, extending that a half hour a week until you are able to wait two and a half to three hours between each bathroom break.[3468] A meta-analysis of thirty-one studies involving more than 1,800 women with urinary incontinence in fourteen countries found that those who were randomized to pelvic floor muscle (Kegel) training were, on average, five times more likely to be cured (and eight times more likely for women suffering stress incontinence).[3469]

A Bit of a Stretch

Physical activity has been associated with lower urinary incontinence risk, but the only interventional studies for exercises not exclusive to the pelvic floor are yoga trials.[3470] Check out see.nf/yogatrials for details, but basically, compared to a strict time- and attention-control group involving nonspecific muscle stretching and strengthening exercises, those randomized to actual yoga saw a significant benefit for stress incontinence but not for urgency incontinence.[3471]

PROSTATE ENLARGEMENT

Urinary symptoms in older men are most commonly caused by an enlarged prostate gland, a condition known as benign prostatic hyperplasia, or BPH. BPH affects millions of men in the United States[3472]—as many as half by the time they're in their fifties and 80 percent of men by their eighties,[3473] making it one of the most common diseases to affect men in Western populations.[3474] The male prostate surrounds the outlet from the bladder, so it can obstruct normal urine flow if it grows too big. This obstruction can cause a weak or hesitant urine stream and inadequate emptying of the bladder, necessitating frequent trips to the restroom. What's more, stagnant urine retained in the bladder can become a breeding ground for infection.

PHARMACEUTICAL AND SURGICAL APPROACHES

Unfortunately, the problem appears to worsen as the gland continues to grow larger. Millions of American men have undergone surgery for BPH, and billions have been spent on drugs and supplements.[3475] Current medical treatments, like finasteride (Proscar), are clinically effective, but their efficacy is compromised by adverse effects and low compliance rates.[3476] Side effects include sexual dysfunction, high-grade prostate cancer, and depression. No wonder men don't like to take it![3477] A study of more than a million American men reported the one-year adherence rate at only 29 percent.[3478]

Sexual dysfunctions linked to finasteride include impotence, decreased libido, ejaculatory disorders, and gynecomastia (male breast enlargement).[3479] In 2021, internal documents from Merck, the drug company that makes Proscar, were made public, thanks to legal action from the Reuters news agency. It turns out that Merck knew as far back as 2009 that its drug appeared to cause persistent erectile dysfunction (even after the drug was stopped), but Merck's "Risk Management Safety Team" decided to basically sit on the information.[3480]

That brings us to the "gold standard" treatment for BPH: surgery.[3481] Procedures involve a slew of different Roto-Rooter-esque techniques with innocent-sounding acronyms, like TUMT, TUNA, and TURP. The *T*s stand for *transurethral*, or going inside and up the penis with an instrument called a resectoscope. TUMT is *transurethral microwave thermotherapy*, in which doctors use an antenna-like tool to essentially tunnel up the penis and, with microwaves, burn out a shaft.[3482] TUNA stands for *transurethral needle ablation*, which involves burning out a column with a pair of heated needles. And these are so-called *minimally* invasive techniques.[3483] In the gold standard procedure, called TURP for *transurethral resection of the prostate*, surgeons use a loop of wire to core out the gland. Side effects include "postoperative discomfort."[3484]

There has got to be a better way.

BPH IS NOT INEVITABLE

Most doctors may assume BPH is just an inevitable consequence of aging since it is such a common condition, but that wasn't always the case. In the 1920s and '30s in China, for instance, a medical college in Beijing reported that BPH affected not 80 percent of male patients but only about 80 *individual cases* over fifteen *years*. The historic rarity of both BPH and prostate cancer in China and Japan has been attributed to the countries' traditional plant-based diets.[3485] Recent studies on Tsimane men, Bolivian subsistence farmers who center their diets around starchy staples like plantains,[3486] found that advanced cases of BPH were almost nonexistent, confirming its noninevitability.[3487]

Population studies suggest that low intake of animal protein and high intake of fruits and vegetables may be protective.[3488] Compared to men eating meat less than once a week, those eating meat on a daily basis had more than twice the odds of suffering from BPH-type symptoms.[3489] In a more granular study, researchers found that poultry and eggs seem to be the worst, along with refined grains, but no association was found for red meat or dairy.[3490] Of all plant foods, eating onions and garlic has been associated with significantly lower BPH risk.[3491] In general, cooked vegetables may work better than raw, and legumes—beans, split peas, lentils, and chickpeas— have also been associated with lower risk.[3492] Men consuming the isoflavones found in just a cup a day of soymilk[3493] also harbored lower risk.[3494] Textured vegetable protein, known as TVP, is a soybean product often used in veggie chilis and pasta sauces. Although I prefer less processed soy foods, I would recommend this type of TVP over the TVP used in urology, which stands for *transurethral vaporization of the prostate*.[3495]

PLANT YOUR PROSTATE

In *How Not to Die*, I detailed a series of experiments by Ornish and colleagues, who pitted the blood of individuals before and after a plant-based diet against cancer cells growing in a petri dish. The blood of men on the standard American diet slowed the growth rate of prostate cancer cells by 9 percent. But, when men followed a plant-based diet for a year, the blood circulating within their bodies could suppress cancer cell growth by 70 percent. Nearly eight times the cancer-fighting power with a plant-centered, rather than meat-centered, menu.[3496] (Similar studies have found that women on plant-based diets appear to dramatically strengthen their defenses against breast cancer in just two weeks.[3497]) What if the same experiment was performed on the type of normal prostate cells that grow to obstruct urine flow?

Within just two weeks, the blood of men eating plant-based diets acquired the ability to suppress the abnormal growth of noncancerous prostate cells. What's more, the effect didn't seem to dissipate over time. The blood of long-term plant-based eaters had the same beneficial effect for up to twenty-eight consecutive years. So, it appears that as long as we continue to eat healthfully, the rates of prostate cell growth will go down—and stay down.[3498] However, some plants may be particularly prostate positive.

Saw Palmetto and a Supplement That Actually Works

Saw palmetto berry is "undisputedly" the most common herbal supplement used for BPH,[3499] but it doesn't work.[3500] One supplement that may help prevent[3501] and treat[3502] BPH is vitamin D. Details on both in see.nf/saw.

GO TO SEED

Flaxseeds can be used to treat BPH. Men given the equivalent of around three tablespoons of flaxseeds daily experienced relief comparable to that achieved with commonly prescribed drugs such as Flomax or Proscar[3503]—but without their side effects. Pumpkin seeds also work,[3504] as detailed in see.nf/seeds, leading the European equivalent of the FDA to conclude that they can be used for the "relief of lower urinary tract symptoms related to an enlarged prostate after more serious conditions have been excluded by a medical doctor."[3505]

Wee Hours of the Night

One of the most burdensome symptoms of BPH is nocturia, frequently having to get up in the middle of the night to pee.[3506] Common sense might tell us to just try to drink less before bed, but, remarkably, there is not a clear association between fluid intake and nocturia.[3507] One study of about 150 men did find a correlation between the frequency of nocturia and nighttime water intake, as well as how much water you drink in the four hours before bedtime,[3508] but another study, with more than one thousand older adults, found no relationship between the amount of bedtime fluids and having to repeatedly get up to urinate.[3509] I was surprised to learn that fluid restriction has never been properly put to the test. There was a study in which a group of older men averaging four pees a night were told to reduce their daily fluid intake from about seven cups to around five cups and were able to shave nightly bathroom trips down to three,[3510] but it and other similar studies[3511,3512] failed to include a control group to really nail down cause and effect.

It's even harder to get people to restrict sodium. Nocturia reviews with titles asking the question "Which Matters Most, the Water or the Salt?"[3513] note that salt intake has been associated with nocturia frequency,[3514] presumably due to increased thirst-driven fluid intake. This has led to recommendations to cut down on salt to control nocturia severity, but sodium restriction is hard to study because compliance is notoriously poor.[3515] You can, however, compare the change in nocturia episodes of those who successfully cut down on salt intake versus those who didn't. Based on that, it appears that even cutting back on as little as a half teaspoon of salt a day may reduce nightly episodes by 40 to 60 percent.[3516,3517]

Evening protein intake may also contribute to nocturia. The main determinant of urine concentration is not sodium but urea, which is a breakdown product of protein excretion. Protein-rich suppers were found to correlate with excess overnight urine production, leading to the as-of-yet-untested conclusion that a "reduction of evening protein consumption may be an effective lifestyle intervention in the management of nocturia. . . ."[3518]

HIT A SOUR NOTE

What other foods have been shown to help? Cranberries were evidently used by Native Americans to treat urinary ailments.[3519] Cranberries can successfully shrink rodent prostates by as much as 33 percent,[3520] but the first human trial, "The

Effectiveness of Dried Cranberries (*Vaccinium macrocarpon*) in Men with Lower Urinary Tract Symptoms," wasn't published until 2010. The dried cranberries weren't those sugary, oily Craisins but rather just straight, whole cranberry powder. Significant improvements in BPH symptoms, quality of life, and all urination parameters studied were noted for about three-quarters of a teaspoon a day of powdered cranberries.[3521]

What about less than a quarter of a teaspoon or even an eighth of a teaspoon? Both of those doses beat out placebos for decreasing BPH symptoms.[3522] The researchers used a branded supplement, but since it was just straight cranberry fruit powder, you might as well buy it in bulk, which is much cheaper, and just throw it into a smoothie or sprinkle it on some oatmeal. An eighth of a teaspoon would cost less than a penny a day.

A pilot study also concluded that cranberries might prevent recurrent urinary tract infections in elderly men with BPH, but the controlled study lacked a placebo or even randomized allocation, making the findings suggestive at best.[3523]

GARLIC AND TOMATOES

What about a berry that's a little tastier? Welch's-funded researchers put purple (Concord) grape juice to the test for BPH, but it failed to show any benefit.[3524] If cranberries are the most effective fruit, what might be the most effective vegetable? I review trials done on tomato paste[3525] and garlic extracts[3526] for BPH in see.nf /garlictomatoes. Unfortunately, they were both before-and-after studies without control groups so the purported benefits offer only suggestive evidence.

PRESERVING YOUR CIRCULATION

A noted seventeenth-century physician was quoted as saying, "A man is as old as his arteries."[3527] Women are, too, though few seem to recognize it. A nationally representative survey of U.S. women found that most considered their greatest personal health risk to be cancer. Only 13 percent correctly identified cardiovascular disease, which is the actual leading killer of women (and men,[3528] and centenarians[3529]). Sadly, between 2009 and 2019, American Heart Association surveys have noted a "concerning decline" in the proportion of women who understood heart disease to be their leading cause of death.[3530]

A recent editorial in the journal *Aging Medicine* rhapsodized that "the blood vessel is the candle of life," boldly asserting that "[a]ll disease stems from vessels."[3531] There's even a microcirculatory theory of aging that suggests the loss of blood vessel density as we age—by as much as 50 percent in some tissues, such as areas of the brain—may be contributing to organ deterioration as the removal of waste and the delivery of oxygen and nutrients are impaired.[3532] You could say that what brings us blood brings us life.

HOW TO BOOST YOUR EPCs

How can we remain young at heart? The capacity of our blood vessels to repair themselves is dependent on endothelial progenitor cells that emerge from stem cells in our bone marrow to patch up any holes in our endothelium, the innermost lining of our blood vessels that keeps our blood flowing smoothly.[3533] Watch see.nf /epc for a demonstration of the power of endothelial progenitor cells[3534] and what we can do to increase their number and function, such as avoiding even secondhand cigarette smoke[3535] and getting regular aerobic exercise,[3536] considered a "first-line" strategy for helping to prevent and treat arterial aging.[3537] What about diet?

A randomized controlled trial showed that reducing intake of saturated fat (mostly butter) significantly elevated endothelial progenitor cell numbers,[3538] consistent with a study on baboons showing that even a few weeks of a high-cholesterol, high-fat diet could cause dramatic, premature endothelial cell senescence.[3539] Individual foods that have been shown to increase circulating endothelial progenitor cells include berries,[3540] onions,[3541] and green tea,[3542] and a diet centered completely around whole plant foods not only showed a boost in endothelial progenitors but an improvement in endothelial function, along with a drop in LDL cholesterol.[3543]

A NORMAL CHOLESTEROL LEVEL IS A DEADLY CHOLESTEROL LEVEL

Scientific consensus panels going back decades established—"beyond a reasonable doubt"—that lowering LDL cholesterol reduces the risk of heart attacks.[3544] Consistent evidence "unequivocally" establishes that LDL causes our number one killer, heart disease. This evidence base includes hundreds of studies involving literally millions of people.[3545] In other words, "[i]t's the cholesterol, stupid," quipped *American Journal of Cardiology* editor in chief[3546] William Clifford Roberts. His CV is more than a hundred pages long, and he's published about 1,700 articles in the peer-reviewed medical literature.[3547] Yes, there are at least ten traditional risk factors for atherosclerosis, but, as Dr. Roberts notes, only one is required for the progression of the disease: elevated cholesterol.[3548] All the other factors, such as smoking, high blood pressure, diabetes, inactivity, and obesity, merely exacerbate the damage caused by high cholesterol.[3549]

Phew! you say, because your bloodwork just came back and your doctor said your cholesterol is "normal." But, hold on. Having a *normal* cholesterol level in a society where it's *normal* to drop dead of a heart attack isn't necessarily something to celebrate. With heart disease the top killer of men and women, we definitely don't want to have *normal* cholesterol levels. We want to have *optimal* levels—and not "optimal" by arbitrary laboratory standards but optimal for human health.

Normal LDL cholesterol levels are associated with the buildup of atherosclerotic plaques in our arteries[3550] even in those with so-called optimal risk factors by current standards: blood pressure under 120 over 80, normal blood sugars, and total cholesterol under 200.[3551] If you went to your doctor with those kinds of numbers, you'd get a gold star. But, when ultrasound and CT scans were used to actually peek inside the bodies of patients boasting those numbers, overt atherosclerotic plaques were detected in 38 percent. Maybe those digits ain't so optimal after all.

Perhaps we should define an LDL cholesterol level as optimal only when it no longer causes disease.[3552] (What a concept!) How would we go about figuring that out?

When more than a thousand men and women in their forties were scanned, most of those with "normal" LDL levels under 130 had frank atherosclerosis. No atherosclerotic plaques were found only when LDL was down around 50 or 60,[3553] which just so happens to be the level most people had before our diets changed to what they are today.[3554] The majority of the global adult population had LDLs around 50 mg/dL. So, average values today are regarded as normal based on a sick society.[3555] What we want is a cholesterol level that is normal for the human species, which is considered to be around 30 to 70 mg/dL (or 0.8 to 1.8 mmol/L).[3556]

Although an LDL level in this range might seem excessively low by modern American standards, it is precisely the normal range for individuals living the lifestyle and eating the diet[3557] for which our ancient ancestors were genetically adapted over millions of years: a diet centered around whole plant foods.[3558] Given that the LDL level our body was designed for is less than half of what is presently considered "normal,"[3559] it's no wonder that we are awash in a pandemic of atherosclerotic heart disease.

Why is there a tendency in medicine to accept small changes in risk factors[3560] when the goal shouldn't be just decreasing risk but *preventing* plaques from forming in the first place?[3561] In that case, how low should we go?[3562]

One noted professor of vascular biochemistry noted: "In light of the latest evidence from trials exploring the benefits and risks of profound LDL cholesterol-lowering, the answer to the question *How low should we go?* is, arguably, a straightforward *As low as you can!*"[3563] How we get there, though, matters. Low may indeed be better, but if we're lowering our LDL with drugs, then we need to balance the benefit with the risk of pharmaceutical side effects.[3564]

There's a reason we don't try to drug everyone with statins by putting them in the water. Yes, it would be great if everyone's cholesterol was lower, but the drugs themselves have countervailing risks.[3565] So, doctors aim to use statins at the highest dose possible to achieve the largest LDL cholesterol reduction possible without increasing the risk of muscle damage the drugs may cause.[3566] Statins also increase the risk of developing type 2 diabetes.[3567] However, when you use healthy lifestyle changes to bring down cholesterol, all you get are the benefits[3568]— including a significant *drop* in diabetes risk.[3569] But, can you get your LDL low enough with only your diet?

Ask some of the country's top cholesterol experts what levels they shoot for, and odds are you'd hear something like an LDL under 70 or so.[3570] Just cutting down on the saturated and trans fats found in meat, dairy, and junk, as well as reducing intake of the dietary cholesterol found mostly in eggs, is unlikely to get most people to the target.[3571] However, those eating completely plant-based diets can *average* an LDL that low.[3572] It's no wonder plant-based diets are the only dietary patterns ever proven to reverse the progression of coronary heart disease.[3573]

Pressure Points

A similar "normal"-as-deadly paradigm exists for blood pressure. We know the leading risk factor for death in the United States is the American diet, with tobacco number two, but killer number three is high blood pressure, also known as hypertension.[3574] It's so deadly because it increases your risk of dying from so many different diseases, from heart disease and stroke to heart and kidney failure.[3575]

Check out my video see.nf/bloodpressure for an evolution of the guidelines, but basically, there is an exponential increase in risk of dying from a stroke or heart disease as our blood pressures go up, starting from around 110 over 70.[3576] Forcing pressures that low with drugs would have unacceptable consequences, though. For example, if high-risk individuals are given enough drugs at high enough doses to lower their blood pressure even down to a top number of 120 or so, more than 100,000 deaths and 46,000 cases of heart failure might be prevented every year. At the same time, this would be expected to cause, for example, 43,000 cases of electrolyte abnormalities and 88,000 cases of acute kidney injury.[3577] You can see the conundrum that guidelines committees face.

On the one hand, lowering blood pressure is good for your heart, kidneys,

(continued)

and brain, but, at a certain point, the side effects from the drugs could outweigh the benefits.[3578] Ideally, we want to get patients' blood pressures as low as possible,[3579] but we may only want to use drugs to do it "when the effects of treatment are likely to be less destructive than the elevated BP [blood pressure]." The problem is that most people who die from heart disease, heart failure, and stroke may be in the borderline range—at risk, but not sufficiently elevated to warrant drug treatment.[3580]

If only there were some way to lower blood pressures without drugs to get the best of both worlds. Thankfully, there are: regular aerobic exercise, weight loss, smoking cessation, increased dietary fiber intake, decreased alcohol intake, consumption of a more plant-based diet, and cutting down on salt. The advantage is not limited to the lack of bad side effects. Lifestyle interventions like plant-based diets can actually work *better* than drugs because you're treating the underlying cause and can actually have beneficial side effects.[3581]

LOWER FOR LONGER

On the standard American diet, atherosclerosis, the hardening of our arteries, can start when we're just teenagers.[3582] Investigators collected about 3,000 sets of coronary arteries and aortas—the main artery in the body—from accident, homicide, and suicide victims aged fifteen to thirty-four and found fatty streaks in teens, which can turn into atherosclerotic plaques when we're in our twenties and get worse in our thirties before they start killing us off.[3583] How many of the teens, though? All of them. One hundred percent of the teenaged victims had fatty streaks building up inside their arteries. All of them had the first stage of the disease, and those streaks were already blossoming into atherosclerotic plaques bulging into the arteries of 55 to 65 percent of those in their early thirties. It's chilling, I know, to realize that most people in their early thirties already have plaques in their arteries. In other words, most of you probably have heart disease—whether you know it or not. The researchers conclude with the line: "Atherosclerosis begins in youth."[3584]

If you had diabetes, would you wait until you started going blind to start treating it?[3585] With heart disease, you can't just wait until you become symptomatic, because your first symptom may be your last. For the majority of Americans who die from heart disease, the first symptom is called "sudden cardiac death."[3586]

An ounce of prevention is worth much more than a pound of cure, because there is no cure for dead.

How do you prevent atherosclerotic heart disease? By lowering your LDL cholesterol through a diet that is sufficiently low in saturated fat and cholesterol—that is, one that restricts meat, junk, dairy, and eggs.[3587] "Is such a radical proposal totally impractical?" asked a review in the *Journal of the American Heart Association*.[3588] It would take an "all-out commitment," but the reviewers evoked the successful public health triumph of slashing smoking rates and lung cancer deaths to argue that anything is possible.

What evidence do we have that a lifelong suppression of LDL will prevent heart disease? There is a genetic mutation of a gene called PCSK9 that about one in fifty African Americans are lucky to be born with because it gives them about 40 percent lower cholesterol levels throughout their whole lives.[3589] This gives them dramatically lower rates of coronary artery disease, a whopping 88 percent drop in risk—despite otherwise ominous risk factors.[3590] Most with the mutation had preexisting conditions such as high blood pressure, being overweight or a smoker, or having diabetes, but that all just goes to show that a lifelong history of reduced LDL cholesterol levels significantly lowers the risk of coronary heart disease even in the presence of multiple other risk factors.

This near 90 percent drop in cardiac events, like heart attacks or sudden death, occurred only at an average LDL of 100 mg/dL, compared to 138 mg/dL in those without the mutation. With drugs or diet, you could easily achieve an LDL even lower than that.[3591] But, wait. Why does the lowering of LDL cholesterol by about 40 mg/dL in those with the lucky mutation reduce the incidence of coronary heart disease by nearly 90 percent, whereas that same forty-point drop with a statin drug would reduce coronary heart disease prevalence by only about 20 percent? The most likely answer is duration.[3592] The longer the arteries are exposed to higher LDL levels in the blood, the more cholesterol can accumulate within the artery wall and inflame it.[3593]

Just as tobacco exposure is measured in pack-years, the amount smoked multiplied over time, an editorial in the *Journal of the American College of Cardiology* introduced the concept of cholesterol-years to take into account the full extent to which our arteries have been bathing in it.[3594] This explains why the indigenous Tsimane, the farmers in Bolivia I mentioned on page 259, are practically free of coronary artery disease at an average LDL of only down around 90. An eighty-year-old Tsimane appears to possess the "vascular age" of an American in their midfifties.[3595] When it comes to lowering LDL, it's not only how low, but how long, and the lower, the longer, the better.[3596]

If you're being treated with drugs later in life, you may have to get your LDL under 70 mg/dL to halt the progression of atherosclerosis.[3597] But if we start early enough in life, it may be sufficient to lower LDL to only about 100 mg/dL, which is consistent with country-by-country data that suggested heart disease would bottom out at a population average of about one hundred.[3598] That's why healthy lifestyle choices may wipe out 90 percent or so of our risk for having a heart attack, whereas drugs may only reduce it by 20 to 30 percent.[3599] But that 90 percent is only if you can keep it down your whole life.

If you're using drugs late in life to try to stop the *progression* of your disease, you have to get your LDL under 70 mg/dL, but in order to *reverse* a lifetime of bad food choices with drugs, you probably have to get it down to around 55. And, if your heart disease is so bad you've already had a heart attack and you're trying not to die from another one, ideally, you might need your LDL to be pushed down to about 30.[3600] Once you get that low, not only would you prevent any new atherosclerotic plaques[3601] but you'd help stabilize the plaques you already have so they'd be less likely to burst open and kill you.[3602]

HOW EFFECTIVE ARE STATINS?

Why cut down on any foods when you can just take a pill? I discuss the efficacy of statin drugs in depth in see.nf/statins. The absolute risk reduction is only 1 percent, so for every hundred people who take a drug like Lipitor for a few years, only one person averts a heart attack.[3603] However, in order to take a cholesterol-lowering drug every day, most say they want an absolute risk reduction at least about twenty-five times higher than that. So, the dirty little secret is if patients knew the truth, if they knew how little these drugs actually worked, nearly no one would agree to take them. A study on patient expectations titled "Are Preventive Drugs Preventive Enough?" concluded that this suggests "at best a lack of discussion and patient education and at worst a degree of misinformation on the benefits of these drugs."[3604]

This sounds terribly paternalistic, but hundreds of thousands of lives are at stake. Quite simply, if patients were told the truth, a lot of people would die. More than thirty million Americans are on statins.[3605] Even if the drugs saved one in a hundred, that could mean hundreds of thousands of lives lost if everyone stopped taking them. As a paper titled "The Preventive-Pill Paradox" concluded: "It is ironic that informing patients about statins would increase the very outcomes they were designed to prevent."[3606]

Are Statins Right for You?

If you have a history of heart disease or stroke, taking a statin drug is recommended. Period. Full stop. If you do not have any *known* cardiovascular disease, then the decision should be based on calculating your own personal risk, which you can easily do online if you know your cholesterol and blood pressure numbers.[3607] See, for example, the American College of Cardiology risk estimator[3608] (see.nf/acc), the Framingham risk profiler[3609] (see.nf/framingham), or the Reynolds Risk Score[3610] (see.nf/reynolds).

I prefer the American College of Cardiology's estimator because it not only gives you your current ten-year risk but also your lifetime risk. Under the current guidelines, if your ten-year risk is below 5 percent, then you should just stick to diet, exercise, and smoking cessation to further bring down your numbers unless there are extenuating circumstances. If your ten-year risk hits 20 percent or higher, the recommendation is to add a statin drug on top of lifestyle modification. Between 5 and 7.5 percent, the tendency is to adhere to lifestyle interventions unless you have risk-enhancing factors, and between 7.5 and 20 percent, most lean toward adding drugs. Risk-enhancing factors your doctor should take into account when helping you make the decision include a family history of heart disease or stroke, really high LDL ($\geq$ 160 mg/dL), metabolic syndrome, chronic kidney or inflammatory conditions, and persistently high triglycerides ($\geq$ 175 mg/dL), C-reactive protein ($\geq$ 2.0 mg/L), or Lp(a) ($\geq$ 50 mg/dL—see page 274).[3611]

If you're still not sure if you should take statins, the American Heart Association guidelines suggest considering getting a coronary artery calcium score,[3612] though the U.S. Preventive Services Task Force has said explicitly that the current evidence is insufficient to conclude that the harms of the test outweigh the benefits (even though the radiation exposure is relatively low these days).[3613]

HOW SAFE ARE STATINS?

Studies show that as many as 75 percent of people stop taking statins prescribed to them.[3614] When asked why, most former statin users cited muscle pain as the primary reason for discontinuing the pills.[3615] Up to 72 percent of all side effects of statins are muscle symptoms associated with the drug.[3616] Taking coenzyme Q_{10} supplements as a treatment for statin-associated muscle symptoms seemed like a good idea in theory[3617] but failed to actually help when put to the test.[3618] Normally, the symptoms go away after you stop the drug, but they can sometimes linger for a year or more.[3619] Muscle-related side effects could also be coincidental or psychosomatic and have nothing to do with the drug. Many clinical trials show that such side effects are rare, though it's also possible that those same trials, funded by the drug companies themselves, under-recorded the side effects.[3620]

However, even in Big Pharma–funded trials that attributed only a small minority of symptoms to statins, researchers found that those taking the drugs were significantly more likely to develop type 2 diabetes than those randomized to placebo pills.[3621] Why? We're still not exactly sure, but statins may have the double-whammy effect of impairing insulin secretion from the pancreas and also diminishing insulin's effectiveness by increasing insulin resistance.[3622] Tragically, this elevated risk persists for years even after statins are stopped.[3623]

What About Red Yeast Rice Supplements?

Red yeast rice supplements, which contain a statin-producing mold, are not recommended,[3624] as "dramatic" variations in the active components have been found (for example, hundredfold differences in lovastatin levels). Also, a third of retail red yeast rice supplements tested were contaminated by a potential kidney-damaging fungal toxin called *citrinin*.[3625] An updated 2021 analysis found citrinin exceeding safety levels in 97 percent of sampled supplements, including supplements labeled "citrinin-free," posing a "serious health concern."[3626]

In view of the benefit of statins in the reduction of cardiovascular events, our top killer, any increase in the risk of diabetes, which is typically our seventh leading cause of death (eighth with COVID),[3627] would be outweighed by the cardiovascular benefits.[3628] Statin users would be expected to develop an extra two cases of diabetes mellitus per thousand patient-years, during which time six and a half cardiovascular events, such as heart attacks or strokes, would be prevented.[3629] Of course, that's a false dichotomy.[3630] We don't have to choose between heart disease and diabetes. We can treat the cause of both with the same diet and lifestyle changes. The diet that doesn't only stop the progression of heart disease but reverses it[3631] is the very same way of eating that can reverse type 2 diabetes into remission.[3632] A healthy enough plant-based diet may prevent further major cardiac episodes in as many as 99.4 percent of patients with significant heart disease.[3633]

What About PCSK9 Inhibitors?

Extrapolating data from graphs from large cholesterol-lowering trials suggests that the incidence of cardiovascular events like heart attacks would approach zero if LDL cholesterol can be brought below 60 mg/dL in individuals who had never had a heart attack and down around 30 mg/dL for those trying to prevent another one.[3634] Is it even safe to have cholesterol levels that low? We didn't really know until PCSK9 inhibitors were invented.[3635]

If you remember, PCSK9 is the gene that gave some people lifelong low LDL.[3636] Drug companies were inspired by the natural mutation to target the gene pharmacologically.[3637] See see.nf/pcsk9 for a full discussion, but basically, on PCSK9 inhibitors, people can achieve an LDL below 40 mg/dL and some even under 15 mg/dL.[3638] The risk of heart attacks falls in a straight line as LDL gets lower and lower, even down below 10 mg/dL without apparent safety concerns, such as impairments of the synthesis of adrenal, ovarian, or testicular hormones that the body makes from cholesterol.[3639]

We can take comfort in the fact that those with extreme PCSK9 mutations, which lead to a reduction in levels of LDL-C to below 20 mg/dL their whole lives, remain healthy and have healthy kids.[3640] There's another type of genetic mutation that leaves people with LDLs of about 30 mg/dL throughout their lives, and they are known to have an exceptionally long life expectancy.[3641] Mutations that affect cholesterol are in fact what cause the so-called longevity syndromes, but that doesn't necessarily mean the drugs are safe.[3642] The bottom line is that we should try to get our LDL cholesterol down as low as we can, but much longer follow-up data are necessary any time a new class of drugs is introduced.[3643] So far, so good, but we're only a few years out. We didn't know, for instance, that statins increased diabetes risk until a decade *after* they had been approved and millions had already been exposed.[3644] It's also worth mentioning that PCSK9 inhibitors cost about $14,000 a year.[3645]

THE GREAT STENT SCAM

Besides personal habits and biases, another reason lifestyle efforts are often neglected may be the preoccupation many cardiologists have with all the fancy gadgets and new procedures out there.[3646] Some might feel as if they had been trained to be highly skilled fighter pilots, ready to go into combat with high-tech weaponry, but then are asked to go on a boring, preventive diplomatic mission instead. Beyond missing an opportunity to treat the underlying cause, certain common cardiology practices have been shown to do more harm than good. This is not to pick on cardiologists. Many current medical practices have been found to offer potential harms with no benefit.[3647] Physicians themselves estimate that about a fifth of medical care is unnecessary.[3648]

My seven-part video series on stents and angioplasty starts with see.nf/stents. The bottom line: During a heart attack, placing stents can be lifesaving, but hundreds of thousands of these procedures are done for stable angina, meaning on a nonemergency basis.[3649] It was thought they would relieve symptoms,[3650] but they don't actually prolong life or reduce the risk of having a heart attack in the future, compared to "medical therapy," which includes lifestyle interventions and taking statins.[3651] As the *Harvard Heart Letter* put it, "Stents are for pain, not protection."[3652] But then it was discovered in a famous double-blind, randomized, controlled trial[3653] that stents may not even help with pain.

Hold on. A double-blind, randomized, controlled trial involving *surgery*? In a drug trial, you can give study participants a placebo sugar pill so they won't know if they're in the active treatment group or the control group, but wouldn't you notice if someone cut into your groin? Not if you got *sham* surgery.[3654] Yes, placebo surgery is a thing. In the study, the researchers cut into every subject, threaded up the catheter, then did or did not place the actual stent. And, those who got the sham surgery experienced the same pain relief as those who got the real surgery.[3655]

If heart attacks are caused by blocked arteries, then why doesn't physically opening them up help? Because most heart attacks are caused by narrowings blocking less than 70 percent of your arteries, so the killer plaques don't tend to show up on angiograms.[3656] Before rupture, these plaques often don't limit blood flow, so they may be invisible to angiography and stress tests.[3657] The most dangerous lesions may therefore not be amenable to angioplasty and stents, which do nothing to modify the underlying disease process itself.

TREATING THE CAUSE

To drastically lower LDL cholesterol, we need to drastically reduce our consumption of the three components that raise it: trans fat, saturated fat, and dietary cholesterol.[3658] Once a common ingredient in processed foods in the United States, trans fat–laden partially hydrogenated oils have since been effectively banned in the country and restricted in dozens of others around the world.[3659] These days, in three-quarters of the countries surveyed, most exposure to trans fats now comes from meat and dairy.[3660] Cholesterol-raising saturated fat is found mainly in animal products and junk foods. Dairy (including pizza) is our top source of intake in the United States, followed by chicken, then pastries, pork, and burgers.[3661] Dietary cholesterol is found exclusively in animal-derived foods,[3662] and, overwhelmingly, eggs are our number one source. Chicken is our second leading source, followed by beef, dairy, and pork.[3663] It is therefore no surprise that the core dietary recommendation from the leading scientific societies of cardiology for cardiovascular disease prevention is to "emphasize the consumption of plant-based rather than animal-based foods."[3664]

Randomized controlled trials involving more than 50,000 people have shown that cutting down on our saturated fat intake leads to a reduction in cardiovascular disease, and the more we decrease saturated fat content, the more our cholesterol drops. The gold-standard Cochrane review concluded: "[T]o lower risk population groups should continue to include permanent reduction of dietary saturated fat."[3665] (Archie Cochrane was an evidence-based medicine pioneer whose legacy is memorialized in an eponymous nonprofit respected for its high-quality systematic reviews.) The American Heart Association got so fed up with "butter-is-back" industry attempts to convince people that butter is not harmful that it released a Presidential Advisory[3666] "to set the record straight on why well-conducted scientific research overwhelmingly supports limiting saturated fat in the diet."[3667]

The proscription against saturated fat extends to tropical oils, which are often used in junk foods, including coconut oil, palm oil, and palm kernel oil,[3668] though animal-derived sources appear to be worse. The Animal and Plant PROtein And Cardiovascular Health (APPROACH) trial randomized people to diets high or low in saturated fats, composed of protein sources from red meat, white meat, or non-meat (bean, grain, and nut). Researchers adjusted the different diets to achieve the same saturated fat intake across all three, tweaking with butterfat for the two meat groups and tropical oils for the nonmeat group. Their findings? At the same saturated fat intake, red meat and white meat both elevated LDL cholesterol higher than plant-based protein sources.[3669] Red meat and white meat appeared to be equivalently bad, which is the case even in randomized controlled trials that didn't normalize saturated fat levels. Swapping out beef for chicken and/or fish doesn't significantly lower LDL cholesterol levels.[3670]

Dietary cholesterol has also long been known to be a significant contributor to atherosclerosis.[3671] A 2020 meta-analysis of more than fifty randomized controlled trials found that egg consumption significantly increases LDL cholesterol.[3672] Even studies funded by the egg industry show that eggs increase our blood cholesterol.[3673] This appears to translate into significantly higher coronary artery calcium scores among those who eat more eggs, which is a sign of atherosclerotic plaque buildup in the arteries[3674] and, most important, to a significantly greater risk of heart attacks and death. Based on a half dozen populations studied in the United States, following tens of thousands of people for up to thirty years, each additional half an egg consumed per day was significantly associated with higher risk of developing cardiovascular disease and dying from all causes put together.[3675] And this higher risk of death persisted even after taking other lifestyle behaviors into account, including overall dietary quality. In other words, it does not appear to be just because those eating more eggs were eating more bacon.[3676]

Despite pressure from the egg industry,[3677] the 2015 to 2020 Dietary Guidelines for Americans explicitly told people to "eat as little dietary cholesterol as possible," as recommended by the Institute of Medicine,[3678] advice that was reiterated in the 2020 to 2025 guidelines: "The National Academies recommends that *trans* fat and dietary cholesterol consumption to be as low as possible,"[3679] using the rationale that any intake above zero increases LDL cholesterol concentration in the blood and therefore increases the risk of our number one killer.[3680]

As noted by J. David Spence, director of the Stroke Prevention and Atherosclerosis Research Centre, "After conviction for false advertising," for suggesting that eggs were safe, "the egg industry has spent hundreds of millions of dollars trying to convince the public, physicians, and policy makers that dietary cholesterol is harmless." In reality, regular consumption of eggs should be avoided by people at risk of cardiovascular disease, Dr. Spence wrote, which "essentially means all North Americans who expect to live past middle age."[3681]

What About Lp(a)?

Lipoprotein(a), also known as Lp(a), is an underrecognized independent risk factor for cardiovascular disease. It contributes to coronary artery disease, heart attacks, strokes, peripheral arterial disease, calcified aortic valve disease, and heart failure. These can occur even in people without high cholesterol[3682] because Lp(a) *is* cholesterol. It's basically an LDL cholesterol molecule linked to another protein,[3683] which, like LDL alone, transfers cholesterol into the lining of our arteries, contributing to the inflammation in our atherosclerotic plaques.[3684] For more on Lp(a) and what we can do about it, check out see.nf/lpa and see.nf/lpadiet. In short, Lp(a) blood concentrations are mostly genetically determined,[3685] but there are some dietary tweaks that can help.

We've known for years that the trans fats found in meat and dairy are just as bad as the industrially produced trans fats found in partially hydrogenated oil in junk food when it came to raising LDL cholesterol levels.[3686] When it comes to Lp(a), though, the trans fats in meat and dairy appear to be even worse.[3687] However, merely cutting out meat and following a lacto-ovo vegetarian diet does not appear to be sufficient.[3688] There are some specific plants that may help a bit, including ground flaxseeds[3689] and amla (dried Indian gooseberry powder).[3690] When study participants were put on a whole food, plant-based diet packed to the hilt with fruits and vegetables, their Lp(a) levels dropped by 16 percent within four weeks. In those twenty-eight days, they also lost fifteen pounds, on average,[3691] but weight loss does not appear to improve Lp(a) levels, so the researchers figured it must have been the food.[3692] In addition to causing weight loss, a month of plant-based eating can dramatically improve blood pressure even as people cut down on their blood pressure medications.[3693] You can also get a twenty-five-point drop in LDL cholesterol and a 30 percent drop in C-reactive protein, as well as significant reductions in other inflammatory markers for a "systemic, cardioprotective effect."[3694]

VEGETARIAN STROKE RISK

Healthy plant-based diets have been associated with lower all-cause mortality,[3695] with up to a 34 percent lower risk of death from any cause over an average of an eight-year period.[3696] If sustained through adulthood, that would translate into more than four extra years of life.[3697] A meta-analysis of a dozen studies prospectively following more than half a million people for up to twenty-five years similarly found significantly lower heart disease and overall death rates among those eating more plant-based.[3698] That's no surprise, a systematic review concluded, given the evidence that plant-based lifestyle programs have "potentially stabilized or even reversed coronary artery disease."[3699]

Those eating plant-based tend to be slimmer and have significantly lower LDL cholesterol, triglycerides, blood sugars, and blood pressures,[3700] as well as less carotid artery wall thickening[3701] and plaque buildup[3702] measured via ultrasound in the neck. Changes in risk factors can happen fast, as evidenced by results from one-[3703] to three-week[3704] ad libitum (eat-all-you-want) plant-based "kick-start" programs. For example, the nonprofit Rochester Lifestyle Medicine Institute created an at-home fifteen-day program, called Jumpstart. Of its first few hundred participants on a whole food, plant-based diet, obese patients lost an average of seven pounds without controlling portions or counting calories; diabetics saw their fasting blood sugars drop by twenty-eight points; those with LDL cholesterol levels over 100 mg/dL experienced a thirty-three-point drop,[3705] which is comparable to some statin drugs;[3706] and hypertensive individuals experienced a seventeen-point drop in systolic blood pressure,[3707] which is better than drugs. All this was achieved within just two weeks on the diet.[3708]

If you compare the artery function of those who don't eat meat to those who do, the healthy ability of arteries to dilate normally and let more blood flow is four times better among those eating vegetarian, and, apparently, the longer, the better. The degree of superior artery function correlated with the number of years eating meat-free. Instead of their artery function worsening over time as they aged, it was getting better the longer they ate more healthfully.[3709]

Studies dating back thirty-five years show that those eating plant-based also have improved blood "rheology," meaning fluidity or flowability,[3710] which may play a role in their cardiovascular protection.[3711] Subsequent interventional studies putting these cross-sectional findings to the test show that switching people to a plant-based diet can improve rheology measurements within just three[3712] to six weeks.[3713] Might the blood of vegetarians flow a bit too well, though? A study of thousands of British vegetarians found that they were at higher risk of hemorrhagic (bleeding) stroke,[3714] but the twelve-part video series I produced on vegetarians and stroke risk triggered by the study (starting with see.nf/vegstroke) was in vain, since, as I note in see.nf/strokeupdate, six subsequent studies[3715,3716,3717] found that, if anything, there is a lower stroke risk among those eating more plant-based.[3718]

LOW-CARB DIETS ARE LOW-LIFESPAN DIETS

While those eating plant-based diets appear to enjoy lower risk of cardiovascular disease and longer lives,[3719] those eating low-carb diets suffer significantly higher rates of cardiovascular disease and shorter lives—a 22 percent increase in overall mortality risk.[3720] So, the side effects of low-carb ketogenic diets may not only include, as a recent review recited, "chronic fatigue, nausea, headaches, hair loss, reduced tolerance to alcohol, reduced physical performance, heart palpitations, leg cramps, dry mouth, bad taste, bad breath, gout, or constipation,"[3721] but premature death as well.[3722]

Low-carb diets have been found to worsen heart disease[3723] and impair arterial function.[3724] Within just three hours of eating a meal rich in saturated fat—even from a plant source like coconut oil—there is significant impairment of artery function.[3725] Artery function worsens on a ketogenic diet,[3726] even after about a dozen pounds of weight loss, and this appears to be the case with low-carb diets in general.[3727]

Lower-carb diners also suffered significantly higher risk of dying from cancer.[3728] This could be due to higher IGF-1 induced by higher animal protein intakes[3729] (see the IGF-1 chapter) or perhaps even greater industrial toxin exposure. Ninety percent of persistent pollutant exposure comes from foods derived from animals,[3730] so it's no surprise that those eating diets that are lower in carbohydrates and higher in protein have higher levels of pollutants circulating throughout their bodies, including mercury, lead, PCBs 118 and 153, DDE (from DDT), trans-nonachlor (a component of the banned pesticide chlordane), and hexachlorobenzene (a banned fungicide). Mediterranean diet scores have also been correlated with elevated levels of PCBs (118, 126, 153, and 209), trans-nonachlor, and mercury, presumably due to the focus on fish consumption.[3731]

A FISH TALE

Thanks in part to the American Heart Association's recommendation that people who are at high risk for heart disease should ask their doctors about omega-3 fish oil supplementation,[3732] fish oil pills have exploded into a multibillion-dollar industry,[3733] yet the most extensive systematic assessment of the evidence found that increasing the intake of fish fats (EPA and DHA) has "little or no effect on deaths and cardiovascular events."[3734] Longevity experiments on mice found no benefits for aging or lifespan either.[3735] Where did we even get this idea that the omega-3 fats in fish and fish oil supplements were good for you? I review the whole saga in see.nf/fishoil and discuss contaminants, rancidity, and the five massive new trials that have been published, randomizing tens of thousands of participants to various formulations of fish oil versus placebo.[3736,3737,3738,3739,3740] It's possible some fish oil formulation will eventually prove to be helpful,[3741] but, for now, meta-analyses "unequivocally demonstrate that there is no cardiovascular benefit" to over-the-counter fish oil supplements.[3742]

SWAP MEAT

What about simply eating fish? In population studies, it's hard to separate the effects of fish consumption with the attributes of fish consumers. People who eat fish tend to smoke less, exercise more,[3743] be in a higher socioeconomic class, and eat fewer prepared meals, more organic foods, less high-fat dairy and meat, more vegetables, and fewer sweets.[3744] When researchers try to tease out some of these other factors, most studies on fish consumption show no association with cardiovascular mortality.[3745]

However, one of the key questions that always needs to be addressed in nutrition studies is, *instead of what?*[3746] For example, are eggs healthy? Compared to sausage links? Yes. Compared to oatmeal? No.[3747] In this way, the inclusion of seafood in the diet may displace foods that are even less healthy.[3748] Surprisingly, randomized controlled trials show that fish is even worse than red meat when it comes to LDL cholesterol.[3749] So, fish may be worse than beef, but it's still better than bacon.

Harvard researchers found that when it comes to sources of protein and the risk of premature death, processed meat was the worst, followed by eggs, whereas plant protein sources were the best.[3750] In essence, they found that eating tuna salad was better than egg salad or a BLT, but a bean burrito beat out the bunch. When it came to all-cause mortality, plant protein beat out every type of animal protein—red meat, chicken, fish, dairy, or egg. Swapping red meat for white meat, such as poultry and fish, would not be expected to significantly reduce mortality rates,[3751] but something like swapping chickpeas for chicken would. Swapping in just 3 percent of calories of plant protein in place of any source of animal protein was associated with a significantly lower risk of all-cause premature death.[3752]

Disappearing Act

Since heart disease is our number one killer, it is the primary determinant of how long we live. Bill Castelli, longtime director of the longest-running epidemiological study in the world—the famous Framingham Heart Study—was once asked what he would do to reverse the coronary artery disease epidemic if he were omnipotent. His answer? "Have the public eat the diet . . . described by Dr. T. Colin Campbell."[3753] In other words, he told PBS, if Americans ate plant-based enough, the whole heart disease epidemic "would disappear."[3754]

PRESERVING YOUR HAIR

In every grade school class photo, I seemed to have a mess of tousled hair on my head. No matter how much my mom tried to tame my hair, it was a little unruly. (I sported the windblown look without even trying.) Later came my metalhead phase, with headbangable hair down to the middle of my back. Sadly, though, like many of the men in my family, it started to thin, then disappear. Why do some lose their hair and others don't? Why do some people go gray earlier than others? How can we preserve the looks of our locks?

GRAYING

The graying of hair is one the most obvious signs of aging.[3755] It's also known by a technical term I had never heard before: *canities*.[3756] (The first time I saw the word I misread it, wondering what gray hair had to do with dentistry.) Evidently, gray hair isn't really gray or even white, but the pale yellowish tinge of the constitutive keratin protein that, like polar bears, looks white by the way light reflects off it.[3757]

WHY DO WE GRAY?

I detail the prevailing "free radical theory of graying"[3758] in <u>see.nf/gray</u>. Basically, free radicals naturally produced in the production of pigment[3759] lead to the deaths of pigment-producing cells[3760] as our antioxidant defenses decline as we age.[3761]

REVERSIBLE AND CONTRIBUTORY CAUSES

The age-related "exhaustion of the pigmentary potential"[3762] is thought to be mainly genetic,[3763] with a family history of premature graying present in up to 90 percent of cases.[3764] But if the rate of graying is caused by oxidative damage, what role might be played by antioxidants and systemic oxidative stress outside the hair follicle? Those with premature graying do seem to have higher circulating markers of oxidative damage and lower antioxidant levels in their blood.[3765] The higher prevalence of premature graying among smokers[3766] also supports this possibility that external free radicals may speed up oxidation in the aging hair follicle.[3767] Obese individuals tend to gray early, consistent with the oxidative stress concept, though drinkers do not.[3768] Alcohol consumption clearly causes oxidative stress,[3769] yet it is not significantly associated with premature graying.[3770]

Those trying to maximize their intake of antioxidants by eating plant-based must deal with the Achilles' heel I noted on page 210—the risk of vitamin B_{12} deficiency for those not actively supplementing their diets with B_{12} or B_{12}-fortified foods.[3771] B_{12} deficiency is one of the rare reversible causes of hair graying through some unknown mechanism.[3772] Thankfully, hair can repigment after B_{12} repletion.[3773] Another reversible cause is hypothyroidism, which can be treated with thyroid hormone replacement.[3774]

Rather than oxidative stress, what about regular stress? In <u>see.nf/hairstress</u>, I cover whether fight or flight can turn hair white, why we evolved to gray in the first place, and whether premature or extensive graying may be a sign of accelerated aging and subsequent risk of age-related diseases.

Do Hair Dyes Cause Cancer?

Since there is typically no way to reverse hair color loss, up to 60 percent of men and women in Western countries choose to use hair colorants, often to cover gray.[3775] Check out <u>see.nf/dye</u> for the entire saga, but basically, in response to FDA-mandated cancer warning labels in 1979, the hair dye industry started reformulating to eliminate its most carcinogenic ingredients.[3776]

(continued)

This led to the drop-off of some cancers[3777,3778,3779] but not others,[3780] leading some scientists to conclude that "exposure to hair colorants should be reduced as much as possible."[3781]

BALDING

Each human head harbors about 100,000 hairs[3782] and normally sheds about 100 a day as old hairs are replaced with new ones.[3783] But, as we age, hair thinning affects at least 50 percent of women by age fifty and 40 percent of men by thirty-five,[3784] rising to a lifetime prevalence of up to 80 percent.[3785] Age-related hair loss is known as androgenic or androgenetic alopecia in the hormone or gynecology literature, or male or female pattern hair loss in dermatology.[3786] Either way, it's characterized by chronic, progressive hair loss, predominantly of the central scalp.[3787]

CAUSE AND CONSEQUENCES

The word "androgenic" hints at the cause of male pattern hair loss. Derived from the Greek *andro-* for "man," androgens, male hormones like testosterone, exert an inhibitory effect on hair follicles in the scalp.[3788] This is ironic, since those same hormones are the principal *drivers* of hair growth[3789] on other areas of the body, such as the face and armpits.[3790] (Hair follicles in eyelashes appear unaffected either way.[3791]) Some knowledge of the role of male hormones dates back at least to Hippocrates, who noted, "Eunuchs do not . . . become bald,"[3792] which indeed appears to be the case. Castration can also halt the progression of hair loss in men, though it doesn't reverse it.[3793] The role of testosterone was nailed down when a Yale pathologist noticed that the castrated twin brother of a bald man had a full head of hair. As an experiment, he administered testosterone to the castrated brother, who subsequently went bald, too.[3794]

(If the ethics of that seem questionable, consider why the guy was castrated in the first place. Castration was recommended for the "feeble-minded" to "mitigate aberrant behavior,"[3795] such as the "nameless habit" of masturbation.[3796] Though the original justification[3797] for removing the testicles and ovaries of "idiot children" in the nineteenth century was in part to rein in "confirmed masturbators," under the refinement of the twentieth century, the rationale switched to eugenics.[3798] Due to eugenics laws in the United States—the first in the world[3799]— mentally handicapped persons were routinely sterilized without their consent or knowledge, a practice upheld by the U.S. Supreme Court in 1927.[3800] In the 1930s, a vocal proponent complained, "The Germans are beating us at our own game."[3801])

Is there some sort of evolutionary advantage to going bald? Though bald men may have more direct scalp exposure to sunlight, they do not appear to have higher "sunshine vitamin" D levels,[3802] but with higher levels of circulating testosterone in their blood, might they possess greater virility?[3803] On the contrary, researchers have found that balding men may be found to be less sexually attractive, averaging fewer lifetime sexual partners.[3804] What the elevated testosterone does get them is increased risk for prostate problems.[3805] While men who are genetically predisposed to have higher lifetime testosterone levels tend to have better bone density and decreased body fat, aside from hair loss, they are also more likely to suffer prostate cancer and high blood pressure.[3806]

The hypertension connection may explain why the brains of balding men are more likely to be littered with traces of ministrokes (white matter hyperintensities) on MRI.[3807] The majority of studies on the question have found that baldness is a risk factor for cardiovascular disease. Researchers suggest signs of balding be used in a clinical setting by doctors as a visible marker to identify men at increased risk of heart disease to target for prevention intervention.[3808] In women, hair loss is associated with a ninefold increased risk of having metabolic syndrome, a cluster of risk factors that include excess body fat around the waist, along with increased blood sugar, pressure, and triglycerides.[3809]

REVERSIBLE HAIR LOSS

The role male hormones play in female hair loss is uncertain,[3810] as only a minority of women with female pattern hair loss exhibit elevated androgen levels in the blood.[3811] Women often thin, predominantly over the top and front, rather than go bald[3812] and, unlike men, may not feel that they have the option of sporting a shaved head.[3813] Female hair loss may also have more varied causes.

Whereas an aging man losing his hair may just be assumed to have male pattern baldness, female hair loss demands a clinical investigation.[3814] For example, as many as one-third of those with hypothyroidism,[3815] an underactive thyroid gland condition that strikes women up to seven times more than men, present with diffuse hair loss.[3816] This is usually irreversible even with thyroid hormone replacement, underscoring the importance of early diagnosis. Oral contraceptive use, crash dieting, and the recent birth of a child can also cause a common type of hair loss called *telogen effluvium*.[3817]

Unlike most of the hair follicles on our body and on our pets, which are in a resting maintenance "telogen" phase, approximately 90 percent of the hair follicles on our scalp are in an active growing "anagen" phase.[3818] In both men and women, stressful events, such as surgery and sickness, can cause a mass reset of the hair cycle, switching follicles into the telogen phase, which only lasts two to three months before the cycle renews.[3819] (COVID-19 was a major cause of this.[3820]) This reset means that a few months after the traumatic event, your hair can start falling out in clumps as the new hairs that are being born all begin to simultaneously push out the established hair, rather than being staggered over time. People tend not to make the connection with their precipitating event and fear they may go bald, but telogen effluvium tends to be self-limiting. The hair loss resolves as the new hairs start growing out over the subsequent months, but it may take a year or longer to experience cosmetically significant regrowth.[3821]

How do you know what kind of hair loss you have? Pattern hair loss can often be distinguished from telogen effluvium with what's called a pull test.[3822] After not washing your hair for at least twenty-four hours, grasp approximately fifty hairs between the thumb, index finger, and middle finger and, slowly and gently, pull them away from the scalp.[3823] Normally, most of your hairs are in an active growing phase, so less than 10 percent of the hairs should come out. If more than that come out and they have a small white bulb on the scalp end (what's referred to as telogen "club hairs"), then you may be experiencing telogen effluvium.[3824]

MODIFIABLE RISK FACTORS

Balding men tend to have not only higher levels of testosterone but higher levels of testosterone receptors in their scalps,[3825] which appears to be mostly genetically determined.[3826] Identical twins show a concordance rate of about 80 or 90 percent, meaning if one twin is balding, eight or nine times out of ten, the other twin is, too.[3827] But what about the 10 to 20 percent who share the same genetics but have discrepant hair loss? What can we learn from them?

No, hair loss is not caused by washing or brushing your hair too much, two of the many myths out there.[3828] In identical twin women, the sister with higher levels of stress, more marriages, more divorces or separations, and more children was more likely to suffer hair loss.[3829] In both identical twin pairs of brothers[3830] and sisters,[3831] wearing hats appeared to be protective, but the results for exercise and caffeine intake were contradictory. Exercise and caffeine were associated with less hair loss in female identical twins but more hair loss in male identical twins. Perhaps this is because interventional trials show that aerobic exercise can increase testosterone levels in men.[3832] Interestingly, caffeinated coffee can increase testosterone in men but decrease levels in women.[3833]

The data on tobacco were consistent. Studies of identical twin pairs of men[3834] and women[3835] found that smoking was a common factor associated with a receding hairline, a factor confirmed in studies of the general population.[3836] This is thought to be due to genotoxic compounds in cigarettes that may damage the DNA in hair follicles and cause microvascular poisoning of their blood supply.[3837] Other toxic agents associated with hair loss include[3838] mercury, which seems to concentrate about 250-fold in growing scalp hair.[3839] Mercury poisoning from his syphilis treatment may have been the reason Shakespeare started losing his hair.[3840] Thankfully, doctors don't give their patients mercury anymore. These days, as the Centers for Disease Control and Prevention (CDC) points out, mercury "enters the body mainly from dietary seafood sources."[3841]

Perimenopausal women frequently seek treatment for what is thought to be hormone-related hair loss, but there are case reports of women with high fish intake and correspondingly high blood mercury levels whose hair loss can be reversed with a fish-free diet. For example, within two months of the elimination of dietary tuna, mercury blood levels can drop as much as a third and hair can not only start growing back but it can completely regrow within seven months. The medical director of the Center for Menopause, Hormonal Disorders and Women's Health suggests doctors should consider screening for mercury toxicity in the face of hair loss, since "[i]nstructing patients to reduce fish intake . . . could offer relief of symptoms" from heavy metal-induced hair loss.[3842] (Though, admittedly, thinking back to glam bands of the 1980s, sometimes heavy metal may lead to too much hair.)

DRUG TREATMENT FOR HAIR LOSS

Historically, recommended treatments for hair loss included sprinkling mouse droppings and the ashes of a donkey's penis on your head.[3843] Julius Caesar reportedly tried a mélange of minced mice, horse teeth, and bear grease.[3844] Treatments today may be less exotic, but apparently no less desperate, as more than $3 billion is reportedly spent every year in the United States to treat hair loss.[3845] Currently, the only two FDA-approved drugs for hair loss are minoxidil, sold as Rogaine, and finasteride, sold as Propecia.[3846] I cover the efficacy and safety of both in see.nf/hairdrugs.

PULL THE PLUG

There are also surgical options, though punch grafts or "plugs" historically gave hair restoration procedures a bad name.[3847] Developed back in the 1950s, small circles of scalp skin from areas where hair is still growing, like the back of the head, were transplanted to bald areas on the top and front.[3848] This left an unnatural cornrow doll's hair appearance.[3849]

Today, there is "follicular unit transplanting," where a long strip of hairy scalp is surgically excised and divided into much smaller punches for transplantation.[3850] The transplanted follicles then retain the androgen resistance native to their original location. For men who are completely bald, hairs can be transplanted from the chest, abdomen, legs, shoulders, or beard.[3851] Most of the grafted hair follicles tend to survive (on the order of 85 percent), and high rates of patient satisfaction have been recorded.[3852] However, cosmetically desirable results require multiple operations, and each carries up to a 5 percent rate of complications,[3853] which can include necrosis at the excision site, excessive scar tissue, and infections, though serious complications are rare.[3854]

PLASMA AND LASERS

What about nondrug, nonsurgical interventions? Autologous platelet-rich plasma therapy has been tried, a process in which concentrated portions of your own blood are repeatedly injected into your scalp. The efficacy may be similar to the available drugs,[3855] but the evidence thus far is considered to be insufficient to recommend it, and it remains unapproved in the United States and Europe for hair restoration purposes.[3856] Botox in the scalp is also not recommended. The thought was that relaxing scalp muscles might prevent hair loss by improving blood flow,[3857] but when it was actually put to the test, it *caused* hair loss in some pilot study participants.[3858] Then, there are lasers.

The FDA cleared the first low-level laser therapy (LLLT) device for pattern hair loss in 2007,[3859] and now there are clinics advertising lasers for everything from tennis elbow[3860] to "scrotal rejuvenation."[3861] As I go through in see.nf/lasers, there have been at least ten randomized controlled trials of LLLT devices for hair loss,[3862] and though there are statistically significant improvements in hair density and thickness, there may be little *clinically* significant improvement.[3863] If you want to give them a try anyway, in the video I offer some safety tips and advice on how to choose between the dozens of FDA-cleared devices currently on the market.[3864]

SUPPLEMENTS FOR HAIR LOSS

Are there nutrient deficiencies that can cause hair loss? After bariatric surgery, hair loss is the most frequently reported nutrient deficiency symptom, but the surgery often involves anatomy rearrangement to purposefully cause malabsorption.[3865] In general, there is little evidence to suggest that vitamin and mineral supplementation benefits people unless they are actually deficient.[3866] This is the case with vitamin C, zinc, iron, and biotin, which can actually do more harm than good.

The details for these studies are in see.nf/hairsupplements. For example, there has not been a single clinical trial demonstrating efficacy of biotin for any kind of hair loss,[3867] unless a deficiency is induced by raw egg white consumption,[3868] and biotin supplements can cause havoc on a bunch of different blood tests.[3869] (See page 464.)

In terms of poor regulation, sloppiness by supplement manufacturers includes accidentally putting two hundred times the intended selenium dose that ended up *causing* hair loss due to selenium toxicity.[3870] The same can happen when getting too much vitamin A[3871] or vitamin E, yet the best-selling hair supplement on Amazon.com contained both A and E vitamins, and the next most popular one contained vitamin A, vitamin E, and selenium.[3872]

What about all the patented hair-growth supplements on the market these days? A dermatology journal review considered the available evidence and concluded that, at least to date, it should be considered a myth that any increase hair growth.[3873] Ironically, such supplements may actually be more expensive than the current medications—up to more than $1,000 a year, compared to $100 to $300 a year.[3874] What about treating hair loss from the inside out with food?

FOODS FOR HAIR LOSS

Population studies have found that pattern baldness is associated with poor sleeping habits and the consumption of meat and junk food,[3875] whereas protective associations were found for the consumption of raw vegetables and fresh herbs,[3876] as well as frequent intake of soymilk. Drinking soy beverages on a weekly basis was associated with 62 percent lower odds of moderate to severe hair loss,[3877] raising the possibility that there are compounds in plants that may be protective.[3878]

There is no shortage of Rapunzel-length boasts of different dietary regimens and other alternative treatments to "cure" hair loss,[3879] but a critical review of the literature shows much of the evidence was obtained on shaved rodents.[3880] Even when clinical studies are done on actual people, sometimes there's no placebo control, so you have no idea if the food had anything to do with it.[3881] Check out see.nf/hairfoods for a remarkable case report of a totally bald man receiving a fecal transplant and regrowing a full head of hair, as well as detail on all the foods shown in a randomized, double-blind, placebo-controlled trial to improve hair loss. These include the hot pepper compound[3882] found in a daily one-half of a habanero pepper[3883] or a teaspoon of medium-hot red pepper,[3884] the daily soy isoflavones[3885] found in three-quarters of a cup of tempeh or just straight cooked soybeans, or a half cup of soy "nuts,"[3886] and the pumpkin seed oil found in about four pumpkin seeds a day.[3887] Unfortunately, the supplement they used wasn't straight pumpkin seed oil but an amalgam of vegetable powders and other ingredients, and the study was financially supported by the product's marketing firm.[3888] But it can't hurt to eat a few pumpkin seeds, perhaps encrusted with cayenne on your tempeh wings.

TOPICAL HERBAL TREATMENTS

If pumpkin seed oil is so anti-androgenic, what about just rubbing it on your scalp? It works on mice,[3889] but what about men or, in this case, women? Pumpkin seed oil (about a quarter teaspoon rubbed onto the scalp once a day) was tested head-to-head against minoxidil foam (5 percent once daily) for three months in women with female pattern hair loss. Both treatments worked, but the minoxidil worked better,[3890] though at about five times the cost.

A similar experiment compared a topical 0.2 percent caffeine solution, which is about five times stronger than coffee, to 5 percent minoxidil, and the researchers found they worked similarly well for balding men.[3891] However, as with the pumpkin seed oil trial, there was no third placebo group to ensure the study participants weren't somehow just improving on their own[3892]—due to seasonal influence, for example, with greater shedding in the fall than in the spring.[3893]

Dripping caffeine on human hair follicles growing in a petri dish enhances hair growth,[3894] and when it was finally put to the test against placebo, it won out for both male[3895] and female[3896] pattern baldness. In the study on men, 85 percent were satisfied after using the caffeine-containing shampoo for six months, compared to only 36 percent in the placebo shampoo group.[3897] EGCG, one of the major constituents of green tea, can also promote human hair growth in vitro,[3898] perhaps via inhibition of 5α-reductase,[3899] and may help balding mice,[3900] but I couldn't find any clinical hair growth trials on green tea.

Pyrithione zinc (1 percent) shampoo, typically used for dandruff, beat out placebo for increasing hair density in balding men after twenty-six weeks, but not enough for the study subjects to notice any difference, and it worked less than half as well as 5 percent minoxidil.[3901]

What about topical herbal treatments used since time immemorial?

Ginger offers a good cautionary tale. Ginger has a long history of traditional use in Asia to halt hair loss and heighten hair growth. Do a quick search for "ginger shampoo" on Amazon.com, and nearly a thousand entries pop up. But when the Natural Science Foundation of China finally put it to the test, researchers were surprised to find that ginger actually *suppressed* human hair growth. Given their results, they suggested that ginger could instead be used for the removal of unwanted body hair.[3902]

Polygonum multiflorum, known in traditional Chinese medicine circles as *he-*

shouwu, is a flowering plant in the buckwheat family popularized as a hair tonic.[3903] Like green tea, there are promising in vitro[3904] and rodent studies,[3905] but no human clinical trials. Rosemary, however, has been put to the test.

Rosemary Oil

In see.nf/rosemaryoil, I detail a series of experiments on successfully treating a patchy form of hair loss called *alopecia areata* with a mixture of essential oils[3906] or, less pleasantly, topical onion[3907] or garlic juice.[3908] In terms of age-related pattern hair loss, rubbing a quarter teaspoon of your favorite lotion premixed with ten drops of rosemary essential oil for each fluid ounce onto your scalp twice a day appears to work as well as the drug minoxidil in balding men.[3909] That much rosemary oil would cost about a penny a week.

PRESERVING YOUR HEARING

For what we can do to preserve our sense of smell—primarily not smoking[3910]—see my video see.nf/smell. Though this can have serious consequences, such as missing gas leaks[3911] or adding more salt to foods,[3912] most people who are affected don't even seem to be aware their sense of smell is impaired, even when directly asked about it.[3913] Hearing loss, however, is considered a major cause of global disability,[3914] ranking among the top chronic conditions affecting older adults.[3915] Yet, for far too long, as a National Academy of Medicine report put it, hearing loss has been "relegated to the sidelines of health care."[3916]

HEARING AIDS FOR AGE-RELATED HEARING LOSS

Age-related hearing loss, also known as *presbycusis* (from the Greek *presbys* for "old" and *akousis* for "hearing"), affects about a quarter of those in their sixties, more than half in their seventies, and 80 percent of those in their eighties in the United States.[3917] More than 95 percent of centenarians were also found to have profound hearing loss.[3918] Because of impaired communication,[3919] this may lead to social isolation, loneliness,[3920] and depression.[3921] It may even threaten one's life due to an associated increase in motor vehicle accidents.[3922]

Hearing aids can help, though they appear to be vastly underutilized, with fewer than one in six hearing-impaired older adults using them.[3923] Barriers include comfort, cosmesis, and cost. Unlike countries like the United Kingdom, which have provided hearing aids to their citizens for free for more than half a century,[3924] in the United States the devices have been prohibitively expensive, averaging between $2,000 and $7,000, and are often not covered by health insurance.[3925] Thankfully, the bipartisan Over-the-Counter Hearing Aid Act was passed in 2017, which gave the FDA three years to allow their sale through traditional retail outlets rather than doctor's offices or specialty shops to increase competition and bring down costs.[3926] The FDA understandably missed their statutory deadline due to COVID-19, but with masking and physical distancing making it even more difficult for the hearing impaired to communicate, the need for affordable options had never been greater.[3927] Thanks in part to pressure from a presidential executive order, over-the-counter hearing aids finally hit U.S. shelves on October 17, 2022.[3928]

How well do they work? Unlike "aural rehabilitation," a collection of coping strategies such as lip reading, which has not been shown to be effective in older adults with hearing loss,[3929] hearing aids have been proven to be effective in improving the ability of adults with mild to moderate hearing loss to understand others and take part in everyday situations.[3930] They are considered the first-line clinical management tool for those seeking help for hearing difficulties.[3931]

Some of the complaints people used to have with hearing aids, such as whistling tones from acoustic feedback, have since been digitally reduced or eliminated in modern devices. Other issues that arise from blocking the ear canal, such as changes in the sound of your own voice or hearing yourself chewing, have been more difficult to rectify.[3932] People like to think that correcting hearing problems with sound amplification is as straightforward as correcting vision problems with eyeglasses, but just because sounds are louder doesn't necessarily mean they're clearer.[3933] Insufficient benefit is one of the leading reasons why some people who have hearing aids just don't wear them.[3934] But, are there benefits beyond symptomatic relief that might change the cost-benefit calculus?

HEARING AIDS FOR COGNITIVE DECLINE

If you visit the websites of leading hearing aid brands, you'll see marketing claims implying that their products can prevent or forestall cognitive decline.[3935] I review the science in see.nf/thinkingaids, but sadly, as a recent World Health Organization review concluded, "There is insufficient evidence to recommend use of hearing aids to reduce the risk of cognitive decline and/or dementia."[3936] Hearing aids may not help your brain, but they can still add significant symptomatic relief of hearing difficulty. What about treating the cause of hearing loss in the first place?

HOW TO REVERSE EARWAX-INDUCED HEARING LOSS

One of the most common, reversible causes of hearing loss is earwax buildup. Earwax is normal, and if it's not causing symptoms, it should be left alone. It doesn't start interfering with hearing acuity until it clogs at least 80 percent of the ear canal. Ironically, hearing aids are a risk factor for excessive earwax, as is anything else you put into your ear, like earplugs, since that stimulates the earwax glands.[3937] For further irony, so, too, may the cotton-tipped swabs that as many as two-thirds of people use to clean out their ears.[3938] So, you may think you're making things better by swabbing out your ears, but you may actually be making things worse.[3939] In fact, just the removal of protective wax can leave your canals dry, itchy, and achy or even lead to "Q-tip otalgia," a term coined in the *Journal of the American Medical Association* to refer to an ear pain syndrome caused by cotton-tipped swabs.[3940] You shouldn't need to clean your ear canals at all because the wax should make its way out on its own.

Ears are self-cleaning. The lining of your ear canal grows outward from your eardrum, so secreted earwax and any dirt that's been trapped is eventually conveyor-belted out. However, this self-cleaning mechanism can fail in one in twenty younger adults and as many as one in three older adults, and it may lead to excessive or impacted earwax accumulation, though those affected may not even be aware of it.[3941] Seventy percent of those surveyed who had both ears completely blocked with wax thought their hearing was good, but when their ears were cleared, they were suddenly able to hear better. Clearing out impacted wax can also improve symptoms of ear irritation, pressure, and fullness,[3942] but what's the best way to do it?

Q-tips and other cotton-tipped swabs are a no-no. Pushing anything into the ear canal can end up making things worse by impacting wax even deeper into the ear or traumatizing the canal, resulting in abrasions,[3943] infections,[3944] or even eardrum perforation in a small percentage of users.[3945] There's even been a case report of a cotton swab causing a brain abscess and fatal meningitis, though the presence of wood splinters suggests the tip had broken off inside the ear.[3946] Cotton swab packaging already cautions users against ear canal insertion, but perhaps warning labels should be made clearer, wrote one clinical medical officer: "[D]o not go near the ear hole or avoid the ear altogether."

What about wax removal ear drops? There are about a dozen different formulations on the market, none of which appears to work any better than any other one or even when compared to just saline (salt water) or even plain tap water. But, five days of treatment does clear earwax in about one in five cases (22 percent) compared to only 5 percent clearing up on their own within that time frame.[3947] At the very least, ear drops may be able to soften wax before bulb syringe irrigation.[3948]

Also called ear syringing, irrigation involves flushing out wax with a low-pressure jet of warm (body temperature) water. It works up to 70 to 90 percent of the time, and if it doesn't, clinicians have fancy devices to manually remove the wax under direct observation.[3949] Irrigation can also be tried at home. Those randomized to use a bulb in the comfort of their own home had about a 50 percent success rate in clearing the obstruction[3950] and, armed with this knowledge, were significantly less likely to subsequently require in-office irrigation.[3951] Significant complications only happen in approximately one in a thousand irrigations.[3952]

You should *not* use an oral water jet. There are scientific papers with titles such as "Catastrophic Otologic Injury from Oral Jet Irrigation of the External Auditory Canal." Even at one-third power, Waterpiks were shown to perforate the eardrums of fresh cadavers. Those who insist on violating this important proscription should, at the very least, choose the lowest setting, use a tip with multiple orifices, and make sure the water stream is directed only against the walls of the ear canal and never straight back toward the eardrum,[3953] but I still strongly caution against it.

What About Ear Candling?

Ear candles (also known as ear cones) are promoted as a low-cost, effective treatment for earwax,[3954] but as I document in see.nf/candling, a series of experiments found that it not only offers no benefit, it can make things worse[3955] and even result in serious injury.[3956]

HEARING LOSS IS NOT INEVITABLE

Earwax is one thing, but what about preventing age-related hearing loss? It's said to be a natural part of the aging process,[3957] but that's what we used to think about pathological conditions like high blood pressure. The vast majority of people eventually develop hypertension, just like the vast majority of people eventually lose their hearing, so it must just be an inevitable consequence of growing old, right?

But then it was discovered that there were rural populations living in Africa,[3958] Asia,[3959] and the Amazon,[3960] who ate and lived more healthfully and did not experience an inexorable rise in blood pressure as they aged. So, it appeared hypertension was a lifestyle choice rather than an aging effect—and the same may be true for hearing loss.

The Mabaan, a tribe living in the Sudanese bush, were found to retain their hearing into old age.[3961] Another study, on the isolated native population on Easter Island, found that exposure to modern environments appeared to undercut their hearing advantages.[3962] What is it about our modern world that seems to lead us to lose our hearing as we grow older?

Age-related hearing loss is a result of the premature death of the sensory hair cells in the inner ear, which turn vibrations into electric signals to the brain.[3963] Once they're lost, they don't grow back, so prevention is critical.[3964] What is killing the sensory hair cells? A study of more than 2,000 twins found that the heritability of age-related hearing impairment was only 25 percent, so most of the risk is due to nongenetic influences.[3965]

Risk factors include smoking, ototoxic (hearing-damaging) medications, and repeated exposure to loud noises.[3966] Noise exposure earlier in life appears to render the inner ear more vulnerable to aging.[3967] Animal studies suggest exposure to low-level yet constant noise over 60 decibels may also be harmful.[3968] This has not been demonstrated in humans, but if you use a white noise generator to sleep, it can't hurt to make sure it's under 50 decibels.[3969] Aminoglycoside antibiotics, such as streptomycin, amikacin, neomycin, and kanamycin, are among the highest-risk medications for sensory hair cell toxicity,[3970] but loop diuretics (for example, furosemide, sold as Lasix) and NSAIDs (nonsteroidal anti-inflammatory drugs like aspirin, ibuprofen, and naproxen) have also been linked to progressive hearing loss.[3971] The key to the preservation of hearing in older Mabaan tribe members, however, may be their diet.

What About Cell Phone Radiation?

Your inner ear may be the organ most frequently and directly exposed to cell phone radiation. Might that have adverse effects on hearing? Long-term cell phone users have been found to have detectable hearing loss compared to nonusers, though not enough to be noticeable. The impairment was measurable in both ears, which may be more consistent with a radiation effect than simply a constant loud-noise-in-one-ear effect.[3972] I explore all the studies in see.nf/phones, but in short, researchers found no effect at thirty minutes of cell phone use, but sixty minutes did appear to immediately impact hearing threshold levels at specific frequencies.[3973] Bluetooth was found to be safer, presumably because it operates at nearly a thousand times lower strength.[3974]

WHAT TO EAT TO SLOW HEARING LOSS

The reason the researchers concluded that the Mabaan tribe's diet likely accounted for their lack of age-related hearing loss is they also appeared to lack something else:

coronary artery disease.[3975] What kills more of us in the industrialized world than anything else doesn't appear to touch them at all.[3976] Their blood pressures are also perfect their whole lives, at about 110 over 70 into their seventies, while the rest of us, on average, become hypertensive starting as early as our forties.[3977] And, it's no wonder. The Mabaan diet is centered around whole grains (sorghum) and "almost free of animal protein." So, the researchers suggested that atherosclerosis clogging the small blood vessels feeding the inner ear may be the underlying cause of age-related hearing loss in most of the rest of the world.[3978]

Indeed, healthier diets are associated with a significantly lower risk of hearing loss, and for all three diet quality scoring systems they used, avoidance of meat was most strongly linked to lower risk.[3979] The Mabaan also do not eat sugary junk, which explains their almost total absence of dental cavities.[3980] A high glycemic diet of refined carbohydrates is also associated with developing age-related hearing loss,[3981] and elevated blood sugars in general may explain why diabetics and prediabetics are at higher risk, too.[3982] Even among whole grains, sorghum has a particularly low glycemic index due to its resistant starch content,[3983] causing about a 25 percent lower rise in blood sugar response compared to whole wheat.[3984]

Impaired blood circulation may also explain how noise damages the inner ear, since loud noises cause constriction of the accompanying blood vessels.[3985] It may also help clarify the link between obesity and hearing loss. Excess weight may just be a proxy for unhealthier diets, but the pro-inflammatory state of obesity can itself lead to vascular dysfunction.[3986] Measures of systemic inflammation seem to directly correlate with age-related hearing loss, as do measures of oxidative stress.[3987]

Details in see.nf/earfoods, but basically, blueberries can actually reverse hearing deficits in rats,[3988] though adding antioxidants to their food[3989] or water[3990] seems to help prevent age-related hearing loss, whereas antioxidant supplements fail to improve hearing in people.[3991] What has been shown to help is folic acid supplementation,[3992] of which the healthiest sources are dark green leafy vegetables and legumes. (Just one cup of cooked lentils has 90 percent of an adult's daily needs,[3993] for example, and a cup of edamame 120 percent.[3994])

WHAT TO AVOID TO SLOW HEARING LOSS

A 2021 broad overview titled "Role of Nutrition in the Development and Prevention of Age-Related Hearing Loss" screened thousands of papers and concluded: "Diets rich in saturated fats and cholesterol have deleterious effects on hearing that could be prevented by lower consumption."[3995] The case of the Mabaan makes for a compelling story, but what exactly are the reviewers basing that conclusion on? It's true that you can prove it in laboratory animals—randomize rats to added saturated fat[3996] or chinchillas to added dietary cholesterol, and scientists can show that atherosclerosis-inducing diets exacerbate inner ear damage and hearing loss—but that doesn't necessarily mean the same is true in people.[3997]

There are cogent epidemiological data. For example, a study of thousands of twins was able to draw a significant link between a diet high in cholesterol and hearing impairment.[3998] In the Blue Mountains Hearing Study, which enrolled thousands of older men and women, dietary cholesterol was the nutritional component most associated with age-related hearing loss. Those eating about two eggs' worth of cholesterol a day had 34 percent greater odds of hearing loss compared to those only getting about a single egg's worth. Consistent with a vascular cause, people on statins and particularly those at higher doses appeared to be at lower risk. The researchers suggest that atherosclerotic inflammatory changes, caused by the high cholesterol diet, in the tiny arteries feeding the inner ear would explain their findings, but how about actually looking at the arteries to see if this is true?[3999]

The extent and severity of coronary artery disease in the heart, as determined by angiogram, were found to be closely correlated to hearing loss.[4000] Since atherosclerosis is a systemic disease affecting the entire arterial tree, this has relevance for the arteries feeding the inner ear. The same connection was found for the amount of atherosclerotic plaque found in the carotid arteries in the neck. The greater the plaque, the poorer the hearing,[4001] and the greater the risk of further hearing impairment measured over the subsequent five years.[4002] We're getting closer, but how about the arteries that directly supply the inner ear? Early autopsy data suggest[4003] and direct imaging studies show[4004] a direct correlation between the degree of hearing loss and atherosclerotic narrowing of those arteries.

Now all we need is an interventional trial to wrap it all up in a bow. Yes, diets high in cholesterol[4005] and high in saturated fat[4006] have been shown to kill off cochlear hair cells and cause inner ear damage and hearing loss in laboratory animals, but it's not as though you can lock up hundreds of people for a few years, force them to eat different amounts of saturated fat, and see what happens to their hearing. Oh, but you can, and they did. Enter: the Finnish Mental Hospital Study. In 1958, one of two mental hospitals near Helsinki changed its menus to decrease its patients' intake of saturated animal fat.[4007] Then, after a few years, the two hospitals switched their menus. It was one of the first interventional trials of its kind and showed you could decrease heart disease deaths by decreasing saturated fat intake.

And their hearing? It followed the exact same pattern.[4008] As their heart disease got worse, so did their hearing.[4009] And, after the hospitals switched their menus, the reverse happened—and not just by a little. Patients in their fifties in the lower saturated fat hospital ended up with significantly better hearing than the group in the control hospital who were ten years younger.[4010] The researchers stated that "our audiological studies lead us to conclude that diet is an important factor in the prevention of hearing loss."[4011]

PRESERVING YOUR HORMONES

The search for a hormonal fountain of youth has a colorful and controversial history. Sigmund Freud recommended that the perimenopausal mother of Prince Philip, Duke of Edinburgh, have her ovaries irradiated with high-intensity X-rays to restore her youthful vitality. During the 1920s and '30s, this was evidently accepted as an energizing "cure" for the symptoms of aging in women.[4012] Mental and physical debilities in men were blamed on "seminal losses" from masturbation, and when injecting semen into the blood of elderly men was deemed too dangerous, an eminent physiologist chose instead to inject the "juice" from freshly crushed dog testicles.[4013] This eventually led to a popular cottage industry of the transplantation of testicular extracts, minced tissues, or entire testicles of goats, guinea pigs, or chimpanzees to "rejuvenate" aging men.[4014] By 1940, more than 10,000 testicular implantations had taken place in human experimentation trials at San Quentin State Penitentiary in California.[4015]

"ANTI-AGING" HORMONES

Millions are spent on hormone treatments to slow aging, but they may do more harm than good.

HUMAN GROWTH HORMONE

Of all of the anti-aging clinic scams and hucksterisms, the selling and administration of human growth hormone has been called "perhaps the most blatant and organized form of quackery today."[4016] As I detail in see.nf/hgh, not only is there no evidence of anti-aging effects,[4017] if anything, growth hormone may actually accelerate the aging process.[4018] Given the risk of cancer and potential for a *shortened* lifespan, one prominent clinician remarked that growth hormone may be a "true anti-aging drug" in that it may prematurely stop you from growing any older.[4019]

Tired of "Adrenal Fatigue"

Many seeking treatment for common nonspecific symptoms are led to believe that they are suffering from some sort of hormonal deficiency.[4020] "Adrenal fatigue" is the prototypical example. Chiropractor-coined in 1998, the invented diagnosis has since been embraced by naturopaths, functional medicine practitioners, and anti-aging doctors,[4021] but the title of a systematic review in an endocrinology journal says it all: "Adrenal Fatigue Does Not Exist."[4022] I do a deep dive in see.nf/adrenal. In sum, hawking unproven tests and treatments for a made-up malady could delay the diagnosis of an actual, treatable condition.[4023]

DHEA

Dehydroepiandrosterone (DHEA) is the most abundant steroid hormone circulating in our blood,[4024] though levels drop with age[4025] after a peak at around thirty.[4026] Heralded as an "anti-aging" "superhormone" "panacea,"[4027] U.S. DHEA had sales of more than $50 million a year[4028] on the premise that replenishing youthful levels might have restorative effects. As I document in see.nf/dhea, early enthusiasm has been replaced by a sober skepticism as the "panacea" repeatedly failed to beat out placebo.[4029] Aside from intravaginal DHEA for vaginal atrophy,[4030] which I'll cover in the Preserving Your Sex Life chapter, the only convincing benefit is the improvement of birth rates of women in their late thirties undergoing in vitro fertilization.[4031,4032] As with any supplement, there are concerns about quality control issues. Some "DHEA" supplements just blatantly lie and contain no DHEA whatsoever,[4033] but there are natural ways to boost DHEA.

Lower protein intake is associated with higher levels of DHEA,[4034] and an interventional trial found that increasing fiber intake actively raised levels,[4035] so what about putting them together? Researchers found that after only five days on an egg-free vegetarian diet, levels of DHEA in the blood increased by nearly 20 percent.[4036] It can also be tested the other way: When study participants already eating a plant-based diet were switched to a conventional diet, their DHEA levels dropped by up to 20 percent.[4037,4038] It seems the bodies of those eating plant-based hold on to the hormone better, excreting less in their urine, which is normally something seen only when fasting.[4039]

Holding On to Eggs by Letting Go of Dairy

What can women do to preserve their fertility in the first place? We used to think that women's ovarian reserve of eggs stayed relatively stable until a rapid decline at around age twenty-seven,[4040] but we now know it appears to be a more steady and gradual loss of eggs over time, starting at peak fertility in one's early twenties.[4041] As I review in see.nf/ovarianreserve, Harvard researchers suggest that the increased dairy consumption corresponding with as much as a decade's worth of accelerated ovarian aging is either because of contamination of milk products by endocrine-disrupting chemicals or the presence of natural reproductive hormones.[4042] Around 60 to 80 percent of dietary exposure to estrogens, progesterone, and other placental hormones comes from dairy products.[4043] (Cows are typically milked while they're pregnant.[4044]) Once inside the human body, these bovine hormones get converted into estrone and estradiol, the main active human estrogens,[4045] which could end up altering the speed of ovarian decline.[4046]

MENOPAUSE

Life after menopause is unusual in the animal kingdom. Females of most species die soon after their reproductive capacity drops off,[4047] which was true even for humans until the last century or so. (The average life expectancy of women in the United States in 1900 was forty-eight.[4048]) These days, though, women may live more than a third of their lives after menopause, so the question becomes, *how can women thrive through this transition and beyond?*

MENOPAUSE ON PAUSE

Since 1970, the proportion of women having their first child after age thirty-five increased nearly tenfold.[4049] This may introduce a "longevity penalty" on their children, as those born to older mothers don't tend to live as long, but women having children later tend to live longer themselves.[4050] I explore this phenomenon in my video see .nf/delaymenopause, along with the diet and lifestyle factors that affect the timing of menopause, including smoking,[4051] marital history,[4052] and plant protein intake.[4053]

MEDICALIZING MENOPAUSE

A woman is considered to be postmenopausal after twelve consecutive months without a menstrual period.[4054] In the United States, the average age at menopause is 51.5. About 20 percent of women escape symptom-free, whereas 20 percent at the other end of the spectrum face severe symptoms from the accompanying hormonal changes. Some get better over time, like hot flashes, but others tend to get worse, like vaginal dryness.[4055] Hot flashes and night sweats typically last about five to seven years[4056] but may exceed a decade in 10 to 15 percent of individuals.[4057] The medical establishment's answer was hormone replacement therapy.

Even the name, hormone replacement, speaks to the medicalization of menopause as a disease. Taking thyroid hormone for an underactive thyroid gland or insulin for type 1 diabetics who don't make any of their own is hormone replacement therapy. In contrast, the drop in hormones like estrogen during menopause is the normal and natural state, so the name for this treatment has since been changed to simply *hormone therapy* or *menopausal hormone therapy*.[4058] It was originally marketed not merely for symptom relief but as a fountain-of-youth formula, preying on older women's self-esteem, vanity, and fear of aging,[4059] as popularized in the cringeworthy 1968 bestseller *Feminine Forever*, written by a Manhattan gynecologist named Robert Wilson.

"The unpalatable truth must be faced that all postmenopausal women are castrates," Wilson wrote. He recommended hormones be prescribed to lift women from their "vapid cow-like" state[4060] and make them "much more pleasant to live with."[4061] It's a little-known fact that Wilson's work promoting the drugs was funded by—you guessed it—the Big Pharma hormone manufacturers themselves,[4062] who ponied up more than a million dollars.[4063] He dismissed the suggestion that hormones like estrogen and progesterone might cause breast cancer as "against all logic," suggesting that, if anything, it would *protect* women from breast cancer. By the 1990s, up to 40 percent of menopausal women in the United States were on these drugs,[4064] raking in billions of dollars a year for the pharmaceutical industry.[4065] But then the revelations of the Women's Health Initiative and the Million Women Study were published, indicating elevated risk for breast cancer, blood clots, and endometrial cancer.[4066] The use of menopausal hormone therapy plummeted by 80 percent,[4067] along with a subsequent sharp and significant reduction in breast cancer rates.[4068]

MORE BREAST CANCER *AND* MORE CARDIOVASCULAR DISEASE

As far back as the 1940s, concerns were being raised that dosing women with estrogens might cause breast cancer,[4069] but it took the bulk of a century before it was decided to definitively study the safety of something prescribed to millions.[4070] I describe the whole saga in my video see.nf/premarin, but basically, the bombshell landed in the summer of 2002. The Women's Health Initiative study found so much more invasive breast cancer in the estrogen and progesterone (PremPro) users that they were forced to stop the study prematurely. Researchers expected that lowered cardiovascular risk would balance this out,[4071] but the women didn't just have more breast cancer; they had more heart attacks, too, as well as more strokes and more blood clots to their lungs.[4072] In 2003, the Million Women Study was published in Europe, confirming breast cancer fears,[4073] and in 2004, the estrogens-only (Premarin) wing of the Women's Health Initiative was also halted prematurely due to elevated stroke rates.[4074]

The news that women treated with hormone therapy experienced more breast cancer, cardiovascular disease, and overall harm "rocked women and physicians across the country."[4075] Before the study, estrogen had been the most prescribed drug in the United States,[4076] but after its publication, the number of prescriptions dropped immediately[4077] and, within a year, so did the incidence of breast cancer[4078] around the world.[4079] The Women's Health Initiative hormone trial cost about a quarter billion dollars to run, but given the number of lives the drop in hormone usage subsequently saved (including more than 100,000 fewer cases of breast cancer alone over the subsequent decade), the net economic return was estimated at $37 billion, a 140-fold return on investment.[4080]

Big Pharma did not go gently into that good night. Even after the findings were published, millions of prescriptions continued to be dispensed.[4081] Mortified at all the cancer his colleagues were causing, one doctor wrote, "How long will it take us to discard the financial gains, to admit that we are harming many of our patients, and to start changing our prescription habits?"[4082] Many physicians continue to cling to the "non-evidence-based perception"[4083] that hormone therapy carries net health benefit despite overwhelming evidence to the contrary,[4084] and that has been blamed on "decades of carefully orchestrated corporate influence on medical literature."[4085] Lawsuits from breast cancer victims unearthed internal documents showing that the drug companies hired PR firms to ghostwrite dozens of skewed reviews and commentaries in medical journals.[4086] It's been said that the "current culture of gynecology encourages the dissemination of health advice based on advertising rather than science."[4087]

After the truth came out, Big Pharma continued to try to distort the medical record by paying to have editorials appear in medical journals to downplay the risks and promote unproven benefits. Of the 110 partisan polemics that were published, only 6 disclosed their financial relationship with the hormone manufacturers.[4088] As pharmacology professor Adriane Fugh-Berman put it, "Women were placed in the way of harm by their physicians, who acted as unsuspecting patsies for the pharmaceutical companies."[4089] If we really wanted to prevent heart attacks in women, instead of being drug industry pawns, doctors could recommend simple lifestyle behaviors that may eliminate more than 90 percent of heart attack risk.[4090]

THE RISKS AND BENEFITS OF MENOPAUSAL HORMONE THERAPY

Where do things stand now with menopause hormone therapy? The U.S. Preventive Services Task Force, echoing other authorities, such as the American Academy of Family Physicians,[4091] American Geriatrics Society,[4092] and American Heart Association,[4093] now recommends against the use of hormone therapy for the prevention of chronic conditions in postmenopausal women with or without a uterus.[4094] Note that the guidance is separate from hormone therapy for the treatment of severe menopausal symptoms for which the American College of Obstetricians and Gynecologists advises "the gynecologist should help the patient to weigh the risks against the benefits."[4095] To make an informed decision, let's run the numbers.

Estrogen is very effective in reducing hot flash frequency and severity, by about 80 percent compared to placebo,[4096] with no difference noted between pills or patches.[4097] Hormone therapy can also decrease the risk of osteoporotic fractures. For women with an intact uterus, if two hundred took hormones for ten years, that would be expected to result in nine fewer fractures. Those are the upsides: symptom relief and fewer fractures.[4098] In the same scenario, those benefits would have to be weighed against four additional heart attacks (fatal or not), two extra strokes, four more cases of dementia,[4099] two more cases of breast cancer, one more case of fatal lung cancer, four extra cases of gallbladder disease, and ten extra blood clots[4100] (though not a single partridge nor pear tree). Unless the menopausal symptoms were debilitating and everything else was tried and failed, it's hard for me to imagine a woman choosing to accept that risk-benefit balance were she given all the facts.

The safety profile is better for younger (recently menopausal) women, those at reduced risk of cardiovascular disease, blood clots, and breast cancer, and those who lack a uterus and can therefore take estrogen-only preparations.[4101] (Otherwise, the risk of uterine cancer is too great.[4102]) Just the estrogen gives the same symptomatic relief,[4103] but eleven fractures would be prevented in two hundred women over a decade and there were no extra heart attacks or dementia and two *fewer* cases of breast cancer up against six extra cases of gallbladder disease, only one extra blood clot case, and those same two extra strokes.[4104] In either case, the FDA recommends estrogens only be prescribed "at the lowest effective doses and for the shortest duration,"[4105] though it's not clear whether lower doses are actually safer or not.[4106]

WHAT ABOUT "BIOIDENTICAL" HORMONES?

The Women's Health Initiative used Premarin because it was the most commonly prescribed form of estrogen; in fact, more than a million prescriptions are still written for it every year in the United States.[4107,4108] It's a mixture of more than fifty different estrogens from horse pee.[4109] ("Premarin" comes from the words "pregnant mare urine." If you're skeptical, try crushing a pill and sniffing it.) The dour findings of the Women's Health Initiative (combined with some high-profile celebrity endorsements) saw interest shift to *bioidentical hormones* made from plants rather than a horse source. As I explore in see.nf/bioidentical, there are now pee-free and FDA-approved bioidentical hormones, but they are expected to carry the same risks.[4110]

So, how can you safely treat menopausal symptoms like hot flashes? The American College of Obstetricians and Gynecologists suggests palliative measures, such as "consuming cool drinks."[4111] Turning down the thermostat, layering clothing, and using fans can offer some relief,[4112] but is there really no way to treat hot flashes without the cancer, clots, and coronaries? Thankfully, there is.

The Risks and Benefits of Mammograms

Speaking of making informed choices about your own body in the face of the confusion generated by the corrupting commercial interests of multibillion-dollar industries, what about mammograms? Contradictory recommendations have been published—for example, getting mammograms from age forty versus fifty, screening annually versus every other year,[4113] or not getting them routinely at all.[4114] Nine out of ten women surveyed vastly overestimated the benefits of mammograms or had no idea how beneficial they are. One survey found that "if women knew how small the real effectiveness of breast cancer screening in preventing breast cancer deaths is, 70% said they would not submit to it."[4115] You may be in that 30 percent, though, and you have every right to decide for yourself.

Decisions with completely one-sided consequences—all risk or all benefit—are easy. For example, should doctors teach women to do breast self-exams? The answer is no. It was put to the test. Hundreds of thousands of women were randomized to perform self-exams or not. Researchers not only didn't find any benefit to doing them, they found harms, including double the number of women who had to get biopsies taken. Self-exams were not shown to decrease the risk of getting breast cancer, dying from it, or catching tumors in earlier stages. That's why the U.S. Preventive Services Task Force came out explicitly recommending against teaching women to do breast self-exams in 2015.[4116]

To be clear, the USPSTF didn't come out against breast self-examination—only against teaching women to do them. That's because reminding women to perform self-exams only appeared to cause harm with no benefit. If you do discover an abnormality, then definitely tell your doctor, but being told to get in the practice of looking seems to do more harm than good. Yet, most doctors continue to teach women to perform self-exams. If self-exams haven't been shown to help and, in fact, have been shown to harm, why do physicians keep calling for them? Because that's just what they've been telling women forever. Medical inertia may trump women's health, even without a multibillion-dollar industry tipping the scales to push for the practice to continue, which brings us to mammograms.

Over the last half century, more than half a million women have participated in ten randomized trials of mammography, each with about a decade of follow-up.[4117] What does the science have to say? Let's imagine that one thousand asymptomatic women at average risk were randomized to either skip mammograms or get screened following the USPSTF recommendations to get mammograms every other year starting at age fifty. Over the next twenty years, we would expect two hundred false alarms (though resulting in only thirty biopsies) and three cancers would be missed, but fifteen gratuitous cases would be found, meaning women would be diagnosed with—and treated for—breast cancer unnecessarily. (A third potential harm, getting radiation-induced breast cancer from the mammogram X-rays, is not included in the model because only rough indirect estimates exist, on the order of one to five cancer cases per ten thousand women.[4118]) On the other side of the scale, thanks to mammograms, two breast cancer deaths would be averted, though no lives would apparently be saved overall.

When surveyed, women think mammograms cut the risk of dying from breast cancer in half, saving the lives of about one in twelve. In reality, about five women in a thousand die per decade from breast cancer without regular mammogram screening compared to four in a thousand dying with screening. Doesn't saving the life of even a single woman in a thousand make it all worth it? But even that may not even be true. None of the ten randomized trials have ever shown an overall mortality benefit, meaning it appears that no lives are actually saved.[4119] How does that make any sense? If a decade of mammograms prevents one in a thousand women from dying from breast cancer, then the only way for no lives to be saved is if mammograms somehow led to the deaths of one in a thousand *healthy* women. This is where the overdiagnosis may come in.

The fact is that some of the tiny tumors picked up on mammograms may have

(continued)

never progressed[4120] and some might have even disappeared on their own.[4121] Autopsy studies of accident victims show that 7 to 39 percent of women aged forty to seventy are walking around with tiny breast cancers, 96 percent of which will never go on to spread or kill them. So, had those tumors not been picked up during screening, the women may have been none the wiser, may have never been affected by them or even known they had them. But, once cancer is detected on a mammogram, you have to treat it because you don't know what it's going to do.[4122] And this treatment comes with all the attendant harms of unnecessary surgery, chemotherapy, and radiation.[4123]

Unnecessary radiation treatments to the chest increase the risk of dying from heart disease and lung cancer,[4124] which could explain why mammograms may kill as many as are saved.[4125] Those who survive become mammography's biggest cheerleaders, thinking mammograms saved their lives.[4126] In actuality, the more likely scenario—in fact, the two to ten times more likely scenario—is that the treatment didn't do anything because the cancer wouldn't have hurt you anyway.[4127] So, you went through all that pain and suffering for nothing. That's the irony about mammograms: The people who are harmed the most are the ones who claim the greatest benefit.

I am not opposed to mammograms. I *am* opposed to the patronizing attitude that women should be pressured into getting them without being fully informed about the benefits and risks. Some women will still choose to get them, but others will not. It's for you to decide.

RELIEVING YOURSELF OF EXCESS ESTROGEN

The general public is so confused about mammograms that most people believe they prevent or reduce the risk of developing cancer.[4128] Of course, getting screened for cancer doesn't change the risk of getting cancer in the first place. The good news is that the same diet and lifestyle changes that can protect against breast cancer can also protect against the leading cause of death, cardiovascular disease, which kills ten times more women in the United States—about 400,000 women dead each year[4129] versus 40,000 for breast cancer.[4130]

In the Harvard Nurses' Health studies that followed more than 150,000 women and their diets for decades, researchers found that those who ate more plant foods and fewer animal foods were significantly less likely to cultivate breast cancer—and that was even after controlling for factors such as body weight, family history, alcohol use, and exercise habits. Furthermore, plant-based eating appeared particularly protective against the deadliest[4131] types of tumors.[4132] The California Teachers

Study, with more than 90,000 women, found similar results, including significantly reduced breast cancer risk associated with a plant-based dietary pattern, particularly for the hardest-to-treat tumors.[4133]

Circulating estrogen levels in both pre-[4134] and postmenopausal[4135] women are strongly associated with breast cancer risk, potentially explaining virtually the entire relationship between excess body fat and breast cancer.[4136] (Estrogen produced by fatty tissue spills over into the bloodstream.[4137]) Does that explain why plant-based eaters, who tend to be thinner on average, have lower breast cancer risk? There are studies finding lower average estrogen levels in pre-[4138] and postmenopausal vegetarians that don't appear be explained solely by their slimmer frames. That may be due to greater fiber intake.[4139]

Our body gets rid of excess estrogen the same way we evolved to get rid of excess cholesterol—by dumping it into the digestive tract, where it expects that there will be a lot of fiber to grab it, hold on to it, and flush it out.[4140] Without fiber, excess hormones (and cholesterol) can just wind up getting reabsorbed into the bloodstream,[4141] but our body just assumes our intestines are going to be packed with fiber all day long because that's the context in which we evolved. We did start eating meat once we developed tools, but plants don't tend to run as fast, so the bulk of our diets was made up of a lot of bulk. Our ancient ancestors got an estimated seven times more fiber than we're getting now.[4142]

Researchers at my medical alma mater published a study in *The New England Journal of Medicine* in which vegetarian and nonvegetarian women were "provided with plastic bags and insulated boxes filled with dry ice for three 24-hour fecal collections." (You've heard of popsicles; these were more like poopsicles.) Vegetarians excrete two to three times more estrogens every day, because they produce two[4143] to three[4144] times greater "fecal output." So, passing on hormone pills is just one way to reduce breast cancer risk. The other is to rid yourself of estrogen excess the way nature intended.

THE BEST AND WORST FOODS FOR MENOPAUSE SYMPTOMS

The lower estrogen levels of plant-based women may protect them from breast cancer, but might they suffer worse menopausal symptoms? It turns out the opposite may be the case, granting them the best of both worlds. Those eating strictly plant-based diets report significantly fewer bothersome symptoms around menopause. This included the vasomotor symptoms, such as hot flashes and night sweats, as well as other physical symptoms of menopause, like muscle and joint aches, fatigue, sleep difficulties, reduced strength and stamina, lethargy, skin changes, weight gain, facial hair, bloating, and urinary frequency or incontinence. The researchers concluded:

"Eating a plant-based diet may be helpful for women in menopausal transition who prefer a natural means to manage their symptoms."[4145]

Which foods may account for the difference in symptoms? Fruits, vegetables, soy, and plant-based omega-3-rich foods, such as flaxseeds, correlated with lesser symptom severity, whereas "total flesh food" (meat), dairy, and fish-based omega-3s were associated with more severe menopausal symptoms. What appeared to be the deciding factors, though, were berries, leafy greens, and vegetable intake more broadly.[4146] In general, according to a 2020 review of dietary intake and menopausal symptoms, those eating higher-quality diets, including more fruits, vegetables, and whole grains, tend to suffer less—not only from vasomotor and physical symptoms but also from psychological symptoms, sleep disorders, and bladder and genital issues. On the other hand, diets high in processed foods, sweets, meats, and saturated fat were linked to more severe symptoms.[4147]

As I note in see.nf/menopausal, both oxidative stress[4148] and inflammation[4149] are associated with menopausal symptoms, but correlation doesn't necessarily mean causation. Interventional studies with control groups are necessary, especially since studies on hot flashes show such a large placebo effect (at least 35 percent relief),[4150] such that some have suggested surreptitiously giving women sugar pills as a treatment.[4151]

The largest dietary interventional trial for menopausal symptoms was within the Women's Health Initiative umbrella. Instead of randomizing women to take hormones, the researchers randomized them to advice to eat a low-fat diet. Adherence was poor, so the women in the low-fat group never actually achieved a low-fat diet,[4152] but they did cut back a bit on meat[4153] and ate at least one more serving a day of fruits or vegetables.[4154] The result? They ended up significantly more likely to eliminate their hot flashes or night sweats. They also lost more weight, but the benefits on vasomotor symptoms of menopause appeared to extend beyond just the weight loss.[4155]

Within a more plant-based diet, those randomized to a vegetarian diet plus daily walnuts, almonds, and flaxseed oil did better than those randomized to the same diet but with the addition of extra-virgin olive oil instead. After sixteen weeks, the meat-free diet rich in plant-based omega-3s reduced hot flash frequency significantly better than the olive oil group.[4156] In fact, even just two daily teaspoons' worth of ground flaxseeds alone can significantly decrease menopausal symptoms. In a head-to-head trial of flaxseeds versus hormone therapy (typically bioidentical estrogen plus a form of progesterone), the flaxseeds reduced menopausal symptoms to about the same extent as the hormone pills.[4157] This may have been due to the phytoestrogens in flaxseeds, though, rather than the omega-3s.

WHY THERE ISN'T A WORD FOR HOT FLASH IN JAPANESE

Hot flashes, also known as hot flushes, are the most common menopausal symptom for which women seek treatment.[4158] They afflict up to 80 to 85 percent of American and European menopausal women[4159] and, along with night sweats, last more than seven years on average.[4160] But as I explore in see.nf/hotflash, these symptoms are not universal nor inevitable.[4161] In Japan, for example, only 15 percent of women may be affected.[4162] In fact, there isn't even a term for *hot flash* in the Japanese language.[4163]

The absence of a Japanese term is all the more remarkable because the language is said to be "infinitely more sensitive" in describing body states than English,[4164] with all sorts of extremely subtle distinctions for somatic sensations.[4165] In Japanese, there are twenty or more words just to describe the state of one's stomach and intestines, but hot flashes appear to be so unusual there that researchers had to come up with ways to describe them in Japanese surveys.[4166] They hypothesized it might be the soy.[4167]

I review the interventional trials on soy foods and isoflavone supplements in see.nf/isoflavones. Dozens of such clinical trials have been performed, and, indeed, the equivalent of about two servings of soy foods a day has been found to reduce hot flash frequency by about 20 percent more than placebo and hot flash severity by around 25 percent more than placebo, compared to more like a 30 to 40 percent net reduction from estrogen hormone therapy.[4168] Soy isoflavones have also been shown to improve other menopause concerns, including vaginal dryness,[4169] bone density,[4170] depression,[4171] memory, and cognitive function more generally.[4172]

The bottom line, wrote one consensus panel of experts, is that soy can be considered a first-line treatment for symptoms of menopausal hot flashes and night sweats.[4173] One convenient whole-food source of soy are soy "nuts" (dry roasted soybeans). Harvard Medical School's Center of Excellence in Women's Health funded a randomized crossover study of a half cup of unsalted soy nuts a day (divided into three or four portions and spaced throughout the day) and achieved a 50 percent reduction in hot flashes within two weeks.[4174] But, what's inconvenient about soy nuts is the formation of AGEs (see the Glycation chapter) in the roasting process, so incorporating canned soybeans into meals would be better.

What if you combined a plant-based diet and soybeans? Two randomized controlled trials found that reduced-fat plant-based diets with a daily half-cup serving of cooked whole soybeans can reduce the number of serious hot flashes by 84 to 88 percent within twelve weeks. Overall, most randomized to the plant-based group ended up free of moderate-to-severe hot flashes, compared to 95 percent still suffering in the control group.[4175,4176]

Soy and Breast Cancer

Contrary to rampant misinformation online, the best available evidence consistently shows a protective effect of soy consumption in the prevention of breast cancer.[4177,4178] Each daily 5 g increase in soy protein consumption—less than a cup of soymilk—is associated with a 12 percent reduction in the risk of dying from breast cancer.[4179] This may help explain why women living in Connecticut, for example, can end up with ten times more breast cancer than women living in Japan.[4180] Review see.nf/soybreast for a discussion of the mechanism and source of the controversy.

It is estimated that one in eight U.S. women will develop invasive breast cancer during her lifetime.[4181] Switching from dairy milk to soymilk would be expected to reduce breast cancer risk by about a third, though this may say more about the breast cancer–promoting effects of dairy milk than the breast cancer–preventing effects of soy. Postmenopausal or premenopausal, women drinking a cup of dairy milk a day appear to have about 50 percent greater breast cancer risk than those averaging less than a cup every two months or so. Researchers suggest that this may be due to the estrogen levels in dairy milk (particularly since about 75 percent of cows in dairy production are pregnant) or the IGF-1 in the milk or provoked by milk protein consumption.[4182]

Are the anti-estrogenic effects of soy foods in the breast enough to actually change the course of the disease? The first human study on soy food intake and breast cancer survival was published in 2009 in the *Journal of the American Medical Association*, suggesting that "[a]mong women with breast cancer, soy food consumption was significantly associated with decreased risk of death and [breast cancer] recurrence."[4183] That study was followed by another one,[4184] then another one,[4185] each with similar findings. That was enough for a wide range of cancer experts offering nutrition guidelines for cancer survivors to conclude that, if anything, soy foods should be beneficial.[4186] Since then, two additional studies have been published,[4187,4188] for a total of five out of five studies that tracked more than 10,000 breast cancer patients, and they all point in the same direction.[4189]

Pooling all the results, soy food intake after breast cancer diagnosis was associated with both reduced mortality and reduced recurrence—that is, a longer lifespan and less likelihood that the cancer comes back. This improved survival was for women with either estrogen receptor–negative tumors or estrogen receptor–positive tumors, and for both younger and older women.[4190] In one study, for example, 90 percent of the breast cancer patients who ate the most soy phytoestrogens after diagnosis were still alive five years later, while half of those who ate little to no soy had died.[4191] Pass the edamame.

IS THERE HOPE FOR HOPS?

Flaxseeds also have phytoestrogens (called *lignans*) that are associated with breast cancer prevention[4192] and survival.[4193] Interventional trials involving before and after biopsies have shown beneficial effects in breast cancer patients randomized to muffins containing flaxseeds versus flax-free placebo muffins.[4194] Higher lignan exposure may reduce breast cancer mortality between 33 and 70 percent.[4195]

Also, like soy, flaxseeds have been shown to improve LDL cholesterol,[4196] artery function,[4197] and blood pressure.[4198] Flaxseeds also lower other cardiovascular risk factors, including C-reactive protein[4199] and Lp(a),[4200] and can improve blood sugar and weight control.[4201] Unfortunately, they do not appear as effective as soy for improving symptoms of menopause.[4202] Meta-analyses of red clover or black cohosh, other sources of phytoestrogens, also proved disappointing.[4203]

The most potent phytoestrogen is found in beer.[4204] Hopein, also known as 8-prenylnaringenin or 8-PN,[4205] is the reason that handling hops causes women to start menstruating.[4206] It may also contribute to feminized features in alcoholic men, like gynecomastia (man boobs) and a "female escutcheon."[4207] (I had to look that one up. "Escutcheon" derives from the Latin word for "shield." It's medical lingo for the shape of one's pubic hair—diamond-shaped for men or triangle-shaped for women.) The pro-estrogenic effects could also help explain why beer drinkers appear to have better bone density.[4208]

What about hops for hot flashes? As I explore in see.nf/hops, a daily teaspoon of dried hop flowers can significantly reduce hot flash symptoms,[4209] but unfortunately, the estrogenic compounds in hops act more like the breast cancer–promoting compounds in pregnant horse urine than the breast cancer–preventing compounds in soy.[4210] That explains why hops are such a common ingredient in so-called breast-enhancing supplements—that is, because they act more like animal estrogen.[4211] That also helps explain why beer may be more carcinogenic to the breast than some other forms of alcohol.[4212]

LAVENDER FLOWERS

Lavender is widely used to help alleviate menopausal symptoms. To my surprise, there were sixteen interventional trials involving more than a thousand women putting it to the test.[4213] One supposedly double-blinded, crossover, clinical trial, for instance, randomized a hundred menopausal women to lavender aromatherapy in which they smelled lavender for twenty minutes twice a day for a few weeks and then switched to sniffing the "placebo" control, which was diluted milk. I don't know how the women could have been effectively blinded given the fragrance (or lack thereof), so the placebo effect can't be discounted, but the hot flash frequency remained about the same during the control weeks yet was cut in half during the weeks sniffing lavender.[4214] Other physical menopause symptoms, along with decreased sexual desire and feelings of anxiety and depression, also improved during the lavender exposure.[4215]

The scent of lavender essential oil did not appear to help postmenopausal women with insomnia, a common complaint.[4216] What about just eating lavender flowers? More than a dozen randomized controlled trials have found that smelling lavender can help with anxiety, and that appears to extend to eating lavender, too.[4217] Eighty-three percent of postmenopausal women randomized to capsules containing 500 mg of lavender flower powder (which I measure out as one teaspoon of dried flowers) twice a day reported a good or very good improvement in anxiety, compared to only 44 percent in the placebo capsule group.[4218] The same team of researchers tried the same dose on postmenopausal women having difficulty sleeping. Seventy-four percent of those unknowingly taking the lavender reported satisfactory improvements on subjective sleep quality compared to only 31 percent of the control group.[4219] It's not clear if the active component(s) are water soluble, so the same effect may or may not be achieved drinking the same amount in the form of lavender tea.

FENNEL SEEDS AND FENUGREEK

The nice thing about studying herbs and spices is that entire servings can be stuffed into pills to perform randomized, double-blind, placebo-controlled trials. In this way, a half teaspoon of ground black cumin powder was found to significantly improve menopausal symptoms compared to placebo, but the effects may be limited to the psychological aspects, such as decreased anxiety, more vitality, and improved mental health.[4220]

Fennel seeds, which aren't actually seeds but the whole little fruits of the fennel plant, can more broadly improve symptoms, including improvements in hot flashes and night sweats, as well as other physical, psychological, and sexual symptoms.[4221] Details in see.nf/fennelfenugreek, along with fenugreek, another galactagogue spice. No, not another sci-fi reboot, a *galactagogue* is something that increases breast milk production in lactating women.[4222] Fenugreek can also, at one and a half teaspoons a day, improve symptoms of early menopause.[4223]

"ANDROPAUSE"

Today, testosterone is mass marketed to aging men for nonspecific symptoms supposedly related to what's been called "andropause," the decline in testosterone levels as men age. Also known as male menopause,[4224] penopause,[4225] viropause, androgen deficiency in aging males (ADAM),[4226] late-onset hypogonadism, or simply "low T syndrome,"[4227] it is considered a classic example of disease-mongering,[4228] a "template" for how to hawk a disease.[4229] Disease-mongering is the selling of sickness by widening the boundary of illness to encompass ordinary life experiences.[4230] The medicalization of menopause made billions for Big Pharma. Why not extend that to the other half of the aging population?

THE "LOW T" TSUNAMI

In 1889, physiologist Charles-Édouard Brown-Séquard, one of the first to postulate the existence of hormones, claimed to have "rejuvenated" himself with injections of extracts of testicles from dogs and guinea pigs. The rejuvenation must not have worked that well, as he died a few years later,[4231] but not before thousands of physicians administered his "Brown-Séquard Elixir."[4232] Recipients included Hall of Fame pitcher Jim "Pud" Galvin, the first to use a purported performance-enhancing substance in Major League Baseball.[4233] This was followed by rich old men opting for testicular transplants from humans, monkeys, and goats before testosterone was finally discovered in the 1930s.[4234]

Testosterone levels do tend to drop, on average, about 0.5 percent a year, but this may be due more to obesity and coexisting medical conditions than to age per se.[4235] In the Healthy Man Study, for example, men reporting excellent health appeared to experience no drop in testosterone between the ages of forty and ninety-seven.[4236] So, it's not inevitable,[4237] but rather mostly a consequence of chronic conditions like hypertension, diabetes, depression, heart disease, liver disease, lung disease, kidney disease,[4238] or simply deconditioning or excess body fat.[4239] Of course, you could try to treat the underlying cause with diet and lifestyle changes, but where's the profit in that?

Big Pharma marketers of "low T" ran a sophisticated, direct-to-consumer ad campaign to lead men to believe that testosterone deficiency could be a cause of generic symptoms such as "low energy, feeling sad, sleep problems, decreased physical performance, or increased fat."[4240] Take the quiz! They came up with consumer tests, encouraging men to ask their doctors about testosterone if they exhibited nonspecific symptoms such as "falling asleep after dinner."[4241] There was so little correlation between the answers and testosterone levels[4242] that the questionnaires had up to a 70 percent false-positive rate,[4243] so 70 percent of those who were found to have testosterone deficiency—according to the quiz, that is— actually did not.

Only two industrialized countries, the United States and New Zealand, even allow predatory direct-to-consumer drug ads, but testosterone hawkers sidestep these prohibitions by running "disease awareness" campaigns that don't mention brands by name.[4244] Anti-aging clinics started touting testosterone replacement therapy,[4245] and regular clinicians were convinced en masse by sponsored CME (continuing medical education, or often more accurately *commercial* medical education)[4246] to an "irrational exuberance in testosterone prescribing."[4247] It worked. The billions spent on advertising[4248] translated into billions in annual sales,[4249] a "global tsunami of testosterone prescriptions"[4250] resulting in a hundredfold increase in testosterone sales.[4251]

TESTOSTERONE "REPLACEMENT" PUT TO THE TEST

There are legitimate reasons to prescribe testosterone, but since the Nobel Prize–winning isolation of testosterone in 1935, there has been only one FDA-approved indication: "classic hypogonadism."[4252] That's low testosterone due to conditions such as missing or damaged testicles or certain genetic anomalies.[4253] In contrast, 25 percent of men prescribed testosterone these days may not have even had their testosterone levels tested.[4254] Or, they may have gotten tested and their levels were normal or even high, but they still got prescriptions.[4255] Why even bother getting a test, though? Most of the "hypogonadal" symptoms bear no relation to testosterone levels in the blood. The exception are a few sexual symptoms, such as "low frequency of sexual thoughts," which do seem to be tied to testosterone levels under 320 nanograms per deciliter (ng/dL), though more than a quarter of men with normal testosterone levels had similar symptoms.[4256]

There are no generally accepted lower limits for healthy testosterone levels in the blood.[4257] Suggested reasonable thresholds range from less than 200 ng/dL (from the American Association of Clinical Endocrinology) to as high as 350 ng/dL (from the European Association of Urology).[4258] When put to the test, though, by first chemically castrating men, then adding back more and more testosterone, researchers only saw definitive changes in sexual desire and function when men's levels sank below 100 ng/dL.[4259] Regardless of the cutoff used, for a hypogonadism diagnosis, the Endocrine Society guidelines require two low-testosterone measurements taken in the morning, preferably four weeks apart,[4260] in the context of consistent symptoms.[4261] (Testosterone levels naturally fluctuate season to season, week to week, day to day, and even hour to hour,[4262] with levels higher in the morning and dropping as much as 30 to 40 percent by midafternoon.[4263])

These guidelines are often ignored.[4264] In the United States, a study of hundreds of thousands of men starting testosterone found that only 10 percent got the recommended second test.[4265] Fifty percent only got one test, and the remaining 40 percent didn't appear to get tested at all. As many as 77 percent of older men may see testosterone levels lower than 300 ng/dL on the first test, but after running a confirmatory second test, that number can drop down to 18 percent and further fall to just 3 percent when other recommended criteria are included, such as a morning blood draw.[4266]

So, the vast majority of men treated with testosterone "replacement" therapy don't actually need it.[4267] But that doesn't necessarily mean that they wouldn't benefit from it. Maybe men have different set points and taking extra testosterone might help even if they don't test as being deficient. You can imagine men feeling better taking testosterone just from the placebo effect, which is why it's so important to put it to the test.[4268] Researchers intercepted older men lining up for testosterone treatment because they or their doctors thought it would help with symptoms, such as reduced energy or libido, and randomized them to a testosterone gel or a placebo gel. The results? Testosterone worked—but so did the placebo, such that there were no significant differences in the end.

Testosterone flopped even for sexual symptoms. But weren't those the one set of symptoms actually correlated with low testosterone? Yes, but that doesn't mean low testosterone is the cause.[4269] Rather than low testosterone leading to sexual disinterest, perhaps sexual disinterest leads to less testosterone. When men have sex, they can get a spike in testosterone levels in their blood,[4270] so much so that their beards may actually grow faster on days they have sex.[4271] Men resuming sex after nonhormonal treatment of their erectile dysfunction—via penile pumps or prostheses, for example—bump up their testosterone level by a whopping average of 450 ng/dL.[4272] (In contrast, interestingly, men don't get a testosterone boost when they masturbate. This may be because testosterone increases with "competitive success," like winning at sports. While sex "is not usually regarded as a competitive event," psychology researchers note, "one's mental state following coitus could nevertheless be something like that of a winner," as opposed to the mental state after masturbation.[4273])

Though the study participants tended to have testosterone levels on the low side, the inclusion criteria for the study were symptoms, not specific blood level cutoffs.[4274] No wonder, perhaps, that testosterone was found to be effectively useless. The researchers were giving testosterone to men who may have already had enough. How about a randomized, double-blind, placebo-controlled trial of symptomatic men filling strict criteria for testosterone deficiency? Enter the Testosterone Trials, funded by the NIH.

THE TESTOSTERONE TRIALS

In 2004, an authoritative report from the National Academy of Medicine concluded that testosterone therapy offered no clear evidence of benefit for any health outcome examined and larger, longer, better studies were necessary to know for sure. In response to this mandate, the NIH funded not one, not two, but seven clinical trials across a dozen academic centers randomizing men to testosterone or placebo for twelve months. The men had to be at least sixty-five with measured and confirmed low testosterone levels (< 275 ng/dL) and exhibiting a symptom like diminished vitality or libido.[4275] What would "correcting" testosterone levels back up to that of young healthy men do for seven clinical endpoints: cognition, vitality, physical function, sexual function, anemia, bone health, and cardiovascular health?

There was great hope testosterone replacement would improve brain function. Population studies had shown a correlation between lower testosterone levels and higher risk of cognitive impairment[4276] and dementia.[4277] Prostate cancer patients receiving long-term androgen deprivation therapy (surgical or chemical castration) seemed to be at higher risk of dementia later on.[4278] But, in the Testosterone Trials, "correcting" testosterone levels failed to improve memory or other cognitive functions,[4279] and the same failure was noted in a meta-analysis of more than a dozen other randomized controlled testosterone studies.[4280] An editorial in the *Journal of the American Medical Association* concluded that these "convincing, unequivocal findings affirm that testosterone treatment does not improve cognitive function in older men."[4281]

Testosterone also failed to improve both physical function and vitality scores.[4282] This is consistent with dozens of other randomized controlled trials that found little to no effect on physical functioning, depressive symptoms, energy, or vitality.[4283] It's no wonder that, within a year, 80 to 85 percent of men who had started testosterone stop taking it. In fact, based on a study of nearly 16,000 patients, about 50 percent stop taking topical testosterone and about 70 percent stop getting injections within three months.[4284] The lack of noticeable benefits makes sense if indeed lower testosterone is a consequence, rather than a cause, of obesity, lack of exercise, and chronic disease.[4285]

However, the Testosterone Trials did find that testosterone improved bone mineral density.[4286] Unfortunately, if you put together all ten of the randomized controlled trials on testosterone therapy and bone health to date, no overall bone benefit was found.[4287] The opposite may be the case, though, for sexual symptoms.

There was a transient increase in sexual function, but by the end of the year, there was no significant difference between the placebo group and those who got the real thing.[4288] In contrast, most high-quality trials (ten out of thirteen) have found that testosterone therapy in men with low levels increases their sex drive, and seven out of twelve firmly found it to improve erectile function.[4289] The size of the effect, however, is small, described as "marginal."[4290] Testosterone replacement may help with mild cases of erectile dysfunction but is only a fraction as effective as drugs like Viagra.[4291] My mind was blown to learn that eunuchs had active sex lives even though they had been castrated when they were boys.[4292] Experimentally, severely hypogonadal men (including bilateral surgical castration) with testosterone levels as low as 25 ng/dL not only got erections when exposed to an erotic film but had longer-lasting erections than men with intact testicles in the control group![4293]

A low libido does, however, seem to be a genuine symptom of low testosterone.[4294] So, men with documented low levels of testosterone who suffer from reduced sexual desire and want to improve their sex drive may be candidates for testosterone after consideration of the associated risks.[4295] There are testosterone pills, patches, topical gels, injections, implanted pellets, and even mucoadhesive tablets you stick to your gums.[4296] The different routes appear to work comparably,[4297] though injections are likely cheapest, costing about $150 a year instead of more than $2,000 for some of the topical preparations.[4298] It's worth noting that it may take weeks for testosterone levels to rise and months for symptoms to reverse, though the placebo effect can kick in immediately.[4299] What are the downsides?

THE RISKS OF TESTOSTERONE THERAPY

I do a deep dive into potential problems in see.nf/trisks, which include sexual infidelity,[4300] an increase in "tit-for-tat" provoked aggression,[4301] and the most ironic side effect: developing low testosterone. The reason bodybuilders develop shrunken testicles is that taking supplemental testosterone instructs the feedback loop in the brain to downregulate natural production, leaving the body in an even greater state of deficiency should the testosterone therapy ever stop.[4302] This creates a vicious but profitable cycle of dependency.[4303]

Testosterone can also stimulate our bone marrow to generate more red blood cells,[4304] which is good if you're anemic,[4305] but sludging up your blood with too many red cells can put you at risk for heart attacks and strokes.[4306] Indeed, the Testosterone in Older Men (TOM) trial had to be cut short because the testosterone group was having ten times more cardiac events than the placebo group.[4307] Since black box warnings have been issued that testosterone presents "a risk of serious and possibly life-threatening cardiovascular (heart and blood vessel) problems,"[4308] prescriptions for testosterone have declined sharply.[4309]

One leading anti-aging journal carried a commentary comparing testosterone replacement therapy to the emperor's new clothes, noting that the topic remains "astonishingly controversial."[4310] What do you expect when there's a billion-dollar industry at stake? An analysis of popular YouTube videos on the subject suggests that mass misinformation persists,[4311] yet a systematic review of more than 150 randomized controlled trials concluded, "We identified no population of normal men for whom the benefits of testosterone use outweigh its risk."[4312]

The Risks and Benefits of PSA Prostate Cancer Screening

Testosterone therapy surprisingly does not seem to worsen symptoms of prostate enlargement,[4313] but what about prostate cancer? We've known about testosterone's role in prostate cancer since the 1940s, when surgical castration was shown to cause a dramatic regression of tumors.[4314] To this day, testosterone suppression is universally accepted as the first-line treatment for symptomatic metastatic disease.[4315] Whether or not testosterone causes prostate cancer or merely accelerates it,[4316] the question is moot since autopsy studies show that as many as about one-third of men in their thirties and two-thirds of men by their sixties already have tiny prostate cancers growing inside them—whether they know it or not.[4317] That's why guidelines recommend rectal exams and PSA screening before starting testosterone.[4318] What about prostate cancer screening in general?

While 64 percent of men develop hidden prostate cancers by their sixties,[4319] the lifetime risk of being *diagnosed* with prostate cancer is only about 11 percent and the risk of dying from it is 2.5 percent.[4320] So, most men die *with* their prostate tumors rather than *from* them. Indeed, most men with prostate cancer spend their whole lives never even knowing they had it. That's one of the problems with screening: Many prostate cancers that are detected during screening may never have led to harm even if they'd continued to go undiscovered.[4321] Nonetheless, not all men are so lucky. Nearly 28,000 die from prostate cancer every year[4322] (at the average age of eighty).[4323] So, should you get a PSA prostate screening test or not?

The U.S. Preventive Services Task Force recommends against routine PSA screening,[4324] as do the American College of Preventive Medicine,[4325] the American Academy of Family Physicians,[4326] and the majority of professional medical societies in developed countries around the world (thirty-six out of forty-two).[4327] In 2018, though, the USPSTF shifted from a summary judgment against routine screening to stating that "the decision about whether to be screened for prostate cancer should be an individual one" for men aged fifty-five to sixty-nine,[4328] which is more in line with the "shared decision making" stance of the American Urological Association,[4329] American College of Physicians,[4330] and American Cancer Society.[4331] In other words, men should be informed about the risks and benefits and decide for themselves. However, men who are on the fence and don't express a clear preference in favor of screening should not be screened, according to the latest USPSTF recommendations.[4332]

More recently, an international panel of experts concluded that clinicians need not feel obligated to systematically bring it up, judging that most men would decide to decline PSA screening given the clear harms and small and uncertain benefits.[4333] That, however, is up to each individual. Let's run the numbers.

Similar to the 92 percent of women who either overestimated the mortality reduction from mammograms by tenfold or more or simply didn't know, 89 percent of men vastly overestimated the benefits of prostate cancer screening or had no idea. Most thought fifty prostate cancer deaths could be prevented out of one thousand men regularly screened,[4334] when in reality it's more like one.[4335] But doesn't even a one-in-a-thousand chance of not dying from cancer make a few blood tests worth it? The downsides are more than inconvenience.

About 1 in 7 men who undergo PSA screening will test positive, yet, in two-thirds of the cases, the subsequent biopsy results will be normal.[4336] So, out of 1,000 regularly screened men, about 150 will have a false alarm and be biopsied unnecessarily, which can cause minor complications like pain and bloody ejaculate, or, in approximately 1 percent of cases, more serious complications, like blood-borne infections that require hospitalization.[4337] The greatest harm, however, is overdiagnosis. Unnecessary biopsies are bad enough, but nothing compared to unnecessary cancer treatment.

Large-scale randomized trials suggest that 20 to 50 percent of men diagnosed with prostate cancer would have never become symptomatic in their lifetime. They never would have been the wiser had they not been screened, but now they may be needlessly heading to the operating table. About three in a thousand men die during radical prostatectomy or soon after the surgery. That may help explain why there appears to be no overall mortality benefit to prostate cancer screening.[4338] For every life saved, another one may be extinguished for a cancer they would never have even known about.[4339]

Another fifty in a thousand end up with serious surgical complications. Even if the surgery goes smoothly, about one in five men develop long-term urinary incontinence requiring use of pads, and most—two out of three—will experience long-term erectile dysfunction. Most men who receive radiation therapy also

(continued)

experience long-term sexual erectile dysfunction, and up to one in six experience long-term bowel issues, such as fecal incontinence. If this treatment was saving your life, it would be worth it, but it may be fifty times more likely that you were instead overdiagnosed with a cancer that would never have bothered you. In that much more likely case, you would be suffering all harms, no benefit.[4340] Yet, it's like with mammograms—the people who have been harmed the most feel as though they've been helped the most.

NATURAL WAYS TO BOOST TESTOSTERONE

To treat low testosterone, the American Urological Association, the European Association of Urology, and the Endocrine Society, the oldest association devoted to hormone research (so old they used to be called the Association for the Study of Internal Secretions),[4341] all recommend lifestyle modifications as the first-line treatment.[4342] In other words, treat the underlying cause.

Obesity and comorbidities underlie most cases of low testosterone in older men,[4343] which is frequently reversible with weight loss.[4344] An enzyme in body fat actually converts testosterone into estrogen.[4345] Even just losing 5 percent of your weight is associated with a significant increase in testosterone levels. Men losing more than 15 percent of their weight bumped up their testosterone by more than 150 points (ng/dL) on average,[4346] and those losing about 30 percent of their weight (through bariatric surgery) experienced around a 250-point increase.[4347]

Exercise may raise testosterone levels,[4348] but it depends on which kind. Despite the popular belief that resistance exercises, such as weight lifting, increase testosterone, a systematic review of training trials of older men found that only aerobic and interval training made a difference.[4349] Interestingly, listening to music while you work out may cause testosterone levels to drop. Within thirty minutes of listening to music, testosterone levels in men decline by 14 percent.[4350] Do all kinds of music have this effect or just some genres? While a half hour of silence had no effect, listening to thirty minutes of Mozart, jazz, pop, or Gregorian chants (no relation) had similar suppressive effects. What about a half hour of people's personal favorites? Testosterone levels were cut in half! What's going on? Since testosterone in men is related to dominance and aggression, we may have evolved using music as a way to soothe the savage beast, like a melodious cold shower to keep everyone chill.[4351]

What else may decrease testosterone? Sleep deprivation. Experimentally restricting men's sleep to five hours a night for one week lowered testosterone levels by 10 to 15 percent.[4352] Alcohol can do it, too. While two or three alcoholic drinks can cause an acute transient increase in testosterone that peaks after about two hours,[4353] randomizing men to three beers a day for three weeks reduced testosterone blood levels by about 7 percent (compared to nonalcoholic control drinks).[4354] Heavy coffee–drinking men appear to have higher testosterone levels,[4355] but when put to the test, those randomized to five small (6 oz) cups a day for eight weeks saw an increase in testosterone at the end of one month, but the effect seemed to disappear by month two.[4356]

What about "testosterone boosting" supplements? An analysis of the top "T-Boosters" sold on Amazon.com found that 70 percent contained components that had either no effect, an indeterminant effect, or even *decreased* testosterone[4357] in as many as 10 percent of such supplements.[4358] One of the few constituents that would be expected to increase levels, however, is fenugreek.

Fenugreek seed has been used historically as an aphrodisiac and for male reproductive issues.[4359] It can increase the testicular weight and testosterone production in rats, but what about people?[4360] Clinical trials of fenugreek with daily dose equivalents as low as a quarter teaspoon[4361] to two-thirds of a teaspoon[4362] were found to raise testosterone levels[4363] by about 10 percent within three months, accompanied by a rise in sex drive and arousal.[4364] Side benefits include an improvement in LDL cholesterol, triglycerides,[4365] and short- and long-term blood sugar control (with actual fenugreek powder working better than fenugreek extract supplements).[4366] It can also make your armpits smell like maple syrup.[4367] (Really!)

TESTOSTERONE LEVELS AND DIET

What about broader dietary changes that might increase testosterone for those who are low and suffering from diminished libido? I do a deep dive in see.nf/tdiet. Acutely, high-fat meals can have a dramatic effect on testosterone levels.[4368] When men ate a McDonald's Sausage & Egg McMuffin breakfast, their testosterone levels plummeted by 25 percent within an hour and stayed down for up to four hours.[4369] It's not just the inflammation,[4370] because the drop in testosterone was found to precede the bump in inflammation from the saturated fat. Testosterone can significantly drop within fifteen minutes of eating a ham and cheese sandwich, which is hardly even time for it to be digested.[4371] This led scientists to focus on digestive hormones like GLP-1,[4372] which is released within fifteen minutes of consuming a high-fat meal[4373] and appears to have a suppressive effect on testicular function.[4374] The researchers suggest that "men should minimise their fat intake . . . in order to optimise testicular function."[4375]

High-protein diets can also suppress testosterone,[4376] contrary to the "flagrant misuse of scientific information" in *Men's Health* magazine.[4377] When overweight men were randomized to a few scoops of whey (dairy) protein powder, their testosterone dropped one hundred points within an hour,[4378] explaining why high-protein, low-carbohydrate diets may cause large decreases in testosterone levels.[4379] That doesn't mean junky carbs are any better, though. Drinking two soda cans' worth of sugar water can also cause testosterone to plummet.[4380]

Can Phytoestrogens Be Feminizing?

I cover the evidence in see.nf/phyto, but even considerably higher doses than the one or two daily servings of soy phytoestrogens that Asian men typically eat do not exert feminizing effects on men,[4381] nor do they affect testosterone levels in people.[4382] What about the phytoestrogens in flaxseeds? Men fed six daily slices of flaxseed-enriched bread containing two tablespoons of ground flaxseed experienced no change in testosterone levels over a period of six weeks, compared to weeks avoiding flaxseed.[4383] There was a case of a man who developed gynecomastia (breast enlargement) after starting a tablespoon of flaxseed oil a day, but he was also on a statin drug, which on its own increases gynecomastia risk.[4384]

TESTOSTERONE AND MORTALITY

Big Pharma framed low testosterone as a serious health problem. "It is one thing to tell men that Low T can make them grumpy," read a commentary in *JAMA Internal Medicine*, but "it is another to say that it can kill them."[4385] Most observational studies have reported associations between low testosterone and increased mortality, which isn't surprising because obesity and chronic illness—even acute ailments like heart attacks or infections—decrease testosterone levels, whereas healthy older men are able to maintain their levels. So, low testosterone can act as a barometer of health[4386] and is much more likely a consequence, rather than a cause, of disease.[4387]

In the largest observational trial of men at high cardiovascular risk who had been given testosterone replacement,[4388] when researchers controlled for these other confounding factors, testosterone takers were found to be at significantly higher risk of heart attack, stroke, or premature death.[4389] Testosterone may help explain why women outlive men by an average of seven years.[4390] This might be expected given that testosterone is a powerful immune suppressant.[4391]

Men have a reduced capacity to fight infections and don't respond as well to vaccinations compared to women. That said, less immune activation may have the advantage of less autoimmune disease. Testosterone may be the reason women have higher rates of diseases like lupus, rheumatoid arthritis, and multiple sclerosis,[4392] but the reason men have more infectious disease morbidity and mortality. Lower infection risk is one reason why neutered cats live years longer than "intact" males.[4393] In fact, there are rare mammals who evolved "semelparous" reproductive strategies in which the males engage in a single, "out with a bang" mating frenzy fueled by surging testosterone before dying shortly thereafter from a total collapse of their immune system.[4394] So, might human eunuchs actually live longer?

Castration does extend the lifespan of rodents.[4395] (Then again, giving them hundreds of 10,000-volt electric shocks can, too, so I'm not being prescriptive.[4396]) A historical study of Korean eunuchs suggested they lived fourteen to nineteen years longer than uncastrated men of similar socioeconomic status, with a centenarian rate more than a hundred times higher than present-day populations.[4397] However, the existence of one eunuch purported to have lived 109 years, close to the longest lifespan ever recorded in men, cast aspersions on the accuracy of the records.[4398] A similar analysis dating back as far as the 1500s of castrati—male singers castrated before puberty to maintain their pitch— found no survival advantage compared to "intact" male singers during the same period.[4399]

More contemporary records can be drawn from the history of American eugenics in which the developmentally disabled were sterilized en masse through the 1930s,[4400] a practice that was sanctioned by the U.S. Supreme Court.[4401] At one Kansas mental institution, the hundreds who were castrated were found to live, on average, thirteen years longer than their uncastrated colleagues. The fact that death from infection constituted the chief difference between the two groups is consistent with the testosterone hypothesis.[4402] Regardless, testosterone replacement therapy is not a viable anti-aging strategy. Sadly, as an editorial published in the *Journal of the American Medical Association* lamented, "Testosterone misuse will not simply disappear for lack of logic or evidence as none was needed to get it started—rejuvenation fantasies thrive on hope without needing facts. . . ."[4403]

PRESERVING YOUR IMMUNE SYSTEM

A decline in immune function is one of the most well-recognized consequences of aging. We see this in increased vulnerability to acute viral and bacterial infections, such as the flu and pneumococcal pneumonia.[4404] In the developed world, infectious diseases are the fourth leading cause of death among the elderly, who suffer triple the mortality rate of acute infections compared to younger adults.[4405] This is exacerbated by a relatively poor response to vaccination, a phenomenon that's been recognized since the dawn of vaccine development.[4406] For example, while flu shots can build up sufficient antibody protection in 50 to 75 percent of younger individuals, that proportion falls to as few as 10 to 30 percent of older adults, who are among those who need the protection the most.[4407]

At the same time, we've known for nearly thirty years that the immune cells of eighty-year-olds produce significantly more pro-inflammatory signals.[4408] As I discuss in the Inflammation chapter, this suggests the worst of both worlds—a decline in the part of the immune system that fights specific infections and an aggravation of nonspecific overreactions that can lead to inflammation.[4409] We saw this play out with COVID-19. Certainly, older adults are more likely to be in tinderboxes like nursing homes and carry comorbidities that make infection more likely and serious, but part of their vulnerability may lie in both declining immune function and the potential for a hyperinflammatory "cytokine storm" immune reaction linked to poorer outcomes.[4410] Since I already covered the inflammaging dimension, I'll concentrate here on immunosenescence, the decline in immune defense with aging, and what we can do about it. (For the too-fantastical-to-be-believed overview on how the immune system actually works, see my Infections chapter in *How Not to Die*.)

LIFESTYLE

How can our daily habits influence our immune function?

WEIGHT LOSS

Obesity can weigh down the efficacy of vaccination,[4411] such that despite flu shots, individuals who are obese can have double the risk of coming down with the flu or flu-like infections compared to healthy-weight, vaccinated individuals.[4412] In fact, one of the reasons obese persons have higher cancer rates may be an impairment of antitumor immunity.

The Swedish Obese Subjects (SOS) trial was the first long-term controlled study to assess the outcomes of thousands of bariatric surgery patients against matched control subjects who began the trial the same weight but then followed a nonsurgical route. Over the next ten to twenty years, the control group's weights remained about the same, while the surgical group maintained about a 20 percent weight loss and also suffered significantly fewer heart attacks and strokes, developed 80 percent less diabetes, and, not surprisingly, had lower overall mortality. They also got less cancer.[4413]

Obesity severely impairs the function of our natural killer cells, critical members of our immune system's rapid-response force, fighting against cancerous and virus-infected cells. But when obese individuals were randomized to a weight-loss program, researchers saw a significant reactivation of natural killer cell function within only ninety days.[4414] An exercise component was included in the program, though, so it's difficult to tease out the impact of just the weight loss since physical activity on its own can boost natural killer cell activity.[4415]

EXERCISE

Exercise can ramp up our immune system by so much that we can reduce the number of sick days we have to take by 25 to 50 percent.[4416] Natural killer cells taken after thirty minutes of cycling killed off 60 percent more cancer cells in a petri dish.[4417] This may be one of the reasons exercise seems to both help prevent cancer and improve cancer survival.[4418] Men and women aged sixty-four and older who were randomized to twenty-five to thirty minutes of vigorous exercise three days a week for ten months before they got flu shots achieved significantly better protection,[4419] though you can't just slouch on the couch all year and jump up for a brisk walk right before your flu[4420] or pneumonia[4421] shot and expect additional protection. For more on what exercise can do to bolster your immunity, and for which infections interventional studies have shown exercise can help prevent, watch see .nf/exerciseimmunity.

Breathing in the Forest

Another way to lower cortisol levels is by forest bathing, surrounding yourself with trees,[4422] which may also elevate natural killer cell activity, as shown in a series of randomized controlled trials I document in see.nf/forestbathing. It turns out, as I explain in my follow-up video see.nf/treefragrance, trees produce aromatic volatile compounds called *phytoncides*,[4423] like pinene, that you breathe into your lungs in the forest.[4424] They enter your bloodstream[4425] and boost natural killer cell activity.[4426]

A combination of wood aromas improved the recovery of mice from stress-induced immune suppression,[4427] but is it really just the fragrance of the forest? Researchers investigated whether that same boost in natural killer cell activity could be achieved by just vaporizing some essential oil from one of the trees into a hotel room overnight—and it worked![4428] Ironically, these phytoncide compounds are part of the tree's *own* immune system, which we may be able to

(*continued*)

commandeer.[4429] Researchers speculate these compounds may be playing some role in the fact that more heavily forested regions in Japan appeared to have lower death rates from breast cancer and prostate cancer.[4430] Being out in nature has been found to be an important coping strategy among cancer patients.[4431] It turns out this could potentially help more than just with coping, thanks to the fragrance of trees.

SLEEP

In mice, sleep deprivation has alternatively been found to undermine vaccine efficacy,[4432] have no effect,[4433] or even bolster protection,[4434] but, consonant with popular wisdom, there is "surprisingly strong evidence"[4435] that sleep enhances immune defenses in human beings. Individuals getting inadequate sleep on the days immediately before and after getting a hepatitis B[4436] or flu vaccine[4437]—for example, fewer than six hours compared to more than seven—tended to end up with significantly fewer protective antibodies. This was confirmed in interventional trials of imposed sleep loss.

In one study, half the participants had to pull an all-nighter after getting a hepatitis A vaccine. The individuals who had been allowed to sleep normally that night after getting the exact same vaccination ended up with twice the antibodies in their bloodstream a month later.[4438] Even one year later, they were significantly more protected—all because of one night's sleep.[4439] Can't you try to make up for it by sleeping longer on subsequent nights? Even then, the die may have already been cast. Those getting a flu shot during a week in which they were restricted to four hours of sleep a night ended up with less than half the antibodies ten days later compared to the regular sleeping group, despite sleep getting extended to twelve hours a night in the sleep-debt group the subsequent week.[4440] Sleep deprivation—whether going to bed too late[4441] or getting up too early[4442]—has also been shown to impair natural killer cell activity.

What about infection rates? In the Harvard Nurses' Health Study II, those averaging no more than five hours of sleep a night appeared to have about a 40 percent greater chance of coming down with pneumonia, relative to those sleeping for eight hours. Those who were both overweight and not sleeping enough were at more than 80 percent higher risk.[4443] In a more direct demonstration, researchers at the Mayo Clinic dripped cold viruses right into people's noses, and those self-reporting sleeping fewer than seven hours a night were about three times more likely to come down with a cold than those who slept for eight hours or more.[4444] Self-reported sleep tends to underestimate duration, so the study was repeated using a wrist accelerometer for objective measurements. Those sleeping no more than six hours a night were four times as likely to fall ill compared to those getting seven hours or more.[4445] Note that infection rates were the same. After all, they had virus instilled directly in their nose. The well-rested group was just able to clear the virus so quickly that they were four times less likely to become symptomatic.[4446]

FOODS

As you can imagine, the upkeep of our immune system takes a tremendous amount of energy.[4447] We churn out millions of new immune cells every day.[4448] This may be why our immune function contracts as we age, paralleling the shrinkage of other energy-demanding organs, such as our muscles. This isn't inevitable, though. Some are able to maintain a fully functional immune system into old age.[4449] Part of the deterioration may be a function of the tendency for dietary quality to decline as we get older.

PRODUCE AISLE PROTECTION

Do people who eat well stay well? Those who eat more fruits and vegetables do appear to have a lower risk of getting an upper-respiratory-tract infection like the common cold. Even just one added apple a day may indeed help keep the doctor away.[4450] In terms of more serious respiratory infections, such as influenza, on a community-wide level, a 5 percent increase in obesity prevalence is associated with a 6 percent increase in flu-related hospitalizations.[4451] The same increase in physical inactivity rates was linked to a 7 percent increase in hospitalizations, and low rates of fruit and vegetable consumption may increase flu-related hospitalizations by 8 percent. Fruit and veggie intake is also linked to all sorts of other healthy behaviors, though. The only way to know if shopping the produce aisle can boost immunity is to put it to the test.

To assess the theory that inadequate nutrition could help explain the loss in immune function as you age, researchers split eighty-three volunteers aged sixty-five and older into two groups. The experimental group ate at least five servings of fruits and vegetables a day, while the control group ate fewer than three. All the participants were then vaccinated against pneumonia, a practice recommended for everyone over the age of sixty-five.[4452] The goal of vaccination is to prime our immune system to produce antibodies against that particular pathogen in case we ever get infected. Compared with those in the control group, the study subjects eating five or more servings of fruits and vegetables had an 82 percent greater protective antibody response to the vaccine. This was after just a single month of eating a few extra servings of fruits and veggies a day.[4453] That is how much control our forks may exert over immune function.

KIWIFRUIT, ECHINACEA, AND ELDERBERRY

Certain fruits and vegetables may give the immune function an extra boost. One that's been put to the test is kiwifruit. Preschoolers were randomized to eat either bananas or gold kiwifruits every day. Compared to the banana group, the kiwi-eating kids appeared to nearly halve their risk of contracting a flu-like illness or cold. (Why *gold* kiwifruits? The study was funded by the company that owns the patent on gold kiwifruits.)[4454] However, about 1 in 130 children may be allergic to kiwifruit,[4455] which may make kiwis the third-most-common food allergen (after milk and eggs),[4456] so they are not for everyone.

A similar experiment was tried on another high-risk group, the elderly. Those in the control group who ate bananas and got an upper-respiratory-tract infection suffered with congestion and a sore throat for about five days, compared to the kiwifruit eaters, who felt better after one or two days.[4457] In contrast, anti-flu drugs like oseltamivir (Tamiflu) may only shorten symptom duration in adults by an average of about seventeen hours.[4458] A 2020 review titled "Food or Medication? The Therapeutic Effects of Food on the Duration and Incidence of Upper Respiratory Tract Infections" noted another advantage: The price of kiwifruit is "much lower."[4459]

Kiwis are technically berries. (They were known originally as Chinese gooseberries before some innovative New Zealand exporters named the fuzzy brown fruit after their fuzzy brown bird.) What about other berries? I cover all the studies on elderberries in see.nf/elderberries. In short, four studies seemed to show positive results, but they were also all funded by elderberry product companies.[4460] Finally, in 2020, an independent (philanthropy-funded) study was published—a randomized, double-blind, placebo-controlled trial of an elderberry extract for the treatment of influenza. In contrast to the industry-funded studies, those randomized to the elderberry seemed to do *worse*, experiencing more aches and pains. Among those not taking Tamiflu, the participants randomized to the elderberry placebo were sick for five days, whereas those randomized to the *real* elderberry were sick for *seven* days.[4461] The accompanying editorial concluded that, based on these results, "we can confidently advise patients not to take elderberry."[4462] As I show in the video, similarly disappointing results have been reported for the herb echinacea.[4463]

Elderberry supplements may not even be safe.[4464] A case report was published about a man taking an elderberry extract suffering an attack of acute pancreatitis (a sudden painful inflammation of the pancreas). What makes the case is that it went away when he stopped the supplement and then reappeared again years later when he tried taking it again, which suggests cause and effect. Why take elderberry extracts, though, when you can just eat the elderberries themselves? Because consuming raw elderberries can cause you to puke your guts out,[4465] as I found out the hard way after foraging a backyard bush for breakfast. Turns out raw elderberry fruit forms cyanide.[4466] Only after recovering did I discover CDC reports like "Poisoning from Elderberry Juice—California" about eight people having to be medevacked out by helicopter after someone brought freshly squeezed elderberry juice to a gathering.[4467] All I can say is, I'm glad my body rejected it. What would they have put on the headstone? *Author of* How Not to Die *killed by a smoothie*.

OTHER BERRIES

What other berries might help us? In see.nf/immuneberries, I go through the whole rundown. Interventional studies show, for example, that blueberries can increase the numbers of natural killer cells,[4468] the aromatic spice cardamom can increase their activity,[4469] and black raspberries appear to do both,[4470,4471] but does this translate into fewer infections? Sea buckthorn berries boost the activity of another type of "first responder" immune cell[4472] but fail to help prevent respiratory, digestive, or urinary tract infections compared to placebo.[4473]

Goji berries do actually appear to have relevant, real-world, beneficial effects on immune function. Older men and women aged sixty-five to seventy were randomized to eat four teaspoons[4474] of powdered goji berries or an identical-appearing placebo powder every day for 90 days. On day 30, everyone received a flu shot. By day 60, the goji group already had a significantly better antibody response such that, by day 90, three times more of the goji group achieved sero-conversion (a sufficiently protective antibody threshold): 28 percent versus only 9 percent in the placebo group.[4475]

Do They Need to Be Organic?

In a review updating the evidence of the implications of pesticides on human health, the body of evidence linking pesticide exposure and cancer is said to be "so huge that the role of pesticides in cancer development can no longer be doubted."[4476] However, most of the data showing DNA damage from pesticides are limited to occupational exposure: among farmers and workers in fields, within the pesticides industry itself, or among those living in high-spray areas.[4477] What about the residues left on conventional produce? I explore that body of literature in my video see.nf/pesticides. In short, those who choose organic

(continued)

produce seem to have lower cancer rates after controlling for confounding factors,[4478] but even if it is cause and effect, the benefits of consuming conventionally grown produce are likely to outweigh any possible risks from pesticide exposure.[4479] So, concerns over pesticide risks should never discourage us from eating as many fruits and vegetables as possible. The potential lifelong damage of any pesticides on produce is estimated to cut only a few minutes off a person's life on average, which is nothing compared to benefits we get from eating fruits and veggies.[4480]

VEGETABLES

A series of experiments involving fruit and vegetable deprivation dramatically demonstrated the impact that healthy foods can have on our immune function. Figuring that their carotenoid pigments may be responsible for the immune-actuating effects, researchers advised volunteers to try to avoid all brightly colored fruits and vegetables. It didn't take more than two weeks for measures of their immune function to plummet. White blood cells taken from the participants became sluggish to proliferate in the face of immune activation. To see how quickly this activity could be recovered, they tried three potential rescue treatments each day: one and a half cups of tomato juice, one and a half cups of carrot juice, or a serving of powdered spinach. Within a week of starting the tomato juice, white blood cell activity started to significantly perk up, but neither the carrot juice nor the spinach seemed sufficient to salvage immune function.[4481] This tells us two things: Remarkably, we can affect our immune function with simple dietary decisions, and not all veggies are alike.

When this study was repeated to look at other immune markers, tomato and carrot appeared more evenly matched. (Spinach was skipped this time.) Both the post-deprivation tomato and carrot juice periods saw a significant increase in natural killer cell activity, for example.[4482] In contrast, tomato extract supplements (Lycomato) failed to result in any improvements in immune defense.[4483] Could something as simple as tomato juice improve immune protection even in those who hadn't been deprived of carotenoid-rich fruits and vegetables? Well-nourished elderly men and women were randomized to a cup and a half of tomato juice or mineral water for eight weeks, and no difference in immune function was found.[4484] So, if you're stuck in a rut of beige food like white potatoes, it doesn't take much to recoup some of your lost immune function, but if you're eating a minimum threshold of healthy produce, it's going to take more than a glass of tomato juice. Either add multiple daily servings of fruits and vegetables like in that flu shot study, or level up your veggies to include some at the top of the heap, like broccoli.

CRUCIFEROUS VEGETABLES

On page 492, I explore how crucifers are critical for intestinal immune function. Broccoli can also boost our natural killers.[4485] Researchers drew blood from study participants before and after they ate broccoli sprouts for just a few days and found that the ability of their natural killer cells to produce *granzyme B* went up. That's an enzyme used to activate what are called "execution caspases" in target cells to initiate a self-destruct protocol and wipe out virus-infected and cancerous cells.[4486] Does this translate into helping us actually fight off infection? Researchers dripped flu viruses into the noses of volunteers to find out.

In a randomized study, compared to the placebo (alfalfa sprouts), about 4 oz of broccoli sprouts eaten on the day before and the day of infection significantly reduced the viral load as well as virus-induced inflammation in the nose in smokers. The researchers concluded that cruciferous vegetables like broccoli may present a "low-cost and low-risk measure for reducing the impact of influenza."[4487] The same was found for reducing respiratory syncytial virus disease in mice[4488] and blocking Epstein-Barr virus in vitro.[4489] Sulforaphane, the purported active component in broccoli and other crucifers, has also been found to restore bacteria recognition and engulfment in macrophages extracted from the lungs of patients with pulmonary diseases like emphysema (COPD).[4490] However, the concentration they used might only be reached in the bloodstream by eating around five cups of broccoli at one sitting,[4491] so we won't know clinical relevance until it's been studied at more modest doses.

NO NEWS IS GOOD NEWS

Nitric oxide—not to be confused with nitrous oxide, aka laughing gas—is best known as the "open sesame" molecule our artery lining releases to enable our blood vessels to dilate, but it also has broad-spectrum antiviral, antibacterial, and antifungal properties. It's secreted into our airways as a first line of defense against respiratory infection,[4492] shooting up more than 500 percent over baseline.[4493] Nitrate-rich vegetables can improve athletic performance,[4494] but what about immune performance? Infusions of spinach leaves have been used since ancient times to treat respiratory symptoms,[4495] but as I explore in see.nf/noimmune, the evidence that this translates into lower infections rates still remains suggestive.[4496]

SEAWEED

What about underwater greens? Billions of pounds of sea vegetables are harvested each year.[4497] Japan has among the highest per capita intake of seaweed, and its consumption is associated with lower disease rates and even lower all-cause mortality,[4498] though it may just be an indicator of following more traditional Japanese dietary customs.[4499] In terms of immune function, wakame, which is the kind you find in seaweed salad, can double[4500] or quadruple[4501] the replication potential of T cells, an important part of our immune defense against viruses like herpes. See my video see.nf/wakame to learn what eating just 2 g a day of wakame can do for those suffering from various herpes infections and how wakame can significantly boost protective antibody responses to flu vaccination.

Soy foods can also boost antibody-producing B cells. Those randomized to three daily cups of soymilk increased B cell populations in the blood by about 35 percent more than those receiving dairy milk.[4502] Japan also has among the highest per capita soy consumption,[4503] so the speculation that seaweed intake may help explain the relatively low rates of HIV[4504] and COVID-19[4505] in the country could also be extended to other traditional Japanese foods.

What about nori, probably the most accessible seaweed? They're the sheets used for making sushi rolls,[4506] but they can also make quick and easy snacks, one of my go-to favorites. It's hard to beat the nutrient density; each sheet has as little as a single calorie.[4507] Study participants randomized to a nori extract for eight weeks experienced an increase in natural killer cell activity.[4508] The dose they were given was equivalent to about seven sheets of nori a day,[4509] though, so it's not clear what the effects of smaller doses might be.

CHLORELLA

About 95 percent of all infections begin in our mucosal surfaces, the moist linings of our eyes, nostrils, and mouth.[4510] To protect these surfaces, our body covers them with a special antibody called *immunoglobulin A* (IgA), which it pumps out to the tune of ten thousand million billion a day (1×10^{19}).[4511,4512] This provides an immunological barrier that neutralizes and prevents viruses from penetrating the body. The IgA in saliva, for example, is a first-line defense against pneumonia, influenza, and other respiratory-tract infections.[4513]

Researchers in Japan found that IgA concentrations in breast milk could be increased by giving mothers chlorella, a unicellular freshwater green algae (essentially, a single-celled plant) sold as powder or compressed into tablets.[4514] What about other parts of the body? Chlorella didn't convincingly improve the immune response to flu vaccination,[4515] but it did increase IgA secretion into the mouth.[4516] Unfortunately, as I cover in see.nf/igachlorella, it's not clear if this translates into fewer illnesses.

Chlorella can also significantly improve natural killer cell activity.[4517] This may play a role in reducing liver damage in chronic hepatitis C virus infection,[4518] with benefits for cholesterol, blood pressure, and blood sugar control,[4519] but as I note in my video see.nf/nkchlorella, there was a concerning case report of apparent chlorella-induced psychosis that makes me wary.[4520]

GARLIC

In World War II, garlic was called "Russian Penicillin" because, after running out of antibiotics, that's what the Soviet government turned to.[4521] Does it actually work? Eating garlic appears to offer the best of both worlds, dampening the overreactive face of the immune system by suppressing inflammation,[4522] while boosting protective immunity, such as natural killer cell activity. Check out see.nf/coldsandcancer for double-blind, placebo-controlled trials of garlic for the prevention of the common cold and cancer. (Garlic supplement users did not appear to be protected from COVID,[4523] but it may take up to fifty-four capsules of garlic extract supplements to obtain the same amount of garlicky goodness found in just one clove of crushed raw garlic.[4524])

What happens if you cook it? If you compare raw chopped garlic to garlic that's been cooked in various methods, you can see dramatic drops in one of the purported active ingredients. You can get a 66 percent drop when you boil it for six minutes, 94 percent less when you simmer it for fifteen minutes, and a full 100 percent wipeout from just one minute of stir-frying it.[4525] What about roasted garlic? Surprisingly, even though roasting is done at temperatures hotter than boiling water, it preserves about twice as much. Raw garlic has the most, but it may be easier for some to eat two or three cloves of cooked garlic than the equivalent (half a clove) of raw.[4526]

In *How Not to Die*, I suggested that the only major caveat against consuming garlic (besides a potential decrease in kissability) is that garlic can have blood-thinning effects, so maybe you shouldn't have any a week before elective surgery.[4527] That was based on a study in which subjects were fed 10 g of garlic every day for two months, which is about three daily cloves.[4528] However, at a more "socially acceptable" dose of one to two cloves a day for a week, no changes in clotting function were noted.[4529] What about garlic breath? Raw apple, raw lettuce, and mint leaves have all been shown to be at least partially effective.[4530]

MUSHROOMS

As I show in my video see.nf/mushrooms, cooked white button mushrooms can also boost IgA production[4531] while potentially tamping down immune overactivity. A randomized, double-blind, placebo-controlled clinical study confirmed an apparent anti-allergy effect of an oyster mushroom component in kids who had a history of recurrent upper-respiratory-tract infections.[4532]

Shiitake mushrooms have also been shown to improve human immune function. Just eating two or three large dried shiitake mushrooms a day for a month resulted in an increase in the proliferation of two types of first-line immune defenders, all while lowering markers of systemic inflammation.[4533] What we care about most, though, is actually preventing infections.

White button mushroom supplementation enhances natural killer cell activity in aged mice, for example, but it doesn't actually protect them against subsequent influenza infection.[4534] Oyster mushrooms seem to work—at least in athletes. After intensive exercise, elite athletes can suffer a 28 percent reduction in natural killer cell activity during recovery.[4535] When they were given about one daily oyster mushroom's worth[4536] of the special beta-glucan fiber found in fungi (sourced from oyster mushrooms), not only did their natural killer cell counts buoy up, but they suffered fewer upper-respiratory-tract symptoms over three months. In the placebo group, 84 percent suffered four or more symptoms, compared to only 12 percent in the mushroom group.[4537]

NUTRITIONAL YEAST

That same immune-activating beta-glucan fiber is found in brewer's, baker's, and nutritional yeasts. Details in see.nf/nooch, but basically, the IgA-boosting effects[4538] of the beta-glucan from a daily heaping teaspoon or so of nutritional yeast can reduce the incidence, duration, and severity of upper-respiratory-tract infections compared to placebo.[4539] And what's the downside—tastier popcorn? Randomized controlled trials have also found it has anti-inflammatory effects[4540] sufficient to improve wound healing,[4541] reduce the severity of canker sores,[4542] and alleviate symptoms in ragweed sufferers, as well as benefit weight loss.[4543,4544] None of the studies reported treatment-related adverse effects,[4545] but I would caution against the use of any kind of yeast for those with two specific autoimmune diseases: Crohn's disease[4546] (see.nf/crohns) and a skin condition known as *hidradenitis suppurativa*[4547] (see.nf/hidradenitis).

GREEN TEA

Our body is always on the lookout for *PAMPs*, pathogen-associated molecular patterns. These are molecules foreign to our body that are associated with infection, such as components of bacterial cell walls. We have immune cells with pattern-recognition receptors that recognize these "nonself" signatures. Not all bacteria are pathogenic, though, so, in order to be more accurate, the name was changed to *MAMPs*, microbe-associated molecular patterns. The beta-glucans in yeast and mushrooms are major MAMPs.[4548] They make up the cell walls of fungi, so they act as nonspecific immunostimulants (as opposed to a specific immunostimulant like a vaccine).[4549] Essentially, when our body detects beta-glucans in our system, to err on the side of caution, it immediately thinks *fungal infection*, not shiitake stir-fry.[4550] We can then benefit from that increased vigilance.

There are also MAMP mimickers in certain plants. Bacteria, fungi, parasites, and tumor cells all release a class of MAMP compounds called *alkylamines*.[4551] Theanine, the unique amino acid that gives tea its savory (umami) taste, is broken down in our gut into an alkylamine called *ethylamine*, which then circulates throughout the body. You can tell if someone is a tea drinker by testing their urine for ethylamine.[4552] There are also preexisting alkylamines in apple peels (*n*-Butylamine),[4553] wine (iso-amylamine),[4554] and healthy vaginal secretions (isobutylamine).[4555]

Alkylamines enhance the proliferation and activity of gamma-delta T cells, a type of first-line defender.[4556] The "priming" of these cells by ethylamine may explain why gamma-delta T cells taken from tea drinkers are more active than those taken from coffee drinkers. Take white blood cells before and after just one week of tea drinking, and you get two to four times the defensive interferon release upon exposure to bacteria in vitro. The day-to-day low-level exposure to ethylamine seemed to maintain their immune cells in a constant ready state. There has even been speculation that primate immune systems evolved to take immune-boosting advantage of the alkylamines and their precursors in plant foods.[4557]

Tea drinkers have been documented to have lower rates of influenza[4558] and as little as half the risk of dying from pneumonia.[4559] A randomized, double-blind, placebo-controlled trial found that those taking concentrated green tea capsules had about one-third fewer days of cold and flu symptoms compared to those randomized to placebo capsules, but the dose equivalent was comparable to drinking ten cups of tea a day.[4560] Subsequently, a similar trial on healthcare workers found that those participants randomized to the equivalent of just one and a quarter cups of green tea a day[4561] for five months were about three times less likely to come down with the flu (4 percent versus 13 percent in the placebo group).[4562] How low can you go? In 2020, researchers tried to push the envelope and found that even the equivalent of half a cup of green tea a day (about one typical teacup's worth)[4563] cut the risk of upper respiratory infection in half, but less than a quarter cup a day did not.[4564]

What About Gargling with Green Tea?

A study that involved swabbing the mouths of volunteers ten, forty, and sixty minutes after they drank some tea found that antiviral concentrations[4565] of tea

(continued)

compounds were retained in the oral cavity even an hour after ingestion.[4566] The studies that I mentioned earlier found a reduction in infection risk even with swallowed green tea extract capsules; they show that direct contact with our throat is not necessary. What about the opposite? What about gargling green tea and spitting it out so there's *only* oral contact?

As I note in see.nf/gargling, acrobatic attempts have been made to present purported tea gargling benefits as statistically significant for upper-respiratory-tract infections[4567] or influenza,[4568] either by folding them in with tea ingestion trials or combining them with observational gargling studies. However, that doesn't change the fact that none of the randomized controlled trials of tea gargling has been found to significantly lower infection risk.[4569] The evidence for water gargling to prevent upper-respiratory-tract infections is also disappointing.[4570]

So, although gargling may work wonders to soothe a sore throat, it may not prevent the sore throat in the first place—unless it's caused by gonorrhea. A single one-minute gargle with an antiseptic mouthwash (Listerine diluted up to 1:4 with water in this case) can significantly reduce the amount of any gonorrhea bacteria you may have in your oral cavity.[4571] Gargling has been found to be superior to simply rinsing out your mouth in terms of reaching the back of your throat. At least twenty seconds is recommended,[4572] but in a study of female sex workers, the average gargle time was only four seconds.[4573]

FIBER-RICH FOODS

In my High in Fiber-Rich Foods chapter in *How Not to Diet*, I relayed the detective story of the search for the keys that fit into two mysterious locks in the body, vital receptors expressed heavily throughout our body—on our nerves, in our gut, and in our immune, muscle, and fat cells.[4574] Spoiler alert: They were the short-chain fatty acids our gut bacteria make when we eat fiber,[4575] constituting a critical line of communication between our gut bacteria and the rest of our body.[4576]

This may explain how fiber is so anti-inflammatory.[4577] For instance, how is it possible that just one high-fiber meal can improve lung function in asthmatics within a matter of hours? We now know that our good gut bacteria turn the fiber we eat into short-chain fatty acids, which then are absorbed into our bloodstreams. They are then free to dock in these receptors found on the inflammatory immune cells in our airways and turn them off.[4578]

Does that mean that people who eat more fiber have better immune systems? How might we determine that? Well, most people have gotten an MMR shot, the measles-mumps-rubella vaccination that's been routinely given to children since the 1970s. Are there measurably more antibodies against pathogens in different dietary groups? Yes, for mumps. All participants had received the same MMR vaccine, but those eating more fiber had significantly higher levels of antibodies against mumps, though not against any of the other bugs.[4579]

To help prove cause and effect, researchers gave volunteers a cocktail of antibiotics to wipe out much of their gut flora as they were getting their annual flu vaccine. Those starting out with low preexisting immunity suffered a striking impairment of their antibody response.[4580] They had much weaker reactions to the vaccine. Conversely, by randomizing people to prebiotics, like fiber, which is what our good bacteria eat, or probiotics, the good bacteria themselves, antibody responses to flu shots can be enhanced.[4581] Does this translate into lower infection risk?

Those with higher levels of fiber-feeding bacteria in their gut were found to be five times less likely to develop viral pneumonia or bronchitis.[4582] Establishing cause and effect, a meta-analysis of randomized controlled trials found that *prebiotics* can reduce the incidence of respiratory tract infections in general.[4583] For probiotics, in children, those randomized to probiotic dairy yogurt, soy yogurt, or supplements experienced both fewer and shorter-lasting upper-respiratory-tract infections,[4584] though, in older adults, only the duration of symptoms appears to be lessened.[4585,4586,4587] Given the potentially negative impacts of probiotics I note in the Prebiotics and Postbiotics chapter, I would suggest instead focusing on feeding the good bacteria we already have, by eating foods naturally rich in dietary fiber.

DO VEGETARIANS MAKE BETTER KILLERS?

As we get older, our natural killer cells tend to lose some of their proliferative capacity and killing power.[4588] What can we do to maintain their function? I reviewed a few plants that appear protective, but what about an entire diet centered around plants? The natural killer cells of vegetarians were pitted head-to-head against those of omnivores in a test to see which could wipe out more leukemia cells, and the vegetarian killer cells were victorious. They were more than twice as effective in killing off cancer. On average, each natural killer cell drawn from the blood of a vegetarian knocked off two cancer cells for every one the nonvegetarian killers succeeded in overtaking. The researchers suggested that "the reduced cancer risk of vegetarians is possibly partially related to the better natural defense system which they seem to have."[4589]

Having more effective immunity doesn't just help protect against cancer by targeting tumors directly. Sometimes infections cause cancers. Take HPV (human papilloma virus). Cervical cancer is now considered a sexually transmitted disease.[4590] It was originally suspected as such, based on cancer rates in "nuns versus prostitutes,"[4591] but we now have DNA fingerprinting proof that virtually all cervical cancer is caused by HPV,[4592] a sexually transmitted virus that also causes cancers of the penis, vagina, vulva, and throat.

HPV is considered a necessary but insufficient cause of cancer. HPV is so common that most young women will contract it, yet most don't get cervical cancer because their immune systems are able to wipe out the virus. Within one year, 70 percent of women clear the infection and more than 90 percent clear it within two years—before the virus can cause cancer.[4593]

Might those with particularly strong immune systems clear the virus even faster? That may explain the finding that vegetarian women had significantly lower HPV infection rates, one of many studies reporting lower risk of HPV infection among those eating plant-based diets.[4594] Greater vegetable consumption alone may even help.

Researchers followed women with cancer-causing strains of HPV infecting their cervix and retested them at three months and nine months, while analyzing their diets. Higher levels of vegetable consumption appeared to cut their risk of HPV persistence in half, doubling their likelihood of clearing this potentially cancer-causing infection.[4595] This may help explain why vegan women have significantly lower rates of all female cancers combined, including cancer of the cervix.[4596] However, a comparison of the natural killer cell activity between vegans and nonvegetarians failed to replicate the earlier study, so other cancer-fighting components or nonimmunological mechanisms may be responsible for the lower cancer rates.[4597]

Plant-Based Pandemic Protection

The COVID-19 pandemic offered a good opportunity to see if eating more healthfully could help stave off infection. Details in see.nf/plantdemic, but basically, Harvard researchers collected data from nearly 600,000 participants and found that those who ate the most healthful plant foods and the least meat, eggs, dairy, and junk not only had a significantly lower risk of suffering a severe course of COVID-19 but they also had a significantly lower risk of getting infected in the first place, even after taking into account comorbidities and other nondietary lifestyle risk factors, such as exercise, smoking, and socioeconomic status.[4598]

SUPPLEMENTS

Are there any supplements that can help protect against infection?

GINSENG

Ginseng is notable for its Latin name, *Panax*, which comes from the word *panacea*, meaning "cure-all."[4599] It can extend the lives of fruit flies[4600] and roundworms[4601] but not mice.[4602] The two main species are American ginseng (*Panax quinquefolius*) and Asian ginseng (*Panax ginseng*), which can be further divided up by processing method. White ginseng is Asian ginseng root that's simply been washed and dried. Red ginseng is Asian ginseng root that undergoes an additional step of steaming before drying.[4603] Various ginseng preparations have been shown to boost populations of B and T cells[4604] and natural killer cell activity,[4605] but what about disease endpoints?

A meta-analysis of randomized, double-blind, placebo-controlled trials found that ginseng appeared to reduce the risk of developing acute upper respiratory infections, but it did not appear to significantly affect the duration of illness. A subgroup analysis, however, suggests that the preventive benefit is limited to Asian ginseng, which cuts infection risk in half compared to placebo, as opposed to American ginseng, which reduced risk by only 14 percent, not reaching statistical significance.[4606]

I cover the downsides in see.nf/ginsengabuse. Aside from the symptoms of "ginseng abuse syndrome" and tissue swelling,[4607] there have been case reports of manic psychosis,[4608] estrogenic effects,[4609] and increased surgical bleeding.[4610] So, some recommend that those with hypertension, hyperthyroidism, a predisposition to mania, estrogen-dependent disease, or upcoming surgery avoid ginseng.[4611]

MULTIVITAMINS

All nutrients play some role in the functioning of the immune system. If you have a nutrient deficiency, then supplementation could certainly improve immunity, but we shouldn't expect that adding extra on top of nutrient sufficiency would necessarily further amplify immune function.[4612] However, many apparently healthy elderly people have been found to have micronutrient deficits,[4613] so what about taking a multivitamin and mineral supplement?

Extraordinary benefits were published in some of the most prestigious journals,[4614] leading reviewers to conclude, "All these reports confirm that immune responses may be enhanced in elderly individuals by the use of micronutrient supplements."[4615] Then, most of the papers were retracted,[4616] one after another.[4617] An earlier paper published by one of the principal authors tipped off investigators.

"Impossible" results from a study purporting to show cognitive benefits of multivitamin and mineral supplements[4618] led to a formal investigation that confirmed the impropriety,[4619] which then led to the cascade of retractions.

Since the debacle, there have been three large randomized controlled trials of multivitamin and mineral supplements for the prevention of infections.[4620] One such study, on noninstitutionalized elders and acute respiratory infections, found no effect on incidence or severity.[4621] Another, on nursing home residents and infections in general, found no fewer cases of infections, though those randomized to the multivitamin and mineral supplements did end up spending fewer days on antibiotics over the eighteen-month-long study.[4622] The third study looked at multivitamin and multimineral supplements separately and found the antibody response to flu vaccines improved on the minerals compared to placebo, while the antibody response to flu vaccines on the vitamins was worse than on placebo.[4623] Neither, however, led to a significant drop in infection rates.

VITAMIN C

Vitamin C has been proposed as a treatment for respiratory infections since its discovery nearly a century ago.[4624] In 1970, Nobel Prize laureate Linus Pauling published an influential book titled *Vitamin C and the Common Cold* that generated tremendous public interest and no doubt helped inspire the dozens of randomized, double-blind, placebo-controlled trials that were to follow to put his endorsement to the test.[4625] Check out see.nf/c4colds for details on what they found, but basically, those under extreme physical stress, such as marathon runners or soldiers on subarctic maneuvers, do appear to benefit from regularly taking vitamin C supplements, cutting their risk of coming down with a cold in half. However, for the general population, daily vitamin C supplementation does not appear to significantly reduce the incidence of infection, though when regular users do get sick, they don't get *as* sick and get better about 10 percent faster. Unfortunately, just starting vitamin C after the onset of cold symptoms doesn't seem to help cut down on cold severity or duration.[4626]

The downside is that vitamin C supplements appear to favor kidney stone formation,[4627,4628] as much as doubling risk. Those taking 1,000 mg or so of vitamin C a day may have a one-in-three-hundred chance of getting a kidney stone every year, instead of a one-in-six-hundred chance, which is not an insignificant risk, given how painful they can be.[4629]

VITAMINS D AND E

Daily vitamin D supplementation appears to reduce the risk of acute respiratory infections in children and adolescents, but it does not seem to make a difference in adults, nor is D effective for boosting antibody responses to influenza vaccination.[4630,4631] Vitamin E, on the other hand, was able to significantly boost immunity to hepatitis B and tetanus vaccinations, though not to diphtheria or pneumonia.[4632] As I detail in see.nf/immunevitamins, the data on vitamin E and infections are mixed, with some studies showing a worsening of infections.[4633] The question appears moot, since randomized controlled trials show vitamin E increases the risk of cancer[4634] and overall mortality.[4635] In other words, those who buy vitamin E supplements may in effect be paying to live a shorter life.

ZINC

In February 2020, a noted virologist told his friends and family, "Stock up now with zinc lozenges" for the coming pandemic.[4636] He based his supposition on the efficacy of zinc for common colds, up to 29 percent of which are caused by coronaviruses.[4637] There's actually a heartwarming backstory to that discovery that I detail in see.nf/zinc, involving a three-year-old girl with cancer who inspired her father to conduct the first randomized, double-blind, placebo-controlled trial on zinc lozenges for the common cold.[4638]

I run through all the studies in the video, but basically, zinc lozenges appear to shorten colds by about three days,[4639] with significant reductions in nasal discharge (by 34 percent), nasal congestion (by 37 percent), hoarseness (by 43 percent), and cough (by 46 percent).[4640] The best way to take zinc for the common cold is lozenges containing around 10 to 15 mg of zinc taken every two waking hours for a few days, starting immediately upon symptom onset as either zinc acetate or zinc gluconate[4641] *without* binders such as citric acid, tartaric acid, glycine, sorbitol, or mannitol.[4642]

Efficacy against more serious infections such as pneumonia may only be present among those with preexisting zinc deficiency.[4643] I was surprised to learn that the essentiality of zinc in humans wasn't established until the 1960s and wasn't formally recognized until 1974.[4644] About 40 percent of men and women in the United States aged sixty and older may not reach the recommended daily intake through their diet.[4645] Unlike some other minerals, such as iron, you can't just get a blood test to tell if you're deficient because zinc levels in the blood aren't a good reflection of overall zinc status in the body.[4646] The best we can do is make sure we get enough in our diet. The healthiest sources are probably legumes, nuts, and seeds, though oysters may be the most concentrated source by far.[4647] (A single oyster has more zinc than a cup of baked beans.[4648])

Zinc supplementation doesn't appear to reduce the risk of getting sick in the first place,[4649] though, and supplementing long-term may actually impair certain aspects of immunity in the elderly. This is perhaps because, at high doses, zinc can interfere with the absorption of other nutrients important to immune function, such as copper and folate.[4650] A month of zinc supplementation did appear to boost the antibody response to tetanus vaccination,[4651] but even two months of zinc supplementation before flu shots didn't appear to have any effect.[4652] Short-term use is considered to be safe, but zinc supplements and lozenges can cause nausea, especially when taken on an empty stomach, and other gastrointestinal symptoms.[4653] You should *never* put zinc in your nose. In the drugstore, you'll find all sorts of intranasal zinc gels, sprays, and swabs, but these have been linked to the potentially permanent loss of one's sense of smell.[4654]

Note there was a happy ending: That three-year-old beat her cancer, never relapsed, and grew up to become a scientist herself.[4655]

VACCINES

Vaccines are considered one of the greatest public health achievements of the last century,[4656] having eradicated smallpox, a scourge that killed hundreds of millions of people, and greatly reducing other major diseases, such as measles and polio.[4657] To this day, vaccines are estimated to save millions of lives each year.[4658]

More than 90 percent of U.S. children get common childhood vaccinations, such as polio and MMR shots, but most adults fail to get their full complement of recommended adult vaccinations. Assuming you got all your childhood vaccinations (and aside from any emergent pandemic needs), the CDC recommends that all adults get annual flu shots, tetanus boosters every ten years (though the World Health Organization doesn't think this is necessary),[4659] shingles vaccination at age fifty, and pneumonia vaccination at age sixty-five. Certain groups need others, such as hepatitis A vaccination for those experiencing homelessness, people with chronic liver disease, or men who have sex with men; or a hepatitis B series for healthcare workers and those who are incarcerated.[4660] Ask your medical professional for a personalized schedule.

How safe are vaccines? In a 2021 systematic review and meta-analysis, the RAND Corporation screened more than 50,000 citations and concluded that routine vaccinations can be considered safe, with only rare serious adverse effects,[4661] such as severe allergic reactions in one to ten individuals in a million. Transient autoimmune syndromes (Guillain-Barré and immune thrombocytopenic purpura) occur in about one to three in a million and ten to thirty in a million for flu shots and MMR vaccines, respectively.[4662]

FLU VACCINE

Each year, influenza typically kills between 4,000 and 20,000 Americans,[4663] though the death toll for the 2017–18 flu season was estimated at 80,000, making it one of the deadliest in the last half century.[4664] Most hospitalizations and 90 percent of flu-related mortality occur in those sixty-five and older.[4665] Mortality rates for the flu at ages seventy-five and older are fifty times higher than for those younger than sixty-five. Nonetheless, the CDC recommends that everyone over the age of six months get a routine flu shot every year,[4666] if for no other reason than to help prevent transmission to the more vulnerable.[4667] As I've discussed, the cruel irony is that older adults—the ones who need protection the most—acquire less robust protection from flu shots due to waning immunity with age.[4668]

Depending on the season, vaccination typically reduces the risk of getting the flu by about 40 to 50 percent.[4669] So, in healthy younger adults, we can say with moderate certainty that we can decrease the risk of getting the flu from about 2 percent each year down to just under 1 percent.[4670] Among older adults, there may be a similar relative risk reduction—from 6 percent down to 2.4 percent—but since the risk is higher and the consequences greater, the absolute benefits are greater, too.[4671]

In the Northern Hemisphere, the flu season can start as early as September and run as late as March.[4672] The problem with getting vaccinated too early is that immunity might wane before the season is over, especially in older adults.[4673] The CDC recommends trying to get vaccinated by the end of October, but getting it at any time throughout flu season is preferable to not getting vaccinated at all.[4674]

Yes, the influenza vaccine can cause Guillain-Barré syndrome, an autoimmune attack on your nerves that can leave you paralyzed for weeks, but so, too, can getting the flu.[4675] As I mentioned, there are only one to three additional individual cases of Guillain-Barré per one million vaccinations versus about seventeen extra cases per million flu episodes.[4676] So, you're much more likely to be temporarily paralyzed by the flu than the flu shot, but since it takes vaccinating about thirty older people to prevent one case of the flu,[4677] getting vaccinated would still be expected to raise your overall Guillain-Barré risk. However, the reason flu shots are recommended is not to lower risk of a rare autoimmune syndrome but to reduce the common—and potentially devastating—impacts of the flu that extend beyond just the respiratory infection.

In the week following a confirmed flu infection, the risk of having a heart attack shoots up to six times higher.[4678] The inflammation of infection can destabilize atherosclerotic plaques, constrict arteries, and make the blood more liable to clot.[4679] So, might flu vaccinations save lives in more ways than one? Those who get their flu shots are indeed less likely to die from cardiovascular disease in a given year as well as all causes put together.[4680] In other words, those who get regular flu shots live longer lives on average. But, who disproportionally gets flu shots? White, married nonsmokers of a higher social class with higher levels of education, higher incomes, and health insurance.[4681] You can't tell if it's truly cause and effect until you put it to the test.

There have been four randomized controlled trials—flu shots versus placebo shots—in those with preexisting heart disease, and, overall, those who got the real shots had a 56 percent lower chance of dying from cardiovascular disease and a 47 percent lower chance of dying from all causes put together. So, flu shots really can be an *extraordinary* lifesaver. Whether the observational data showing fewer deaths across the board—even including those without preexisting heart disease[4682]—similarly pan out is, as of yet, unknown.[4683]

Given the benefits, overcoming vaccine hesitancy should be as simple as correcting misinformation, but, sadly, debunking vaccine myths can actually backfire. Busting the myth that inactivated flu shots (the type given to older adults) can give you the flu surprisingly makes people even less likely to get it.[4684] Similarly, correcting the falsehoods that MMR vaccines cause autism[4685] or that pertussis vaccination causes as many side effects as people think, paradoxically, makes people less inclined to vaccinate.[4686] The researchers conclude that "correcting vaccine myths may not be an effective approach to promoting vaccination."[4687]

PNEUMONIA VACCINE

"Pneumonia may well be called the friend of the aged," wrote Sir William Osler, the "Father of Modern Medicine,"[4688] in 1898. "Taken off by it in an acute, short, not often painful illness, the old man escapes those 'cold gradations of decay' so distressing to himself and to his friends."[4689] The thought was that pneumonia mercifully killed those who would soon die anyway from a potentially more protracted and painful illness. But these days, healthy older adults hospitalized with pneumonia are not significantly more likely to die in the subsequent two years than younger adults in the same situation. Because of comorbidities at older ages, though, pneumonia is the fourth leading cause of death in the world[4690] and the ninth leading cause in the United States.[4691]

The most common cause of community-acquired pneumonia (as opposed to hospital-acquired) is a bacteria known as pneumococcus (*Streptococcus pneumoniae*).[4692] In addition to pneumonia, pneumococcus can cause inner ear infections, sinusitis, and pink eye. It gets serious when it starts to invade the bloodstream, which can result in meningitis (infection of the brain), endocarditis (infection of the heart valves), or sepsis (a life-threatening organ dysfunction caused by blood poisoning).

Thankfully, we have vaccines against pneumococcus. The first was developed more than a century ago, but it fell out of favor after penicillin was discovered and it was thought that antibiotics would eliminate the threat.[4693] Unfortunately, these days, up to 40 percent of pneumococcal infections are resistant to at least one antibiotic,[4694] and, despite our miracle drugs, mortality rates of invasive pneumococcus in the elderly stand at around 15 to 30 percent.[4695] According to randomized controlled trials, pneumococcus vaccines can reduce the risk of those sixty-five and older getting pneumococcal pneumonia by 64 percent and, even more important, the risk of *invasive* pneumococcal disease by 73 percent.[4696] Like the flu vaccine, population studies have found that pneumonia vaccines appear to reduce both the risk of heart attacks and the overall risk of dying, but unlike the flu vaccine, there aren't randomized controlled trials to confirm these bonus benefits.[4697]

SHINGLES VACCINE

A major issue hampering the uptake of shingles vaccination is the lack of awareness of the disease.[4698] Shingles is caused by a reactivation of the chicken pox virus later in life. After your body beats back chicken pox, the virus hides in your spinal cord, waiting for an opportunity to strike again.[4699] When your defenses are down, the virus can surge forth, traveling along the path of a nerve branching off the spinal cord and wrapping around one side of the body to the front, producing skin blisters in a characteristic belt-like pattern that does not cross the midline.[4700] (Both *shingles* and the name of the virus, *zoster*, are from the Latin and Greek, respectively, for "belt."[4701])

The blistering rash can be intensely painful and leave behind scarring or discoloration, but it usually disappears on its own in a few weeks. However, approximately 30 to 50 percent of those with shingles suffer "postherpetic neuralgia," persistent pain that can last for a year or more and sometimes be debilitating. It usually affects nerves around the trunk, but, in 10 to 25 percent of cases, it can erupt across your face and lead to permanent facial muscle weakness, hearing loss, or blindness.[4702] As if all that isn't bad enough, having shingles as much as quintuples your odds of having a stroke over the subsequent few weeks,[4703] a risk that gradually declines over the following six to twelve months.[4704]

It's surprising that more people don't know about this, since the lifetime risk of getting shingles is 30 percent, meaning nearly one in three of us will get it sometime in our lives. Young adults only have about a one-in-a-thousand chance of getting it every year, whereas it climbs to closer to one in a hundred per year for older adults. That comes out to a million cases of shingles annually in the United States.[4705] Thankfully, there is a shingles vaccine.

The first (Zostavax) became available in 2006, using a live, weakened strain of the virus. The efficacy was only about 50 percent, though, and it couldn't be administered to immunocompromised individuals, such as those with HIV or on immunosuppressive drugs, such as chemotherapy. In 2017, however, a recombinant shingles vaccine was approved (Shingrix) with a 90 to 97 percent efficacy for preventing an outbreak. It requires two separate injections two to six months apart[4706] and is expensive ($280), but it's covered by Medicare Part D and most private insurance plans. It can also cause transient systemic symptoms, such as muscle aches, fatigue, headache, fever, and chills, about 10 percent of the time,[4707] but Shingrix is considered to be so much more effective that it's recommended for everyone starting at age fifty, even if you were previously immunized with Zostavax.[4708] Given that the new vaccine is only about five years old, we don't yet have longer-term safety and efficacy data—they're still coming in[4709]—but so far, so good.[4710] I recently turned fifty and lined right up for mine.

PRESERVING YOUR JOINTS

Osteoarthritis, the most common joint disease in the world,[4711] develops when the cartilage that cushions the lining of our joints breaks down faster than our body is able to build it back up.[4712] Affecting more than twenty million Americans, osteoarthritis is the most frequent cause of physical disability among older adults. The average age of diagnosis is fifty-five,[4713] and the most common presenting symptom is pain, most often in the knees, hands, hips, and spine.[4714] In the United States, 40 percent of men and 47 percent of women will develop osteoarthritis within their lifetime.[4715]

PILLS

Acetaminophen (Tylenol) is widely recommended as the first-line painkiller for osteoarthritis,[4716] but it shouldn't be.[4717] Why not? Because it doesn't work. Although acetaminophen can provide *statistically* significant improvements in pain and physical function over placebo, the benefits are not *clinically* significant—the equivalent of just three points better on a hundred-point pain scale compared to placebo.[4718] The minimum change that is deemed clinically relevant is ten points.[4719] Now, this is not to say that Tylenol doesn't *appear* to work; it can drop pain scores by twenty-six points. But it just doesn't work compared to placebo, a sugar pill, which on its own drops pain scores by twenty-three points.

Acetaminophen overdose is the leading cause of sudden liver failure,[4720] but, even at recommended doses, it can still cause liver damage. While acetaminophen is definitely safer than most over-the-counter or prescription pain pills,[4721] those taking it for conditions like osteoarthritis were found to be nearly fourfold more likely to develop liver function abnormalities compared to placebo.[4722]

Traditionally, osteoarthritis was considered to be a prototypical "wear and tear" disorder,[4723] but we now know that inflammation plays an integral role in the disease's process.[4724] So, what about using anti-inflammatory drugs? Most patients with osteoarthritis in the United States are prescribed nonsteroidal anti-inflammatory drugs (NSAIDs), such as over-the-counter ibuprofen (Advil) or naproxen (Aleve), or prescription-only celecoxib (Celebrex).[4725] Unfortunately, primary care practitioners often lack sufficient awareness of the gastrointestinal, cardiovascular, and kidney risks associated with these drugs.[4726]

Side effects from NSAIDs may be one reason why those with osteoarthritis tend to live shorter lives. The drugs do work for osteoarthritis pain,[4727] but 10 to 30 percent of people who regularly take NSAIDs develop stomach ulcers.[4728] NSAIDs also increase the odds of a heart attack by about 50 percent,[4729] which translates into one extra heart attack per one hundred to two hundred users every year[4730] and appears to double the risk of sudden kidney injury in those over fifty.[4731] The risks are considered so great at older ages that the American Geriatrics Society recommends opioid drugs over NSAIDs for chronic pain in those older than seventy-five.[4732]

The cardiovascular, kidney, and gastrointestinal risks are similar for ibuprofen and naproxen.[4733] Prescription-only celecoxib has similar cardiovascular risk to both, but it seems to cause fewer kidney problems than ibuprofen and has significantly lower gastrointestinal risk than either of the over-the-counter drugs.[4734] Given the risks associated with this class of drugs, the consensus is that, if their use is deemed necessary, the lowest effective dose should be taken for the shortest possible duration.[4735]

GELS

The best pharmacological option may be topical NSAIDs,[4736] which just became available over the counter in the United States in 2020.[4737] They appear to have a similar efficacy to oral NSAIDs in terms of pain management[4738] and have a better safety profile since they have lower systemic absorption.[4739] They can cause (mostly) mild skin reactions, but they don't seem to raise the risk of gastrointestinal issues any more than placebo.[4740] They also appear safer in terms of kidney[4741] and cardiovascular risk.[4742]

INJECTIONS

The "nonsteroidal" in NSAID is to differentiate them from anti-inflammatory steroids, like cortisone, which can be injected directly into the joint. A Medicare sample of a half-million patients with osteoarthritis in their knees found that about a third were treated with at least one corticosteroid injection.[4743] This can help with pain in the short term,[4744] but it makes the condition worse in the long term.[4745]

Those getting steroid injections can end up with a worsening of pain, stiffness, and disability with accelerated joint deterioration and progression to total knee replacement surgery.[4746] This is in addition to complications that include osteonecrosis (bone rot) and rapid joint destruction.[4747] In a randomized controlled trial, two years of steroid injections for knee osteoarthritis sufferers led to a significantly greater loss of cartilage volume—and, ironically, no better pain relief—than a placebo injection of saline (basically water).[4748] The study may have been the "final nail in the coffin" for the practice.[4749]

See see.nf/injections to learn about other injections, but in sum, both hyaluronic acid and PRP (platelet-rich plasma—or, perhaps more accurately, *profit-rich placebo*) "cannot be recommended."[4750]

SURGERY

In 2003, a courageous study was published in *The New England Journal of Medicine*, putting the most common orthopedic surgery—arthroscopic surgery of the knee—to the test. Billions of dollars are spent sticking scopes into knee joints and cutting away damaged tissue in osteoarthritis and knee injuries, but does the procedure actually work? Knee pain sufferers were randomized to get the actual surgery versus a sham surgery in which doctors actually sliced into people's knees and pretended to perform the procedure, complete with splashing saline, but never actually did anything within the joint.[4751]

The trial caused an uproar. How could you randomize people to fake surgery? Professional medical associations questioned the ethics of the surgeons and the sanity of the patients who agreed to be part of the trial.[4752] But, guess what happened? The surgical patients got better, but so did the placebo patients who had undergone sham surgery.[4753] Indeed, the surgeries had no actual effect. Currently, rotator cuff shoulder surgery is facing the same crisis of confidence.[4754]

Surgical research has long been ridiculed as a "comic opera,"[4755] as most peer-reviewed surgery publications were just filled with presentations of series of individual cases or airings of professional opinions. Unlike drugs, which must be demonstrated to have a certain safety and efficacy, there is no such requirement for new surgical procedures, which can be introduced without regulatory oversight. Only about one in five surgical procedures performed in all of orthopedics is supported by at least one good randomized controlled trial showing it to be superior to a nonsurgical alternative.[4756] In the fifty-three trials in which surgeries of all stripes were put to the test against sham operations, the majority of surgeries were themselves the shams, unable to beat out the placebo procedures.[4757]

A subsequent systematic review and meta-analysis of arthroscopic surgery for middle-aged or older patients with knee pain, with or without osteoarthritis, concluded that, although there may be a small, transient "inconsequential" benefit, the surgery does not outweigh the harms. Complications of arthroscopic surgery include blood clots (deep venous thromboses) in 1 in 250 procedures, which can travel to the lung, cause an infection, and, extremely rarely, result in death.[4758] What is especially tragically ironic is that those with osteoarthritis who underwent arthroscopic surgery appeared to be three times more likely to end up having to undergo total knee replacement surgery in that same knee within the ensuing nine years.[4759]

PLACEBOS

To be clear, arthroscopic surgery works. It just doesn't work better than fake surgery.[4760] People tend to feel better either way, which may help explain why surgery has been referred to as the "ultimate placebo." So, arthroscopic surgery works like going to a witch doctor works. It even has many of the same components—the journey to the healing place, fasting, and anointment with a purifying liquid (skin prep) before your audience with the masked healer.[4761]

It's been estimated that, across different therapies for osteoarthritis, about 75 percent of pain relief, 71 percent of improvement in function, and 83 percent of stiffness improvement are due to the placebo effect.[4762] This has led to the proliferation of all manner of bogus treatments, such as "low-dose" radiation therapy involving pulsing the joint with 60,000 chest X-rays' worth of radiation.[4763] That treatment does work, but only as well as it does when the equipment is covertly turned off and a recording is played of the *sound* of the machine working.[4764]

A rich literature explores the placebo effect. It's hard enough to believe that a sugar pill could have a clinical effect, but that's just the beginning. Taking two sugar pills has a stronger effect than taking just one,[4765] and green and blue sugar pills have a different effect than red and orange ones.[4766] Sugar pills labeled *Bayer aspirin* help headaches more than sugar pills labeled *generic aspirin*,[4767] which isn't so surprising since patients who were told their tablets were obtained at full cost felt they worked better than those who were told theirs were obtained at a discount.[4768] And a needle is better than a pill.[4769]

The placebo power of administering a shot is so potent that, unbelievably, giving osteoarthritis sufferers placebo injections offers clinically important pain relief that lasts for three months and clinically significant improvements in function and stiffness that last for six months.[4770] This introduces the so-called efficacy paradox. Hyaluronic acid injections are not administered because they don't beat out placebo injections, whereas NSAIDs *are* given because they do have a real effect beyond just the placebo effect. That makes sense, but ready to have your mind blown? Because needles have a greater placebo effect than pills, injecting joints with hyaluronic acid—the treatment that is *not* recommended—works better than the recommended treatment of taking NSAID pills[4771] and would probably be safer, too! So, why not just stick needles into people if that works so well? We do. It's called acupuncture.

There's actually a way to test acupuncture against a placebo. There are "sham acupuncture devices" that look and feel exactly like real acupuncture needles. In actuality, though, the needle tip is blunted and retracts into the hollow shaft like a magic trick. Then, when it's bandaged in place and sticking out, you can't tell if you're getting real acupuncture or fake acupuncture, where there's no "puncture" at all.[4772]

So, what happens when you test acupuncture on knee osteoarthritis? It works! But the fake acupuncture works, too. That's why the American Academy of Orthopaedic Surgeons makes a strong recommendation against it.[4773] Nevertheless, if acupuncture "works" and is relatively safe, why not do it?

Adverse side effects from prescription drugs alone are estimated to kill more than 100,000 Americans every year, making medications a leading cause of death.[4774] Whatever you may think of doctors prescribing placebos, at least they aren't killing people. If there are conditions like osteoarthritis where placebos have been proven to be effective, why don't doctors actively deceive patients by prescribing them?

They do.

Different surveys of medical professionals have found that 17 to 80 percent of physicians and 51 to 100 percent of nurses have given patients "pure" placebos, meaning they didn't just uselessly prescribe antibiotics for the common cold, for instance, but actually gave people an intentionally bogus treatment, like an injection of saline.[4775] There are all sorts of placebos on the market you can even buy for yourself, with brand names like Obecalp[4776] ("placebo" backward), Magic Bullet, and Fukitol. (I'm not kidding!)

Defense of the occasional indispensable medical lie dates back to Plato, who wrote in the *Republic*, "[A] lie is . . . useful only as a medicine to men. . . ."[4777] Thomas Jefferson called it the "pious fraud."[4778] In the medical literature, it's been referred to as the "humble humbug." While some doctors decry giving placebos as quackery,[4779] others, specifically in regards to osteoarthritis, ask, "Why not use it to our advantage?"[4780] *The American Journal of Medicine* published a review on the "Ethics and Practice of Placebo Therapy," which argued that "deception is completely moral when it is used for the welfare of the patient," questioning why the "dwellers in ivory towers decry the use of placebos." Some patients can be sensitive, though, the review warns, so they "should never be told that their precious medicine was a hoax."[4781]

WEIGHT LOSS

Twin studies suggest that about half of osteoarthritis risk is genetic.[4782] What can we do about the other half? Thankfully, there are successful treatments that don't involve capsules, needles, scalpels, or falsehoods.

Obesity may be the main modifiable risk factor for osteoarthritis,[4783] offering an explanation why a study of thousands of skeletal remains from prehistoric hunter-gatherers to modern-day city dwellers found a dramatic rise in incidence over the last half century or so. Compared to healthy-weight individuals (BMI < 25), the incidence of knee osteoarthritis is three times as high among obese individuals (BMI ≥ 30) and five times as high among those with class II obesity (BMI ≥ 35).[4784] Fatty tissue in general[4785] and even right inside our joints—like in the fat pad under the kneecap—can be a source of pro-inflammatory chemicals that have been shown to increase cartilage degradation.[4786]

Losing around just one pound a year over a ten-year period may reduce our odds of developing osteoarthritis by more than 50 percent.[4787] Once you have it, MRI studies show that even just a 5 percent weight loss in overweight sufferers can significantly lower the degree of cartilage degeneration.[4788] As I detail in see .nf/kneereplacement, obese osteoarthritis sufferers who had been randomized to lose weight went on to improve their knee function as much as those undergoing knee surgery, and they did so within just eight weeks. Researchers concluded that losing twenty or so pounds of fat "might be regarded as an alternative to knee replacement."[4789]

This is especially important considering that nearly one in two hundred knee replacement patients dies within three months of surgery. About 700,000 of these procedures are performed every year in the United States. Given its widespread popularity, an editor of an orthopedics journal suggested that "people considering this operation are inadequately attuned to the possibility that it may kill them."[4790]

EXERCISE

Smokers tend to be leaner than nonsmokers,[4791] so that may explain why some studies have found a protective association between osteoarthritis and tobacco use.[4792] Smokers with osteoarthritis, though, tend to have more severe pain and sustain greater cartilage loss than nonsmokers.[4793] Ironically, another potential explanation for lower rates of osteoarthritis among smokers is that they're less likely to play sports.[4794]

Athletic injuries to the knees are a well-established risk factor for osteoarthritis later in life.[4795] At the same time, physical inactivity can put your knees at risk, not only because weakened muscles make for less stable joints but because cartilage also has a "use it or lose it" characteristic. People with paralyzed legs exhibit marked cartilage thinning in their knees,[4796] whereas people who do weight-bearing exercise may have thicker cartilage.[4797] Both extremes of inactivity and excessive activity may be detrimental.[4798]

What about exercise as treatment? There have been four dozen randomized controlled trials of exercise for knee osteoarthritis, involving a total of thousands of patients.[4799] Exercise was found to be so consistently effective for pain relief that some researchers have suggested that no future studies of the question are deemed necessary.[4800] Direct comparisons in trials comparing high and low intensity of aerobic or resistance exercise conclude that intensity doesn't seem to matter, but frequency does. Exercise programs requiring at least three sessions a week were most effective, as were regimens that concentrated on the quadriceps muscles.[4801] Although most were short-term trials,[4802] there have been some showing clinically significant improvements at least one year out with no adverse effects reported.[4803] National and international best-practice guidelines for osteoarthritis emphasize the importance of both weight control and exercise.[4804] What about diet?

DIET

The best-practice management of osteoarthritis is said to include "optimal nutrition" as a first-line intervention. As a prime example, reviewers in the journal *Arthritis* cite the "China Study," which is shorthand for the China-Cornell-Oxford Project, which in turn is short for the "China-Oxford-Cornell Study on Dietary, Lifestyle and Disease Mortality Characteristics in 65 Rural Chinese Counties," a large study summarized by principal investigator T. Colin Campbell, the same Dr. Campbell who coined the term *whole food, plant-based diet*, and his son in the lay book *The China Study*.[4805] What evidence do we have that a plant-based diet might help?

The National Institutes of Health Osteoarthritis Initiative, the largest-ever prospective study of osteoarthritis patients over time, found that higher fat intake was associated with accelerated progression of the disease (as determined by cartilage loss on X-ray).[4806] Upon further analysis, though, it was only the saturated fat that appeared to increase risk. That's the kind of fat found mostly in meat, dairy, and junk, not the monounsaturated or polyunsaturated fats concentrated in nuts, seeds, and vegetable oils.[4807] Just dripping saturated fat on human cartilage cells in a petri dish can increase cartilage matrix degradation.[4808] Cholesterol has the same in vitro effect.[4809]

Both saturated fat[4810] and dietary cholesterol[4811] accelerate the progression of trauma-induced osteoarthritis in mice. Even without trauma, though, animal fat can produce typical osteoarthritis-like lesions in the knee joints of rats.[4812] What about people? Osteoarthritis sufferers tend to have higher cholesterol levels in the blood[4813] and also within their joints, both in aspirated joint fluid[4814] and in the cartilage itself.[4815] Exposing human cartilage to cholesterol has been shown to worsen the inflammatory degeneration,[4816] helping, perhaps, to explain why the higher people's cholesterol, the worse their disease.[4817]

So, might lowering cholesterol with statin drugs help? The data are mixed.[4818] Some studies suggest that statins help,[4819,4820] some found no relationship,[4821,4822] and others indicate that statins could make things worse.[4823,4824] Meta-analysis reviewers suggest that the side effects of statins, in terms of muscle weakness and pain, may mask any protective effects of cholesterol-lowering on reducing osteoarthritis symptoms.[4825] In contrast, a healthy enough plant-based diet may offer the best of both worlds, dropping cholesterol as much as a starting dose of a statin drug within a single week,[4826] while lowering blood pressure and facilitating weight loss.[4827] But, what about direct effects on osteoarthritis?

In a study at Michigan State University, men and women with osteoarthritis were randomized to follow a whole food, plant-based diet or continue their conventional lifestyle. Compared to the control group, the plant-based group experienced a significant improvement in physical function and energy/vitality within one week and a significant reduction in pain within two weeks. Of course, they also lost significantly more weight, but improvements were noted even in some who didn't. Because the control group didn't do anything special, one can't disentangle any placebo effects, but, given the ancillary benefits, eating plant-based may be worth a try.[4828]

The researchers suggest that the plant-based pain benefits may be due to the reduced intake of arachidonic acid, a pro-inflammatory omega-6 fat[4829] found primarily in eggs and chicken.[4830] NSAIDs like aspirin reduce pain by blocking the cascade of inflammatory mediators our body makes from arachidonic acid.[4831] By cutting down on consumption of chicken and eggs, the thinking goes, less of the pain-inducing compounds may be produced in the first place.[4832] (The poultry industry has proposed genetically manipulating chickens to have less arachidonic acid in their muscles to decrease human health risk, but this has yet to be implemented.[4833])

Or maybe the anti-inflammatory nature of plant foods was responsible for the rapid pain relief.[4834] Pro-inflammatory diets are associated with higher osteoarthritis pain intensity,[4835] as well as increased risk of developing the disease in the first place.[4836] So, what about fiber, the most anti-inflammatory dietary component?[4837] As we know, when we eat whole-grain barley for dinner, for instance, our good gut bacteria have it for breakfast the next morning and the short-chain fatty acid butyrate is released into our bloodstream,[4838] which exerts a wide range of anti-inflammatory effects.[4839] Dripping butyrate on cartilage carvings taken from the leg bones of those undergoing joint replacement surgery has been shown to significantly suppress inflammatory cartilage loss in vitro.[4840]

In a study titled "Dietary Fiber Intake in Relation to Knee Pain Trajectory," nearly 5,000 men and women were followed for an average of eight years. Researchers found that those getting at least the recommended minimum fiber intake of about 25 g a day were at significantly lower risk of developing moderate or severe knee pain over time."[4841] What's more, two Framingham cohorts found that a higher intake of fiber was associated with a lower risk of having symptomatic osteoarthritis in the first place.[4842] The provision of extra fiber protects mice from osteoarthritis,[4843] but it has yet to be interventionally tested in people.[4844]

BEVERAGES

Free radicals may also play a role in joint-lining inflammation and cartilage loss.[4845] Observational studies have correlated higher intake of certain antioxidants with a lower prevalence of cartilage deficits or osteoarthritis progression,[4846] but, when antioxidant supplements were put to the test, the results have been largely disappointing.[4847] (They didn't make things worse, though, as did vitamin C in an animal experiment of osteoarthritis.[4848])

On the other hand, when green tea was added to the drinking water of mice, it was found to reduce the incidence of arthritis[4849] and slow the progression of osteoarthritis.[4850] It can also protect human cartilage explants in vitro.[4851] The first and only clinical trial to date was published in 2016. Knee osteoarthritis patients were randomized to either the equivalent of about three cups' worth of green tea a day plus an NSAID or just the drug on its own.[4852] Within four weeks, there was significant improvement in osteoarthritis symptoms in the green tea group, especially with regards to improved physical function. Unfortunately, it was an open-label study, meaning that the participants knew which group they were in, so placebo effects can't be discounted.[4853] Similarly, those drinking two cups a day of spearmint tea for sixteen weeks reported improved osteoarthritis symptoms, but, again, with no placebo control, we can't be confident that the effect was real.[4854]

Other beverages that have been studied in relation to osteoarthritis include soft drinks and milk. Independent of body weight, soda intake has been associated with increased progression of knee osteoarthritis, but only in men, which calls the relationship into question.[4855] Similarly, milk was associated with less disease progression, but only in women, while cheese was linked to greater progression in a U.S. study.[4856] In a Dutch study, though, cheese (but not milk) was found to be cross-sectionally associated with less osteoarthritis.[4857]

One interventional study comparing soy protein to dairy protein reported that soy edged out dairy, suggesting soymilk might be preferable for osteoarthritis sufferers, though we don't know if this arose from superior soy benefits or potential dairy harms.[4858] A study in Iran sought to answer this question. Half the dairy-drinking, osteoarthritis-suffering participants were randomized to try to stop their dairy intake, and those who were successful experienced a significant reduction of pain within three weeks. (A more rigorous study design would have involved switching to an indistinguishable nondairy milk control, though.)[4859]

STRAWBERRIES

If antioxidants play a protective role, what about berries? Strawberries decrease the levels circulating in the blood of an inflammatory mediator known as *tumor necrosis factor*, but that doesn't necessarily translate into clinical improvement.[4860] For example, drinking cherry juice can lower C-reactive protein, another sign of inflammation, but failed to help with osteoarthritis.[4861] Tart cherry juice "provided symptoms relief," but not significantly more so than a cherry-free placebo drink (Kool-Aid). Cherries may help with gout, another kind of arthritis, but failed when it came to osteoarthritis.[4862] Similarly, pomegranates may help with rheumatoid arthritis,[4863] but pomegranate *juice* failed to even beat a do-nothing control group for osteoarthritis[4864] even though pomegranate extracts appeared to protect cartilage in a petri dish.[4865]

Pomegranate juice doesn't lower C-reactive protein levels in the bloodstream, though,[4866] and strawberries do. When people with diabetes were given strawberries for six weeks, not only did their diabetes get better, but their C-reactive protein levels dropped by 18 percent.[4867] Strawberries can even downregulate pro-inflammatory genes to the point of reversing precancerous growth.[4868] Even just a single meal can help.[4869] So, can strawberries improve pain and inflammation in confirmed knee osteoarthritis? Yes.

Obese men and women with osteoarthritis were randomized to the equivalent of a pint and a half of strawberries a day (in the form of freeze-dried strawberry powder) or a control group getting a placebo powder matched for the color and flavor of strawberries for twelve weeks. Inflammatory markers plummeted in the real strawberry group *and* they experienced significant reductions in constant pain, intermittent pain, and total pain. Concluded the researchers, "[O]ur study suggests that simple dietary intervention, i.e., the addition of berries, may have a significant impact on pain, inflammation, and overall quality of life in obese adults with OA [osteoarthritis]."[4870]

The strawberries cut the levels of the inflammatory mediator tumor necrosis factor (TNF) in half,[4871] but strawberry efficacy may not be an anti-TNF effect, since blueberries may also suppress TNF[4872] but failed to beat out placebo when put to the test in a similar randomized, double-blind, placebo-controlled osteoarthritis trial.[4873]

ROSE HIPS

When you think about what fruits may be beneficial for osteoarthritis, you probably don't think of rose hips, the fruits of the rose bush. Commonly steeped into tangy tea, rose hips are sold dried and often in bulk at natural foods stores.

There have been three randomized, double-blind, placebo-controlled trials of rose hips for osteoarthritis. Hundreds of men and women suffering mostly from osteoarthritis of the knee were randomized to three to four months of 5 g a day of rose hip powder, which is about one and a third teaspoon, or a look-alike placebo powder. Those unknowingly taking the real rose hips experienced a significant reduction in pain over placebo,[4874] close to that seen with NSAIDs,[4875] but without any reported side effects.[4876]

BROCCOLI

What about vegetables? Broccoli holds some promise. Sulforaphane, the cruciferous compound thought to play a key role in the benefits we can get from broccoli family vegetables, protects human cartilage from destruction in vitro, but how do we know if sulforaphane even makes it into our joints?[4877] We didn't—until a group of British researchers had knee replacement patients eat broccoli for two weeks before surgery and, during the operation, found it in their synovial (joint) fluid (compared to surgical patients told to avoid cruciferous vegetables).[4878]

Sulforaphane has been shown to decrease the severity of osteoarthritis in mice, but it is only now being tested in people.[4879] The Broccoli in Osteoarthritis (BRIO) study is randomizing participants to broccoli soup as we speak, and we should have the results soon.[4880] Even just ten days of broccoli consumption can cut C-reactive protein levels in smokers by 40 percent, but we don't yet know if this translates into decreased knee pain and dysfunction.[4881] However, there are some foods that have been shown to get at the root: ginger and turmeric.

GINGER

In see.nf/ginger, I review the randomized controlled trials showing that as little as an eighth of a teaspoon of ginger powder can reduce knee osteoarthritis pain,[4882] working as well as ibuprofen[4883] but with gastrointestinal lining protection[4884] rather than damage.[4885] Ginger has evidently been applied externally to painful joints for a thousand years,[4886] though the only controlled study of topical ginger to date involved men applying slices to their scrotum. But the researchers were on the ball: Inflamed testicles healed three times faster in the ginger group.[4887]

TURMERIC

After study participants consumed a daily teaspoon and a half of ginger powder for seven days, researchers drew their blood and dripped it onto cells in a petri dish. They found that the release of inflammatory mediators like TNF is suppressed, compared to when blood taken before the week of ginger was used. The same anti-inflammatory effects can be had with the spice turmeric, but at a small fraction of the dose—less than a tenth of a teaspoon per day.[4888]

There have been sixteen randomized controlled trials of various turmeric formulations for knee osteoarthritis, starting at the equivalent of about half a teaspoon a day for up to sixteen weeks. Eleven of the studies compared turmeric to placebo, and the other five pitted the spice head-to-head against NSAIDs. The turmeric extracts significantly reduced knee pain and improved physical function compared to placebo and had similar effects to the NSAIDs, but with a better safety profile.[4889] In 2020, a study published on topical treatment involving the application of a turmeric extract mixed with Vaseline reported a significant reduction in pain. It was purported to be a double-blind trial, but the placebo was straight Vaseline, so the color difference alone likely tipped off both the participants and the assessors as to which subject was in which group.[4890] So if you're going to make some kind of turmeric-y pumpkin pie smoothie like my Okinawa-inspired concoction on page 196 (maybe with a little ground ginger thrown in), I'd suggest drinking it rather than rubbing it in.

TOPICAL TREATMENTS

We've covered how to help preserve our joints from the inside out, but what about from the outside in?

SESAME SEEDS

With only good side effects—improving blood pressure,[4891] cholesterol, and antioxidant status—sesame seeds are certainly worth a try.[4892] Refer back to page 97 for the randomized controlled trial of a quarter cup of sesame seed for osteoarthritis.

What about topical sesame oil? In a double-blind, placebo-controlled clinical trial, a hospital in Iran randomized patients with traumatic limb injuries to rub the oil drained off tahini (sesame seed paste) onto their affected limbs. Compared to the placebo control of conventional cooking oil, the sesame group experienced prompt pain relief that was significant within forty-eight hours, and the sesame oil even helped prevent skin discoloration from bruising. So, what about rubbing sesame oil onto osteoarthritic knees?

When topical sesame oil was tested head-to-head against the leading topical NSAID, a 1% diclofenac sodium gel, such as Voltaren, the sesame oil was found to work similarly for pain and some measures of function, but the NSAID gel did better at reducing stiffness.[4893]

FLAXSEEDS

What about other topical treatments? Researchers in Turkey tried randomizing people with osteoarthritis of the hands to a warm flaxseed poultice. A warm mixture of flaxseeds and water was applied to participants' hands, which were then wrapped snugly with gauze and covered with a towel and hot water bottle for twenty to thirty minutes once a day for a week. Compared to those in the control group who did nothing, the flax group experienced a significant improvement in pain and function. How do we know the benefit was from the flax and not just the heat and compression? There was a third arm to the study. Sufferers were randomized to the flax compress, a hot compress without any flax, or a control group, and the flax group experienced a significant improvement in pain and function compared to the hot compress group as well.[4894]

What about flaxseed oil, which has been used medicinally for more than a millennium? One hundred patients with mild to moderate carpal tunnel syndrome were randomized in a double-blinded manner to rub five drops of flaxseed oil or placebo onto the front of their wrists twice a day. Compared to those who got the placebo, the flaxseed oil group experienced significant improvements—not only in pain and functional status but also in nerve conduction velocity, indicating an alleviation of nerve damage. This was at a cost of perhaps a dollar a month.[4895] Time to rub flaxseed oil on some arthritic knees!

In another double-blind, randomized, placebo-controlled clinical trial, participants rubbed twenty drops of flaxseed oil or a paraffin-oil placebo onto their knees three times a day for six weeks. Once again, the flax beat out the placebo on every measure—total symptoms, pain, quality of life, and daily life activities as well as sports and recreation function. The topical use of flaxseed oil for soothing joint pain was recommended in traditional Persian medical texts, such as the *Canon of Medicine*,[4896] which was completed around the year 1012.[4897] It just took a thousand years for it to finally be put to the test.

EXTRA-VIRGIN OLIVE OIL

The ascription of "remarkable anti-inflammatory activity" to olive oil is based on laboratory rodents,[4898] but a systematic review and meta-analysis failed to find any anti-inflammatory effects for olive oil.[4899] In people, as I review in see.nf/oliveoil, extra-virgin olive oil may be no better than butter when it comes to inflammation, and even worse than coconut oil.[4900] But, that's for olive oil taken orally. Topically, it may be a different matter.

Knee osteoarthritis sufferers were randomized to topical virgin olive oil versus an NSAID gel for a month. The olive oil group was instructed to apply just 1 g of oil, which is less than a quarter teaspoon, three times a day. So, that would cost less than three cents a day, and it worked![4901] The virgin olive oil rub worked significantly better than the drug in reducing pain. A similar conclusion was reached in a trial for rheumatoid arthritis, where topical extra-virgin olive oil seemed to beat out rubbing on an NSAID gel or nothing at all (a "dry massage" control).[4902]

Low Back Pain

Low back pain became one of the biggest problems for public health systems in the Western world during the second half of the twentieth century.[4903] The lifetime prevalence of low back pain is reported to be as high as 84 percent, and chronic low back pain is present in about one in five, with one in ten being disabled. It's an epidemic fueled, in part, by the obesity epidemic.

Carrying excess weight is a risk factor not only for low back pain[4904] but also for sciatica[4905] and lumbar disc degeneration[4906] and herniation.[4907] As with arthritis, it may be due to the combined effects of heavy loads on our joints and the inflammation and cholesterol associated with being heavier.[4908] Autopsy studies

(continued)

show that the lumbar arteries feeding our spine can become clogged with athero-sclerosis and then starve the discs in the lower back of oxygen and nutrients.[4909]

In see.nf/backpain, I cover the topic in depth, complete with visuals of the cholesterol-laden plaques obliterating the openings to the spinal arteries.[4910] To get you back into circulation, it may help to get circulation into your back. Un-fortunately, it's never been put to the test. Clinical trials have demonstrated the dietary reversal of the progression of coronary artery disease in the heart,[4911] peripheral arteries in the legs,[4912] and pelvic arteries for erectile dysfunction,[4913] but, unfortunately, there has yet to be a randomized controlled trial on the rever-sal of disc degeneration or back pain with diet and lifestyle changes.

SUPPLEMENTS

There has been a dramatic increase in cannabis use among older adults in recent years.[4914] So far, there don't appear to be any signs of adverse cognitive or mental health effects in the population for low-dose, short-term medical cannabis use.[4915] Certainly the evidence for the harms of alcohol use is much stronger.[4916] But is cannabis effective? Can a joint help your joints?

There was a small, transient effect of oral cannabidiol (CBD) oil noted in a case report of osteoarthritic pain that might have just been a placebo effect.[4917] There were no randomized controlled trials of CBD for osteoarthritis until 2021. Unfor-tunately, researchers found that it offered no benefit for pain, compared to placebo, nor for sleep quality, depression, or anxiety.[4918]

Fish oil is another common supplement that fails to move the needle. A system-atic review and meta-analysis of the five randomized controlled trials concluded that it had no statistically significant effect.[4919] However, the most commonly used supplement for osteoarthritis is glucosamine.[4920]

GLUCOSAMINE

I do a deep dive into glucosamine supplements in see.nf/glucosamine. Basically, there are marked inconsistencies in the clinical research literature as to whether it works at all,[4921] with industry funding the most potent predictor of trial outcomes, leading the current American College of Rheumatology guidelines to strongly rec-ommend *against* the use of glucosamine.[4922]

CHONDROITIN

As I note in see.nf/chondroitin, the American College of Rheumatology also strongly recommends against the use of chondroitin,[4923] with the best studies showing "minimal or nonexistent" benefit.[4924] The only trial ever published of pharmaceutical-grade, prescription-only preparations of both chondroitin and glucosamine found that they made the pain of osteoporosis significantly *worse* compared to placebo.[4925]

COLLAGEN

Nearly a millennium ago, a medieval nun suggested eating gelatin to reduce joint pain.[4926] Unfortunately, when collagen was put to the test in multicenter, randomized, double-blind, placebo-controlled trials, it didn't seem to work.[4927] (Gelatin is basically just cooked collagen.[4928]) I review all the studies in see.nf /collagenjoints. The few that have shown benefits[4929] have come under fire from critics.[4930]

A comprehensive systematic review published in 2022 suggested that the reason there haven't been more studies done may be the high incidence of adverse side effects attributed to collagen supplements.[4931]

Randomizing people to even a single meal of a gelatin-based protein drink can lead to memory impairments within hours due to "acute tryptophan deletion." This is presumably due to a drop in the brain of serotonin, which is made from tryptophan.[4932] (As I note on page 73, collagen is an incomplete protein, missing the essential amino acid tryptophan entirely.) Another reason more studies haven't been done is simply that the collagen companies may not be confident they'd get positive results.[4933]

But, since then, the biggest study yet, with more than 150 people, has been published. Collagen company–funded researchers found a significant drop in knee pain and a significant improvement in knee function among those random-ized to collagen supplements.[4934] However, they also found a significant drop in knee pain and improvement in knee function in those randomized to the placebo, with no real difference between them. So, the fact that a sugar pill effectively worked as well as the collagen supplements suggests that collagen doesn't work at all.

PRESERVING YOUR MIND

In *How Not to Die*, the exhilaration of my paternal grandma Greger's miraculous recovery from heart disease was counterbalanced by the horror story that was my mom's mother's descent into Alzheimer's disease. When our own mom first started to show the same symptoms, my brother and I steeled ourselves for the inevitable years of heartbreak and loss. The cruel irony of my father's battle with Parkinson's—hand tremors in a photojournalist—was matched by the mockery of my mother losing her mind. She had double-majored in English and chemistry, earned straight A's throughout nursing school, and was always surrounded by stacks and stacks of library books. Then she lost the ability to read, then to write, and eventually she lost her *self*. Given the family history, the neurologist we first took her to lazily diagnosed Alzheimer's. As did the second opinion and the third. But the fourth neurologist—eliciting an early symptom that I had missed, urinary incontinence—suggested a rare condition known as normal pressure hydrocephalus, an abnormal buildup of fluid within the brain.

There are only a few types of *reversible* dementia. Vitamin B_{12} deficiency is one, medication side effects are another, and normal pressure hydrocephalus is a third. Could it be? I took her in for a diagnostic spinal tap where a few tablespoons of cerebrospinal fluid would be drawn to see if any of the symptoms would change. When I placed her down on the table, she couldn't walk, she could hardly talk, and she didn't know who I was. The fluid dripped out of the needle in her back into a cup, then, incredibly, the lights came back on. Within a span of minutes, my mom was back, walking and talking and hugging. She had been there all along, but the excess fluid had been bearing down on her brain. It was and will likely forever be the happiest moment of my life. But then, in the ensuing hours as the fluid built back up, her mind retreated back into the darkness, like Charlie's in *Flowers for Algernon*. With the diagnosis confirmed, she was scheduled for surgery, a drain was inserted into her brain to permanently siphon off excess fluid, and, just like that, she was back in our lives (and the library).

The moral of the story is to seek out every possible treatable, reversible cause before accepting a terminal diagnosis.

OUT OF MIND

Dementia is one of the most pressing public health challenges of our time.[4935] The single most common keyword in the healthy aging research literature is *Alzheimer's disease*.[4936] Dementia is one of our fastest-growing epidemics, affecting one in ten individuals older than sixty-five and up to 40 percent of individuals older than eighty-five.[4937] "Benign forgetfulness," like frequently misplacing your keys, is even more common. Dementia is much more serious, of course, as it affects daily function. You don't just forget about appointments you have that day; you forget about appointments you *had* that day.[4938]

Alzheimer's is the most common type of dementia and perhaps the most feared disease associated with getting older.[4939] In my clinical practice, I dreaded giving that diagnosis even more than cancer. What weighed so heavily on me wasn't just knowing the psychological toll that was to come for the patient but also the emotional toll that would be placed on their family. The Alzheimer's Foundation of America estimates that more than fifteen billion unpaid hours are supplied annually by more than ten million friends and family members who care for loved ones who may not even recognize them.[4940] Alzheimer's is the single most expensive disease in the United States and around much of the industrialized world.[4941]

We still have neither a cure nor an effective treatment for this disease that invariably progresses to death, despite billions of dollars spent on research. More than 100,000 research articles have been published on Alzheimer's over just the past decades. Nevertheless, very little clinical progress has been made in treating or even understanding the disease. And a total cure? That's likely impossible, since patients with Alzheimer's may never be able to regain lost cognitive function because of fatal damage to their neuronal networks. Nerve cells, once they are dead, cannot be brought back to life. Even if drug companies could manage to figure out how to halt the progression of the disease, the damage has already been done for many patients, and their personality may be forever lost.[4942]

Alzheimer's disease cannot be diagnosed definitively until after death,[4943] when characteristic brain pathology involving microscopic plaques and tangles can be picked up on autopsy.[4944] Some who die with dementia have pristine brains, though, and others who die with normal cognition have all the distinguishing marks of Alzheimer's. In fact, 39 percent of the brains of nonagenarians and centenarians without dementia fulfilled Alzheimer's pathology criteria, so murkiness can remain even after death.[4945] About 30 percent of people who are clinically diagnosed with Alzheimer's are actually misdiagnosed.[4946]

After Alzheimer's dementia, the second most common type is vascular dementia, representing 15 to 20 percent of all dementia cases.[4947] It can develop after a full-blown stroke or a lot of little ministrokes. Sometimes, blood clots only clog a tiny artery for a moment—not long enough to notice, but still long enough to kill off a tiny portion of your brain. These "silent strokes" can multiply and slowly reduce our cognitive function until full-blown dementia develops.[4948] However, despite medicine's attempt to fit different dementias into discrete categories, most brain autopsies of dementia patients reveal multiple pathologies—for example, evidence of both Alzheimer's and vascular lesions.[4949]

THE MYTH OF THE MYTH OF THE MYTH OF SENILITY

Before COVID-19 knocked it down to killer number seven in 2020,[4950] Alzheimer's disease was the sixth leading cause of death.[4951] The average time between a dementia diagnosis and dying is about five years.[4952] While people may not die of dementia per se, it can directly lead to life-threatening complications, such as aspiration pneumonia due to swallowing difficulties that the family may eventually decide not to treat.[4953] The good news is that dementia is not an inevitable consequence of aging.[4954]

The "myth of senility" is echoed across geriatric textbooks: Dementia is a disease, not a normal part of growing old. This is countered in the medical literature by papers about the "myth of the myth of senility."[4955] With the prevalence of dementia reaching 45 percent by the time we're in our late nineties, it's nearing becoming more likely than not. Indeed, various centenarian studies peg the prevalence of dementia anywhere from 27 to 79 percent, yet there are those who reach extreme ages with their cognition intact.[4956] In the autopsy report "No Disease in the Brain of a 115-Year-Old Woman," Hendrikje van Andel-Schipper, who was the oldest person in the world at the time of her death, had almost no atherosclerosis throughout her body, including her brain, and almost no brain plaques or tangles. When she was tested at age 113, her cognitive performance was above average for those nearly half her age.[4957] Had she had not died from stomach cancer, she could have kept on thriving.

We may have about eighty-five billion neurons, or nerve cells, in our brain.[4958] Autopsy studies in the 1970s and 1980s estimated that we lose about 1 percent of them a year, ending up with as few as half as many when we hit old age. The discovery of this apparent inexorable decline was even suggested to play a role in the spike in suicidality among the elderly around that time. But it turns out it was all a mistake, a technical artifact of different patterns of shrinkage upon brain fixation at different ages. In old age, our brains have about 96 to 98 percent as many neurons as we had when we were young.[4959] How can we keep them healthy?

BRAIN DRUGS

"Successful cognitive agers" are considered a product of a healthy lifestyle.[4960] A commonly held misconception is that we have no control over whether or not we develop dementia.[4961] To underscore the primacy of prevention, allow me to first run through the currently available treatment options. I think it will offer new appreciation for the importance of averting the disease in the first place.

ARICEPT AND NAMENDA

Until recently, there were two main types of treatment: the most common, cholinesterase inhibitors like the drug donepezil (Aricept),[4962] as well as memantine (Namenda).[4963] One of the changes seen in Alzheimer's brains is the destruction of nerve cells that use a neurotransmitter called *acetylcholine* to communicate with one another. By inhibiting cholinesterase, which is the enzyme that breaks down this messenger molecule, the drop in acetylcholine levels can be mediated. This can help with some of the symptoms, but it doesn't affect the underlying destruction. The memantine mechanism is less intuitive. People with Alzheimer's lose NMDA (N-methyl-D-aspartate) receptors, yet memantine, an NMDA blocker, also seems to help with symptoms.[4964] Unfortunately, neither tends to improve symptoms enough to make much of a difference.

A meta-analysis of more than five dozen randomized clinical trials concluded that the symptomatic relief from either treatment was so small as to be "not clinically relevant."[4965] Cases of at least moderate improvement occurred uncommonly, but at no higher rate than those getting the placebo.[4966] So many trials have been done on so many patients that it is now "statistically conclusive that no pharmacological intervention achieves a clinically significant improvement of dementia symptoms and functioning in patients with AD [Alzheimer's disease]."[4967] But, that was before there was a new kid on the block: aducanumab (Aduhelm).

THE ADUCANUMAB FARCE

Aducanumab is the first new drug to be approved for Alzheimer's treatment in nearly twenty years.[4968] The FDA's approval of aducanumab proved to be one of the most controversial in recent memory.[4969] Not only has the drug been considered to be clinically ineffective,[4970] a third of patients getting aducanumab suffered swelling or bleeding in the brain.[4971] Not a single member of the FDA expert advisory panel voted in favor of its approval,[4972] and three of the committee members resigned in protest,[4973] one calling it "probably the worst drug approval decision in recent US history."[4974] The response from the scientific community may best be summed up by a commentary written by the head of the American Geriatrics Society titled, "My Head Just Exploded. . . ."[4975]

Check out the whole fascinating saga in see.nf/aducanumab. A congressional investigation concluded the approval of aducanumab was "rife with irregularities," raising "serious concerns about FDA's lapses in protocol and [the drug company] Biogen's disregard of efficacy."[4976] That didn't stop the FDA from its 2023 accelerated approval of a similar antibody, lecanemab (Leqembi), of similar questionable efficacy and safety.[4977]

AMYLOID HYPOTHESIS QUESTIONED

The development of aducanumab was based on the proposal that Alzheimer's dementia is a result of the accumulation and aggregation of sticky, misfolded protein fragments called *amyloid beta*, which form plaques that lead to neuronal cell death and neurodegeneration.[4978] Compelling evidence for this "amyloid cascade hypothesis" comes from rare, inherited forms of Alzheimer's that are caused by gene mutations that specifically result in an elevation in amyloid beta.[4979] However, the vast majority of cases—more than 95 percent—of Alzheimer's disease are "sporadic," not known to be caused by a specific gene,[4980] so it's unclear if they share the same mechanism.[4981]

Skepticism of the amyloid cascade hypothesis centers around a series of disconnects. First, amyloid plaques can build up for decades before symptoms arise. Second, the amount of plaque correlates poorly with the severity of disease.[4982] As I mentioned before, as many as half the autopsies of individuals without dementia score as "probable" Alzheimer's disease and a third as bearing "definite" Alzheimer's pathology, based on plaque burden.[4983] And, third, the areas of the brain with the greatest neuron loss are not in the same places where there is the most amyloid deposition.[4984] In fact, Dr. Alzheimer himself, five years after his groundbreaking discovery, wrote, "So we have to come to the conclusion that the plaques are not the cause of senile dementia. . . ."[4985]

A 2022 investigation into a seminal paper implicating amyloid alleged "shockingly blatant" data fraud, which has further tarnished the reputation of the theory.[4986] Perhaps amyloid buildup is just a manifestation of disease rather than the cause, just as skin lesions were a defining feature of smallpox but not the lethal pathology.[4987] Some posit that amyloid beta may even be protective, churned out by the brain as a defense mechanism. This could be consistent with the increased amyloid deposition found after head trauma.[4988] Regardless, the most damning failure of the amyloid cascade hypothesis is that amyloid-busting therapies like aducanumab don't work.[4989]

Dozens of different amyloid-targeted drugs have failed to slow cognitive decline.[4990] Those sticking to their guns, derided by skeptics as devout members of the "Church of the Holy Amyloid,"[4991] speculate that anti-amyloid drugs fail because they're given too late in the progression of the disease.[4992] After all, amyloid plaques can start forming as early as our late thirties.[4993] This finding has profound implications for the prevention of dementia.[4994]

CAUSAL THEORIES

Drug development for Alzheimer's disease has suffered a 99.6 percent failure rate, the worst of any therapeutic area,[4995] and the few we do have mostly just treat the symptoms.[4996] The good news, as a senior scientist at the Center for Alzheimer's Disease Research titled a review article, is that "Alzheimer's Disease Is Incurable but Preventable."[4997] Diet and lifestyle changes could potentially prevent millions of cases a year.[4998]

PRESERVING YOUR BRAIN'S BLOOD SUPPLY

There is an emerging consensus that "what is good for our hearts is also good for our heads"[4999] because clogging of the arteries inside the brain with atherosclerotic plaque is thought to play a pivotal role in the development of Alzheimer's disease.[5000] In my video see.nf/alzheimers, I trace this connection, dating back to Dr. Alzheimer's first case.[5001] With no energy reserves of its own, the brain is very sensitive to nutrient deprivation.[5002] Interrupting that blood supply even for just a few minutes—for instance, by having a stroke—may double the risk of developing dementia and speed its onset by as much as a decade.[5003]

Autopsy studies have shown repeatedly that Alzheimer's patients tend to have significantly more atherosclerotic plaque buildup and narrowing of the arteries within the brain,[5004,5005,5006] particularly those leading directly to the memory centers.[5007] In light of such findings, some experts have even suggested that Alzheimer's be reclassified as a vascular disorder.[5008] Those with a total cholesterol of 225 mg/dL or higher have up to twenty-five times the odds of ending up with amyloid plaques in their brains ten to fifteen years later (compared to 224 mg/dL or less).[5009] Too much cholesterol in our blood is now universally recognized to be a risk factor for the development of Alzheimer's disease.[5010]

As I explore in see.nf/cholesteroldementia, cholesterol doesn't just help generate atherosclerotic plaques within our brain arteries; it may help seed the amyloid plaques that riddle the brain tissue of people with Alzheimer's.[5011] Under an electron microscope, we can see the clustering of amyloid fibers on and around tiny crystals of cholesterol.[5012] Drug companies have been hoping to capitalize on this connection to sell cholesterol-lowering statin drugs to prevent Alzheimer's, but statins themselves can sometimes cause cognitive impairment, including short- and long-term memory loss.[5013] For people unwilling to sufficiently change their diets, the benefits of statins outweigh the risks,[5014] but it's better if you can lower your cholesterol levels naturally by eating more healthfully to help preserve your heart, brain, and mind.

The number one recommendation of a 2022 consensus panel of experts for the prevention of cognitive decline centers around the concept that "brain health equals heart health."[5015] It is not surprising, then, that the dietary centerpiece of the "Dietary and Lifestyle Guidelines for the Prevention of Alzheimer's Disease" published in the journal *Neurobiology of Aging* was: "Vegetables, legumes (beans, peas, and lentils), fruits, and whole grains should replace meats and dairy products as primary staples of the diet."[5016]

Dietary Oxidized Cholesterol

Total brain cholesterol levels of Alzheimer's victims on autopsy are highly variable and not necessarily higher than in people who died from other causes.[5017] But, *oxidized* cholesterol levels are a different story.[5018] Levels have been shown to dramatically increase in the brains of people with Alzheimer's,[5019] as well as creep up in the spinal fluid of those with mild cognitive impairment.[5020] This adds to a constellation of evidence that oxidized cholesterol may be "the driving force behind the development of Alzheimer's disease."[5021] See the Oxidation chapter for how to reduce your exposure.

TAKING THE PRESSURE OFF

The first trial to showcase an effective strategy for the prevention of age-related cognitive impairment was published in 2019. Earlier, a study of three hundred Alzheimer's patients found that treating vascular risk factors, such as high cholesterol and blood pressure, may slow the progression of the disease but not stop it.[5022] That's why prevention is the key. The Systolic Blood Pressure Intervention Trial (SPRINT) randomized more than a whopping 9,000 older men and women with an average age of sixty-eight with high blood pressure to one of two treatment goals: drugs to push down the top blood pressure number (systolic) to under 140 or more drugs at higher doses to force systolic blood pressure below 120, which is closer to normal blood pressure. The study was planned to last for six years, but the more intensive drug regimen saved so many more lives, reducing overall mortality by 27 percent, that the trial was stopped halfway through.[5023] Were minds saved, as well?

The SPRINT MIND study followed the cognition of the SPRINT participants throughout the trial and for about two subsequent years. The 17 percent reduction in dementia in the intensive blood pressure–lowering group wasn't statistically significant, but the 19 percent drop in the risk of developing mild cognitive impairment was.[5024] Lowering blood pressures therefore appears to prevent cognitive decline. The downsides were the side effects from the numbers and doses of drugs needed to attempt to normalize blood pressures. Yes, there were fewer cases of heart failure in the intensive treatment group, but there were more cases of kidney failure, fainting, and electrolyte abnormalities.[5025] A healthy diet and lifestyle would offer the best of both worlds: lower blood pressures plus a bounty of side benefits.

The arteries in the brain are designed to act not only as a conduit but also as a cushion.[5026] The elastic rebound of artery walls acts as a shock absorber for the pulsations of blood pumping up from our hearts. However, when the artery walls become stiffened with age, the pressure from the pulse can damage small vessels in our brain.[5027] This can cause "microbleeds" in the brain, which are found at about triple the frequency in people with high blood pressure, even if they have never been diagnosed with a stroke.[5028] High blood pressure is also associated with so-called lacunar infarcts,[5029] from the Latin word *lacuna*, meaning "hole." On CT scan, it looks as though your brain has been hole-punched.

These holes appear when little arteries in the brain get clogged and result in the death of a pea-sized region of the brain. Up to a quarter of the elderly have these little ministrokes, and most don't even know it.[5030] They are referred to as "silent infarcts" since they lack clinically overt stroke-like symptoms but are still associated with subtle deficits in physical and cognitive function and can double the risk of dementia.[5031] High blood pressure is also associated with brain shrinkage, specifically in the memory center of the brain.[5032] No wonder elevated blood pressure in midlife is associated with elevated risk of cognitive impairment and Alzheimer's dementia later on, even more so than having the so-called Alzheimer's gene.[5033]

Fourteen of fifteen cross-sectional studies correlated increased arterial stiffness with impaired cognitive performance, and six of the seven longitudinal studies found that arterial stiffness appeared predictive of cognitive decline.[5034] How can we reduce artery stiffness? Reduce our sodium intake. High sodium intake causes excessive arterial fibrosis, the accumulation of scar tissue in the walls of our arteries, resulting in stiffening.[5035] A meta-analysis of eleven randomized controlled trials found that cutting salt intake by less than a teaspoon a day can significantly reduce artery stiffness,[5036] in addition to lowering blood pressure.[5037]

The artery stiffness caused by excessive sodium intake is in fact one of the mechanisms by which too much salt raises blood pressure.[5038] However, excess salt intake is now recognized as a risk factor for dementia independent of blood pressure effects by impairing artery function as well.[5039] In mice, a high-salt diet directly leads to cognitive impairment[5040] and the development of hallmark Alzheimer's brain pathology.[5041]

DIET TRUMPS GENETICS

Few appear to be aware of the good news that much of Alzheimer's risk is modifiable.[5042] For example, one study found that only about a quarter of respondents were aware that high cholesterol and blood pressure increase the risk.[5043] A scoring system was developed for predicting the likelihood of a dementia diagnosis within the next twenty years based on a few factors within our control. Using the scoring system, a fifty-year-old man who didn't finish high school, is physically inactive and obese, and has high blood pressure and cholesterol can be more than *fifty* times more likely to develop dementia compared to a fifty-year-old man who is more educated and active, not obese, and has normal blood pressure and cholesterol, suggesting that we have an enormous influence on risk.[5044]

However, much of the popular press today treats Alzheimer's as a genetic disease, saying it's our genes, rather than our lifestyle choices, that determine whether or not we'll succumb. However, as I cover in depth in my Brain Diseases chapter in *How Not to Die*, when you examine the vastly varying distribution of Alzheimer's disease around the world, that argument begins to crumble.

The lowest validated rates of Alzheimer's disease are found in rural India,[5045] where people eat traditional, plant-based diets centered on grains and vegetables.[5046] A recent study in Taiwan found that vegetarians developed dementia at only two-thirds the rate of nonvegetarians.[5047] In the United States, one study found that those who don't eat meat (including eschewing poultry and fish) appear to cut their risk of developing dementia in half. And, the longer meat is avoided, the lower the dementia risk may fall. Compared to those eating meat more than four times a week, individuals who have eaten vegetarian diets for thirty years or more had three times lower risk of developing dementia.[5048]

See the box below for the good news about how much control we have over the "Alzheimer's gene" *APOE* ε4. Too often, doctors and patients have a fatalistic approach to chronic degenerative diseases, and Alzheimer's is no exception.[5049] "It's all in your genes," they say, "and what will happen will happen." Research shows that although you might have been dealt some poor genetic cards, you may be able to reshuffle the deck with diet.

The Single Most Important Gene for Longevity

Complex genetic mapping techniques, like genome-wide association analysis comparing the DNA of centenarians versus noncentenarians, for example, can identify genes associated with longevity. In my video see.nf/gwas, I describe how the whole process works and what researchers have found. A review of all such studies for lifespan only found one gene confirmed in multiple independent meta-analyses: *APOE*, the "Alzheimer's gene."[5050] Beyond just determining dementia risk, *APOE* is the single most important gene when it comes to having a long and healthy life (though, that's not necessarily saying much).[5051]

What does this gene do to have such a powerful impact on our health and longevity? It codes for the primary cholesterol carrier in the brain[5052] and plays a major role in packaging and transporting LDL ("bad") cholesterol throughout the body.[5053] The good news is that diet can trump genetics. In the video, I explain the so-called Nigerian paradox: how the population with the highest rate of the

"Alzheimer's gene" has one of the lowest rates of Alzheimer's disease, thanks to their extremely low blood-cholesterol levels, due to a diet low in animal fat.[5054] Humans appear to have evolved to sustain an LDL level of around 25 mg/dL.[5055] The average in the Western world is approximately 120 mg/dL. Perhaps it's no wonder that heart disease is the leading cause of death in higher-income countries, and dementia, according to the World Health Organization, is killer number two.[5056]

THE ROLE OF INFLAMMATION

More than a dozen theories have been published on the cause of Alzheimer's, and the "inflammation hypothesis" is one of them.[5057] I review the evidence favoring and opposing in see.nf/braininflammation. I conclude that inflammation may play a role, but you may have to catch it early.[5058]

Alzheimer's manifests as a disease of the elderly, but like heart disease and most cancers, it's a disease that may take decades to develop. Most Alzheimer's sufferers aren't diagnosed until they're in their seventies,[5059] but we now know that their brains began deteriorating long before that. Based on thousands of autopsies, pathologists seemed to detect the first silent stages of Alzheimer's disease—what appear to be tangles in the brain—in half of people by age fifty and even 10 percent of those in their twenties.[5060] The good news is that the clinical manifestation of Alzheimer's disease may be preventable.

THE ROLE OF OXIDATION

Is our brain just rusting? In see.nf/brainoxidation, I contrast the failed antioxidant supplement trials[5061] with the long-term population studies correlating the intake of brain-accessing antioxidants with lower rates of dementia. For example, in the most comprehensive and longest-running cohort to address the question, those averaging the anthocyanins in a single tablespoon of blueberries had a 76 percent lower risk of dementia compared to those getting the anthocyanins in less than a teaspoon or so of daily blueberries.[5062] (Sadly, the number one source of anthocyanins for those in the study was not blueberries but rather blueberry muffins.[5063])

Beyond their antioxidant activity, polyphenols like anthocyanins have been shown to protect nerve cells in vitro by inhibiting the formation of the plaques[5064] and tangles[5065] that characterize Alzheimer's brain pathology. In theory, they could also "pull out"[5066] metals that accumulate in certain brain areas that may play a role in the development of Alzheimer's and other neurodegenerative diseases.[5067]

WHAT ABOUT ALUMINUM?

The "aluminum hypothesis" for the cause of Alzheimer's dates back to 1965, when the inadvertent injection of aluminum into the brains of rabbits induced cognitive deficits along with what initially looked like Alzheimer's disease tangles. Then, in the 1970s, it was first reported that the aluminum content of Alzheimer's brains was higher than that of control brains on autopsy.[5068] Following that, there was a rash of fatal dementia cases linked to dialysis fluids contaminated with aluminum.[5069] This trio of findings led researchers to suggest that aluminum, the third most abundant element on Earth (after oxygen and silicon),[5070] may play a role in the development of Alzheimer's disease.[5071]

The aluminum hypothesis came under heavy fire in the scientific community. Only later did we learn that the most vocal critics were secretly paid hacks for the aluminum industry.[5072] In hindsight, that was probably unnecessary, as the tide of evidence eventually turned against the role of aluminum,[5073] as I review in see.nf /aluminum. What convinced me was a meta-analysis that failed to find a connection between Alzheimer's[5074] and regular antacid use—the most important source of aluminum exposure.[5075]

As I explore in see.nf/aluminumpots, just because aluminum doesn't cause Alzheimer's doesn't mean that aluminum intake is necessarily benign. Those who cook and store acidic foods like yogurt and tomato in aluminum cookware suffer significantly more DNA damage, leading some regulators to recommend that consumers avoid the use of aluminum pots or dishes for acidic or salted foodstuffs.[5076]

In see.nf/antiperspirants, I note how European safety authorities and the FDA also specifically advise against using aluminum antiperspirants on damaged or broken skin,[5077,5078] which may even include avoiding them after shaving.[5079] As a "metalloestrogen,"[5080] aluminum absorption may explain why breast cancer may occur as much as twenty years earlier in women using antiperspirant and shaving their armpits more than three times a week.[5081]

You can also avoid high dietary sources by choosing nonaluminum baking powder for baking and avoiding processed cheese. Aluminum salts can give cheese "desirable slicing properties,"[5082] but that means a single grilled cheese sandwich can end up exceeding the World Health Organization's provisional tolerable daily intake of aluminum by more than 200 percent.[5083]

IRON IN THE FIRE

If aluminum doesn't cause Alzheimer's disease, why does the metal-removing drug deferoxamine seem to help? A remarkable study published more than thirty years ago of the metal-chelating (binding) drug deferoxamine is one of the few clinical trials ever to suggest a change in the course of Alzheimer's.[5084] Details in see.nf

/deferoxamine, but basically, the researchers attributed the halving of the rate of cognitive decline in the deferoxamine group to the ability of the drug to bind aluminum, but deferoxamine was designed as an iron chelator.[5085] Deferoxamine's affinity for iron is six times greater than for aluminum, and iron is a thousand times more abundant in the brain.[5086] Might the dramatic effects be due to ridding the brain of excess iron?

I review the evidence in the video, but iron does seem to co-localize to Alzheimer's plaques;[5087] however, it only appears to accelerate plaques in people with preexisting amyloid buildup, so excess iron just seems to hasten the disease rather than initiate it.[5088] As I explore in see.nf/copper, copper also seems to co-locate with brain pathology,[5089] though it may only present a problem in those who consume too much saturated fat. In the Chicago Health and Aging Project, elderly Chicagoans who got the highest copper doses—largely from multivitamin and mineral supplements—were only at greater risk of cognitive decline when high copper intake was combined with a diet high in saturated fats. In that case, they lost cognition as if they had aged nineteen years during the six years of the study. The researchers proposed that the saturated fat led to the initiation of amyloid plaque buildup, and copper then enhanced disease progression.[5090] The practical implications could be to eat a lot of fruits and vegetables, given the natural metal-chelating effects of many polyphenols, and avoid copper-containing supplements, as well as excessive intake of iron and saturated fat.[5091]

FATHEADED

Attention started to be paid to saturated fat and cholesterol in relation to Alzheimer's disease in the 1990s with the discovery of the role of the "Alzheimer's gene" protein apoE4, the principal cholesterol carrier in the brain.[5092] High saturated fat consumption (sourced predominantly from dairy, meat, and processed foods) is linked to poorer memory[5093] and accelerated cognitive decline. In the Harvard Women's Health Study, for example, higher saturated fat intake was associated with a significantly poorer trajectory of cognition and memory. Women with the highest intake of saturated fat had a 60 to 70 percent greater chance of cognitive deterioration over time, while women with the lowest saturated fat intake had the brain function of women six years younger.[5094]

Meta-analyses of all such studies have found that higher saturated fat consumption is associated with a 40 percent increased risk of cognitive impairment,[5095] a 46 percent increased risk of Alzheimer's disease, and more than twice the risk of developing dementia in general.[5096] A recent review concluded that the link between saturated fat intake and Alzheimer's appears to be "conclusive and detrimental."[5097] How can we cut down on saturated fat? By cutting down on the top sources in the

American diet: cheese, cake, ice cream, and chicken, followed by pork, burgers, and then beef in general.[5098]

There are a number of indirect mechanisms by which saturated fat could contribute to dementia risk, including insulin resistance, high blood pressure, inflammation, or a clogging of cerebral blood vessels,[5099] but it may also make the brain vasculature leaky. Saturated fat may increase Alzheimer's disease risk by disrupting the blood-brain barrier.

The permeability of the blood-brain barrier can be quantified by injecting a dye into people's veins and seeing how much of it leaks into the brain on MRI scan.[5100] Those with Alzheimer's or vascular dementia tend to have leakier brain vessels than age-matched controls.[5101] These disease processes can cause a breakdown of the blood-brain barrier, but this leakiness appears to precede the dementia.[5102] Leakage rates have been found to be elevated in mild cognitive impairment and cerebral small vessel disease, the prodromal syndromes for Alzheimer's disease and vascular dementia.[5103]

Even in healthy individuals, blood-brain barrier leakiness tends to get worse with age,[5104] especially in regions of the brain particularly vulnerable to age-related deterioration, suggesting that the barrier disruption may play a role in run-of-the-mill cognitive decline.[5105] What can we do to maintain the integrity of our blood-brain barrier? Being overweight or obese in middle age correlated with degraded blood-brain barrier function twenty-four years later.[5106] In terms of dietary factors, saturated fat and cholesterol[5107] or just dietary cholesterol alone[5108] can worsen blood-brain barrier permeability. Saturated fat can cause a thirtyfold increase in blood-brain barrier dysfunction in mice and dietary cholesterol a sevenfold increase, both of which can be blocked by a cholesterol-lowering drug.[5109] This may represent a double whammy, since eating saturated fat can increase the production of the amyloid precursor protein from the intestine that's turned into amyloid beta in mice, as well as increase its secretion into the bloodstream.[5110] A single meal high in saturated (dairy) fat can cause a sevenfold increase in amyloid protein levels in the blood.[5111] Combined with blood-brain barrier leakiness, this could explain the proliferation of plaques in fat-fed animal models.[5112] In reference to the burgeoning science in this area, one recent biology journal primer was titled, "Amyloid Beta Emerges from Below the Neck to Disable the Brain."[5113]

WHAT A SINGLE FATTY MEAL CAN DO TO OUR BRAINS

In my Anti-Inflammatory chapter in *How Not to Diet*, I review a litany of studies showing how just a few days on a high-fat, ketogenic diet can blunt cognition,[5114] which may take weeks to recover from.[5115] Even a single high-saturated-fat meal has been shown to impair cognitive performance in people within five hours.[5116]

This might be due to brain inflammation. Saturated fat fed to lab animals crosses their blood-brain barrier, accumulates in the center of the brain, and triggers inflammation. The original studies on animals used lard-based diets, but it appears butterfat causes similar results.[5117] The scenario can also be re-created in a petri dish. When the main saturated fat in a typical American diet (found mostly in dairy and meat)[5118] is dripped onto neurons in vitro, inflammation can be turned on like a light switch.[5119] Fortunately, it is possible to reverse this. When the animal subjects were once again fed their regular low-fat food, the inflammation in their brain disappeared.[5120]

Granted, extrapolating data from animal studies is infamously fraught with difficult challenges.[5121] For starters, the diets are not comparable. High-fat, lard-based rodent food may be around 60 percent fat,[5122] for instance, but even bacon is only about 40 percent lard.[5123] So, we could eat a bacon-only diet and still not get the fat intake of the rodent diet. Saturated fat has been put to the test in people, though.

Researchers covertly increased the saturated fat intake of study participants in randomized crossover trials and found it reversibly induces negative changes in inflammation, mood, brain function, and resting metabolic rate, and even appears to undercut motivation to exercise.[5124,5125] Study subjects became 12 to 15 percent less physically active when they were on diets high in saturated fat compared to low–saturated fat ones.[5126] Note that the researchers used palm oil, which is a saturated *plant* fat that can be found in some vegan spreads, nondairy cheeses, and other processed foods. So, an anti-inflammatory diet is not only more plant-based in general; it is specifically centered around whole, unprocessed plant foods.

POLLUTING YOUR BRAIN

Besides saturated fat and oxidized cholesterol, what else might be in the meat supply to account for meat eaters having up to two to three times the risk of developing dementia compared to vegetarians?[5127] In the Glycation chapter, I discussed the role of advanced glycation end products in baked, broiled, grilled, fried, and roasted meat in age-related cognitive decline,[5128] brain shrinkage,[5129] mild cognitive impairment,[5130] and the development[5131] and progression of Alzheimer's disease.[5132] Persistent pollutants, like chlorinated pesticides, may be another factor.

Among U.S. elders, DDT and its breakdown product, DDE, are associated with increased risk of accelerated cognitive decline,[5133] as well as the diagnosis and severity of Alzheimer's disease.[5134] See see.nf/ddtdementia for details. The toxins are still in our body because they're still in our food supply. Samples were collected from supermarkets across the United States, and fish, other meats, eggs, and dairy had five to ten times higher levels of dioxins and PCBs than the plant foods that were tested.[5135]

ENDOTOXINS

Recently, endotoxins have been proposed as an underlying mechanism for the link between saturated fat and cognitive impairment.[5136] I review the evidence in see .nf/endotoxins, but basically, there are two ways to cut down on endotoxin bursts after meals. One is to not eat so many in the first place. (See page 85.) But, if you do eat meat, the addition of fiber-rich foods can blunt the endotoxin surge. As I show in the video, eating a Sausage and Egg McMuffin with a high-fiber cereal significantly reduced bloodstream endotoxins compared to a McMuffin alone. The fiber also reduced the associated oxidative stress, clearly showing "profound effects on metabolic and inflammatory events after the meal."[5137]

LIFESTYLE

Advanced age is the strongest known risk factor for declining cognition,[5138] but 40 percent of dementia cases appear to be attributable to modifiable risk factors that we can control.[5139] In addition to cleaning up our diets, we can reduce dementia risk by preventing head injuries, not smoking (quitting or not starting to begin with), avoiding secondhand smoke and other sources of air pollution, limiting alcohol use, getting sufficient sleep, reducing obesity, and keeping physically active.

HEAD INJURIES, AIRBORNE POLLUTANTS, AND ALCOHOL

Up to 30 percent of all traumatic brain injuries are sports-related.[5140] That may be why former professional soccer players appear to be five times more likely to die from Alzheimer's disease than matched controls,[5141] especially among those playing field positions characterized by executing more "headers."[5142] A study of former National Football League players suggests American football also places athletes at risk.[5143] Boxers even have their own term—"dementia pugilistica"—to describe the punch-drunk syndrome of former prizefighters.[5144] Less than 1 percent of dementia cases globally are probably attributable to traumatic brain injury, but it's still worth taking precautions.[5145] Bicycle helmets may reduce the risk of serious head injury by as much as 60 percent compared to unprotected cyclists.[5146] Protective headgear is also recommended for high-risk impact sports,[5147] as are policies eliminating body checking in youth ice hockey.[5148]

In contrast, as many as 14 percent of global Alzheimer's disease diagnoses are potentially attributable to smoking.[5149] Tobacco is a major risk factor for stroke, which itself increases dementia risk, as well as having a direct effect of increased brain amyloid burden and oxidative stress.[5150] The good news is that the risk of ex-smokers is similar to that of never-smokers.[5151] Interventional studies of smoking cessation to prove cause and effect are, like studies entailing major dietary change, hard to do because of the lack of long-term compliance. One can, however, show that the cognition of successful quitters is significantly better over time compared to those in cessation trials who failed to stop smoking.[5152] Even secondhand smoke exposure has been associated with increased risk of Alzheimer's and other forms of dementia.[5153]

Dementia and cognitive decline have also been consistently associated with exposure to ambient air pollution. Interest in the impact of air pollutants was sparked twenty years ago by the paper "Air Pollution and Brain Damage,"[5154] in which Alzheimer's-type pathology was found in the brains of dogs raised in cities with high pollution versus low pollution.[5155] In the human brain, the presence of magnetite nanoparticles suggests pollutants from traffic exhaust may be traveling directly to the brain through olfactory nerves from inside the nose,[5156] though pollutants could also indirectly lead to brain injury through systemic inflammatory effects.[5157]

Alcohol-related dementia has been referred to as a silent epidemic.[5158] Excess alcohol consumption may contribute to as many as 24 percent of cases of dementia. What about light drinking?[5159] Hopes that low-level alcohol consumption might even be beneficial for cognition[5160] were dashed by a Mendelian randomization study that found, if anything, alcohol consumption causes earlier onset of Alzheimer's disease.[5161] The good news is that those quitting even heavy drinking followed by prolonged abstinence can experience a recovery of lost brain volume and cognitive function.[5162]

Don't Kiss Your Memories Goodbye

Another risk reduction strategy is being careful who you smooch. Amyloid beta is strongly conserved throughout evolution. The human variant dates back at least four hundred million years and today can be found in most vertebrate species.[5163] So it must have some sort of beneficial function. Historically, survival of the fittest has been less about the dynamics of predator against prey than about the starkest us-versus-them—the microbial threats that prey on us all. Amyloid beta may be part of our immune system, an antimicrobial peptide that protects us against brain infections. It has been shown to be antibacterial, antifungal, and antiviral against a range of common pathogens. For example, temporal lobe samples from Alzheimer's brains are better at killing off *Candida* yeast, a cause of fungal meningitis, than samples from the same part of the brain from those who died of other causes.[5164]

(continued)

Amyloid beta also binds to herpes simplex virus 1 (HSV-1), leading to protective viral entrapment.[5165] HSV-1 is the virus that normally causes cold sores (also known as fever blisters) but it can also infect the brain. Is it possible that infection with this common virus could trigger amyloid deposition in our body's attempt to suppress it but thereby, inadvertently and eventually, lead to Alzheimer's disease?

I was surprised to find about a hundred scientific publications linking HSV-1 infection to Alzheimer's disease.[5166] In one study, for instance, researchers followed tens of thousands of individuals and found that those with either oral herpes (HSV-1) or genital herpes (HSV-2) were more than twice as likely to develop dementia during the sixteen-year follow-up period. Even more convincing (and offering a dose of good news) is that those with HSV who took antiviral medications (like acyclovir) appeared to be 90 percent less likely to develop dementia compared to those with untreated HSV.[5167] Unfortunately, there are not yet licensed vaccines to prevent getting infected in the first place, but you can reduce your risk of HSV-1 by avoiding kissing or sharing utensils, cups, water bottles, towels, or lip balm with those who have an active oral infection (though asymptomatic viral shedding can also occur).

GETTING BRAINWASHED EVERY NIGHT

Sleep is a great mystery. A trait shared across animal species, sleep must be of vital importance to survive natural selection pressures to eliminate such a vulnerable state.[5168] Indeed, cringeworthy experiments have shown that keeping animals awake long enough can be fatal within eleven to thirty-two days.[5169] One function of sleep that has been elucidated in recent years is the clearance of toxic waste byproducts[5170] through a newly discovered drainage system in the brain.[5171] This may explain why PET scans show that even a single all-nighter can cause a significant increase in accumulation of amyloid beta in critical brain areas.[5172] Find out more about this brain-wide fluid transport network termed the glymphatic system in my video see.nf/brainwash.

Unfortunately, this brain filtration system appears to decline with age.[5173] See see.nf/glymphatic for the role that sleeping position could potentially play. (Teaser: Sleeping on our right side could theoretically maximize brain drainage.[5174])

Might Melatonin Help?

What about using melatonin to improve sleep quality, in the hopes of clearing out extra debris?[5175] There was an interesting case report of identical twins. Both had

Alzheimer's disease, but only one was treated with melatonin. The treated twin not only appeared to sleep better but also had milder memory impairment.[5176] Melatonin has been shown to improve the memory of aging-accelerated rats considered to be laboratory models for Alzheimer's disease,[5177] but what about in people?

A total of seven randomized, double-blind, placebo-controlled trials of melatonin for Alzheimer's disease have been performed on hundreds of patients, lasting between ten days and twenty-four weeks. Those randomized to melatonin appeared to sleep better, but, sadly, melatonin had no effect on improving cognitive abilities.[5178]

EXPANDING WAIST, SHRINKING BRAIN

Overweight individuals have about one-third higher risk of developing dementia, and those who are obese in midlife seem to have about 90 percent greater risk.[5179] I explore this large body of data in my video see.nf/obesitydementia, including how excess body fat can impair cognition at any age,[5180] which correlates with structural brain differences.[5181] The brain appears to shrink as the waist expands,[5182] perhaps due to the inflammation and oxidative stress, both related to obesity.[5183] Based on a meta-analysis of twenty studies, mental performance across a variety of domains can be significantly improved with even modest weight loss, though no studies have yet been done to determine if this then translates into a normalization of Alzheimer's disease risk.[5184]

EXERCISE YOUR BRAIN

The improved cognition in weight-loss studies may also be confounded by exercise.[5185] I review all the key interventional studies in see.nf/exercisebrain. Added exercise tends to improve the cognition of adults with normal cognition[5186] or mild cognitive impairment.[5187] Based on a meta-analysis of nearly a hundred randomized controlled trials, more important than session duration, weekly frequency,[5188] program duration, or intensity[5189] may be total training time—a total of about fifty-two total hours of exercise to establish a cognitive benefit.[5190] Unfortunately, an exercise intervention failed to slow cognitive decline once dementia was diagnosed.[5191]

Boosting BDNF with Exercise

How does exercise work exactly? Neurotrophins are a family of growth factors that promote the development, function, and survival of neurons (the nerve cells in our brain).[5192] The most abundant neurotrophin is called *brain-derived neurotrophic factor*, or BDNF,[5193] the levels of which appear to correlate with integrity of the hippocampus, the memory center of the brain.[5194] On autopsy, most studies show decreased BDNF in the brains of people with Alzheimer's.[5195] Since it crosses the blood-brain barrier, BDNF levels in the brain can be estimated by measuring its levels in the blood.[5196] Compared to healthy controls, those with Alzheimer's have significantly lower BDNF blood levels.[5197]

Given the neuroprotective properties of BDNF, it would make sense that low levels might contribute to the disease,[5198] but how do we know that the Alzheimer's isn't just leading to a drop in BDNF instead of the other way around?[5199] The Framingham Heart Study, a longitudinal study that followed thousands of people over time, found that having higher BDNF blood levels appears to cut in half the risk of developing Alzheimer's over the next decade.[5200] And, once you have the disease, higher levels of BDNF seem to predict a slower cognitive decline.[5201] Bolstering the causal case, people born with genetic variations that naturally lead to lower BDNF secretion do appear to suffer impairments of cognitive function and brain health.[5202]

Thankfully, boosting BDNF is as easy as lacing up our walking shoes. Physical activity is the best studied factor for boosting BDNF.[5203] Based on twenty-nine trials involving more than a thousand subjects, single sessions of exercise, regular exercise, and especially acute exercise in the context of regular exercise have been shown to increase BDNF levels.[5204] Cycling at 70 percent maximal work rate for just ten minutes, for example, can significantly elevate levels.[5205] The greater the workout intensity, the greater the rise in BDNF,[5206] but even among elderly individuals with limited ambulation, a physical therapy intervention using progressive dynamic resistance training seemed able to boost BDNF blood levels.[5207]

So, is BDNF one of the reasons exercise boosts brain power? Yes, at least in rodents. Researchers have clearly shown that blocking BDNF blocks the memory-enhancing effects from exercise in rats and mice, effectively proving the role of BDNF in mediating the exercise benefit. In people, the best we can do is try to see if the level of exercise-induced improvement in BDNF corresponds with the level of exercise-induced improvement in memory performance. This only seems to be the case in four of the ten studies on the matter, though, so the answer is less clear.[5208]

Boosting BDNF with Calorie Restriction

Fasting has been espoused as a way of rejuvenating the body as well as the mind,[5209] but after fasting for just eighteen hours, you can start to get really irritable.[5210] Remarkably, after a few days of fasting, you may experience a sometimes euphoric mood enhancement,[5211] for which BDNF may play a role. I explore this phenomenon in my video see.nf/fastingbdnf. Fasting, by definition, is unsustainable, though. What about more modest caloric restriction?

Cutting 25 percent of calories from our daily diet has been shown to cause a 70 percent rise in BDNF after only three months.[5212] Over that same time period, just a 10 percent or so reduction in calories can improve memory performance.[5213] Is there anything we can *add* to our diets to boost BNDF levels so we can get the benefits without the hunger?

Boosting BDNF with Food

Caloric restriction studies can sometimes be confounded by changes in dietary quality.[5214] For example, one study in which those on low-calorie diets had higher BDNF levels involved not just eating less but also eating more healthfully—less saturated fat and sugar, and more fruits and veggies.[5215] A single high-fat meal can suppress our BDNF levels within hours. We know it's the fat itself because researchers see the same response after injecting fat straight into people's veins.[5216] This may help explain why increased consumption of saturated fats in a high-fat diet may contribute to brain dysfunction, including neurodegenerative diseases, long-term memory loss, and cognitive impairment.[5217]

In my video see.nf/foodbdnf, I compare it to the Soviet fasting trials for schizophrenia. After the patients were fasted for up to a month, they were put on a diet that excluded meat and eggs. When the researchers reported remarkable effects even years later, that was for the patients who stuck with the diet. Those who broke the diet evidently relapsed, whereas the closer the diet was followed, the better the effect.[5218] Since we know from a randomized controlled trial that removing meat and eggs can improve mental states within just two weeks,[5219] it's hard to know what role the initial fasting itself played in the reported improvements.

In the video, I go through all the foods that have been shown to boost BDNF. These include high-flavonoid fruits and vegetables,[5220] nuts,[5221] turmeric,[5222] and cocoa powder. For example, researchers randomized older men and women to a daily high-flavonoid chocolate drink (containing the flavonoid content of about two and a half tablespoons of natural cocoa powder) or a low-flavonoid chocolate drink (equivalent to around two tablespoons of Dutched cocoa).[5223,5224] Those randomized to weeks of more flavonoids experienced significant increases in BDNF levels and global cognitive function.[5225] One food is capable of boosting BDNF after just a single meal: rye groats.

Healthy young adults were randomized to a late-evening meal of either a whole-grain bread containing intact rye kernels or regular white bread. Before breakfast the next morning, more than ten hours after eating their evening meals, their blood was drawn. Those who had eaten the whole intact rye the night before had 33 percent higher BDNF levels. Given the timing, this is suspected to be a microbiome effect, bolstered by a corresponding 30 percent increase in butyrate levels in the blood. Remember, butyrate is a good bacteria by-product of the gut fermentation of fiber and other prebiotics,[5226] and it increases BDNF expression in mice.[5227] The administration of probiotics—the good bacteria themselves—did not seem to affect BDNF levels,[5228] so it may be better to pamper the good bugs we already have.

MIND YOUR MICROBIOME

BDNF is just one of the ways fiber-derived butyrate may contribute to brain health. Elderly individuals with higher levels of butyrate in their blood tend to have lower levels of amyloid in their brains on PET scan. In vitro, butyrate inhibits the neurotoxic clumping of amyloid beta.[5229] In rats, it acts as a cognitive enhancer in those with impaired memory function,[5230] and, in a mouse model of Alzheimer's, butyrate profoundly reduces amyloid levels in the brain and improves cognitive function[5231]—even at a late stage of the disease.[5232] Butyrate may even prevent amyloid beta in the blood from even getting into the brain in the first place.[5233]

"Germ-free" mice raised Bubble Boy–style in a sterile environment have a leaky blood-brain barrier, which is normally meant to wall off the brain from any toxins circulating in the bloodstream.[5234] Butyrate maintains and repairs the barrier function of the gut,[5235] so perhaps the mice's lack of good gut bugs could explain the leaky brain. Indeed, researchers proved it was the butyrate by restoring the germ-free mice's blood-brain barrier function with butyrate or just by seeding their guts with fiber-eating bacteria.[5236]

The release of butyrate is not the only way our good gut bugs can interact with our brain. There is a big nerve—the vagus nerve—that goes directly from our gut straight up into the brain. There are certain Bifidobacteria[5237] and Lactobacillus[5238] probiotics that can be fed to mice that ameliorate anxiety- or depression-related behaviors, as well as reduce their stress hormone levels, but they only work in animals with an intact vagus nerve. When the nerve is cut, so is the line of communication between their gut bugs and their brains, and the effects are abolished. In humans, in what sounds like science fiction, stimulating the vagus nerve with an electric current was found to significantly enhance memory retention,[5239] but eating fiber-rich foods is probably more pleasant than surgical electrode implantation.

Our microbiome can also modulate inflammation in the body.[5240] Most of the variation in gut bugs between people is attributable to differing diets,[5241] and switching from a fiber-rich, plant-based diet to an animal-based one not only significantly reduces butyrate levels within days but it fosters the growth of pro-inflammatory bacteria.[5242] This is consistent with cross-sectional data that find that those eating more plant-rich diets typically have an anti-inflammatory microbiome, whereas those eating more animal-rich diets tend to have more pro-inflammatory species.[5243]

Researchers were able to prove the role of bad gut bugs by performing fecal transplant studies with mice. They replicated the same kind of brain inflammation and dysfunction seen in lard-fed mice by just transferring the gut bacteria fostered by lard-eating mice into other mice that had not eaten lard.[5244] The closest we've come in people is showing that feeding mice feces from obese humans impairs their memory (compared to being fed fecal matter from normal-weight humans). If bad gut flora contribute to cognitive dysfunction, how about treating Alzheimer's patients with antibiotics in an attempt to wipe out the bacteria? A pilot study of an antibiotics cocktail suggested that there was enough potential benefit to run a more rigorous trial.[5245] Unfortunately, the follow-up study failed to show any significant effect.[5246]

There have been more than twenty randomized trials on probiotics and cognition in mostly healthy adults, with no overall benefit found across the board.[5247] (One study even found probiotics impaired memory, compared to placebo.[5248]) But, just looking at five studies done on those affected by mild cognitive impairment or Alzheimer's disease, a variety of *Lactobacillus* and / or *Bifidobacteria* species for twelve weeks did appear to move the needle and improve cognition compared to the control group.[5249]

BRAIN SUPPLEMENTS

Over the last twenty years, Big Pharma has invested more than half a trillion dollars into dementia treatment research, so far to little avail.[5250] In light of this, many have turned to supplements. An AARP-commissioned survey found that 36 percent of people seventy-four and older take a supplement for brain health,[5251] to the tune of billions of dollars a year.[5252] The most commonly marketed brain supplement is one I'd never heard of before (a consequence, I guess, of never having owned a television): Prevagen.[5253]

JELLYFISH STING

Prevagen contains a protein derived from a luminescent jellyfish that the company claims has been "clinically shown to improve memory,"[5254] but even its own study failed to show significant improvements in any of the nine measured cognitive tasks that were tested,[5255] leading the AARP to accuse the company of "deceiving millions of aging Americans."[5256] Prevagen may be more than just a waste of money, as the manufacturer was cited for failing to report more than a thousand adverse events relayed by consumers to the FDA.[5257] More on this shameful story in see.nf /prevagen.

A 2019 survey by the Pew Charitable Trusts found that more than half the respondents believed that the FDA requires supplements to be tested for safety, but this isn't true.[5258] One study of dozens of supplements sold as cognitive performance boosters found that most (71 percent) claimed an ingredient on the label that wasn't actually in the supplement, and, even worse, 38 percent contained ingredients that are not even allowed to be in supplements, such as prohibited drugs.[5259] Another study of a dozen "brain health supplements" similarly found that eight out of twelve were misbranded (missing an ingredient promised on the label), and ten out of twelve were deemed adulterated (containing unlisted compounds— for example, caffeine in a product that explicitly highlighted "DECAFFEINATED" on its label). Only one out of twelve supplements was genuinely third-party certified and contained what its label said it did.[5260]

GINKGO

Ginkgo biloba is one of the most common "brain health" supplements,[5261] with as many as 2 percent of Americans taking it.[5262] Over the last few decades, an extract of gingko leaves has become one of the most widely used herbal treatments for dementia.[5263] Details in see.nf/ginkgo, but the bottom line is that a Cochrane review concluded that the "evidence that Ginkgo biloba has predictable and clinically significant benefit for people with dementia or cognitive impairment is inconsistent and unreliable."[5264]

GINSENG, ROSEMARY, SAGE, AND LEMON BALM

Ginseng is another herbal remedy that's been tested in randomized controlled trials, and, sadly, most such studies flopped.[5265] What about culinary herbs you can actually eat?

In *Hamlet*, Ophelia notes that rosemary is for remembrance,[5266] an idea that goes back at least a few thousand years to the ancient Greeks, who claimed that the fragrant herb "comforts the brain . . . sharpens understanding, restores lost memory, awakens the mind. . . ."[5267] Even just sniffing rosemary may have an effect, as suggested by a study of cognition in a room infused with rosemary essential oil (compared to lavender essential oil or no odor at all).[5268] Furthermore, the boost in performance has been correlated with the amount of a rosemary compound that made it into their bloodstream, presumably through their lungs or nasal passages.[5269] What about just eating it?

Older adults with an average age of seventy-five were given two cups of tomato juice with either about a half teaspoon of powdered, dried rosemary (an amount one might use in a typical recipe), a full teaspoon, two teaspoons, more than a tablespoon, placebo pills, or nothing at all. Compared to placebo, memory speed improved after the lowest dose, but *worsened* after the highest dose, suggesting that more isn't necessarily better.[5270]

Sage and lemon balm are two other herbs in the same botanical family prized in folk medicine for their purported brain benefits.[5271] Cognitive benefits were also found within hours of consuming a teaspoon of dried sage or a tea bag's worth (1.6 g) of dried lemon balm.[5272] Note, however, that a trial using rosemary, sage, and lemon balm *extracts* showed no memory enhancement, suggesting consuming the herbs whole is preferable.[5273] Note also that these studies just tracked the acute effects of single doses in healthy individuals. Are there any herbs or spices that can be used to actually improve cognition over time?

Aromatherapy

The bump in cognitive performance from sniffing rosemary essential oils was demonstrated in young, healthy volunteers,[5274] but what about those who really need it? A group of Japanese researchers posed a pie-in-the-sky notion that certain smells could lead to "nerve rebirth" in people with Alzheimer's.[5275] Twenty-five years ago, simply raising such a possibility as a hypothetical was heretical. Everybody knew that dead neurons cannot be replaced.[5276] That's what we were all taught, until 1998.

Patients with terminal cancer volunteered to be injected with a special dye that gets incorporated into the DNA of new cells. On autopsy, researchers then went hunting for nerve cells that lit up and there they were: New nerve cells were found in the brain that did not exist months or even days before, demonstrating that "the human brain retains the potential for self-renewal throughout life."[5277] The accompanying editorial was titled "Take Comfort in Human Neurogenesis."[5278]

Of course, that doesn't mean smells can cause such revitalization. An aromatherapy regimen of rosemary, lemon, lavender, and orange essential oils was attempted with Alzheimer's patients for a month,[5279] and the trajectory of their steady decline in cognitive function appeared to reverse over that period. Week-long before-and-after studies of both lavender oil and a combination of rosemary and lemon oils appeared to show similar effects.[5280] But, the studies all lacked a control group. Even with a control, though, how do you eliminate the placebo effect?

(continued)

To test the power of expectancy effects, volunteers were given a memory test and then asked to repeat the test while exposed to sage essential oil. Some were randomly told that sage has a positive influence on memory, while others were told that sage impairs memory. You can probably guess what happened. Those expecting the sage to help did better, and those expecting the sage to hurt did worse.[5281] It would seem that our psychological expectations are able to trump any actual physiological effects. However, researchers have tried to come up with some creative solutions.

In one study of patients with dementia, researchers alternated months of applying a lavender-scented oil to the participants' faces versus an unscented oil to their feet, or vice versa. So, everyone was getting the care and attention of the oil massage, but if there really was some benefit to breathing in lavender, then one would presume they would do better during the months they have the lavender on their face rather than on their feet. But they didn't, which suggests lavender doesn't help.[5282] Most aromatherapy trials for dementia similarly flopped,[5283] but there was one notable exception I detail in see.nf/lemonbalm.

Two studies have subsequently been published to try to replicate the remarkable results I review in that video. In the first, there was a 38 percent reduction in agitation and aggression, a 50 percent reduction in depression and dysphoria (the opposite of euphoria), and a significant improvement in neuropsychiatry symptoms overall. But, pretty much the same was found in the unscented control group.[5284] In other words, just a minute or two of touch and social interaction can make a big difference, but there did not seem to be any specific benefit from the lemon balm. The second study did not clarify matters. Lemon balm appeared to reduce agitated behavior in participants without dementia but not in those with dementia, while lavender seemed to have the opposite effect, improving behavior in participants with dementia but not those without it.[5285] Obviously, more research needs to be done, especially given the safety and simplicity of aromatherapy interventions. But who's going to fund such studies—Big Balm?

TURMERIC

In see.nf/turmericdementia, I relay a remarkable case series in which the symptoms of three Alzheimer's patients dramatically improved after being treated with turmeric.[5286] The investigators concluded that this was the first demonstration of turmeric as an "effective and safe drug" for the treatment of Alzheimer's. Of course, it's not a drug at all. Turmeric is just a spice you can buy inexpensively at any grocery store. The researchers had given study participants around a quarter teaspoon a day, which would come out to less than five cents.

I review the available evidence in see.nf/curcumind, but ultimately, though there may be a small cognitive benefit for curcumin supplementation in older adults without dementia,[5287] the two randomized, double-blind, placebo-controlled trials of curcumin in patients with Alzheimer's both failed to show cognitive benefits.[5288,5289] Why didn't researchers see the same dramatic results with curcumin supplements that were reported in the case reports of those given turmeric? Perhaps those cases were total flukes. On the other hand, perhaps turmeric, the whole food, may be greater than the sum of its parts. Curcumin is just one of hundreds of phytochemicals found in turmeric.[5290] In response, some researchers have suggested creating a blend of components that "represents turmeric in its medicinal value better than curcumin alone."[5291] But why concoct some artificial mixture when Mother Nature already packaged it all in turmeric? Because a common spice can't be patented, and if you can't patent it, how are you going to charge more than five cents?

SAFFRON

Although there were intriguing anecdotes of recovery using the spice turmeric,[5292] the best data we have on spice-based interventions for Alzheimer's are for saffron, with three double-blind trials (detailed in see.nf/saffron) showing promise. Saffron does not appear to improve cognition in individuals without dementia, however.[5293]

The three trials were funded by noncommercial public grants, not supplement or spice companies.[5294] However, they were all conducted in Iran, which controls about 90 percent of the world's saffron crop.[5295] So, promoting saffron consumption may be of national interest, which reminds me of the New Zealand government funding research on kiwifruit. But who else is going to fund studies on a simple spice?

Each saffron flower only produces a few threads, such that you need 50,000 flowers to make a single pound of spice. That's enough flowers to fill a football field. No wonder it's the most expensive spice in the world, retailing for about $200 an ounce. It doesn't take much, though. The cognition studies used as little as 0.125 g a day, which is only about four small pinches of fifteen threads each.[5296] Side effects may include an elevation of mood, as eleven randomized trials have found that, overall, saffron benefits mild to moderate depression significantly better than placebo[5297] at doses as little as a single pinch a day (30 mg).[5298] Daily doses are considered safe up to 1.5 g a day (fifty pinches).[5299]

(Saffron is typically sold in containers holding 1 or 2 g.) Taking 5 or more grams a day can cause serious reactions, and overdoses involving 12 to 20 grams a day may be fatal.[5300]

VITAMIN D

As of 2019, vitamins such as vitamin D replaced *Ginkgo biloba* as the most common component of "brain health" supplements.[5301] Observational studies have found that those with lower vitamin D levels have poorer cognition over time[5302] and are more likely to develop dementia.[5303] There are so many confounding factors when it comes to the sunshine vitamin, though. For example, those with lower levels are more likely to be less physically active, smokers, and obese,[5304] and each one of those may independently affect the brain. Randomized controlled trials have found that vitamin D can improve cognition in diseased rats[5305] and mice, but what about us?[5306]

An interventional trial finding no effects of vitamin D on young adults was published in 2011, but it wasn't until 2018 that a trial was conducted on elderly people with mild cognitive impairment. A randomized, double-blind, placebo-controlled trial showed that 400 IU of vitamin D a day for twelve months significantly improved cognitive function over placebo.[5307] The next year, a similar trial was published, but with 800 IU a day for those with full-blown Alzheimer's. That worked, too.[5308]

The best dosing is uncertain.[5309] An ambitious trial comparing 600 IU, 2,000 IU, and 4,000 IU a day for a year in overweight older women with low vitamin D blood levels found that those taking 2,000 IU a day performed better in learning and memory tests than those taking only 600 IU, whereas the 4,000 IU group did worse in one measure (reaction time). However, other trials of relatively healthy adults comparing 2,000 IU versus 800 IU[5310] or 4,000 IU versus 400 IU[5311] found no clear differences in overall cognitive performance.

ANTIOXIDANTS, MULTIVITAMINS/MINERALS, AND SOUVENAID

Oxidative stress is implicated in the development of Alzheimer's and further brain deterioration. Might antioxidants help? I review the interventional evidence in see.nf/brainvitamins. Supplementation with vitamin E, selenium, or both failed to prevent Alzheimer's, but the data on treating the disease are mixed, with two studies suggesting vitamin E supplementation made things better,[5312,5313] and one finding that it may make things worse.[5314]

Similarly disappointing outcomes have been reported for other antioxidants,[5315,5316] the multivitamin and mineral supplement Centrum Silver,[5317] zinc,[5318,5319] calcium,[5320] or Souvenaid, a nutritional drink branded as Fortasyn Connect, as I document in my video see.nf/centrum.

B VITAMINS

For background on what homocysteine is, what it does, and all the preclinical and epidemiological evidence linking it to dementia, check out my video see.nf /homocysteine. In short, it's a toxic metabolite naturally formed in the body that can then be detoxified using three vitamins: folate, vitamin B_{12}, and vitamin B_6.[5321] A number of recent systematic reviews and meta-analyses of randomized controlled trials of B-vitamin supplements have found no effect on global cognitive function for healthy[5322] or impaired individuals,[5323] nor do they appear to slow cognitive decline.[5324] Normally, this would close the case, but a deeper dive suggests the situation may be more complicated.

The concern is that B-vitamin deficiencies give rise to homocysteine, which in turn causes brain dysfunction. If B-vitamin supplements are given to people who don't have B-vitamin deficiencies and don't have high levels of homocysteine, then negative results don't really help to answer the question at hand. In the VITACOG trial, for example, hundreds of men and women with mild cognitive impairment were randomized to placebo or the B vitamins that detoxify homocysteine—folic acid (the supplement form of folate), B_{12}, and B_6—for two years. No overall cognitive benefit was found. But, when the analysis was restricted to only those who needed the supplementation, that is, those who started out with higher-than-average homocysteine levels, then researchers saw a significant benefit in global cognition and some measures of memory.[5325] Even more remarkable was the reduction in brain shrinkage.

As we age, our brains slowly atrophy. The brains of those aged ninety and older weigh about 10 percent less than brains of those in their fifties. That comes out to a loss of about 5 oz of brain.[5326] Shrinkage is much accelerated in patients suffering from Alzheimer's disease, while an intermediate rate of shrinking is found in people with mild cognitive impairment. In the VITACOG study, the rate of brain atrophy in those with high homocysteine levels who were randomized to the B-vitamin supplements was cut in half.[5327] In regions especially vulnerable to the Alzheimer's disease process, the B-vitamin supplements reduced shrinkage by as much as seven-fold.[5328] The researchers concluded, "We show that a simple and safe treatment that targets homocysteine can slow down the accelerated rate of brain atrophy found in mild cognitive impairment."[5329]

Sufficient B-vitamin status can only account for a fraction of failed trials, though; the vast majority of studies involved those with elevated homocysteine levels greater than 12 μmol/L.[5330] A wider-ranging issue is the lack of baseline measurements of cognitive function. They are missing from about three-quarters of participants in the trials.[5331] This is because most of the large B-vitamin supplementation trials were originally set up to investigate the effects of lowering homocysteine levels not on cognition but on cardiovascular disease, and researchers merely added in cognitive measurements at the end as a secondary outcome.[5332] Why do we care about baseline cognitive measurements? If the participants were randomly assigned to B vitamins or placebo and then, months or years later, ended up with the same brain scores, doesn't that effectively prove the B vitamins had no cognitive benefit? Not if there was no decline in either group. If there was no measurable cognitive decline in the placebo group, then there's nothing for the B vitamins to thwart. "In other words," a pair of reviewers wrote, "you cannot prevent something that is not occurring."[5333]

The Alzheimer's Disease Cooperative Study fulfilled both criteria necessary to properly put B-vitamin supplementation to the test—high homocysteine levels at baseline and a decline in mental functioning in the placebo group. Eighteen months later, there was no overall difference in cognition between the two groups.[5334] However, a planned subgroup analysis did find a significant slowing of cognitive decline in the B-vitamin group among those with mild dementia, just not for those further along. What about preventing the nutrient deficiencies in the first place?

HOW TO LOWER HOMOCYSTEINE

Most people get enough B_{12} and B_6, but the reason the elderly individuals may be stuck at a homocysteine level of 11 μmol/L[5335] is that they aren't getting enough folate.[5336] That should come as no surprise since folate is found concentrated in beans and greens, and 96 percent of Americans don't even get the minimum recommended amount of beans or dark green leafy vegetables.

Since folate tends to be the limiting B vitamin for the general population, the FACIT trial randomized more than eight hundred older men and women to folic acid supplements or placebo for three years. Those in the folic acid group dropped their homocysteine from an average of 13 down to 10, yielding demonstrable cognitive benefits—and not just by a little. The researchers estimated the extra folic acid gave people the performance of someone 4.7 years younger for memory, 1.7 years younger for sensorimotor speed, 2.1 years younger for information processing speed, and 1.5 years younger for global cognitive function.[5337] All that for a cost as low as two cents a day.

So, should all older adults take folic acid supplements? Everyone needs to get enough folate, which is one of many reasons I recommend people eat dark green leafy vegetables and legumes every day, but, as I noted on page 53, folic acid is not folate and may carry safety concerns. So, the best way to get folate may be from food.

Even just one week on a plant-based diet can drop elevated homocysteine levels by 20 percent, from around 11 µmol/L to 9 µmol/L,[5338] which is a normal level for those replete with B vitamins.[5339] This may be directly due to the folate-rich vegetables and beans or indirectly due to the fiber in the plants. Every 1 g of daily fiber consumption may increase folate levels in our blood by nearly 2 percent, perhaps by boosting folate production in the colon by all our friendly gut bacteria.[5340]

Another explanation for the rapid improvement could be from the decreased intake of methionine, an amino acid that comes mostly from animal protein. Homocysteine is a breakdown product of methionine. After eating bacon and eggs for breakfast and a steak for dinner, for example, homocysteine levels spike in the blood.[5341] Thus, decreased methionine intake on a plant-based diet may be another factor contributing to lower, safer homocysteine levels.

The irony is that those who eat plant-based diets long-term can develop terrible homocysteine levels. Meat eaters may average 11 µmol/L, but vegetarians can be at nearly 14 µmol/L and vegans at 16 µmol/L.[5342] Why? Vegetarians and vegans get a lot of fiber and folate, but not enough vitamin B_{12}, which in modern times is only found dependably in animal products, fortified foods, or supplements. As I noted on page 211, a regular, reliable source of vitamin B_{12} is critical for anyone eating a plant-based diet. (It's possible Leonardo da Vinci's stroke might have been from his non-B_{12}-fortified vegetarian diet elevating his homocysteine levels.[5343]) However, when vegans take B_{12}, their homocysteine levels drop below 5 µmol/L.[5344] Why not just down to 11 µmol/L like the rest of the population? The reason the general public may be stuck up at 11 µmol/L is presumably due to a lack of folate. Once vegans got enough B_{12}, they could finally fully exploit the benefits of their fiber- and folate-rich plant-based diets and achieve the lowest levels of all.

Cognitive Stimulation, Music Therapy, and Cryostimulation

There are a few common nondrug, non-supplement, non-lifestyle approaches to dementia treatment, such as "use-it-or-lose-it" mental stimulation,[5345] group social activities,[5346] music therapy,[5347,5348,5349] and cryotherapy,[5350] that I profile in see.nf/cog. All unfortunately offer little or no lasting cognitive improvement but may provide some peripheral benefits.

BRAIN FOODS

Given what we've learned about the beneficial effects of plant food constituents, like polyphenols and fiber, and the detrimental effects of animal and junk food components, like salt and saturated fat, it should come as no surprise that a systematic review and meta-analysis of diet quality and dementia found that healthier diets are associated with significantly lower risk of developing Alzheimer's disease and dementia in general. Healthier dietary patterns were typically defined as being higher in fruits, vegetables, legumes, and whole grains, and lower in meats.[5351] In a cohort study that followed more than 5,000 adults with an average age of fifty-one for sixteen years, a healthier diet was also associated with the small minority (4 percent) who achieved "ideal aging," meaning they were free of chronic disease and had peak performance in physical, mental, and cognitive tests. (Some of the ideal aging criteria were easier to attain than others. The first on the list was "Being alive.")[5352]

The World Health Organization Guidelines for reducing the risk of cognitive decline and dementia encourage eating a diet centered around "[f]ruits, vegetables, legumes (e.g. lentils, beans), nuts and whole grains," while limiting added sugars, salt, saturated fat, and the trans fats found in processed foods and, naturally, in meat and dairy.[5353] Certain plant foods, however, may stand out.

Using the largest twin registry in the world, researchers concluded that "greater fruit and vegetable consumption may lower the risk of dementia and Alzheimer's disease."[5354] The reason it's so useful to study twins is that we can get special insight into environmental and dietary influences if one gets Alzheimer's and the other doesn't, since, genetically, twins are so similar. A meta-analysis of all such observational studies found that each additional serving (100 g) of fruits or vegetables a day was associated with a 13 percent reduction in the odds of cognitive impairment and dementia.[5355] Of the half dozen cohort studies that followed tens of thousands of people for up to thirty years, those in the highest category of fruit and vegetable consumption had a 43 percent lower risk of developing Alzheimer's disease compared to those who ate the least.

Any fruits and vegetables in particular? In a recent state-of-the-art review on preventing Alzheimer's disease specifically, the directors of Loma Loma Linda University's Alzheimer's Prevention Program laid out seven "key takeaways":[5356]

1. Reduce processed sugars.
2. Reduce fats, especially saturated fat.
3. Reduce animal products.
4. Reduce processed foods.
5. Consume more plants of all varieties, especially greens and beans.

6. Increase consumption of fruits, especially berries.
7. Reduce salt consumption.

Note that berries and greens were singled out, the brain foods of the fruit and vegetable kingdoms. Eating strawberries and spinach can mitigate age-related cognitive decline in rats.[5357] What about in people?

BLUEBERRIES

There are 8,000 different kinds of polyphenols found ubiquitously in foods of plant origin,[5358] but berries are packed with them.[5359] There is a subset of polyphenols called anthocyanins that are natural red, blue, and purple pigments capable of crossing the blood-brain barrier and localizing in brain regions involved in learning and memory.[5360] Given their powerful antioxidant and anti-inflammatory properties, aging researchers started feeding berries to rodents.

Older rats fed blueberries or strawberries experienced a reversal in age-related decrements of cognitive performance.[5361] The first experiments on older humans weren't published until 2010, starting with a small pilot study. Older men and women suffering from memory complaints were given either the juice equivalent of a whopping four to six cups of wild blueberries or a placebo drink each day for twelve weeks.[5362] The apparent cognitive improvements after the three months of the study were sufficient to inspire a more rigorous trial with a more modest daily serving size. Healthy men and women between the ages of sixty and seventy-five were randomized to the equivalent of one cup a day of regular (non-wild) blueberries (in freeze-dried powder form) or placebo (a blueberry-flavored and colored powder with the same calories, but no actual berries). Compared to placebo, the real berry group again experienced improvements in certain cognitive measures. The researchers concluded, "These findings show that the addition of easily achievable quantities of blueberry to the diets of older adults can improve some aspects of cognition."[5363]

The participants in the follow-up study were cognitively intact. Is it possible that one cup of regular blueberries is sufficient to boost cognition in healthy people, but five cups of wild blueberries are needed for the cognitively impaired? A study using a single cup of regular blueberries for mild cognitive impairment wasn't published until 2020. The randomized, double-blind, placebo-controlled trial found significant cognitive enhancement over placebo after a few months.[5364]

Even a single meal can do it. Multiple randomized controlled trials have shown that kids do significantly better on executive function and memory performance tests (but not reading) in the hours immediately following the consumption of the equivalent of about one and a half cups of wild blueberries compared to placebo.[5365,5366,5367,5368] Similar acute cognitive benefits within hours of consumption of a single dose of wild blueberries (one cup's worth) have also been demonstrated in adults, particularly in the context of more demanding tasks and cognitive fatigue.[5369]

Dairy Buries Berries

In the one trial that did not show clear beneficial effects of blueberry consumption, the berries were blended in milk.[5370] We've known for fifteen years that adding milk to black tea can completely blunt the positive effects of tea on artery function. The researchers blamed casein—a protein in milk that binds polyphenols and can prevent their absorption.[5371] The one plant-based milk that's been tested (soymilk) did not show the same irreversible binding.[5372] But eating milk chocolate or dark chocolate with a glass of milk blocks the absorption of about half of select cocoa polyphenols.[5373] Similarly, adding milk to coffee results in fewer than half of the chief polyphenols making it into your system,[5374] and the same happens with berries and cream.[5375]

Mixing strawberries with water causes a nice spike in strawberry anthocyanins in our blood over the next three hours, but that spike is cut by about half if the same strawberries are mixed with milk.[5376] It's the same with blueberries, as laid out in a study titled "Antioxidant Activity of Blueberry Fruit Is Impaired by Association with Milk." Researchers found that the total antioxidant capacity of our bloodstream shoots up within an hour of consuming a cup and a half of blueberries with water, and it remains elevated five hours later. With milk, one might expect less of a bump, but study participants ended up even worse than when they started. After eating a whole bowl of blueberries, they had *less* antioxidant capacity in their body—because they ate them with milk.[5377] That could explain the lack of clear cognitive benefit in the berries and milk study, as well as the heterogeneity in blueberry blood pressure–lowering studies. The studies that used water showed a significant benefit, but the ones that incorporated milk or yogurt did not.[5378]

Aside from the milk study, fourteen out of fifteen randomized controlled trials of blueberries and mental performance found a significant improvement in at least one cognitive domain.[5379,5380] Four out of five interventional studies on improving artery function also found a blueberry benefit.[5381,5382] This may help explain some of the cognitive effects, as functional MRI scans have found blueberry consumption can improve blood flow to critical regions of the brain.[5383]

Most of the blueberry cognition studies were done on children or younger adults, but a few tried out berries on older populations. One found that taking fish oil alongside blueberries appears to eliminate any memory enhancement for some reason.[5384] Another suggested protection from postoperative cognitive dysfunction. General anesthesia can muck with the minds of the elderly. As many as one in four to one in three people over the age of sixty suffer a reduction in cognitive function after being put under on the operating table, and this can last for weeks or months.[5385] However, when older individuals were randomized to get a little more than a pint of blueberries' worth of blueberry juice a day for two weeks before getting elective major surgery, they suffered significantly less postoperative memory disturbance, compared to participants who got nothing.[5386] But, as we know, with a do-nothing control group, placebo effects cannot be ruled out. Some are of the opinion that it is too early to draw "definitive conclusions"[5387] and that blueberries are not ready to be "administered in routine clinical practice,"[5388] but what level of evidence do you need when we're talking about a food that's healthy anyway?

OTHER BERRIES

In rats, raspberries can ameliorate some of the learning and memory impairments induced by a high-fat diet,[5389] but cherries can also boost rat cognition,[5390] yet when put to the test in people, tart cherry juice failed to significantly improve outcomes compared to control beverages[5391] after taking into account the sheer number of variables tested.[5392] Cranberry juice also flopped.[5393] As I detail in see.nf/mindberries, a bunch of different berries were able to improve cognition in both the young[5394] and the old,[5395] though the longest interventional trial period has only been twenty-four weeks.[5396]

To see if short-term improvements in cognition translate into affecting the course of brain aging, we must look to observational trials that follow subjects for multitudes for years. For example, one study followed the cognition of hundreds of twins over a decade and found that the anthocyanins in less than a quarter cup of blueberries a day or around a daily cup of strawberries seemed to slow cognitive aging by four years.[5397] These results suggest that simply eating a handful of berries every day, an easy and delicious dietary tweak, may slow your brain's aging by years. That's one of the reasons I have them every day at breakfast.

VEGETABLE NITRATES

Of eighteen different food groups, consumption of vegetables was associated with the least brain volume loss over time.[5398] In cohort studies large enough to get even more granular, of all categories of vegetables, dark green leafies showed among the strongest protective association against cognitive decline.[5399,5400] Those eating green vegetables every day had 78 percent lower odds of suffering from cognitive impairment.[5401] The Rush Memory and Aging Project compared the cognitive decline over five years in men and women with an average age of eighty-one who ate green leafy vegetables every day versus those eating less than a serving a week and made an extraordinary discovery. Are you sitting down? Quoting from the study: "The rate of decline among those who consumed 1–2 servings per day was the equivalent of being 11 years younger compared with those who rarely or never consumed green leafy vegetables."[5402] So *now* are you sitting down . . . to a big salad?

In the Harvard Nurses' Health Study, the only category that appeared to beat out green leafies for cognitive function were cruciferous vegetables, like broccoli, cabbage, and cauliflower; veggies like kale and collards got double billing, straddling both groups.[5403] Broccoli sprout juice[5404] or straight sulforaphane,[5405] the compelling cruciferous component, shows a broad range of neuroprotective effects in vitro against everything from arsenic and carbon monoxide to pesticides and memory-erasing drugs. Sulforaphane has also been shown to be directly protective in various rat and mouse models of Alzheimer's disease,[5406] but it wasn't put to the test in people until recently.

The 2021 study involved randomizing older men and women to the amount of sulforaphane precursor found in three cups of broccoli[5407] each day for twelve weeks. It provided the first direct evidence that cruciferous vegetables may improve working memory and processing speed.[5408] However, given that population studies also single out non-cruciferous greens—spinach, for example, has even been referred to as an "anti-Alzheimer plant"[5409]—might other components in greens also play a role? For instance, what about nitrates?

As we age, our cerebral blood flow drops, which may influence cognitive decline and the development of neurodegenerative disease.[5410] This reduction in the amount of blood flowing through our brain may be due to an age-related decrease in the production of nitric oxide, that "open sesame" molecule that dilates our blood vessels, causing them to widen and thereby increasing blood flow. But production of nitric oxide can be boosted by the consumption of nitrate-rich vegetables, like leafy greens and beets, which is one of the reasons they can improve athletic performance. What about cognitive performance?

Check out see.nf/braingreens for all the studies, but basically, nitric oxide can not only improve brain function but maybe even structure—the development of connectivity networks more closely resembling those of younger adults. This was taken as evidence of the potential enhancement of neuroplasticity in older brains with nitrate-rich vegetables.[5411]

A PIGMENT OF YOUR IMAGINATION

Dark green leafy vegetables are also one of the most concentrated sources of carotenoids[5412] and vitamin K.[5413] Higher levels of the plant-based vitamin K (*phyl-loquinone*, or vitamin K_1) are associated with higher cognitive function in centenarians, but that is not the case with higher levels of an animal-based form of vitamin K (*menaquinone-4*, a type of vitamin K_2). So, the higher levels of K seen in more cognitively intact centenarians may have just been a proxy for greens consumption. For example, blood levels of plant-based vitamin K were highly correlated with the levels of lutein,[5414] a carotenoid in greens that concentrates in the human brain.[5415]

Our brain is especially vulnerable to free radical attacks, due to its high fat content and cauldron of high metabolic activity.[5416] We certainly don't want our brain to go rancid. In my video see.nf/brainlutein, I review the importance of lutein for brain health, based in part on autopsy studies. If only there were a way we could physically look into the living brain with our own two eyes. There is—with our own two eyes!

The retina, the back of our eyeball, is actually an extension of our central nervous system. It's an outpouching of the brain during development, and, right in the middle, there's a yellowish spot. This is what doctors see when we look into your eye with that bright light. That spot, called the macula, is our HD camera, where we get the highest-resolution vision, and it's packed with lutein (from the Latin *luteus* for "yellow").[5417] Since levels in the retina can correspond to brain levels, our eyes can be a window into our brain, and indeed the amount of "macular pigment," which consists of lutein and other carotenoids in greens, like zeaxanthin, correlates with cognitive test scores[5418] and improvements of brain function[5419] and structure.[5420]

Where is lutein found? The avocado and egg industries like to boast about how much of these macular pigments is in their products, but the real superstars are dark green leafy vegetables. A half cup of cooked kale has fifty times more lutein than a hard-boiled egg; a spinach salad would offer more lutein than a fifty-egg omelet.[5421] Even Avocado Board–funded studies couldn't show guac-related benefits,[5422,5423] but adding as little as 60 g of spinach, which is like one-fifth of a 10-oz package of frozen spinach, can significantly boost macular pigment in most people within a month.[5424]

As you can see in see.nf/luteintrials, lutein/zeaxanthin supplements can improve vision[5425] and cognition,[5426] but while they can help both prevent and treat a leading cause of age-related vision loss[5427] (see the Preserving Your Vision chapter), supplements do not appear to improve the cognition of those already stricken with Alzheimer's disease.[5428]

Lion's Mane Mushroom

Small studies on about 1 to 3 g a day of powdered lion's mane mushroom (known, less palatably, as bearded tooth fungus) found some cognitive benefits for those with normal cognition[5429] and mild cognitive impairment,[5430] but not early Alzheimer's, though there was an improvement in the ability to perform activities of daily living, a measure of independence. Details on these studies and more in see.nf/mane.

COFFEE AND TEA

In the Adventist Health Study-2, the largest prospective study of plant-based eaters to date, I was surprised to see the average dietary polyphenol intake of nonvegetarians was *higher* than the vegetarians and vegans. Why would this be? Mainly because the nonvegetarians drank more coffee,[5431] which is the leading source of polyphenols in the United States.[5432] Is coffee consumption good for the brain? It's complicated, as I detail in see.nf/coffeetea, but basically, an apparent lack of overall association between coffee drinking and dementia may be obscured by deleterious effects of high coffee consumption[5433] potentially balancing out protective effects of low coffee consumption.[5434]

Data on green tea, however, appear to have a linear dose-response, meaning that any green tea consumption is better than none when it comes to risk of cognitive deficits, and the more, the better.[5435] Interventional studies have found that *black* tea can acutely improve attention and alertness,[5436] but population studies did not find it related to the risk of dementia or cognitive decline.[5437]

BRAIN-BOOSTING SPICES

Garlic compounds[5438] and extracts[5439] have been shown to ameliorate age-related cognitive dysfunction and reduce Alzheimer's neuropathology in rodents. To test garlic in people, young healthy volunteers were randomized to five weeks of twice-a-day capsules containing just an eighth of a teaspoon of straight garlic powder, like you would find at any grocery store. Compared to placebo capsules matched for color, texture, size, shape, and even smell, those getting the pinches of garlic powder experienced significantly improved memory and attention.[5440] As I detail in see.nf/brainspice, ginger may help in middle age,[5441] and as little as a quarter teaspoon of ground black cumin seeds can have positive cognitive impacts in both the young[5442] and the old.[5443]

KEEN AS A BEAN

The association between legume consumption and improved cognitive performance[5444] has been used to try to explain why dementia prevalence is lower in

East Asia, where people eat ten to forty times more soybean products compared to those in the West.[5445] I review the conflicting population data in see.nf/brainsoy, but in terms of interventional evidence, there have been sixteen randomized controlled trials involving more than a thousand participants, and, overall, soy or soy compound interventions have been found to improve overall cognitive function and memory.[5446] For example, disguising soybeans in chili to randomize people to higher soy diets resulted in significant improvements in short- and long-term memory within ten weeks.[5447]

Some Are More Equol Than Others

There has been one randomized, double-blind, placebo-controlled trial of soy isoflavones in Alzheimer's patients. After six months, no cognitive benefits over placebo were found for a few daily servings of soy foods' worth;[5448] however, there was preliminary evidence of benefit among those who were equol producers.[5449] Among elderly Japanese, equol producers also had less than half of the white matter brain lesions on MRI, compared to nonproducers.[5450] Check out see.nf/equol for details, but basically, some people benefit from soy even more than others since they have gut bacteria that can soup up an isoflavone in soy into an even more beneficial compound called equol.[5451]

About half of Japanese and Korean people can produce equol, but only about one in seven Americans can.[5452] Excessive use of antibiotics can wipe out our good bugs and turn an equol producer into a nonproducer, but how can we acquire the right bugs in the first place?[5453] There is a group of Westerners with high equol production rates: vegetarians, perhaps because they eat more fiber,[5454] or less dietary fat[5455] or cholesterol.[5456] Whatever it is about those eating plant-based diets, they may soon be the only remaining majority equol producers, as Asian populations continue to westernize their diets.[5457]

WHOLE GRAINS FOR WHOLE BRAINS?

Based on cross-sectional studies of thousands of men and women older than the age of fifty, high whole-grain intake is positively associated with the Successful Aging Index, a measure representing not only the avoidance of disease and disability but also the maintenance of cognitive function and engagement in physical, social, and productive activities.[5458] This was determined after attempts to control for various other dietary and lifestyle factors, but it's impossible to control for everything. When mice were randomized to barley instead of white rice, they lived significantly longer, suffered less hair loss, achieved a glossier coat, were better able to balance on a rod and hang upside down for longer, and retained better long-term spatial memory.[5459] In contrast, as I document in see.nf/braingrain, the human interventional evidence to date is underwhelming.

BRAIN HEALTH NUTS

Frequent nut eaters tend to live longer[5460] and think better,[5461] but that doesn't mean the nuts necessarily have anything to do with either. In see.nf/nutbrains, I address some of the factors confounding population studies on nut consumption. The bottom line is that evidence from interventional studies on nuts for cognition has been underwhelming, though a substudy of PREDIMED suggested that if you're eating half a handful of nuts a day, it may be worthwhile to go up to a full palmful, and if you're using regular olive oil, it may be worth the switch to extra-virgin.[5462]

FISH OIL FAIL

What about fish oil for brain health? A review of dementia risk reduction strategies compiled a list of common attributes of purportedly brain-healthy diets. People are encouraged to limit their intake of meat, including poultry, and fatty, sugary, and salty processed foods, as well as eat a predominantly plant-based diet rich in fruits and vegetables (especially berries and greens), legumes, and whole grains. But, there is also a tendency to encourage people to eat fatty fish.[5463]

Recommendations for fish consumption are based on observational data finding, for example, a significantly lower risk of Alzheimer's (but not dementia more broadly) in fish eaters,[5464] a significantly lower risk of dementia (but not Alzheimer's disease specifically) in fish oil supplement takers,[5465] and greater hippocampal volume associated with higher levels of omega-3s in the blood.[5466] Fish eaters also tend to eat more greens and berries, smoke less, exercise more,[5467] and have higher education levels than non-fish-eaters.[5468] Fish oil supplement takers also appear to eat more fruits and vegetables, smoke less, and exercise more than those who don't take those supplements, and they also tend to have higher socioeconomic status.[5469] To see if the apparent benefits of aquatic omega-3s from population studies are real and not just due to associated confounding factors, researchers have performed dozens of randomized, controlled, interventional trials.

There have been three randomized, placebo-controlled trials of omega-3s for Alzheimer's disease over periods of six, twelve, and eighteen months, and, unfortunately, they failed to show a cognitive benefit.[5470] Maybe the study participants' disease had progressed so much by the start of the study that it was too late by then?[5471] The World Health Organization funded the latest and largest comprehensive review of long-chain omega-3s (from algae or fish) for cognitive outcomes, and researchers found no significant protection from cognitive impairment or dementia and only "clinically unimportant" effects on global cognition. The reviewers conclude: "People concerned about their cognitive health should be advised that taking long-chain omega-3 supplements is not helpful for cognition. . . ."[5472]

IS THERE A THRESHOLD EFFECT?

The concept of vitamins was first described by none other than Dr. Funk.[5473] In his landmark paper in 1912, he discussed the notion that there were complex compounds our body couldn't make from scratch, so we had to get them from our diet.[5474] By the mid-twentieth century, all the vitamins had been discovered and isolated,[5475] but it wasn't until the 1960s that we realized that certain fats were essential, too,[5476] including omega-3 fats concentrated in foods like flaxseeds and walnuts that our body can elongate into the long-chain omega-3s DHA and EPA, which we can also get preformed from algae or fish sources.[5477]

The fact that it took so long and under such extreme circumstances to demonstrate the essential nature of omega-3s (see.nf/essentialfats) illustrates how hard it is to develop overt omega-3 deficiency. Of course, the amount required to avoid deficiency is not necessarily the optimal amount for health. (See my scurvy example on page 211.) There doesn't appear to be any cognitive benefit of long-chain omega-3 supplementation for the general public, but what about for those who don't eat fish?

Consider the famous Multidomain Alzheimer Preventive Trial, in which more than a thousand elderly individuals with memory complaints were randomized to DHA and EPA (in fish oil) or placebo for three years. Overall, the DHA and EPA had no significant effect on the rate on cognitive decline.[5478] However, most of the subjects were eating fish and thereby already getting preformed DHA and EPA in their diets. So, perhaps there is a threshold for protection and they all started out above it. Finding no benefit in general population studies like this cannot fully inform us about the role of long-chain omega-3s in brain health. That would be akin to giving half of these people oranges, finding no difference in scurvy rates (zero in both groups), and concluding that vitamin C plays no role in scurvy.

What if you sifted back through the Multidomain Alzheimer Preventive Trial data and just looked at what happened to those who had low levels of fish consumption (as estimated by low blood levels of long-chain omega-3s)? That's exactly what the researchers did, and they found that for at least one measure of executive function, there was significantly less decline in the fish oil group compared to placebo.[5479] One always has to be careful with post hoc analyses, so the results are considered exploratory rather than conclusive. Nonetheless, this could potentially explain why clinical trials of long-chain omega-3s have so often failed. Perhaps it's because the studies were not focused on those who could benefit most—that is, those who start out with low levels in the first place.

OMEGA-3 SUPPLEMENTS

So, should people who don't eat fish consider taking DHA and EPA for optimal brain health? That's the question I address in see.nf/dhabrain. Jumping straight to the interventional evidence, a randomized, double-blind, placebo-controlled trial of cognitively intact elderly found both a significant improvement in executive function and significantly less brain shrinkage after about six months of long-chain omega-3 supplementation compared to placebo.[5480] A similar twelve-month trial of algae-based DHA in cognitively impaired elderly showed significantly improved cognitive function (including full-scale IQ) and volume of the hippocampus—that seat of memory in the brain—compared to placebo.[5481] So, having sufficient EPA and DHA long-chain omega-3s may be important for preserving brain function and structure, but what's "sufficient" and how do we get there?

As I describe in the video, those who don't eat fish tend to fall below a tentative omega-3 threshold that can be reached by taking 250 mg of a mix of pollutant-free (algae-derived) EPA/DHA. Technically, the only omega-3 that is truly essential is ALA, the plant-based, short-chain omega-3, because we can make DHA and EPA from it.[5482] However, the efficiency of this conversion varies and may decline with age.[5483] So, while most DHA supplementation trials in the general population fail to abate cognitive decline,[5484] until we know more, non-fish-eaters should consider supplementing[5485] with 100 to 300 mg of DHA a day.[5486]

WHY NOT JUST EAT FISH?

The comprehensive World Health Organization review that failed to find appreciable cognitive benefits to long-chain omega-3 supplementation suggested that perhaps any upsides are counterbalanced by the potential neurotoxic contamination of fish and fish oil products with heavy metals, organochlorines, polychlorinated biphenyls, and polycyclic aromatic hydrocarbons.[5487] This may help explain studies that have found higher fish consumption predicting *worse* cognitive function.[5488] Most such findings have emerged from studies of children, but higher omega-3 levels have also been associated with higher levels of cognitive impairment and dementia in older adults.[5489]

Watch see.nf/fishbrain for details on the actual studies, but here's an illustrative case report: A ninety-one-year-old man with years of progressive memory loss was diagnosed with Alzheimer's disease. Cognitive testing showed he had dementia, and his friends and family assumed he was nearing the end of his life. However, a detailed history revealed that he had consumed swordfish once or twice a week for several years, and he was subsequently found to have severely elevated mercury levels. But, within ten months after high-mercury fish was removed from his diet, his mercury levels dropped to normal, his memory bounced back, and cognitive testing showed he no longer had dementia.[5490] So, it seemed he didn't have Alzheimer's disease after all but rather mercury poisoning from a handful of monthly meals of contaminated fish.

A systematic review and meta-analysis of toxic metals and Alzheimer's disease found that blood levels of mercury and another heavy metal, cadmium, were significantly elevated in Alzheimer's patients compared to controls.[5491] Switching to a plant-based diet can cut cadmium (and lead) levels in half within just three months, and lower mercury levels by 20 percent, as measured in hair samples, but the heavy metal levels bounce back when an omnivorous diet is resumed.[5492] Whether this helps account for the data showing two to three times lower dementia rates in vegetarians[5493] is unclear. Although blood levels of mercury are correlated with Alzheimer's risk, brain mercury levels, assessed on autopsy, do not correlate with brain pathology.[5494]

Perhaps mercury blood levels are just markers for fish consumption and the real culprit is one of the other pollutants, like PCBs, that can get stuck in our body for decades.[5495] In that case, what about purified fish oil? The methods fish oil supplement manufacturers use, like distillation, leave considerable amounts of PCBs and other pollutants in the products, so much so that when taken as directed, salmon, herring, and tuna oils would exceed the tolerable daily intake for toxicity.[5496] Thankfully, one can get the benefits without the risks by getting DHA from algae instead,[5497] which is where the fish get it for themselves.[5498] So, we can cut out the middle-fish and get DHA at the bottom of the food chain, directly from the source.

BMAA in Seafood

Famed neurologist Oliver Sachs and colleagues solved a convoluted puzzle of a mysterious cluster on some exotic tropical isle of what seemed like three neurodegenerative diseases wrapped into one: ALS parkinsonism dementia complex.[5499] Affected natives were eating flying fox fruit bats who ate the seeds of the fruit of a tree that concentrated a neurotoxin called BMAA from blue-green algae that grow in its roots.[5500] As I document in see.nf/alsfish, BMAA gained global concern when it was then found in the brains of Floridians who died from Alzheimer's disease[5501] and in Florida seafood at levels comparable to the contaminated fruit bats.[5502]

(continued)

In my follow-up video see.nf/alsdiet, I note that some researchers consider BMAA to be a strong contender as a major contributor to Alzheimer's disease,[5503] especially after monkeys fed BMAA-spiked food developed Alzheimer's-type pathology in their brains.[5504] The greatest strike against the theory, however, is that some of the autopsy studies—including the most comprehensive one—found no trace of BMAA in Alzheimer's brains at all,[5505] part of an ongoing debate about the sensitivity of different testing methods.[5506] Until the matter is settled, some consider it prudent to try to limit exposure.[5507]

In addition to fish and crustaceans,[5508] BMAA is found concentrated in shark products and certain algae supplements. Shark fins (used for soup)[5509] have among the highest BMAA levels recorded,[5510] and fifteen out of sixteen shark cartilage dietary supplements were found to be contaminated.[5511] Of eighteen blue-green algae (*A. flos-aquae*) and spirulina supplements, eight contained toxins at levels exceeding the tolerable daily intake values, but only two contained BMAA.[5512] However, of five protein powder supplements containing spirulina that were tested, four turned up contaminated.[5513]

EAT FOR YOUR BRAIN'S HEALTH

Knowing what components or specific foods we should—or shouldn't—include to help protect our brain function is critical, but what is the best overall diet for preserving our mind?

GIVEN THE FINGER

Given the apparent efficacy of various individual lifestyle interventions, what if we combined some of them? The first large, randomized, controlled trial of a multidomain, lifestyle-based intervention for at-risk older adults was the Finnish Geriatric Intervention Study to Prevent Cognitive Impairment and Disability (or FINGER, for *FINnish GERiatric*), published in 2015.[5514] More than a thousand men and women in their sixties and seventies were randomized to either a combination of nutritional guidance, exercise, cognitive training, and vascular risk factor management or a control group receiving only regular general health advice. After two years, the improvement in cognition was significantly better in the lifestyle intervention group, though the effect size was small (0.13).[5515] (Effect size can be quantified as a "standardized mean difference" [SMD]. An SMD of 0.2 is considered small, 0.5 moderate, and 0.8 large.) On a population scale, even small effects can have important public health implications, but why wasn't there a greater impact?

The rather modest results of interventional trials like FINGER have been used to argue against a major role for lifestyle behaviors in the prevention of dementia, but it may actually be because they didn't go far enough. For example, the recommended "brain-healthy diet"[5516] in the FINGER trial was no more than advice to eat four servings of fruits and vegetables a day, for example, and to choose lower-fat meat and dairy. It's true that the more participants stuck to the diet recommendations, the better they did, but small changes may only beget small results.[5517]

MEDITERRANEAN DIET

What about broader sweeping changes, like a Mediterranean-style diet? There have been dozens of observational studies following a total of nearly 100,000 people for three years up to twelve years that found those scoring higher on a Mediterranean diet index tended to have less of a decline in global cognitive function. However, the effect size was again relatively small,[5518] and there was no discernible reduction in the rates of incident dementia or mild cognitive impairment.[5519] About a dozen randomized controlled trials of Mediterranean-style diets have reported on seventy-two cognitive test outcomes, but only a small percentage—eight out of seventy-two—showed a statistically significant advantage.[5520,5521]

To see how the Mediterranean diet could be improved, researchers tried to tease out its protective components. Fish consumption showed no benefit, and neither did moderate alcohol consumption. The two critical pieces appeared to be vegetable consumption and the higher ratio between unsaturated fats and saturated fats, essentially the balance between plant fats and animal fats.[5522] Of all the dietary features of Mediterranean diet scoring, the one most linked to better cognitive performance and greater total brain volumes is reduced meat consumption.[5523]

MIND DIET

To devise a diet tailored to protect the brain, researchers at Rush University Medical Center chose components that reflected the most compelling evidence to create their Mediterranean–DASH Intervention for Neurodegenerative Delay (MIND) diet. The DASH diet, which stands for Dietary Approaches to Stop Hypertension, was originally designed for cardiovascular defense. From it, they took its emphasis on reducing saturated fat, sweets, and meats (including fish). From the Mediterranean diet, they took dairy restriction and the emphasis on beans and nuts, but, instead of potatoes, the MIND diet took as its centerpiece the consumption of green leafy vegetables at least six times a week. And, instead of fruit in general, it specifically emphasized berry consumption. The MIND diet also gave people points for reducing their intake of fast food or fried foods to less than once a week.[5524] "Combining the two diets," the Academy of Nutrition and Dietetics summarized, "the MIND diet emphasizes natural, plant-based foods, specifically promoting an increase in the consumption of berries and green leafy vegetables, with limited intakes of animal-based and high saturated fat foods."[5525]

Watch see.nf/mind to see what it can do. In short, there have been about a dozen studies on the MIND diet, and they all found that greater adherence to it was associated with benefit to at least some aspect of cognition, with seven of the nine trials that measured global cognitive function finding benefits across the board,[5526] including up to a 53 percent lower risk of developing Alzheimer's disease.[5527] And, the side effects may include a longer life. Compared to the bottom third of MIND diet scores, those of an average age of seventy achieving the upper third had a 37 percent lower risk of dying in the subsequent twelve years.[5528] However, as of yet, there has only been one randomized controlled trial to properly test the diet. So far, so good, with the three-month pilot trial finding that those randomized to advice to follow the MIND diet had significant improvements in six out of eight cognitive measures.[5529]

The Harvard Nurses' Health Study was large enough to try to tease through the MIND diet's components to see what was predominantly driving the apparent benefit, and the researchers concluded it was the reduction in saturated and trans fats.[5530] If the key factor in the Mediterranean diet is meat reduction and the crux of the MIND diet seems to be cutting down on the saturated fat and trans fats in butter and junk, then what about trying whole food, plant-based nutrition?[5531]

WHOLE FOOD, PLANT-BASED DIET

In my video see.nf/antiaging, I explore the possible reasons why longtime vegetarians are as much as three times less likely to develop dementia.[5532] It could be because they're exposed to less saturated fat,[5533] cholesterol,[5534] animal protein,[5535] or AGE gerontotoxins.[5536] However, though just moving away from animal foods without regard to the healthfulness of plant-based replacements appears to protect from cognitive impairment,[5537] MIND diet scoring more closely aligns with cognitive performance than just scoring for reduction of animal products, suggesting that there may be benefits to the emphasis on healthy plant foods, like greens and berries.[5538]

So maybe it's also because plant-based diets protect against oxidative stress and inflammation.[5539] Dietary factors may also influence the effect of stress on cognitive decline. Diets characterized by high intake of animal proteins, saturated fats, and added sugars, along with low intake of plant-based foods, can increase the release of corticosteroid stress hormones like cortisol from the adrenal glands, which may promote the development of dementia.[5540]

The key takeaways for preventing Alzheimer's with diet are: Reduce added sugars, added salt, saturated fat, animal products, and processed foods in general, and eat more plants (especially greens and beans) and fruits (especially berries).[5541]

THERE ARE NO RANDOMIZED CONTROLLED TRIALS OF PARACHUTES

After reading this chapter, you might be surprised to see conclusions from systematic reviews on what we can do to prevent cognitive decline like this one: "The current literature does not provide adequate evidence to make recommendations for interventions."[5542] Researchers cite the lack of sufficient randomized controlled trials as a basis for these kinds of conclusions.[5543] Randomized controlled trials are undeniably the gold standard for testing new medications. The highest level of evidence is necessary because drugs kill an estimated 100,000 Americans every year. I'm not talking about overdoses, medication errors, or illicit drugs. Regular, FDA-approved prescription drugs are the sixth leading cause of death in the United States.[5544] So, you'd better make absolutely certain the benefits of new drugs outweigh their potentially life-threatening risks.

However, if you're talking about healthy lifestyle behaviors, the side effects are all essentially good, so we arguably don't need the same level of evidence to prescribe them. In my video see.nf/rctdementia, I profile a "modest proposal" published in the *Journal of Alzheimer's Disease* for a series of randomized controlled trials for dementia prevention. I mean, how can we *really* know that traumatic brain injury raises dementia risk unless we randomize folks to get beaten in the head with baseball bats? Until we have randomized control data, how can we physicians recommend patients not get hit in the head? While we were at it, we could chain thousands to treadmills versus couches for a few decades or hook thousands on cigarettes.[5545] The editorial concluded: "It is time to realize that the ultimate study . . . in regard to lifestyle and cognitive health in aging *cannot be done*. Yet the absence of definitive evidence should not restrict physicians from making reasonable recommendations based on the evidence that is available."[5546]

Having said that, as I'm writing this in 2023, a randomized controlled trial to see if a whole food, plant-based diet and lifestyle program can slow down, stop, or even reverse the course of Alzheimer's disease is currently wrapping up. Dr. Dean Ornish and colleagues have randomized fifty-one patients with early Alzheimer's to essentially the same diet and lifestyle program he used to reverse the progression of heart disease, type 2 diabetes, hypertension, high cholesterol, and early-stage prostate cancer.[5547] With the recognition that this book would probably be published after their initial results were released, Dean gave me an exciting sneak peek at their preliminary findings—and what do you know: It looks like plant-based lifestyle changes are going to end up beating the new $50,000 biotech infusions for efficacy without causing your brain to swell and bleed.[5548]

PRESERVING YOUR MUSCLES

A loss in muscle mass is a characteristic of aging found in every species studied so far.[5549] In people, muscle mass tends to start to decline after age thirty,[5550] accelerating after age fifty to a loss of 1 to 2 percent every year.[5551] By eighty, approximately 50 percent of the fibers in the muscles of our limbs are lost.[5552] The annual loss of muscle strength can be even more dramatic, suggesting a loss of muscle *quality* as well as quantity.[5553] This is not just because people tend to become less active with age.[5554] Even among master athletes like marathon runners and weight lifters who remain fit throughout their lives, performance tends to decline after about forty, dropping in half by age eighty.[5555]

A POUND OF FLESH

Excessive age-related loss of skeletal muscle mass, strength, and function is termed *sarcopenia*, from the Greek *sarx* for "flesh" and *penia* for "loss." Approximately 25 percent of us suffer from sarcopenia by our late sixties and 40 percent by the time we're eighty,[5556] with rates running as high as nearly 70 percent in those seventy and older living in nursing homes.[5557]

Sarcopenia is associated with not only an increased risk of falls but an overall shorter lifespan.[5558] The loss of muscle strength may be even more important, though, as it is tied to mortality regardless of muscle mass.[5559] This applies to both upper and lower body strength,[5560] though hand grip strength is commonly used as a proxy for total body strength.[5561] Every kilogram of force decline in annual grip strength is correlated with a 33 percent increased risk of mortality. Even grip strength in middle age is highly predictive of late life disability twenty-five years later.[5562]

Frailty is a closely related concept. Though recognized for centuries, its definition wasn't standardized until 2001.[5563] Frailty is defined as having at least three of the following five criteria: weakness (as measured by grip strength), unintentional weight loss (of ten pounds or 5 percent of body weight in the past year), exhaustion (self-reported), slow walking speed (based on the time to walk fifteen feet), and low physical activity.[5564] Individuals meeting one or two of the criteria are classified as "pre-frail."[5565] About one in forty are frail by age sixty-five, one in four after age seventy-five,[5566] and one in three of those older than eighty-five.[5567]

The heritability of muscle mass and strength may be as high as 50 to 60 percent.[5568] What can we do for the rest over which we may have some control?

USE IT OR LOSE IT

A study following sedentary Americans over the age of sixty-five for twelve years found that they lose about 1 percent of their muscle mass every year.[5569] In contrast, a similar study in Japan found age-related decreases in muscle mass "were trivial."[5570] Why the difference? In the Japanese study, the participants were informed of their results, so they often tried to improve through strength training before their next check-in. This was especially true among the middle-aged men, who got so competitive that their muscle mass may have actually *increased* with age, which shows that the steady loss of muscle mass with age is not inevitable. You just have to put in some effort.

Although we have yet to work out the best "dose"—timing, frequency, and repetitions[5571]—resistance exercise is considered the most effective strategy to prevent age-related muscle weakness,[5572] treat muscle loss,[5573] and improve physical function.[5574] For example, older men and women with an average age of seventy on a generic twenty-four-week strength training program with three sessions a week experienced about a 10 percent increase in leg muscle mass, a 40 percent increase in lower and upper body strength, and about a 20 percent decrease in sit-to-stand time,[5575] which is a measure of physical function that can predict fall risk.[5576] Exercise interventions are considered the key to maintaining the independence of frail and pre-frail individuals,[5577] but they can also reverse their frailty designation. Frail men and women with an average age of eighty were randomized to a program that combined endurance, strength, coordination, balance, and flexibility exercises for an hour a day, five days a week. All forty-nine of the individuals in the control group started out frail, and they remained frail. But sixteen of the fifty-one individuals in the exercise group (31 percent) reversed their frailty status within six months.[5578]

On the other hand, inactivity—or even a drop in activity levels—can actively make matters worse. Anyone would lose muscle mass after lying in bed for days at a time, but older adults on bed rest appear to lose muscle mass six times faster than younger people. Within just ten days of being on bed rest, older study subjects (average age sixty-seven) lost two pounds of lean leg mass,[5579] which is more than younger subjects (average age thirty-eight) lost in an entire month of bed rest.[5580] Immobilizing one leg in a knee brace for four days caused a similar drop (about 10 percent) in muscle strength in young and old individuals, but, a week later, the strength of the subjects in their twenties was fully recovered, whereas the strength of those in their sixties still remained relatively impaired.[5581] This helps explain why 30 to 60 percent of elderly patients may lose some independence in basic activities of daily living in the course of a single hospital stay.[5582]

Even a milder form of disuse can lead to muscle atrophy. Elderly men and women were asked to reduce their activity by dropping their daily step counts from their moderately active 6,000 steps a day down to around 1,400 daily steps. Within just two weeks, they lost about 4 percent of the lean mass in their legs, about 1.3 pounds. The investigators concluded, "This superficially 'benign' intervention of simply reducing daily steps demonstrates just how deleterious a period of inactivity . . . can be for older persons."[5583] This is especially worrisome given that older adults have such difficulty even with heavy strength training to recover muscle losses due to disuse and neglect. Use it or lose it—sometimes for good.

DEFUELING THE FLAMES

In the step-reduction study, the decline in activity was accompanied by an increase in markers of inflammation. For example, researchers found a 25 percent rise in the subjects' C-reactive protein levels within two weeks of reducing their step counts.[5584] The muscle wasting in cancer is mediated by inflammation; what about the muscle wasting of aging?[5585] Those suffering from sarcopenia,[5586] pre-frailty, and frailty[5587] do indeed tend to have higher levels of systemic inflammatory markers, such as C-reactive protein, which are independently associated with lower muscle mass and diminished upper and lower body strength.[5588] This has led to suggestions that anti-inflammatory diets may help.[5589]

Meta-analyses of observational studies, including a representative sample of the U.S. population,[5590] have found up to twice the odds of sarcopenia[5591] and frailty[5592] for those eating more pro-inflammatory diets. Eating high on the Dietary Inflammatory Index has also been associated with low grip strength, low walking speed,[5593] and impairment in the activities of daily living. This has all led to the proposal that chronic inflammation is a "key underlying mechanism" of frailty, but observational studies can't prove cause and effect.[5594]

An inflammatory trigger would help explain why saturated fat—the single most pro-inflammatory component of the Dietary Inflammatory Index[5595]—is associated with greater risk of sarcopenia.[5596] Compared to those getting about 8 percent of their calories from saturated fat—which meets the U.S. federal recommendation of less than 10 percent[5597] but exceeds the American Heart Association's advice to stay below 6 percent[5598]—those getting twice as much (16 percent) lost the amount of lean mass that you generally see with ten years of aging.[5599] This may help explain why the leg muscles of CrossFit trainees eating a ketogenic diet may shrink by as much as 8 percent.[5600] However, a more likely explanation is that without enough of the preferred fuel (carbohydrate), their bodies started burning more of their own protein.[5601] What about all the protein they were eating, though?

HUMAN PROTEIN REQUIREMENTS

In my video see.nf/proteinhistory, I trace the saga of enthusiasm for protein in the nutrition world,[5602] peaking with what was called the Great Protein Fiasco,[5603] followed by a massive downward recalculation of human protein requirements by the 1970s.[5604] To this day, however, some still obsess about protein.[5605] For example, those promoting Paleolithic diets try to make the case for protein from an evolutionary perspective.[5606]

One food, however, has been fine-tuned over millions of years to contain the perfect amount of protein just for us:[5607] human breast milk, which may actually have the lowest protein concentration compared to any other animal in the world, at less than 1 percent protein by weight.[5608] This is one of the reasons why dairy milk can be so dangerous for babies.[5609] Although the protein content in breast milk has been described as "extremely low," it's exactly where it needs to be—at the natural, normal level for our species.

The "low" protein level in human breast milk (about 6 percent of calories) doesn't mean that's all that adults need. At that level, elderly individuals would not be able to maintain their muscle mass.[5610] Adults can weigh ten times more than infants, but we only eat about four or five times more than babies do, so our food needs to be more concentrated in protein. Nevertheless, people tend to get about twice as much as they need.[5611] The recommended dietary allowance (RDA) is 0.8 g of protein per kg of body weight per day for all adults regardless of age, which is about your ideal weight in pounds multiplied by four and then divided by ten. So, someone whose ideal weight is 100 pounds may require up to 40 g of protein a day. On average, they probably only need about 30 daily g of protein, which is 0.66 g per kg, but we round it up to 0.8 g because everyone's different and we want to capture most of the bell curve.[5612] As I'll detail in the Protein Restriction chapter, people may be more likely to suffer from protein excess than protein deficiency.[5613]

Some advocate for protein intake for older individuals in excess of the official recommendations. Among them, not surprisingly, are consultants for the National Cattlemen's Beef Association and members of the Whey Protein Advisory Panel for the National Dairy Council.[5614] They argue that age-related muscle loss may be a consequence of "anabolic resistance" among the elderly, a diminished muscle-building response to weight training or protein intake, but most studies have failed to detect such a phenomenon.[5615] Indeed, the most comprehensive[5616] study on the protein needs of healthy adults found no difference in protein requirements with age,[5617] and authorities in the United States,[5618] the EU,[5619] and globally[5620] agree. However, just because the elderly don't *require* more protein doesn't necessarily mean they wouldn't benefit from more. And what about *unhealthy* adults already suffering from frailty or sarcopenia?

DOES EXTRA PROTEIN INCREASE MUSCLE MASS OR STRENGTH?

I do a deep dive in see.nf/muscleprotein, but basically, when all the studies on protein or amino acid supplementation for older men and women were put together, overall, there was no significant improvement in lean body mass or upper or lower body muscle strength.[5621] Even the term "lean body mass" can be misleading.[5622] Because high protein intake alone can cause liver and kidney swelling,[5623] an increase in total body lean mass may just be a reflection of "increased visceral organ size"[5624] or water retention.[5625]

In nonfrail older adults, extra protein or essential amino acid supplementation appears to have little[5626] or no[5627] effect on muscle mass, strength, or performance when taken alone or added to an exercise regimen. What about in those who really need it—sarcopenic, pre-frail, or frail individuals? One of the first things doled out by doctors is a "nutrition shake" like Ensure, typically an ultraprocessed sugary mess of corn syrup, oil, and protein concentrates, often laced with artificial colors, flavors, and sweeteners. Though Big Pharma giants like Abbott Laboratories (makers of Ensure) spend millions of dollars a year in lobbying and campaign contributions to help make these products medicine's go-to choice,[5628] a systematic review and meta-analysis of randomized clinical trials on such drinks for the management of frailty published in 2021 found no discernible benefit for any measured outcomes—muscle mass, muscle strength, muscle function, frailty status, cognitive function, or mortality.[5629]

Researchers have been trying to find effective ways to treat sarcopenia for decades, and, so far, only resistance exercise has consistently yielded benefits.[5630] One of the largest and most rigorous studies to treat pre-frail and frail adults was published in 2021. Hundreds were enrolled to test the effects of leucine, whey protein, soy protein, creatine, and a combination of creatine and whey versus a placebo control (cornstarch) in the context of a sixteen-week resistance training program. The strength training itself worked, increasing muscle mass and function, but everything else flopped. No added benefit to frail or pre-frail individuals taking any of those supplements compared to taking the cornstarch placebo.[5631]

IN HARM'S WHEY

I was surprised that neither milk[5632] nor milk protein[5633] was able to bulk up people more. After all, milk is naturally designed to put a few hundred pounds on a baby calf within just a few months. Of all proteins, the milk protein whey stimulates the greatest response in terms of short-term muscle protein synthesis, likely due to its high concentration of leucine, the amino acid that triggers mTOR. (If you remember from the mTOR chapter, that's the enzyme that accelerates growth but may also accelerate aging.) Straight leucine supplements also fail to add muscle.[5634] If leucine stimulates muscle protein synthesis, why doesn't this translate into greater muscle mass?

Muscle tissue is in constant flux.[5635] Every day, our entire musculature undergoes about a 2 percent turnover rate. Giving people a bolus of specially tagged protein, researchers were able to follow it through the body. About 10 percent of it gets socked away in our muscles within hours after consumption.[5636] In other words, we are what we just ate. Surprisingly, though, there is no correlation between these acute changes in muscle protein creation and long-term changes in muscle mass,[5637] as verified by MRI scans.[5638]

We used to think protein timing was important and that there was a narrow window of opportunity right after exercising to boost muscle growth, but again, the short-term measures don't predict long-term results. Instead, strength training appears to increase overall muscle protein-making capacity for whenever the protein is available.[5639] This realization led to the busting of another protein myth—the thought that it was better to spread protein intake throughout the day since muscle protein synthesis maxes out at a certain dose.[5640] If anything, when actually put to the test, the opposite result was found.[5641,5642,5643,5644]

This also explains why plant proteins can accrue muscle on par with animal proteins.[5645] For example, even though the acute muscle protein synthesis to whey protein is greater than soy protein in the immediate hours after consumption,[5646] the accretion of muscle mass and strength is the same. Even beef studies funded by the National Cattlemen's Beef Association weren't able to show a difference,[5647,5648] just as American Egg Board–funded studies failed to find muscle benefits from adding eggs.[5649,5650] However, JUST Egg, a plant-based egg patty made out of mung beans, did seem able to improve muscle strength, at least in what appeared to be a post hoc analysis of an eight-week randomized controlled trial.[5651]

So, in the end, whey protein may just leave one to suffer added mTOR activation side effects.[5652] Superficially, this includes the acne endured by whey-supplementing athletes[5653] and bodybuilders.[5654] More important, dermatologists editorialized that restricting dairy could help "prevent more serious mTOR . . . -driven diseases of civilization like obesity, diabetes and cancer."[5655] In a bid to slow muscle wasting in cancer, for example, researchers tried giving leucine to cancer-ridden mice but only ended up doubling the growth of their tumors.[5656] The isoflavone phytoestrogens in soy may do the opposite—suppressing mTOR, at least in mice[5657]—while alone boosting human lean mass independent of the protein in a randomized, double-blind, placebo-controlled trial.[5658] Just the isoflavones alone boosted fat-free limb mass at a daily dose equivalent of about three-quarters of a cup of tempeh, two-thirds of a cup of boiled soybeans, or a half cup of soy nuts.[5659]

PLANT PROTEIN PREFERRED

The association between plant-based dietary patterns and muscle mass, strength, and function is inconsistent,[5660] but some studies have shown that plant protein in particular is linked to a lower risk of sarcopenia,[5661] pre-frailty, and frailty,[5662] improved physical performance,[5663] and more successful aging, as measured in scales that take into account functional impairments, self-reported vitality, mental health, chronic diseases, participation in social activities with friends and family, and the number of yearly excursions.[5664] Researchers suggest it might be due to differences in the protein itself, such as the lower methionine content benefit in plant proteins I'll cover in the Protein Restriction chapter, but it could also be from the nutritional baggage that accompanies protein from animal sources.[5665]

Food is a package deal. If you go to the Harvard School of Public Health's web page on protein, you'll see that it emphasizes the source rather than the amount of protein as being most consequential for health. This is because foods present a "protein package," which can contain saturated fat and sodium on one hand, or antioxidants and fiber on the other. This is why its number one tip for making the best protein choices is "Get your protein from plants when possible."[5666]

Aren't Plant Proteins Inferior and Incomplete?

All nutrients come from the sun or the soil. Vitamin D, the "sunshine vitamin," is created when skin is exposed to sunlight, and everything else comes from the ground. Minerals originate from the earth, and vitamins from the plants and microorganisms that grow from it. The calcium in a cow's milk (and in her two-hundred-pound skeleton) came from all the plants she ate, which drew it up from the soil. We can cut out the middle-moo, though, and get calcium directly from the plants.

Where does protein come from? Protein is made up of an alphabet of amino acids, most of which we can make from scratch, but some are "essential," meaning our body can't make them so they're essential to get from our diet. But other animals don't make them either. All essential amino acids originate from plants and microbes, and all plant proteins have all the essential amino acids.[5667] The only truly "incomplete" protein in the food supply is gelatin, which is missing the amino acid tryptophan, so the only protein source you couldn't live on is Jell-O.[5668]

Those eating strictly plant-based diets average about 20 percent more protein than the recommended daily allowance.[5669] Those who don't know where to get protein on a plant-based diet *don't know beans*. (Legumes like beans, split peas, chickpeas, and lentils are the protein superstars of the plant kingdom, but protein is found in all whole plant foods to varying degrees.) That's protein quantity, though. What about protein *quality*?

The concept that plant protein was inferior to animal protein arose from studies performed on rodents more than a century ago. Scientists found that infant rats don't grow as well on plants.[5670] However, infant rats don't grow as well on human breast milk either. Does that mean we shouldn't breastfeed our babies? Of course not! Rat milk has ten times more protein than human milk[5671] because baby rats grow about ten times faster than baby humans.[5672]

It is true that some plant proteins are relatively low in certain essential amino acids. So, almost fifty years ago, the myth of "protein combining" came into vogue—literally, in the February 1975 issue of *Vogue* magazine. As I detail in see .nf/combining, this fallacy was refuted decades ago.[5673] Outdated concerns about plant protein digestibility have also been effectively debunked based on updated human data.[5674] We know from muscle biopsies, DXA scans, ultrasound imaging, and strength testing that both vegans and omnivores have comparable muscle gains in response to resistance exercise.[5675]

ANTIOXIDANTS FOR AGE-RELATED MUSCLE LOSS?

Antioxidants could be one muscle-preserving component of the plant protein package. Oxidative stress is suggested to play a central role in the onset of sarcopenia.[5676] For example, mice missing a major antioxidant enzyme suffer a dramatic acceleration of age-related muscle loss,[5677] and some epidemiological studies have tied higher antioxidant intake with increased grip strength and faster walking speed.[5678] Human muscles are certainly highly responsive to vitamin C intake. Even half a kiwifruit can triple muscle concentrations. That's where an estimated two-thirds of our body's vitamin C is pooled.[5679]

Vitamin C is necessary as an enzyme cofactor for the synthesis of both collagen and carnitine, and thereby plays a key role in muscle structure and function.[5680]

However, the observational data relating vitamin C intake and/or blood levels with muscle outcomes are mixed. Three of the five studies on vitamin C and muscle mass measures, including the largest one, found a protective association,[5681,5682,5683] while the other two studies found no association either way.[5684,5685] The hand grip data are similarly split,[5686,5687,5688,5689] though all three of the frailty studies found a protective association,[5690,5691,5692] but so did only one[5693] of the four studies on vitamin C and the prevalence of sarcopenia.[5694,5695,5696] I couldn't find any interventional trials on treating frailty or sarcopenia with antioxidants, but there have been randomized controlled trials using vitamin C and/or vitamin E supplements to boost resistance training gains in lean mass, muscle strength, or performance over placebo, but they all universally failed.[5697] The more consequential component of the plant protein package may be fiber.

FIBER FOR FRAILTY

There seems to be a microbiome "signature" of frailty. Fecal samples from frail individuals show a striking lack of bacterial diversity[5698] and, in particular, a deficit of fiber-eating "good bacteria"[5699] such as *Lactobacillus*.[5700] Fecal transplant studies I feature in see.nf/musclefiber peg it as a cause, just not a consequence, of the condition, and interventional studies show that randomizing people to fiber-rich foods,[5701,5702] prebiotics,[5703] or certain probiotics can improve performance.[5704] I conclude it's probably preferable to foster the growth of our own fiber feeders by feeding them fiber, which has the dual benefit of also cutting down[5705] on protein putrefaction toxins like indoxyl sulfate[5706] thought to play a role in muscle wasting.[5707]

CAUGHT OFF BASE

As we age, the ability of our kidneys to excrete acid declines.[5708] To buffer the acid, our kidneys produce the base ammonia from the amino acid glutamine, which it can effectively pull from our muscles.[5709] As acid levels rise, our adrenal glands release stress hormones like cortisol, which degrade our muscle proteins,[5710] releasing glutamine and other amino acids our liver can turn into glutamine, which then allows our kidneys to generate ammonia to neutralize the acid.[5711] So, part of the muscle breakdown as we age may be our body's attempt to maintain its pH (acid/base) balance.[5712] Potassium bicarbonate supplements have been shown to improve muscle performance,[5713] but as I detail in see.nf/muscleph, the best way to keep our kidneys from dipping into the protein stores from our musculature may be to eat an acid-neutralizing (alkaline, or base-forming) diet.[5714]

HOW TO REDUCE YOUR DIETARY ACID LOAD

Note in the below figure that not all plant foods are alkalinizing and not all animal foods are equally acidifying. Fish, including tuna, is the single most acid-producing food, followed by pork, poultry, cheese, then beef. (Actually, eggs are more acid-producing than beef on a gram-for-gram basis, but people tend to eat less of them at one sitting.) Some grains can be a little acid-forming, such as bread and rice, but, interestingly, not pasta. Beans are significantly acid-*reducing*, but not as much as fruits are, even tart ones like citrus. Vegetables are crowned as the most alkaline-forming foods.[5715] However, beans and other legumes are the only major sources of protein that are alkaline-forming instead of acid-forming.

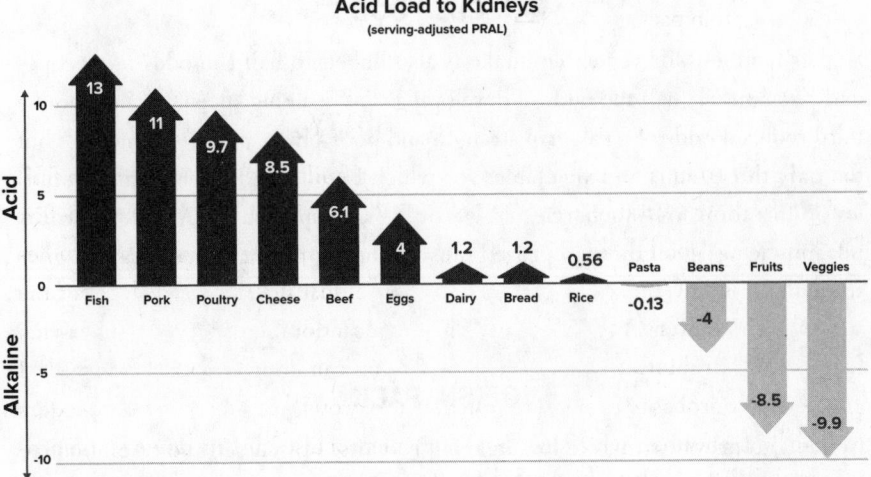

Acid Load to Kidneys
(serving-adjusted PRAL)

A strictly plant-based diet can flip our diet from acid-forming to net alkaline and significantly raise urine pH, whereas eating plant-based just a few days a week has been found to reduce the acid load but not eliminate it.[5716] Vegans have to actually eat their vegetables, though.

Salt intake also appears to increase stress hormone production through an acid/base mechanism,[5717] potentially explaining why high-salt diets are associated with reduced muscle function.[5718] So, we should also aim to cut down on processed foods, which are the source of about 75 percent of sodium intake in the United States.[5719]

Drop Acid

Our dietary acid/base imbalance doesn't only affect muscle health. For millions of years before we learned how to hunt or mine salt, our ancestors ate a

(continued)

net neutral or alkaline-generating diet.[5720] The shift to an acid-generating diet has been implicated in a wide range of disorders, including osteoporosis, type 2 diabetes, high blood pressure, kidney stones, depression, anxiety,[5721] gout,[5722] and renal failure.[5723] When mice were given alkaline water to drink, their telomeres elongated[5724] and their survival increased compared to controls,[5725] leading to editorials like "Is $NaHCO_3$ [baking soda] an Antiaging Elixir?"[5726] In see.nf/bakingsoda, I explain why it's preferable to alkalinize from the produce aisle.

MUSCLE FOODS

Higher fruit and/or vegetable intake is also linked to half the odds of sarcopenia,[5727,5728] nearly half the odds of developing slow walking speed,[5729] and about a third reduced odds of weak grip strength and poor physical performance,[5730] but the only three fruits and vegetables for which I could find interventional studies on this topic are blueberries,[5731] garlic,[5732] and spinach.[5733] As I detail in see .nf/musclefoods, all three improved muscle quality, performance, mass, and/or strength.

JOE SIX-PACK

Coffee also prevents muscle loss in aging rodents. I discussed the role of coffee boosting autophagy in the Autophagy chapter. Muscle tissues have one of the highest autophagy rates, which is considered essential for muscle integrity.[5734] Mice deficient in autophagy develop a severe loss of muscle mass and strength,[5735] so the "autophagic failure" of aging may play a role in our age-related decline in muscle mass.[5736] This led researchers to try putting diluted coffee in the water bottles of aged mice. Compared to the mice randomized to drink plain water, those that stopped and smelled (and drank) the coffee ended up with 13 percent greater muscle mass in their hind limbs and 18 percent greater grip strength after a single month. I know what you're thinking: The caffeinated mice must have been buzzing on the exercise wheel. But, no. The muscle gains occurred without changes to their activity levels.[5737]

Epidemiological studies have tied greater coffee drinking with higher physical performance[5738] and a greater muscle mass index,[5739] less functional disability at two or more cups a day,[5740] and less sarcopenia at three or more daily cups.[5741] But reverse causality often cannot be excluded in observational studies. Maybe those with reduced mobility are less likely to buy or prepare coffee, or perhaps they have fewer opportunities to drink it socially.[5742] That's where interventional studies come in.

An analysis of more than twenty meta-analyses on caffeine and exercise performance found caffeine to be ergogenic (performance-enhancing) for aerobic activity and muscle strength, power, and endurance,[5743] based on studies going back more than a century.[5744] However, most of the studies have been performed on young men after a single acute dose, typically the amount of caffeine found in two cups of coffee taken around an hour before the activity.[5745] Caffeine does seem to improve functional fitness,[5746] balance, and endurance[5747] in older men and women, as well, but this again was following an acute dose. When young people drank three cups of coffee a day for a month, though, their fat-free mass went up by about a pound while their fat mass dropped one to two pounds.[5748] Coffee can bulk up mice,[5749] but no word yet on older humans.

A POWDER KEG

Cocoa beans may help, too. Three tablespoons of cocoa powder a day significantly improves walking performance.[5750] Unfortunately, as I explore in see.nf /cocoamuscles, the tastiest cocoa doesn't work. Researchers randomized older adults to either natural cocoa, highly Dutched (alkalinized) cocoa, or placebo, and the Dutched cocoa didn't help any better than placebo. Some of the bitter compounds that are removed in the Dutching process are the flavonoid phytonutrients thought responsible for the beneficial effects. But older men and women given a tablespoon of natural, unprocessed cocoa a day for twelve weeks experienced a significant improvement in muscle mass index, grip strength, and all four physical function tests.[5751] And, refreshingly, the study was *not* funded by Hershey, as were many of the others.

CREATINE

I address the shortcomings of HMB (ß-hydroxy ß-methylbutyrate), magnesium, omega-3s, and vitamin D supplements for age-related muscle loss in my video see .nf/hmb, but there is a supplement that may help: creatine.

Creatine is a compound formed naturally in the human body that is primarily involved with energy production in our muscles and brain.[5752] It's also naturally formed in the bodies of many other animals, including those we may consume, so when we eat their muscles, we can take in some extra creatine through our diet.

(The compound was named after *kreas*, the Greek word for "meat," in which it was first isolated.[5753]) We need about 2 g a day, so those who eat meat may get around 1 g from their diet and their body makes the rest from scratch. There are rare birth defects where you're born without the ability to make creatine, in which case you have to get it from diet,[5754] but, otherwise, our body can make as much as we need to maintain normal concentrations in our muscles.[5755]

When people cut out meat, the amount of creatine floating around in their bloodstream goes down,[5756] but the amount in their brain remains the same, because our brain just makes all the creatine it needs.[5757] The level in vegetarians' muscles is lower,[5758] but that doesn't seem to affect performance, as both vegetarians and meat eaters respond to creatine supplementation with similar increases in muscle power output. If the creatine in vegetarians' muscles was insufficient, then presumably it would have had an even bigger boost.[5759] So, basically, when you eat meat, your body just doesn't have to make as much.[5760]

If creatine muscle content dropped as we grew older, that might help explain age-related muscle loss, but that doesn't seem to be the case. Biopsies taken from the muscles of younger and older adults show no difference in creatine content.[5761] Still, if it improves performance, maybe more would help. According to the International Society of Sports Nutrition, creatine monohydrate is the single most effective ergogenic supplement available to athletes for increasing exercise capacity and lean body mass during training.[5762] It's no wonder surveys show that 70 percent or more of athletes have used creatine supplements.[5763,5764] What can it do for older adults?

Without exercise? Nothing. Most studies on creatine supplementation alone show no benefits for muscle mass, strength, or performance.[5765] This makes sense, given the mechanism. Creatine supplementation delays muscle fatigue, which enables people to work out longer and harder. It's that additional volume and intensity that lead to the muscle benefits. So, creatine alone doesn't help, and creatine taken in the context of the same training that's carefully controlled and deliberately equalized doesn't help either.[5766] But, when older people are allowed to exercise as much as they can, most studies on the prevention and treatment of sarcopenia with creatine supplementation show augmented lean mass,[5767] as it does in young adults.[5768]

Adding 3 to 5 g of creatine a day and two to three days of resistance training a week led to an additional three pounds of lean mass over an average duration of about four months.[5769] Some of this lean mass may be water weight, though, not muscle. Creatine causes water retention that can show up as lean mass,[5770] but, compared to placebo, creatine combined with resistance exercise increases muscle strength, as well.[5771] And, the additional gains in mass and strength can persist at least twelve weeks after stopping the creatine in older adults, as long as the resistance training is maintained.[5772]

A reason I never advocated for creatine supplementation in older adults for muscle preservation was that systematic reviews up through 2017 concluded that adding creatine to training increased muscle mass and strength, but this did not appear to translate to improved functioning.[5773] However, in 2019, an updated meta-analysis found a significant improvement over placebo in sit-to-stand test performance,[5774] which is a decent predictor of reduced falls risk.[5775] Again, this was only when accompanied by strength training. There have still been no consistent benefits discovered for supplementing with creatine alone. So, creatine should always be prescribed with a progressive strength-training regimen.[5776]

The Society on Sarcopenia, Cachexia and Wasting Disease convened an expert panel who, despite the lack of long-term trials, suggest creatine be used for the management of sarcopenia.[5777] The recommended dose to achieve muscle saturation is 3 g a day.[5778] Within a month at that slow and steady rate, you achieve the same muscle levels as loading with 120 g over a period of a week.[5779] Note, though, that for older adults, it takes at least twelve weeks of creatine-supplement resistance training to see a significant additive effect.[5780] Recent evidence suggests that taking creatine after exercise might be slightly preferable to taking it before, but this has yet to be verified.[5781]

Are there any side effects? Well, if one can extrapolate from mice, one side effect may be longevity. The average healthy lifespan of creatine-fed mice was found to be 9 percent longer than control mice, and those on creatine performed better on neurobehavioral tests, especially improved memory skills.[5782] But, is taking creatine safe? That's the question I explore in detail in see.nf/creatinerisk.

In short, the only serious side effects appear to be among those with pre-existing kidney impairments or those taking whopping doses of 20 g or more a day for four weeks or longer,[5783] though as many as half of creatine supplements exceeded the maximum level recommended by food safety authorities for at least one contaminant.[5784] One third-party supplement testing outfit that checked for impurities chose as its top pick the BulkSupplements brand, which also happened to be the cheapest at about ten cents per daily 3-g serving, which is about a level teaspoonful.[5785]

Essential Tremor

In How Not to Die, I extensively address Parkinson's, since it's one of our leading killers, but the most common movement disorder is what's called essential tremor—affecting one in twenty-five adults over the age of forty and up to one in

(continued)

five of those in their nineties.[5786] In addition to the potentially debilitating hand tremor, there can be other neurological manifestations, including cognitive impairment, depression, and sleeping problems.[5787] As I explore in see.nf/tremor, most of the attention has focused on a class of tremor-producing chemicals called *beta-carboline alkaloids*,[5788] a type of heterocyclic amine, the class of carcinogens that are formed in a high-temperature chemical reaction between some of the components of muscle tissue.[5789]

For those reluctant to reduce their meat consumption, different marinades have been tested to reduce the formation of these compounds. Hibiscus extracts failed to alter levels[5790] and red wine made things nearly ten times worse,[5791] but a Caribbean marinade[5792] and a variety of berry extracts helped. For example, marinating camel meat in strawberry juice for twenty-four hours before frying can reduce the formation of one beta-carboline alkaloid as much as 40 percent.[5793]

Are there any dietary treatments once you already have the disease? Vanillin—the primary fragrant compound in vanilla extract—was found to be beneficial against tremors induced by these chemicals in rats, but there have yet to be any clinical studies.[5794]

PRESERVING YOUR SEX LIFE

There is a stereotype of older adults as asexual, but this is ageist and inaccurate.[5795] Sex is a valued part of our full adult lives, as evidenced by the fact that the vast majority (85 percent) of surveyed nursing homes report residents engaging in sex acts.[5796] However, sexual activity does tend to decline with age. Though some blue zone nonagenarians continue to be able to "honestly vouch" for their active sex lives,[5797] a national U.S. survey of thousands of older adults found a progressive decline in sexual activity with age, from 73 percent of people between the ages of fifty-seven and sixty-four down to just 26 percent of those aged seventy-five to eighty-five.[5798] Of that 26 percent, most (54 percent) had intercourse two to three times a month, but 23 percent had sex at least once a week. The drop in sexual activity may have less to do with age per se and more to do with declining health.[5799]

The number one reason given for lack of sexual activity among older adults was their or their partners' physical health problems or limitations. This implies that general body upkeep can help keep people actively engaged in all life has to offer, but approximately half of older men and women report specific issues, most often low sexual desire in women and erectile difficulties in men.[5800] Although only a minority appear distressed by these sexual problems,[5801] sexual dysfunction can be a canary in the coal mine for broader health issues.[5802]

In a study in which more than 2,000 men and women were followed for about six years, those with a higher frequency of sexual activity had a significantly lower risk of dying. Those having sex fifty-two or more times a year (approximately weekly) seemed to have only half the mortality rate compared to those having sex once or less a year, even after controlling for physical activity and health conditions, such as obesity, high blood pressure, diabetes, or heart disease. Even though sexual activity may just be an indicator of general health, it might also have protective physical and mental health benefits.[5803] For example, endorphins—feel-good chemicals released during sex—have been shown to improve natural killer cell function.[5804]

Researchers suggest that the reduction in premature death risk may be because sex is a form of exercise, but people may overestimate their exertions in bed.[5805] One of the "Seven Myths About Obesity" identified in *The New England Journal of Medicine* is that a bout of sexual activity burns a few hundred calories.[5806] So, you may think, *Hey, I could get a side of fries with that!* If you hook people up (literally *and* figuratively) and actually measure their oxygen consumption during the act (assuming they don't get too tangled up in all the wires and hoses), having sex only turns out to be the metabolic equivalent of bowling. The average bout of sexual activity may only last about six minutes, and a young man might expend approximately twenty-one calories during intercourse. Because of baseline metabolic needs, he would have spent roughly one-third of that just lounging around watching TV, so the incremental benefit is plausibly on the order of fourteen calories.[5807] So, maybe he can have one fry with that.

Whether a cause or consequence of ill health, sexual difficulties can be improved with lifestyle changes. Smoking cessation, exercise, and a healthier diet—for example, higher fruit and vegetable intake—have been associated with lower risk of both male and female sexual dysfunction.[5808] An interventional trial randomizing diabetic men and women to a more Mediterranean-type diet confirmed that dietary changes can slow the deterioration of sexual function in both sexes[5809] and cut the emergence of new sexual dysfunction in half.[5810]

Passing the Sniff Test

Love may be at first sight and beauty in the eye of the beholder, but vision is not the only sense associated with physical attractiveness and romantic partner preference. Body odor signals a variety of information on matters such as eating

(continued)

habits, hygiene, health, and more.[5811] In a survey of heterosexual college students, men rated visual information as being most important for selecting a lover, while women considered smell to be the single most important physical feature. In other words, women ranked body odor as more important for attraction than "looks."[5812]

Men may be more discriminating in this department than they think. For example, heterosexual men can unconsciously discriminate between body odor samples from pregnant women versus ovulating women. Functional MRI scans show the two different samples light up different areas of men's brains.[5813] How do postmenopausal women smell? What about older men?

As we age, men and women both begin developing a distinctive body odor. The Japanese even have a name for it: *kareishu*.[5814] It appears to be due to a chemical we start producing as early as age forty called *2-nonenal*, which has an unpleasant grassy and greasy odor, caused by the oxidation of omega-7 fats that are increasingly exuded from our skin.[5815]

What can we do to make ourselves smell better? Eat mushrooms. Researchers in Japan carried out a randomized, double-blind, placebo-controlled trial of three different doses of a champignon mushroom extract on the breath odor, pillow odor, pajama odor, and fecal odor of older men and women. Testers sniffed for bad breath one handsbreadth away from the study subjects' mouths as they talked for a minute or two, smelled their used pillowcases and pajamas, and evaluated their fecal odor; the "cooperating person evaluated the smell after the subject used the toilet."

Every dose of the mushroom extract beat out placebo for every test. Within two to four weeks, the mushrooms improved the smell of the participants' breath, bedding, clothing, and poop.[5816] I had never heard of champignon mushrooms. Would they have to be ordered from some rare and exotic mushroom shop? I was pleasantly surprised to learn that champignon is just another name for regular white button mushrooms, the cheapest, easiest-to-find mushrooms you can get just about anywhere. To pit it against a placebo, the researchers had to use an extract they could stuff into a capsule. They didn't describe the extraction process, but if it were just dried mushroom powder, the biggest dose they used would only translate into about a single small mushroom a day.[5817]

What else can we try? In my video see.nf/bodyodor, I show how eating chlorophyll can help, reducing underarm odor at doses on the order of 100 mg a day,[5818] the amount of chlorophyll you could get in about a dozen leaves of spinach.[5819] So, before slathering aluminum onto your armpits, I recommend first trying to deodorize from the inside out by eating a big salad every day, which may improve your body odor two ways: by hitting the chlorophyll threshold and improving your health.[5820]

As I explore in the video, the induction of inflammation with injections of endotoxin (see page 86) gives people an aversive body odor compared to those getting placebo injections.[5821] So, does eating meat make people smelly? The *kareishu* elderly person smell is thought to arise in part from "high animal fat–containing modern diets," but there's only one way to find out. Czech researchers decided to put it to the test, publishing their results in "The Effect of Meat Consumption on Body Odor Attractiveness."[5822] Not just body odor, mind you, but body odor *attractiveness.*

For two weeks, male "odor donors" were placed on a diet that either included or excluded meat and, during the final twenty-four hours, had pads taped into their armpits to collect their body odor. Then, thirty women assessed "fresh odor samples"—hot off the pits—for their pleasantness, attractiveness, masculinity, and intensity.

A month later, the study was repeated with the same men, but this time they followed the opposite diet. The same women were used as judges. The men, incidentally, were paid 2,000 in Czech currency for their time and "potential inconvenience caused by the prescribed diet." And the women who had to sniff all of those armpit pads? They were not paid, though they did receive a chocolate bar for their participation.[5823]

So, whose body odor was the most pleasant, the most attractive? The results showed that the "odor of donors when on the nonmeat diet was judged as significantly more attractive, more pleasant, and less intense." No differences were noted for masculinity.[5824] The researchers concluded that meat may have a "negative impact on perceived body odor hedonicity."[5825] In other words, those eating more plant-based evidently smell perceptively more pleasurable.

FEMALE SEXUAL FUNCTION

The most frequently reported sexual symptom among older women is low libido, followed by poor lubrication and pain during intercourse.[5826] Though there are safe, natural solutions, Big Pharma has money-grabbed women's privates.

MEDICALIZING WOMEN'S LIBIDO

In a textbook case of disease mongering, the pharmaceutical industry has promoted female sexual dysfunction as a mental disorder,[5827] harkening back to the first edition of the *Diagnostic and Statistical Manual of Mental Disorders*—psychiatry's diagnosis manual—which listed frigidity as a mental disorder, along with homo-sexuality.[5828] The latest manifestation is "hypoactive sexual desire disorder," a dis-ease invented by drug companies. There are certainly women troubled by low libido, but that doesn't make it a medical condition. In fact, even women with a normal libido can get diagnosed with hypoactive sexual desire disorder: "A woman who is highly interested in sex, just not with her current partner, can still qualify for a diagnosis"—and the drug. Even a "woman who is happy with her sex life may still qualify for a diagnosis of hypoactive sexual desire disorder if her partner is dissatisfied. . . ."[5829]

I review the shameful saga of the approval of flibanserin (sold as Addyi) in my video see.nf/hsdd. Clinical benefits are marginal, and the side effects significant.[5830] Combining it with alcohol, for example, can cause dangerously low blood pressure and fainting, problems so serious that the FDA put a black box warning—its most serious safety alert—on the drug insert hardly anyone reads.[5831] Even without al-cohol, it can cause severe drops in blood pressure and "sudden prolonged uncon-sciousness."[5832] As pharmacology professor Adriane Fugh-Berman put it, these types of serious side effects "might be acceptable in a cancer drug, but they are entirely unacceptable in a drug given to healthy women for an invented condition."

GET YOUR JUICES FLOWING

Eating more healthfully can extend not only your life but also your love life. Gen-erally speaking, heart-healthy lifestyle changes are sex-healthy lifestyle changes because of the critical role blood flow plays in the sexual responses of both men and women.[5833] For example, researchers can use MRI techniques to measure clitoral engorgement within minutes of exposure to an erotic video.[5834] This helps explain why sexual function in women is significantly affected by the presence of vascular diseases caused by the atherosclerotic narrowing of blood flow[5835] and arterial dys-function.[5836] Rabbits made to be atherosclerotic by being fed dietary cholesterol suffer a decrease in induced clitoral erections.[5837] (Yes, all female mammals have clitorises, as do some birds and reptiles.[5838])

Cholesterol doesn't just build up inside the arteries that feed our heart mus-cle, but inside all our blood vessels. In the heart, atherosclerosis can cause a heart attack, and in the brain, it can cause a stroke. In our legs, it can cause peripheral vascular disease and result in debilitating cramping, and in our vertebral arteries, it may cause disc degeneration and lower back pain. And clogs in our pelvic ar-teries can lead to sexual dysfunction, including decreased vaginal engorgement and "clitoral erectile insufficiency syndrome," defined as "failure to achieve clitoral tumescence," or engorgement. This is thought to be an important factor in female sexual dysfunction.[5839]

Women with higher cholesterol levels report significantly lower arousal, orgasm, lubrication, and sexual satisfaction. The same appears to hold true for women with high blood pressure.[5840] The Framingham Risk Score incorporates both cholesterol and blood pressure, and women with a score indicating even a 2 percent ten-year risk of developing heart disease have nearly twice the risk of sexual dysfunction.[5841] No wonder women randomized to a plant-rich diet experienced a significant improvement in overall sexual function.[5842]

Lubrication is all about blood flow, too. The hydrostatic pressure from all the additional pelvic blood flow in a sexually aroused vagina forces fluid to leak onto the surface wall of the birth canal as vaginal lubrication.[5843] How can we improve blood flow? If you remember from the Preserving Your Mind chapter, the flavonoid phytonutrients in cocoa can help open up arteries, peaking at about ninety minutes after consumption.[5844] So, might that Valentine's Day chocolate make a difference? Women who eat chocolate were found to have higher female sexual function index scores, but the effect disappeared once age was taken into account.[5845] So, chocolate appeared to flop as an aphrodisiac, perhaps because its fat and sugar counteract the benefits of the flavonoids in straight cocoa powder.

What are some whole-food sources of flavonoids? Onions are a major source. "Fresh onion juice" was found to enhance copulatory behavior . . . in rodents. For those of us less interested in how to "increase the percentage of ejaculating rats"[5846] and looking for something other than onion juice for our hot date, apples are the next largest source of flavonoid intake in the United States.

A study out of Italy found that women who ate apples on a daily basis scored significantly higher on an index of overall female sexual function than women consuming less than an apple a day.[5847] Note that the researchers only counted women who ate unpeeled apples, because the phytonutrients are concentrated in the peel, so we don't know if there's a link with peeled apples. Either way, as an observational study, all that could be demonstrated is a correlation between apple eating and improved sexual function. If proven to be cause and effect, the research suggests this could lead to "identifying new compounds and food supplements to use in female sexuality recovery." Or, you can just try eating an apple.

SHOT DOWN IN FLAMES

Women randomized to an increased intake of fruits, vegetables, nuts, and beans with a shift from animal to plant sources of fat experienced a significant increase in sexual function.[5848] The same was found for men and erectile function.[5849] The largest study on diet and erectile dysfunction (ED) found that each additional daily serving of fruits or vegetables may reduce the risk of ED by 10 percent.[5850] This could be due to increased circulation, as well as decreased inflammation.

A review on inflammation and sexual dysfunction concluded that men and women should switch to a diet high in fruits, vegetables, whole grains, nuts, and seeds, and low in sodium and saturated fat.[5851] As I reviewed in the Inflammation chapter, fiber is the most anti-inflammatory dietary component and saturated fat the most pro-inflammatory one. A two-year interventional study that found a significant improvement in the sexual function of men and women randomized to a healthier diet also noted a significant reduction in levels of C-reactive protein, a marker of systemic inflammation. Even the same diet in smaller portions can help. Overweight diabetic women with sexual dysfunction randomized to around a fifteen-pound weight loss through portion control over a year,[5852] which is enough to drop C-reactive protein levels by about 40 percent,[5853] were more than twice as likely to regain normal sexual function.[5854]

You don't have a wait a whole year, though. Changes in inflammation in the blood can occur hour to hour, based on what we just ate. Researchers fed subjects sausage-egg-butter-oil sandwiches versus cheeseless pizza with whole-wheat crust.[5855] There is a pro-inflammatory signaling molecule in our body called *interleukin 18*, which is thought to play a role in destabilizing atherosclerotic plaque. As such, the level of interleukin 18 in the blood is a strong predictor of cardiovascular death.[5856] Within hours of eating the sausage sandwich, interleukin 18 levels rose about 20 percent. In contrast, those eating the whole food, plant-based pizza had about a 20 percent *drop* in interleukin 18 levels within hours of consumption, reinforcing dietary recommendations to eat a diet high in fiber and low in saturated fat.

But the billions in profits are in pills,[5857] not plants, which is why the pharmacology of the female orgasm has been studied ever since 1960, when a researcher at Tulane University implanted tubes deep within the brain of a woman "of borderline defective intelligence" so he could inject drugs directly into her brain to induce repetitive orgasms. A man who had electrodes placed into similar parts of his brain was given a device for a few hours that allowed him to press the button himself to stimulate the electrode. He pressed the button 1,500 times.[5858]

Toying with Phthalates

Phthalates are hormone-disrupting chemicals found in PVC plastics linked to a number of adverse health effects, such as disturbing infant and child genital and behavioral development.[5859] Data have shown, for example, "incomplete virilization in infant boys"[5860] and reduced "masculine play" as they grow up,[5861] and, for girls, an earlier onset of puberty.[5862] In adults, phthalates can affect our sex lives, as I explore in see.nf/phthalates.

In addition to increasing breast cancer risk,[5863] they may impair testosterone production in men[5864] and decrease libido in women.[5865] Most phthalates come from food, based on fasting studies,[5866] but we can get similar drops from simply eating a plant-based diet for a few days.[5867]

The highest levels are found in meats, fats, and dairy.[5868] Poultry consistently comes out as being the most contaminated across the board with some of the highest levels ever reported.[5869] Diets high in meat and dairy may exceed the allowable daily intake set by the U.S. Consumer Product Safety Commission.[5870]

Even during total fasting, a few cases of phthalate urine spikes were noted after showers, suggesting contamination in personal care products.[5871] This may be avoided by choosing unscented products, since phthalates are used as a fragrance carrier.[5872] Certain phthalate levels are now banned from children's toys,[5873] but not from toys for adults. "Jelly"-based sex toys are often made from a plasticized vinyl material loaded with phthalates. Although opting for water-based lubricants may reduce phthalate transfer a hundredfold, such sex toys may still have opposite the intended effect.[5874]

TESTOSTERONE "REPLACEMENT" FOR WOMEN

Testosterone is linked with sexual desire in both men and women.[5875] Women normally produce testosterone throughout the life cycle. Although postmenopausal ovaries continue to produce testosterone,[5876] levels naturally decline with age—falling by approximately 50 percent by age fifty.[5877] This is thought to play a role in the decline in libido (using masturbation frequency as a partner-independent proxy).[5878]

A syndrome of "female androgen deficiency" symptoms has been popularized, but there is no evidence that testosterone "replacement" helps with mood, well-being, or hot flashes, nor bone, cardiovascular, or metabolic health.[5879] The only evidence-based reason to try testosterone in postmenopausal women is for the treatment of low sexual desire that's causing distress,[5880] though as I detail in see.nf/t4women, efficacy is insufficient to warrant FDA approval, especially given the uncertainty about long-term side effects.[5881] DHEA, which can convert into testosterone within the body, fails to significantly improve desire and sexual function,[5882] but natural ways to raise testosterone levels in women are listening to music[5883] and avoiding mint tea.[5884]

Smell to High Heaven

What else can older women do to improve their sexual desire if they so choose? There are two aromatherapy regimens that may help. Women randomized to smell the aroma of lavender for twenty minutes twice a day for twelve weeks experienced a significant improvement in menopausal symptoms, including sexual desire, compared to sniffing the control, which was diluted milk.[5885] Neroli oil, also known as bitter orange, appeared to work even faster. Just five minutes twice a day for five days led to a significant increase in sexual desire at even just a 0.1 percent concentration of the essential oil, compared to instead sniffing the carrier (almond) oil alone.[5886] It's hard to rule out placebo effects, since the controls were not matched for intensity. A better research design might have incorporated synthetic fragrances, but they still may be worth a try.

THE ROOTS OF THE MATTER: GINSENG, MACA, AND ASHWAGANDHA

What about other dietary supplements, such as three roots, ginseng, maca, and ashwagandha? For details, see see.nf/roots, but essentially, ginseng flopped for female sexual dysfunction,[5887] though one small trial of about three-quarters of a teaspoon of maca powder suggested benefit.[5888] Ashwagandha (from *ashwa*, meaning "horse," and *gandha*, meaning "smell,"[5889] because the roots evidently possess the "distinctive smell of a wet horse"[5890]) may also help[5891] but cannot be recommended due to rare cases of liver toxicity. (What else should we expect from a plant with the nickname *poison gooseberry*?[5892])

VAGINAL MOISTURIZERS

Typically starting about four to five years after their last period, about half of postmenopausal women suffer from what they used to call *vulvovaginal atrophy*,[5893] but now referred to by the name *genitourinary syndrome of menopause* (GSM). The Vulvovaginal Atrophy Terminology Consensus Conference Panel of the North American Menopause Society decided that the term GSM was more "publicly acceptable." Not that the original descriptor wasn't accurate, but the panel felt the word "atrophy" had "negative connotations" and the word "vagina" was "not a generally accepted term for public discourse or for the media." The panel likened it to the parallel shift from "pejorative" impotence to "erectile dysfunction."[5894]

Whatever it's called, it involves changes to the vulva (external genitalia), vagina (birth canal), and bladder, caused by menopausal changes in hormone levels. Symptoms include vaginal dryness, burning, itchiness, and irritation, pain

DHEA suppositories for pain during intercourse due to GSM.[5925] It is converted locally into estrogen and does not significantly affect systemic hormone levels.[5926] The downside is that it has to be administered nightly, whereas estrogen preparations are typically used twice a week and vaginal rings only every few months.[5927] For those who would rather have an oral treatment, there's ospemifene, a tamoxifen-type drug that has pro-estrogenic effects on the vaginal lining. However, it actually increases the rate of hot flashes and urinary tract infections in the short term, and insufficient data are available on long-term safety.[5928]

SOY JOY

Japanese-American women have the lowest rates of hot flashes in the United States, as well as the lowest rates of vaginal dryness.[5929] Might it be due in part to their greater soy consumption? There have been a few studies on topical application of soy isoflavone vaginal gels[5930] showing a significant improvement in dryness and pain with intercourse over placebo gels,[5931] roughly on par with estrogen cream in a head-to-head test,[5932] but it's unlikely that these women are applying soy products topically. (A whole new meaning to the term "extra-firm" tofu?) What about just eating soy foods? Feeding isoflavones to older mice increases vaginal blood flow.[5933] What about in people?

Most oral soy supplements flopped,[5934] but as I explore in see.nf/soygsm, the three studies on soymilk and GSM symptoms show promise.[5935,5936,5937] A case report out of New York suggests that it may be possible to overdo it, though. A forty-four-year-old woman presented to her gynecologist with an "increase in desire that required her to self-stimulate to orgasm approximately 15 times daily." A month before, she had started an almost exclusively soy-based diet, eating in excess of four pounds of soy foods a day. Within three months of cutting back, her desire cooled to the point that she "engaged in satisfying sexual activity only twice daily."[5938]

FENNEL AND FENUGREEK

Fennel seeds, which are actually whole little fruits, have been shown to have hormonal effects, for example, offering significant relief from painful periods[5939] comparably to ibuprofen-type drugs.[5940] After menopause, fennel oil extract supplements didn't show any benefit for GSM symptoms,[5941] but whole fennel seeds, powdered into capsules to pit them against placebo in a double-blind, controlled trial, significantly improved menopausal symptoms at a dose of just a teaspoon a day.[5942]

Topical fennel creams are even more impressive. Within eight weeks, about 90 percent of those randomized to a vaginal fennel cream went from experiencing severe pain during intercourse to none, whereas pain didn't go away in any of those on the placebo cream. Vaginal dryness, itching, and pallor also completely disappeared in the fennel group.[5943] These extraordinary results were recently replicated successfully.[5944] Other studies have also found significant benefits to fennel vaginal creams for desire, arousal, lubrication, orgasm, and sexual satisfaction.[5945]

Fenugreek seeds are also hormonally active, as I document in see.nf /fenugreek. Men randomized to capsules containing fenugreek got significant gains in body composition and upper (bench press) and lower (leg press) strength compared to placebo,[5946] along with a significant boost in total blood testosterone[5947] and a doubling of the frequency of morning erections.[5948] And the only side effect? It can make your sweat and pee smell like maple syrup.[5949] (Sounds like a bonus!)

What about sexual function in women? While the estrogen hormone estradiol stimulates vaginal lubrication and blood flow, facilitating a woman's capacity for sexual arousal and orgasm, it's the testosterone that's linked with sexual desire in both men and women. Fenugreek raises the levels of both estradiol and testosterone, resulting in an increase in sexual desire and function, translating into about a doubling of sexual activity compared to placebo.[5950] That was in premenopausal women, but the same dose was subsequently shown to improve sexual symptoms in postmenopausal women as well.[5951] However, it was not found to be as effective as estrogen cream in a head-to-head comparison.[5952]

MALE SEXUAL FUNCTION

"Sex is important to health," reported the *Harvard Health Letter*, noting "[f]requent sexual intercourse is associated with reduced heart attack risk."[5953] However, for men, this seems to be the perfect case for reverse causation. But low frequency of sexual activity appears to predict cardiovascular disease in men even independently of erectile dysfunction.[5954]

"SEX IS KICKING DEATH IN THE ASS WHILE SINGING."
—CHARLES BUKOWSKI

Do men who have more sex actually live longer? I review the evidence in my video see.nf/sexlife, but in a nutshell, the researchers found that men with "high orgasmic frequency" appeared to cut their risk of premature death in half and, apparently, the more, the better: There was a 36 percent drop in mortality odds for every additional one hundred orgasms a year[5955]—but, apparently, not if you cheat. Extramarital sex in men was associated with higher cardiovascular risk for reasons laid out in the video.[5956]

When done right, though, love may protect your lover's life.[5957] Given the purported benefits of sexual activity, the authors of the orgasm study suggested a public health initiative should be launched, similar to the *at least five a day* fruit and vegetable campaign aimed at increasing consumption of produce, though, they acceded, "the numerical imperative may have to be adjusted."[5958]

ED = EARLY DEATH

Up to thirty million men in the United States and approximately one hundred million men worldwide experience erectile dysfunction (ED), the recurrent or persistent inability to attain or maintain an erection for satisfactory sexual performance.[5959] Hold on. The United States has less than 5 percent of the global population yet up to 30 percent of world's impotence? We're number one!

ED is considered to be an important cause of decreased male quality of life[5960]—so much so that one early theory suggested that it may explain the link between impotence and heart attacks. Depression is a risk factor for coronary heart disease, and the thought was that men who couldn't get erections became *so* depressed that they die of a broken heart.[5961]

The real reason the United States is the world leader in ED may be our artery-clogging standard American diet. One in five ED cases may be psychological in origin, but most are "vasculogenic," meaning due to impaired penile blood flow.[5962] Every part of the body needs sufficient blood to function properly. Cholesterol can clog arteries in our inner and outer organs, causing aneurisms, heart attacks, strokes, kidney failure, spinal degeneration, and sexual dysfunction.[5963] Up to three-quarters of men with cholesterol-narrowed coronary arteries have some degree of erectile dysfunction.[5964] But Americans have red, white, and blue pills like Viagra. The problem is that those pills are just a stopgap measure to cover up the symptoms of vascular disease; they do nothing for the underlying pathology—the artery-clogging atherosclerosis that threatens one's life, along with one's love life.

Read my erectile dysfunction section in *How Not to Die* for further details, but basically, men in their forties with erection difficulties have up to a fiftyfold greater risk of having a cardiac event like sudden death.[5965] We used to think of ED in men under forty as being "psychogenic," all in their heads, but we are now realizing that the condition is more likely an early indicator of vascular disease. Over the age of seventy, only a minority of men surveyed describe being bothered by their ED,[5966] but they may not realize the broader implications for the health of their arteries. Some experts contend that a man with ED—even if he does not have any cardiac symptoms—"should be considered a cardiac . . . patient until proved otherwise."[5967]

SURVIVAL OF THE FIRMEST

Given the underlying cause of physiological erectile difficulty, it's no surprise that an artery-healthy diet may be the cornerstone to prevent it. In a 2022 *Urology* paper titled "Consumption of a Healthy Plant-Based Diet Is Associated with a Decreased Risk of Erectile Dysfunction," researchers noted that the 500 percent increase in the number of Americans consuming a plant-based diet in recent years may be accompanied by an improvement in male sexual function. Note that this was apparent only with the consumption of *healthy* plant foods.[5968] Just cutting down on animal products but continuing to down soda with your french fries would not be expected to improve matters in the bedroom. Whole plants for swole pants.

This is consistent with findings from the Harvard Health Professionals Follow-Up Study that followed more than 20,000 men for a little over a decade, from the average age of sixty-two until seventy-three. The study found that those following healthier diets were significantly less likely to develop ED.[5969] A study of Canadian men with diabetes found that each additional daily serving of fruits or vegetables correlated with a 10 percent reduction in ED risk.[5970] This connection appears to extend to younger men, with fruit and vegetable consumption associated with lower ED risk even in men under forty.[5971]

Erectile function may be such a sensitive indicator of cardiovascular health that it may explain why men lost the bone in their penis.[5972] I produced a video on the subject, see.nf/baculum. Without a bone, only genuinely healthy males could "present a really stiff erection," evolutionary biologist Richard Dawkins wrote, "and the females could make an unobstructed diagnosis."[5973]

Bottling Up Your Feelings

A recent study found that men eating organic foods tended to be less likely to have ED.[5974] Interest in the role of pesticides in sexual function dates back more than fifty years[5975] to a report titled "Impotence in Farm Workers Using Toxic Chemicals," published in the *British Medical Journal*.[5976] Agricultural workers frequently exposed to pesticides have up to eight times the odds of a "flat erectile pattern" (lack of nocturnal erections), but it's not clear if there is any effect caused by the traces of pesticides left on conventional produce.[5977] The lower risk among organic consumers may be due to the fact that those eating organic also tend to eat less processed foods and more fresh foods.[5978]

The plastics chemical BPA is associated with declining male sexual function—decreased sexual desire, more difficulty having an erection, lower ejaculation strength, and lower level of overall satisfaction with sex life.[5979] Though we inhale some from dust and absorb some through our skin when touching BPA-laden receipts, 90 percent of our exposure to BPA is from our diet.[5980] In see.nf/bpa, I describe ways to limit our exposure: Reduce our use of polycarbonate plastics, which are usually labeled with recycle codes three or seven, and opt for fresh and frozen foods over canned goods, especially when it comes to tuna and condensed soups. If you do use plastics, don't microwave them, put them in the dishwasher, leave them in the sun or a hot car, or use them once they're scratched.[5981] Using glass, ceramic, or stainless steel containers may be even better,[5982] though, as it's not clear if BPA-free plastics like Tritan are any better.

SOFT PEDALING IT

There are other lifestyle behaviors that impact male sexual function. Smoking may almost double the risk of developing ED, and even secondhand smoke has been implicated.[5983] Experimentally, five of six dogs exposed to just ten or so minutes of cigarette smoke could not achieve erections.[5984] It's hard to rigorously study smoking cessation because of frequent noncompliance, but successful quitters do show significantly improved erectile function. For example, in one six-month study, 54 percent of men who quit smoking regained erectile function compared to 28 percent of persistent smokers.[5985] Cannabis use is also associated with ED. A meta-analysis capturing data from thousands of men found that the prevalence of ED in cannabis users (69.1 percent) was about twice as high as in nonusers (34.7 percent).[5986]

Obesity can cause profound sexual dysfunction,[5987] which can be reversed with sufficient diet-[5988] or surgery-induced[5989] weight loss. Physical inactivity may also cause sexual inactivity,[5990] while regular aerobic exercise can improve erectile function[5991] almost as much as the latest generation of Viagra-type drugs.[5992] At least forty minutes of moderate to vigorous intensity aerobic exercise four times per week for at least six months is recommended for ED recovery.[5993] However, caution must be exercised when it comes to prolonged cycling.

In reference to the Scythians, a group of horse-riding people, Hippocrates wrote that "the great majority among them become impotent."[5994] What about Pelotons and other modern steeds? There are fifty million cyclists in the United States alone,[5995] and there is concern about the repeated compression of the pudendal nerves, which branch off the spine, loop down between the legs, then up into the genitals. At first glance, cyclists appear to have the same rates of ED as non-cyclists, but since cyclists tend to be younger, one has to adjust for age. Once you do that, effectively comparing same-age cyclists to non-cyclists, a systematic review and meta-analysis involving more than 3,000 cyclists found them to be at significantly higher risk.[5996]

What about bicycle seats with a cutout in the middle to relieve perineal pressure? They may actually make things worse! The pudendal nerve and artery don't travel along the midline but rather in Alcock's canals, along either side, and the decreased sitting surface area of cutout saddles can aggravate rather than relieve the pressure.[5997] Cyclists using cutout saddles have up to six times the risk of ED, but this seems limited to those who experience concurrent perineal numbness.[5998] What can you do? The greatest pressure in the critical region comes from leaning forward. Cycling upright was found to result in 40 percent better penile oxygenation than cycling at a sixty-degree angle leaning forward.[5999] You can also regularly switch to standing up on the pedals during prolonged rides.[6000]

VIAGRA: A HARD SELL

Though cholesterol-lowering statin drugs have been shown to help with ED,[6001] the first-line treatment for medical management is the Viagra-type class of drugs known as phosphodiesterase type 5 inhibitors.[6002] They relax the muscle fibers in the penis that normally stanch the influx of blood. Until the "lecture that changed sexual medicine,"[6003] erections were thought to arise from the constriction of blood outflow rather than the expansion of blood inflow.[6004] The lecture, given by Professor Giles Brindley at the annual meeting of the American Urological Association in 1983, involved a visual aid. Before taking the podium, he injected his own penis with a muscle relaxer. Halfway through the lecture, to drive home his point, he proceeded not only to whip it out but then to waddle and waggle down to the front row, pants around his knees, to offer further inspection.[6005] The organizers were "not happy . . . as there were a fair number of wives in the audience."[6006]

Viagra works through a similar mechanism in oral form, originally starting out as a failed chest-pain drug with a serendipitous billion-dollar side effect.[6007] However, rates of discontinuation after about one or two years of use range from 32 to 69 percent in the United States.[6008] So, about half of men decide that the cons outweigh the pros,[6009] due to ineffectiveness,[6010] cost, or side effects,[6011] the most serious of which is non-arteritic ischemic optic neuropathy (NAION). As I detail in see.nf/naion, NAION typically manifests as waking up blind with usually temporary, but sometimes permanent, loss of vision in one or, rarely, both eyes.

For men who don't like drugs, there's always surgery—the implantation of penile prosthetics.[6012] Unbelievably, penile implant usage evidently dates back to the sixteenth century. Early experiments involved transplanting patients' rib cartilage or even their actual rib into their penis.[6013] The rib cage implants left men in a "permanently erect state," but the "Flexirod" technology in the 1960s, which allowed men to keep their ribs intact, had a hinge in the middle so the device could be bent down in half "for improved concealment." Of course, proper sizing is important: If the implants are too small, there can be drooping at the tip, leading to a "supersonic transport (SST) deformity"[6014] (because of its "resemblance to the nose of Concorde" jet). Overlong implants can also be a problem, with the semirigid rods eroding through the glans (tip) of the penis.[6015] Ouch.

Now, there are inflatable devices, and perhaps one day there will be "expandable foams that respond to external magnetic fields" or metal-mesh technology "that could expand and retract in a cage-like fashion."[6016] (Try getting *that* through airport security.)

Getting Under Your Skin

Of the half dozen Viagra-type drugs presently on the market, sildenafil (Viagra) itself may have the greatest efficacy, but it also may have the highest rate of side effects.[6017] Acutely, it's remarkably safe. For instance, one man swallowed sixty-five tablets in a failed suicide attempt.[6018] However, now that Viagra has been around for more than two decades, some *chronic* effects may be cropping up. This includes glaucoma, one of the leading causes of blindness. It involves the degeneration of the optic nerve,[6019] and those using Viagra in the long term have up to nearly ten times the odds of developing it. But it's cancer that has the medical community rethinking the safety of this class of drugs.[6020]

I review the evidence in my video see.nf/viagra, but basically, one of the ways melanoma becomes invasive is through a gene mutation[6021] that downregulates the enzyme phosphodiesterase-5,[6022] which is what Viagra-type drugs do, perhaps helping to explain why those taking drugs like Viagra, Cialis, or Levitra do seem to be at significantly higher risk for this potentially deadly form of skin cancer.[6023]

GETTING STIFFED

An analysis of internet-ordered Viagra found that only 18 percent were authentic. Some of the pills contained a variety of contaminants, such as commercial-grade paint and other drugs, including amphetamines.[6024] On the flip side, "natural" sexual enhancement supplements are among the dietary supplements most tainted with pharmaceuticals.[6025] More than a dozen deaths have been attributed to taking sexual performance supplements laced with diabetes drugs that crashed dozens into hypoglycemic comas.[6026] Hold on. What about supplement manufacturers who say they have independent, third-party certification of purity? There is a practice called *dry labbing*, a dirty little secret of the supplements industry, where quality assurance laboratories just rubber-stamp fake documents.[6027] For a litany of other supplement industry malfeasance, see see.nf/supplements.

The story of BMPEA is a particularly egregious example, as documented by STAT,[6028] one of my favorite sources of medical journalism. A researcher at Harvard published a paper replicating prior research from the FDA detecting a designer amphetamine–like stimulant in various supplements sold in the United States.[6029] In response, one of the offenders, Hi-Tech Pharmaceuticals, the manufacturer of supplements with names like Black Widow and Yellow Scorpion,[6030] sued the Harvard researcher for libel, slander, and product disparagement,[6031] originally to the tune of $200 million in damages.[6032]

The head of Hi-Tech openly admitted that he was "hoping that we were able to silence this guy."[6033] While ultimately unsuccessful in court, Hi-Tech's lawsuit effectively sent a warning to other researchers. Hi-Tech's CEO is attributed as saying that he "hope[s] that the long and costly legal battle will scare away other academics from investigating the supplement industry."[6034]

A BONE TO PICK WITH ED SUPPLEMENTS

Are there any supplements that have been shown to work? I review the available evidence in see.nf/edpills. Vitamins A,[6035] B$_3$,[6036] C,[6037] and E[6038] flopped, and studies on vitamins B$_6$[6039] and D[6040] for ED had no control group to rule out the placebo effect or even to document that they were superior to doing nothing.

One of the most popular ingredients in sexual enhancement supplements[6041]—and one of the most extensively studied[6042]—is ginseng. A meta-analysis of a half dozen randomized controlled trials found that four to twelve weeks of 1,800 to 3,000 mg a day of Korean red ginseng significantly improved erectile function compared with placebo.[6043] Of course, this is assuming there's actually ginseng in your "ginseng." Testing the authenticity of more than five hundred commercial ginseng products across a dozen countries in six continents, 24 percent were found to be adulterated.[6044]

Some natural "aphrodisiacs" are considered too risky. These include yohimbine, Spanish fly, mad honey, and Bufo toad, the latter of which has been banned by the FDA for its potential lethality.[6045] Death has also been attributed to yohimbine, though since it was purchased online, it may have been adulterated with other substances.[6046]

GYM MEMBER

Currently, recommended treatments for ED do nothing to treat and reverse the underlying cause of the problem, whether oral drugs, surgical penile implants, vacuum erection devices, intraurethral (pee hole) suppositories, or intracavernosal (into the shaft) injections.[6047] While the American Urological Association at least encourages physicians to inform patients about the importance of lifestyle change,[6048] the European Association of Urology guidelines go a step further, mandating that lifestyle changes "must precede or accompany ED treatment."[6049] And for good reason. In see.nf/edlifestyle, I detail interventional studies showing how effective exercise[6050] and healthy dietary changes can be in improving erectile function.[6051]

The Atkins Diet: Trouble Keeping It Up

Erectile dysfunction and heart disease can be two different manifestations of the exact same root problem: diseased arteries—inflamed, oxidized, cholesterol-clogged blood vessels.[6052] Thankfully, atherosclerosis in both organs can be reversed with lifestyle changes that include anti-inflammatory, antioxidant, cholesterol-lowering foods.[6053,6054] I profile an illustrative case report in my video see.nf/atkins. The fellow started out pretty healthy, a fifty-one-year-old man with decent cholesterol, no measurable coronary artery plaque, and a working penis. He went on the Atkins Diet and lost a few pounds—and the ability to have an erection. Then he nearly died with a 99 percent blockage to his heart, before a return to a healthier diet was able to reopen blood flow throughout his body.[6055]

I wrote a book about the diet nearly twenty years ago. The Atkins Corporation threatened to sue me, but I kind of won by default, because it declared bankruptcy six months later. You can read the whole book, as well as my rather amusing back-and-forth with Atkins's lawyers, at atkinsfacts.org.

NUT UP

Consumption of at least one serving of vegetables a day and more than two servings of nuts a week was associated with a more than 50 percent decrease in the probability of ED in a snapshot-in-time cross-sectional study.[6056] The first interventional nut study on ED was published in 2011. As I detail in see.nf/pistachios, men eating three to four handfuls of pistachios a day for just three weeks experienced a significant improvement in blood flow through the penis, accompanied by significantly firmer erections.[6057]

But a fourteen-week, randomized, controlled trial of mixed nuts improved sperm counts[6058] and marginally increased orgasmic function and sexual desire but had no effect on erectile function.[6059] As I note in see.nf/mixednuts, the discrepancy is likely due to differences in study populations. The men in the pistachio study were in their forties and fifties, already plagued with chronic ED,[6060] whereas the average age in the mixed nut study was twenty-four years, so the younger men may have started out with near-maximum circulation, leaving them without much nut wiggle room.[6061]

JUST BEET IT

What about vegetables? As discussed, the nitric oxide that allows blood vessels to relax can also be made directly from the nitrates concentrated in vegetables, such as greens and beets. Attempts were made to try to apply nitrates topically on the penis (in the form of a nitroglycerine gel normally used for chest pain), but it caused headaches in both the user and, unless used only under a condom, their partners.[6062] The benefits of vegetable nitrates may explain why eating greens is associated with not only reduced rates of heart disease[6063] but also a longer life-span,[6064] not to mention the potential for a "veggie Viagra" effect. (See a list of the top ten sources on page 495.) That could explain the link between vegetable consumption and improved sexual function[6065] and improved blood flow to the most important organ of the body, the brain.[6066] The only side effect of beeting out your brain may be adding a little extra color to your life—in the form of red stools and urine that is pretty in pee-nk.

Fruit-wise, pomegranate juice flopped (see.nf/pomegranate), but watermelon stood firm (see.nf/watermelon). Watermelon contains a compound called *citrulline*, which turns into arginine inside the body. Straight arginine can improve erectile function,[6067] but it can also cause gastrointestinal distress.[6068] Five daily servings of red watermelon's worth or that found in a single daily wedge of yellow watermelon (one-sixteenth of a modest-sized melon)[6069] can improve erection hardness.[6070] If this is news to you, it may be because the advertising budgets of drug companies like Pfizer, which rakes in billions of dollars annually from the sale of ED drugs, are about a thousand times[6071] that of the entire budget of the National Watermelon Promotion Board.[6072]

POSH SPICE

A half dozen studies have found that the spice saffron beat out placebo or rivaled medications like Prozac in the treatment of depression.[6073] It may be the red pigment, crocin, since that alone (in a dose equivalent to about a half teaspoon of saffron a day) beat out placebo as an adjunct treatment, significantly decreasing symptoms of depression, symptoms of anxiety, and general psychological distress.[6074]

If the spice works as well as the drugs, one could argue that the spice wins,[6075] since it doesn't cause sexual dysfunction in the majority of men and women like most prescribed antidepressants do.[6076] Popular SSRI drugs like Prozac, Paxil, and Zoloft cause adverse sexual side effects in about 70 percent of people taking them,[6077] which can persist even after stopping the drugs.[6078] (Now that's depressing!) Not only is this not a problem with saffron; the spice may even be able to treat antidepressant-induced sexual dysfunction in both men[6079] and women,[6080] as I document in see.nf/crocin.

What about saffron for just regular ED? It was actually a saffron trial that inspired me to suggest the RigiScan engorgement-measuring machine for use in the documentary *The Game Changers*. Suggestive benefit for both oral[6081] and topical[6082] (rubbed on the penis) saffron was found, with caveats summarized in my video see .nf/saffroned.

Costs vs. Benefits

A review on diet and sexual health expounded on the pros and cons of various eating patterns. The benefits of continuing to eat the standard American diet were "[r]elatively affordable and easy to obtain," and downsides were "[i]ncreases risk of total mortality, cardiovascular disease, obesity, metabolic syndrome, stroke, chronic kidney disease, and breast, colon, and prostate cancer."[6083] Thankfully, eating more healthfully is becoming more and more convenient and may be among the cheapest ways to eat.[6084] A meat-free diet, for example, could save individuals an estimated $750 a year.[6085]

PRESERVING YOUR SKIN

The skin is the fastest-growing[6086] and largest organ in our body—about twenty square feet, accounting for about 10 percent of our body weight.[6087] It acts as the most conspicuous mirror of the aging process. As our skin becomes thinner, it is more easily damaged, loses volume and elasticity, and can sag and wrinkle.[6088]

The three main constituents that make up the bulk of our skin are collagen, hyaluronic acid, and elastin. Collagen,[6089] which makes up about 75 percent,[6090] contributes strength and firmness, hyaluronic acid maintains moisture in the skin by trapping water,[6091] and stretchy elastic fibers containing elastin make up about 1 to 2 percent of our skin and help it bounce back into shape.[6092]

As we age, the synthesis of collagen and elastin decreases by about 1 percent a year,[6093] as does overall skin thickness.[6094] The turnover rate of our skin can slow considerably, from every twenty-eight days in the young to forty to sixty days in the elderly.[6095] Our skin's microbiome also changes, in fact, so predictably that people's age can be guessed within about a four-year range just from a swab of the bacteria on their skin.[6096] We don't yet know enough about these bugs to assess their role in the skin aging process, though, which seems to revolve around oxidative stress. That's what causes age spots, also known as liver spots, clumps of oxidized fat and proteins known as age pigment or lipofuscin[6097] (from the Latin *lipo-* and *fuscus*, meaning "dark fat").

NOTHING NEW UNDER THE SUN

As little as 3 percent of skin aging is due to genetic factors, so-called intrinsic aging, and the rest—extrinsic aging—is from our lifestyle, that is, from what we do to our skin.[6098] You can get a sense of the difference by comparing the aging of skin from typically protected areas to skin that's been exposed to the sun— the skin on your tush or the inside of your upper arm, for instance, compared to the skin on your face or hands.[6099] Intrinsic aged skin does lose elasticity and develops fine wrinkles, but it is generally otherwise smooth and unblemished, with pigment diminishing toward pallor. Extrinsic aged skin, on the other hand, can become leathery, bumpy, blotchy, and mottled, with coarse wrinkles and furrows.[6100]

Between 80[6101] and 90[6102] percent of facial aging among people with lighter skin tones is due to sun exposure. Those with darker skin are also affected, though they're relatively protected due to their built-in melanin sunscreen.[6103] That's why dermatologists now agree that there is nothing more important to slow the signs of aging than to protect your skin from the sun.[6104] To illustrate, a dramatic photo of a trucker who spent decades getting more sun on the left side of his face through his driver's side window was published in *The New England Journal of Medicine*,[6105] making him look a bit like a Batman villain. You can check it out at see.nf/trucker. Factors like sun exposure and smoking can make people look eleven years older. Cosmetic surgery, on the other hand, can make people look up to eight years younger.[6106] A healthy lifestyle may work even better at maintaining a youthful appearance.

Protecting our skin from the sun should be a lifetime endeavor. This can involve sunscreen, wearing sun-protective clothing, hats, and sunglasses, and avoiding direct sunlight during the peak hours of 10:00 a.m. to 4:00 p.m., instead seeking shady, covered areas.[6107] Sunbathing is frowned upon, even with sunscreens like zinc oxide or titanium dioxide, which offer broad-spectrum protection against both UV-A and UV-B rays.[6108] We now know that other wavelengths not covered by sunscreens, such as near infrared, also contribute to skin aging.[6109] Men and women who use tanning beds appear significantly older than those who don't, and those who sunbathe appear years older than they actually are, comparable to what is seen with smoking.[6110]

SOMETHING IN THE AIR

Beyond the oxidizing effects of rays of the sun are the oxidizing effects of oxygen in the air, as well as cigarette smoke, automobile exhaust, and other environmental pollutants.[6111] Cigarette smokers develop a distinctive pattern of prominent wrinkles known as "smoker's face."[6112] The effects are so significant that illustrating these aging effects can help smoking teenagers quit. Compared to only one out of eighty teens quitting in a control group, eleven out of eighty teens who had been shown digital aging software presenting their future faces with and without smoking were successfully able to quit.[6113] A similar study presenting the deleterious effects of UV rays of facial images appeared to affect sustained behavioral change in regard to sun-tanning practices.[6114]

Even ambient air pollution has been correlated with signs of skin aging.[6115] Poor air quality index is significantly linked with age spots, increased wrinkling, and skin sagging.[6116] This is blamed on polycyclic aromatic hydrocarbons (PAHs).[6117] These combustion by-products coat diesel exhaust particles and are also formed when coal is burned, tobacco is smoked, and meat is grilled.[6118]

Tobacco smokers get about half their exposure to PAHs from cigarettes and the other half or so from food. For nonsmokers, though, 99 percent of their PAH exposure may come from their diet. The highest levels of these chemicals are found in meat, with pork apparently worse than beef,[6119] but even dark green leafy vegetables can get contaminated by pollutants in the air. So don't forage your dandelion greens next to the highway and make sure to rinse your greens under running water.[6120]

Since PAHs are fat-soluble, absorption of these chemicals may be diminished by eating foods that are lower in fat.[6121] However, they do not appear to build up in our body. Unlike persistent pollutants like PCBs, which may take fifty to seventy-five years to clear from the body after regularly eating farmed Atlantic salmon, for example,[6122] PAHs can pass through us in a single day. After eating a meal of barbecued chicken, a big spike in these chemicals can be seen in the diners' systems—up to a hundredfold increase. However, the body can detoxify most of the PAHs away within about twenty hours.[6123] Instead of detoxing, wouldn't it be better not to "tox" in the first place? A recent dermatology review article ended with this summary: "In conclusion, when patients inquire about a diet that might contribute to younger-looking skin, evidence supports the recommendation to follow a WFPB [whole food, plant-based] diet."[6124]

MEDICAL SKIN TREATMENTS

Anti-aging medicine is one of the fastest-growing medical specialties[6125] and often targeted at women, who are urged to restore their youthful appearance by "any and all available means."[6126] Ninety-two percent of cosmetic procedures are performed on women, most commonly Botox, fillers, and laser or chemical peel skin resurfacing. Each year, millions in the United States undergo cosmetic surgery, including hundreds of thousands of face-lifts, known technically as *rhytidectomies*.[6127]

LOSING FACE

In see.nf/faceliftsbotox, I detail what we know about face-lifts. Basically, none of the techniques has been shown to be definitively better than others,[6128] and they're considered to be relatively safe when performed by a board-certified plastic surgeon.[6129] In the video, I discuss all the complication rates[6130] and the importance of tempering expectations.[6131]

HITTING THE HEADLINES

In the same video, I also cover Botox injections, the most common nonsurgical cosmetic procedure.[6132] In sum, adverse effects are transient and self-limited,[6133] but the increase in injections administered by nonmedical personnel[6134] raises concerns about a potential rise in extremely rare cases of respiratory failure and death occurring hours or even weeks after injection.[6135]

FILLING YOUR FACE

In see.nf/fillers, I cover the second most common cosmetic procedure, volumizing injections of soft tissue fillers.[6136] Adverse outcomes occur in about one in forty procedures, most commonly bruising,[6137] discoloration, swelling, or unsightly lumps and bumps.[6138] The most devastating filler complication is permanent blindness due to an accidental injection into an artery.[6139] More about that in the video, along with similar concerns about the increasing administration of fillers in spa-type (rather than medical) settings[6140] that may use illegal (non–FDA approved) fillers. There have been reports of injections with everything from rubber cement to Fix-a-Flat tire repair sealant, resulting in disfigurement and even death.[6141]

PEEL OUT

Another common cosmetic procedure is the chemical peel. About a million are performed every year, along with another million laser skin "resurfacings"[6142] to provide a "controlled injury to the face."[6143] The reasoning is that the regeneration, repair, and remodeling of the damage caused to the skin can result in a more tightened appearance,[6144] but peels and laser resurfacings may or may not actually help with wrinkles.[6145] The inflammation caused by these types of facials causes edema (fluid retention) in the face, which, because of the swelling, can cause a transient improvement in the appearance of fine wrinkles but, in the end, may do more harm than good.[6146] Short-term side effects include bruising, swelling, itching, crusting, redness, infection, acne, and milia (little white cysts).[6147] Long-lasting side effects can include persistent redness, pigmentation changes, and scarring.[6148]

DIETARY SKIN TREATMENTS

Some animals use diet to increase their sexual attractiveness. Great tits, distinctive olive-and-black songbirds ubiquitous throughout Europe and Asia, tend to prefer carotenoid-rich caterpillars, which make their breast plumage brighter yellow to become more appealing to potential mates.[6149] Might there be a similar phenomenon in humans?

TANNING BED OF GREENS

When researchers showed study participants digital photographs of Asian, African, and Caucasian women and men and asked them to turn a dial to manipulate the skin tone of their faces until they felt the healthiest-looking color was reached,[6150] both female and male subjects preferred the yellow "golden glow" that can be achieved through "dietary carotenoid deposition in the skin."[6151] As I review in see.nf/glow, the healthier you eat, the healthier you may look, but the increase in facial attractiveness from eating more fruits and vegetables[6152] may drop within weeks once you stop,[6153] so you have to keep it up.

There's an entire tanning industry predicated on the belief that darker Caucasian skin appears to be healthier and more attractive, but research suggests that the perceived improvement in appearance from tanning is due to the associated increase in skin yellowness. When you separate out the shade from the hue, study participants actually preferred lighter—but yellower—skin.[6154] When high "kale" models were pitted against high tan models, the golden glow from consuming carotenoid phytonutrients won out.[6155] So, may I suggest the produce aisle to get a good, healthy tan . . . gerine?

SAVE YOUR SKIN

I am not above appealing to vanity, especially for younger individuals for whom surveys suggest eating to improve appearance trumps eating for better health.[6156] So,
I'm always excited when I see articles embrace studies with headlines like "Greens
to Be Gorgeous."[6157] Fruits and vegetables don't just change our hue, though. As I
document in see.nf/internalsunscreen, skin biopsies from women effectively randomized to a daily spinach salad showed a significant increase in collagen production,
accompanied by an increase in skin elasticity and a decrease of facial wrinkles.[6158]
This may have been due in part to an "inside-out" sunscreen effect, as less DNA
damage was noted after the same degree of UV radiation. Kale,[6159] apple,[6160] and
a combination of rosemary and grapefruit extracts[6161] had similar effects. Even just
ten weeks before swimsuit season (but not four), eating a lot of an antioxidant-rich
food, such as tomato paste, can reduce the redness of a sunburn by 40 percent.[6162]

Topical sunscreens and dietary photoprotection with foods like greens[6163] and
sweet potatoes[6164] naturally complement each other for safeguarding our skin. Sunscreens have the advantage of working almost immediately and offering much stronger shielding, while *produce* protection builds up slowly over weeks and only achieves
an SPF of 4, compared to 10 to 40 or even higher with typical sunscreens. On the
other hand, sunscreens have to be deliberately applied, in sufficient amounts, with
sufficient coverage—including all the hard-to-reach places—and then can still rub
off, wash off, or be sweated off, whereas the protection from plants is ever-present
and built-in all over.

ANTIOXIDANT DYNAMICS

Antioxidant levels in our skin are ever-changing hour to hour. Remember that
argon laser study from page 117? Similar technology has been used to show a tight
correlation between low antioxidant levels in the skin and the presence of facial
furrows and wrinkles.[6165] This is consistent with data showing significantly less skin
aging over a fifteen-year period among those eating high-antioxidant versus low-
antioxidant foods.[6166] This constantly fluctuating balance between the antioxidants
we deposit in our skin from our diet and the onslaught of daily oxidant stresses
sapping our reserves can provide insight into some other lifestyle behaviors that
can affect skin health.

For instance, don't forget your beauty sleep. Compared to individuals getting
eight hours of sleep, participants who were kept up for thirty-one consecutive
hours and allowed only five hours of sleep were rated as having redder eyes, more
swollen eyes, darker circles, hanging eyelids, paler skin, more fine lines and wrinkles, and droopier corners of their mouths.[6167] Those who are sleep-deprived are
also perceived as being more tired (duh), less healthy, and less attractive than the

well-rested.[6168] Over time, the oxidative stress associated with sleep deprivation could potentially translate into long-term differences in skin aging parameters.[6169]

Psychological stress may also affect skin aging.[6170] Higher stress hormone levels are associated with increased perceived age.[6171] Think how U.S. presidents look before and after one or two terms in office.[6172] In an aging study out of Boston, hundreds of participants had photographs taken over a ten-year time span. Those under financial stress, even after controlling for income (and health and attractiveness), were rated as looking significantly older than they were at baseline and aging significantly worse over time.[6173]

Antioxidant dynamics may also explain why alcohol consumption is linked not just to digestive tract malignancies but to skin cancer, too.[6174] As I note in see.nf /sunalcohol, after drinking about three shots of vodka, the level of carotenoid antioxidants in the skin drops dramatically within *eight minutes*,[6175] which translates into sunburn susceptibility that can be mediated by drinking it with orange juice.[6176] But berries are even better, so a strawberry daiquiri may lessen burn risk even more than a screwdriver.

Alcohol consumption does not appear to affect skin aging, though. One study found a significant correlation between skin wrinkles and alcohol consumption,[6177] but ten others found no significant associations in either direction.[6178] What about other beverages?

SKIN DRINK

Perhaps not surprisingly, whole-body dehydration is associated with dry eye syndrome,[6179] a condition that disproportionally affects the elderly.[6180] What about hydration and dry skin? A systematic review found that studies show drinking an extra one or two liters (quarts) of water a day for four to seven weeks may improve skin hydration and decrease symptoms of skin dryness and roughness.[6181]

What about tea or coffee? Skin biopsies taken before and after drinking tea show that green tea compounds are deposited in human skin, but to what effect?[6182] The drinking of coffee[6183] or both tea and coffee[6184] is associated with fewer pigmented spots on the faces of Japanese women, but interventional studies are either absent (in the case of coffee) or disappointing (in the case of tea).

Skin biopsies show that a combination of oral and topical green tea increases the elastic tissue content of skin compared to placebos within eight weeks, but not enough to be noticeable to the naked eye.[6185] EGCG, one of the active components of green tea, can reduce UV-induced skin damage in rats,[6186] but when put to the test over three months in people, green tea supplements with the EGCG equivalent of eleven cups of tea a day showed significant photoprotection,[6187] though the equivalent of five daily cups of tea did not.[6188] Maybe the study period just wasn't long enough? A two-year, double-blind, randomized, placebo-controlled trial found a significant improvement in overall solar damage, redness, and telangiectasias (spider veins) on the sun-exposed arm skin of women randomized to consume the equivalent of about two and a half cups of green tea a day, but the same was also found in those randomized to the placebo group. In other words, just being part of the clinical trial may have led the women to change their sun exposure activities and benefit regardless.[6189]

In see.nf/topicaltea, I cover an extraordinary case report that suggested the topical application of green tea could prevent skin cancers,[6190] presumably due to decreased UV-induced DNA damage,[6191] but for those not at particularly high risk of skin cancer, topical green tea is considered to be too irritating to be used routinely.[6192] Once you already have a basal cell carcinoma, applying a 10 percent green tea ointment doesn't seem to help.[6193]

An herbal tea that may help is a soothing South African infusion called honeybush (*Cyclopia*). After it was found to protect the skin of "nude" (hairless) mice from UV damage,[6194] water extracts of honeybush were tested in a randomized, double-blind, placebo-controlled trial. Rather than coming up with a placebo tea that looked and tasted the same, the honeybush tea was dried and powdered into capsules to pit against indistinguishable placebo pills. So, it's not clear how much tea was actually being tested, but after twelve weeks, it decreased eye wrinkle volume by about 28 percent more than placebo.[6195]

The other anti-wrinkling beverage may surprise you: hot cocoa. After drinking a beverage with about two and a half teaspoons of natural cocoa powder, subjects had a significant increase in blood flow within the skin within two hours.[6196] Drink it every day for six weeks, and the redness to the same UV dose is down by 15 percent and, after twelve weeks, by 25 percent. Skin thickness, density, and hydration also improved compared to the placebo, a cocoa from which most of the flavanols had been removed. No change was found in wrinkle severity after twelve weeks,[6197] but a twenty-four-week study found a significant improvement in skin elasticity and a decrease in wrinkle depth[6198]—just from adding less than a tablespoon of cocoa powder to their daily diet.

"Wrinkles Should Merely Indicate Where the Smiles Have Been." —Mark Twain

Wrinkles occur where fault lines develop in aging skin,[6199] a process comparable to breaking in leather gloves.[6200] Over time, the skin folding caused by everyday facial expressions etches the temporary grooves into permanent wrinkles.[6201] In see.nf/wrinkleformation, I cover the roles of Botox, "antiwrinkle" pillows and adhesive strips, genetics, and even the light emitted by smartphone screens. Of course, kids can scrunch up their faces all they want because the architecture of their skin has yet to be irreparably damaged, so the key to preventing wrinkles is preventing the underlying structural damage that makes your skin susceptible to them via choices such as tobacco avoidance and regular sun protection.[6202]

AN ANTI-WRINKLE DIET

If you already have some wrinkles, is there any diet that might reduce them? While a predominantly meat-and-junk eating pattern was associated with more wrinkles,[6203] both a fruit-dominant diet and one with more fruits, vegetables, and nuts were associated with significantly less wrinkling.[6204] I run through all the specific foods associated with more or less wrinkling in see.nf/antiwrinkle, as well as the interventional data on almonds, flax, soy, and mangos—yay,[6205] yay,[6206] yay,[6207,6208] and nay,[6209] respectively.

The paucity of interventional trials limits the confidence one can put into recommendations, but the best approximations were summed up in a 2020 dermatology review titled "An Anti-Wrinkle Diet." Dietary defense strategies included antioxidant-rich foods (see the Oxidation chapter), anti-inflammatory foods (see the Inflammation chapter), anti-glycation foods (see the Glycation chapter), fiber-rich foods for our microbiome, foods like broccoli that boost DNA repair, and foods shown to be able to block collagen- and elastin-munching enzymes (at least in vitro), such as garlic, turmeric, and ginger. In other words, the best approximation for an anti-wrinkle diet is one that's centered around whole plant foods.[6210]

VEGAN VULNERABILITIES

One would expect that plant-based diets might be ideal for preventing and reversing skin aging,[6211] but there are a series of studies that expose some potential vulnerabilities. For example, the skin of vegan patients was found to be more vulnerable to inflammation in a study of phototherapy for psoriasis. Phototherapy typically involves the combination of light-sensitizing drugs with a UV lamp or laser light. After eight weeks of treatments, significantly more vegans (42 percent) ended up suffering severe redness as a side effect when compared to vegetarians (17 percent) or omnivores (10 percent). Why might that be? Because the vegans came preloaded with *furocoumarins*, photosensitizing compounds found naturally in certain fruits and vegetables, such as parsley, parsnips, celery, and citrus. The vegans in the study were reportedly eating 1.3 pounds (600 g) of parsley a week. (That's six cups of parsley in seven days!) They also ate ten pounds of citrus, including two pounds of lemons, and pounds of parsnips and celery each week. It's great that they were getting such healthy produce, but these furocoumarin-rich foods could certainly make your skin more sensitive to getting sunburned.[6212]

Another phototherapy study, this time to destroy precancerous skin lesions, also found more severe skin inflammation in the vegan participants, as well as prolonged healing times. In the omnivores, the average healing time to wound closure was about ten days, which is considered normal. Complete skin healing in the vegans, however, took more than twice as long, twenty-two days.[6213] A protraction of healing and poorer results were also found in both laser tattoo removal in vegans (average healing time of twenty-three days) compared to omnivores (average healing time of nineteen days)[6214] and ablative laser skin resurfacing.[6215] This could be due in part to excess photodamage from eating more photosensitizing produce, but vegans also seem to have delayed healing of wounds unrelated to light exposure.

In a comparison of postsurgical scars from excision of skin cancers between vegans and omnivores, the vegans didn't seem to heal as well. Reduced collagen synthesis was suspected. Collagen is not only the major component of skin in general, but it's also the main connective tissue directly involved in wound healing.[6216] Impaired collagen synthesis could also explain why cosmetic fillers are longer-lasting in omnivores, since the mechanical stress of filler injection works to boost collagen synthesis,[6217] and why micro-focused ultrasound skin treatments seem to work better. Intense focused ultrasound is used to treat sagging skin by generating temperatures up to 140°F (60°C) to trigger a repair process that involves new collagen formation. The researchers suggested that less collagen production would explain why vegan patients experienced significantly less improvement.[6218]

Do those eating plant-based diets really make less collagen? Apparently so. Collagen synthesis rates appear to be about 10 percent lower in vegetarians.[6219] The question is *why*. In every single one of the aforementioned studies that measured vitamin B_{12} levels, the vegan participants were found to be deficient (averaging < 200 pg/mL),[6220,6221,6222,6223,6224] and both human and animal studies show that B_{12} is important for collagen synthesis[6225,6226] and wound healing.[6227,6228] Homocysteine, a toxic by-product of B_{12} deficiency, appears to impair collagen cross-linking,[6229] which confers connective tissue mechanical integrity.[6230] It's critically important that everyone consuming plant-based diets include a regular, reliable source of vitamin B_{12}. (See page 211.)

Another potential contributor is increased protein needs during wound healing. For example, for those trying to heal pressure-induced skin ulcers, recommended protein intake goes from 0.8 g a day per kg of body weight (approximately 0.4 g per lb) up to 1.25 to 1.5 g/kg (about 0.6 to 0.7 g/lb).[6231] This explains why most of a dozen studies of protein supplementation for pressure ulcers found a greater reduction in ulcer size with supplementation.[6232] Vegans average about 1.0 g/kg a day, which is more than enough protein for day-to-day needs,[6233] but omnivores average about 1.3 g/kg, so they may already be getting the excess protein that could be helpful during wound healing.[6234] So, while recuperating from their next tattoo removal, I would recommend vegans up their legume intake.

COLLAGEN SUPPLEMENTS

Oral collagen supplementation has become quite the trendy treatment for skin aging,[6235] available in an array of pills, powders, and products from bars and gummies to collagen-fortified coffee and beer.[6236] Social media is said to be "inundated with paid ads marketing unsubstantiated claims."[6237] What claims, if any, can be substantiated?

I review all the studies on collagen supplementation for skin aging in my video see.nf/collagen. In short, most of the studies have been funded by collagen supplement manufacturers,[6238] and the overall quality of evidence has been considered by reviewers to be "limited, contradictory,"[6239] or "not particularly robust."[6240] A 2022 review titled "Myths and Media in Oral Collagen Supplementation for the Skin, Nails, and Hair" in the *Journal of Cosmetic Dermatology* concluded, "Dermatologists should be aware of the unsubstantiated proclamations of collagen made by companies . . . [that] surpass any evidence currently supported by the literature," and, given the insufficient evidence, "collagen cannot be routinely recommended. . . ."[6241] The evidence is considered "particularly unconvincing," another review determined, when compared to methods more definitely shown to have a positive effect on skin collagen, such as sunscreen use, smoking cessation, and a healthier diet.[6242]

In see.nf/collagendiet, I describe how to stimulate your own collagen synthesis, for example, by ensuring a daily vitamin C intake of at least 95 mg,[6243] which is higher than the current recommendations.[6244]

Though we don't have evidence that collagen is superior to other proteins for skin aging,[6245] if you do want to try it, consumers are advised to contact the manufacturers to clarify sources. Most collagen supplements don't disclose this information—and for good reason.[6246] Terrestrial sources of collagen can include a witch's brew of duck feet, frog skin, kangaroo and rat tails, alligator bones, and horse tendons.[6247] Aquatic sources are mainly from the skins, bones, heads, scales, fins, and entrails of fish.[6248]

Recommended questions for manufacturers include, "What measures were used to protect against contamination or adulteration? If sourced from fish, were low-mercury fish used? If sourced from cows, what steps were taken to ensure that no brain or nervous system matter was included, in order to prevent prion disease?"[6249] In the United States, collagen is exempt from FDA prohibitions against using risky tissues, like brains, that are intended to protect consumers against bovine spongiform encephalopathy (mad cow disease).[6250]

For food safety, religious, ethical, and allergy reasons, there have been calls for non-animal sourcing.[6251] For example, 2 to 4 percent of the population is allergic to bovine collagen.[6252] To solve the mad cow conundrum, there have been calls to genetically engineer cattle without prions to "offer a safe source of collagen-based materials," but why not just get plants to make it? A technique has been developed to produce collagen from plants,[6253] but it has not yet reached commercial viability. It's hard to beat the cost of feet.

TOPICAL SKIN TREATMENTS

Over-the-counter "anti-aging" products constitute a billion-dollar industry.[6254] There is a "psychological effect from spending more," noted a review on the myths of anti-aging skin care, but "don't be seduced by fancy packaging and high prices."[6255] Many products advertise dramatic results that are frequently exaggerated and misleading[6256] and are rarely supported scientifically.[6257] An independent product testing institute questioned the efficacy of anti-aging creams generally, finding that beneficial effects could only be picked up using sensitive instruments without becoming clinically detectable and suggested these products may not work any better than typical moisturizers.[6258]

Cross-sectional studies of Chinese[6259] and British women found that those who regularly used facial moisturizers were guessed to be about two years younger than women of the same age who didn't. However, a third, larger (Dutch) study did not. Regardless, snapshot-in-time studies can never establish cause and effect.[6260] Studies on moisturizers are limited, but they can improve the appearance of dry skin, which can otherwise look discolored, flaky, and rough.[6261] Moisturizers can hydrate the skin and may reduce the appearance of fine lines by 15 to 20 percent, called "the oldest trick [in] the cosmetic industry," but they may not do anything to treat the underlying cause.[6262]

DAILY SPF 15 FACIAL MOISTURIZER

Whether facial foundation, night cream, or anti-aging "serum," the formulations of most skin products are basically a moisturizer combined with purported active ingredients for marketing appeal.[6263] Which ingredients are *actually* active anti-aging agents? I bet you can guess which is the single most effective skincare component out there when I offer as a hint the reminder that up to 90 percent of the visible aging of someone's face is due to sunlight.[6264] From an anti-aging standpoint, the most biologically active ingredient in skin products is sunscreen.[6265]

Considered the single most important practice for maintaining youthful skin is the daily application of sunscreen and employing other protective measures, like wearing a hat. Everything else you can do for your skin pales in comparison, especially for those with pale skin.[6266] UV-A rays are primarily responsible for skin aging, whereas UV-B are the rays that cause sunburn. A broad-spectrum sunscreen covering both is recommended since both types of UV contribute to cancer risk.[6267] To prevent skin cancer, the American Academy of Dermatology recommends sunscreen with an SPF of 30 or higher,[6268] but an SPF of 15 can prevent skin aging.[6269] How do we know? Because it's been put to the test.

Nine hundred adults were randomized to years of recommended daily sunscreen use or continuing with their own discretionary use. (It was considered unethical to withhold protection by giving people placebo sunscreen.) In the end, 77 percent in the recommended daily sunscreen group applied sunscreen at least three to four days per week compared with only 33 percent in the discretionary use group. Would that be enough of a difference to make a difference? Yes, there was significantly less skin aging in the instructed daily use group. In fact, they suffered no detectable increase in skin aging over the four-and-a-half-year study. The researchers concluded, "Regular sunscreen use retards skin aging in healthy, middle-aged men and women."[6270]

Although sunscreens are primarily intended to prevent further facial aging rather than reverse preexisting photodamage,[6271] some in the daily sunscreen use group did show an improvement in skin texture. The results are all the more striking given that the control group was told to continue to use sunscreen and hats whenever they thought it would be needed, suggesting people are poor judges or planners for excess UV exposure when left to their own devices. So, a daily facial moisturizer with an SPF 15 is recommended, even if it is cloudy or raining outside.[6272] Considered the "gold standard" for anti-aging skin care: "daily use of sunscreens in the daytime and retinoids at night. . . ."[6273]

NIGHTLY RETINOIDS?

While sunscreen can prevent further skin photoaging, tretinoin can reverse some of what's already been done. Also known as all-trans retinoic acid and sold under a variety of brand names, including Retin-A, tretinoin is a prescription-only form of vitamin A that can visibly improve mild to moderate photodamage, including fine and coarse wrinkles, freckles, and other pigmentation, and improve overall skin texture after months of regular use,[6274] though it can cause redness, stinging, burning, itching, and peeling in a high proportion of patients.[6275] There are gentler, less potent, over-the-counter topical retinoids: retinaldehyde, retinol, and retinyl esters (acetate, palmitate, or propionate). I compare and contrast them in see.nf /retinoids.

Of all the nonprescription retinoid options, retinol may be the preferred choice,[6276] but tretinoin has by far the most robust track record of efficacy,[6277] so why not ask your doctor for a prescription? Because, as I detail in the video, long-term topical tretinoin use may increase your risk of an even more stinging side effect: premature death.[6278]

TOPICAL NICOTINAMIDE

What other skin cream components have been shown to help with skin aging? While placebo-controlled trials are the standard in most medical research, they are still all too rare for cosmetic products.[6279] This raises efficacy questions, so many are left with simply buying "hope in a jar."[6280] This also raises safety concerns. To this day, cosmetics contain an array of toxic chemicals. Of the more than 12,000 synthetic compounds used in cosmetics, less than 20 percent have been recognized as safe.[6281] Of course, this doesn't mean *natural* ingredients are necessarily harmless. Poison ivy is as natural as you can get, but you wouldn't want to rub it on your face.[6282] However, there are some relatively safe natural options with varying degrees of efficacy.

Topical nicotinamide, also known as *niacinamide*, is a form of vitamin B$_3$ that is nonirritating[6283] and has been described as "one of the best studied cosmeceutical ingredients for anti-aging,"[6284] but it looks like there are only three placebo-controlled human studies,[6285] which gives you an idea of the state of cosmeceutical science.

Skin photoaging is largely mediated by UV-induced free radical formation. One of the consequences of excess sun exposure is the oxidation of sugars and proteins in the skin into yellow-brown pigment that gives aging skin a yellowing, sallow appearance. Since nicotinamide is a precursor to two potent antioxidants, the hope is that this process could be interrupted,[6286] as revealed in the first study, titled "Topical Niacinamide Reduces Yellowing, Wrinkling, Red Blotchiness, and Hyperpigmented Spots in Aging Facial Skin."[6287]

It was a twelve-week, double-blind, placebo-controlled, split-face, randomized clinical study of middle-aged women. In a split-face study, each subject is her own control. The active formulation (in this case, 5 percent nicotinamide in moisturizer) is rubbed on one side of her face and the placebo (straight moisturizer) on the other half, though neither she nor the researchers know which side is which until the code is broken at the end. This controls for skin type and administration technique, since different people apply facial products differently. However, people often use the same hand to apply creams to both sides of their face. So, unless specified that different gloves be worn or hands washed in between, there can be cross-contamination.[6288]

At the end of twelve weeks, there was a small (5 percent) reduction in wrinkles and fine lines and a slowing in the development in blotchiness, spots, and sallowness on the nicotinamide side of the face.[6289] A subsequent publication noted an improvement in skin elasticity as well.[6290] The magnitude of the effects may only be one-third to one-fifth as good as for tretinoin,[6291] but there were no reports of excess skin irritation.[6292]

The other two studies were similar split-face trials, but with 4 percent nicotinamide products. One study found no significant effect on facial wrinkles compared to placebo,[6293] but the other, which was limited to crow's-feet wrinkles around the eyes, found significant improvements in both subjective and objective measures by the end of the eight-week study. Sixty-four percent of the nicotinamide-side eye wrinkles underwent moderate or marked improvement compared to zero percent on the placebo side.[6294]

TOPICAL VITAMIN C

If skin aging is mediated by oxidative stress, why not just directly apply antioxidants like vitamin C? Topical application of antioxidants can lead to levels in the skin that are ten times what is achieved with oral dosing (at least in the skin of mice).[6295] According to a recent review on topical anti-aging skin care by a prominent Beverly Hills plastic surgeon, "At a minimum, patients should be encouraged to use daily sunscreen, a topical retinoid every night, and a topical antioxidant daily."[6296] But which antioxidant? Only one has been clearly shown to work.

Despite its ubiquity in skin care products, there is no evidence to support any role for topical vitamin E in skin aging, whether for wrinkles, discoloration, or texture,[6297] and the one study on topical CoQ_{10} found that it also failed to work significantly better than placebo.[6298] There is, however, one type of vitamin C that has been shown to help.[6299]

Skin biopsy studies show that the topical application of a 5 percent solution of L-ascorbic acid (also known as ascorbic acid, the type of vitamin C found in food) significantly increases the expression of collagen in human skin compared to placebo, suggesting "functional activity of the dermal [skin] cells is not maximal in postmenopausal women and can be increased."[6300] A split-face study involving the application of three drops of a 10 percent L-ascorbic acid solution for three months found significant improvements over the placebo side of the face in fine and coarse wrinkles, sallowness, and skin tone (firmness).[6301] Not knowing which side was which, sixteen out of nineteen (84 percent) patients correctly guessed the vitamin C side as the one showing improvement.

Unfortunately, L-ascorbic acid is unstable in creams. It turns an unsightly brown when it oxidizes, limiting its shelf life.[6302] So, instead, the skin care industry uses more stable vitamin C esters or derivatives such as ascorbyl palmitate, ascorbyl stearate, magnesium ascorbyl phosphate, or ascorbic acid sulfate.[6303] Unfortunately, there is no evidence that these compounds have comparable effects, likely because they are poorly absorbed and only minimally convert to the active form. The good news is that you can make your own.

Although vitamin C concentrations as low as 3[6304] and 5[6305] percent have been shown to have anti-wrinkle effects in split-face or split-neck and arm studies, at least 10 percent is recommended. The 10 percent solution used in the aforementioned split-face study retails for a ridiculous $127 per ounce.[6306] You can make a DIY solution by simply buying L-ascorbic acid in bulk and mixing 3 g into 30 g of water at a cost of about a nickel per ounce, thousands of times cheaper. You can mix it in an eyedropper bottle. Drip just four or five drops on the palm of your hand, and use your fingertips to apply it over your face, neck, and upper chest daily. Be careful not to get it in your eyes, though.

Alpha Hydroxy Acids

There is a reason there's a long historical use of fruit purees as facial masks.[6307] Alpha hydroxy acids, also known as fruit acids, are used at high-strength concentrations in chemical peels, but lower concentrations are sold over the counter as exfoliants.[6308] I review the four placebo-controlled studies in see.nf/alpha. In sum, alpha hydroxy acids can help with past photodamage, but they may make future damage worse by increasing skin photosensitivity.[6309]

SKIN CANCER

More than a million new cases of skin cancer are diagnosed every year, affecting about one in three Americans in their lifetimes.[6310] Risk increases with age[6311] and the incidence has been on the rise.[6312] Should we get screened for skin cancer by getting periodic full-body exams? The Skin Cancer Foundation recommends annual physician exams,[6313] but the official U.S. Preventive Services Task Force position is that there is insufficient evidence to support any interval of skin screening.[6314] This is based in part on a national experiment in Germany.

In 2003, a total body skin exam screening campaign was started in the German state of Schleswig-Holstein. By 2008, melanoma mortality rates had dropped by nearly 50 percent.[6315] Given the apparent resounding success, the program was expanded nationwide in 2009. Sadly, five years later, there was no significant change in melanoma mortality. In fact, national rates had even crept up a bit, and the apparent gains in Schleswig-Holstein vanished back to baseline.[6316] Was the original drop just due to chance?[6317] More nefariously, some have suggested that German doctors, motivated by the financial incentive—a per-screening bonus of €15 (about $20)—started intentionally or unconsciously underreporting melanoma on death certificates to make the program appear effective.[6318] Either way, skin screening has not yet been shown to save lives.[6319]

Note that the USPSTF's lack of endorsement for regular medical skin screening is only in reference to the mass screening of asymptomatic healthy individuals. If you have a suspicious mole or are otherwise at heightened risk due to a personal or family history of skin cancer, you should definitely bring it up with your healthcare provider. The ABCDEs of mole suspiciousness for melanoma, the deadliest form of skin cancer, are A for asymmetry, B for border irregularity, C for multiple colors, D for diameter (larger than a pencil eraser), and E for evolving, a change in size, shape, color, elevation, or symptoms (such as bleeding, itching, or crusting). Basically, any lesion that is new, changing, or unusual (compared to other moles) is suspect.[6320]

SLIP, SLOP, SLAP, SEEK, SLIDE

If universal screening isn't going to save us from skin cancer, what will? The same and best way to reduce the risk of all common cancers: primary prevention. In other words, preventing the cancer from emerging in the first place. Here's another mnemonic, Australia's SunSmart 5 S's program (featuring Sid the Seagull): slip on clothing, slop on sunscreen, slap on a hat, seek shade, and slide on sunglasses.[6321]

A single blistering sunburn on a child may double the risk of developing basal cell or squamous cell skin cancers later in life,[6322] whereas regular use of sunscreen during childhood has been estimated to reduce the incidence of these cancers by 78 percent.[6323]

Ideally, protective clothing should fully cover the arms and legs.[6324] For regular clothes without an ultraviolet protection factor (UPF) tag, densely woven, thicker, and darker cloth tends to be more protective. (Hold a garment up to the light and see whether it shines through.)[6325] Hats should shade the whole head.[6326] Wrap-around sunglasses can better shield the delicate skin around the eyes that may not be protected by sunscreen, and lip products with at least 30 SPF should be applied generously to fully cover the lips.[6327]

Oral Nicotinamide

After decades of use in the cosmetics industry to prevent skin aging,[6328] researchers decided to put nicotinamide to the test for skin cancer prevention. Normally, it would be difficult to fund studies on nonpatentable products that only cost a few cents a day, but preliminary findings[6329] were so extraordinary that ONTRAC was born. Oral Nicotinamide to Reduce Actinic Cancer was a publicly funded, phase III (efficacy-determining) trial randomizing hundreds of people with personal history of skin cancers to 500 mg of nicotinamide or placebo twice a day for a full year. By the end, there were 463 new skin cancers in the placebo group versus 336 in the nicotinamide group. About 25 percent fewer cancers with no significant side effects, for just pennies a day.[6330] Details in see.nf/cancernic.

WHAT ABOUT SENSIBLE SUN EXPOSURE?

The UV rays in sunlight are considered to be a complete carcinogen, meaning they can not only initiate cancer but also promote its progression and spread.[6331] The incidence of melanoma, the scariest kind of skin cancer,[6332] has tripled over recent decades[6333] in part likely due to the increased use of tanning salons.[6334] Tanning beds and their UV rays are considered to be class 1 carcinogens, like tobacco, asbestos, plutonium, and processed meat.[6335] For more on tanning, check out see.nf/tanning.

Unlike natural sunlight, tanning bed lights emit mostly UV-A, which is the worst of both worlds: cancer risk without any vitamin D production.[6336] Sunlight supplies 90 to 95 percent of vitamin D for most people.[6337] In fact, as I detail in see.nf/sun, modeling studies suggest that low vitamin D levels from sunlight avoidance may kill more people[6338] than the skin cancer from sun overexposure.[6339] So, on balance, the benefits of "sensible sun exposure"[6340] might outweigh the risks, but why accept any risk at all when we can get all the vitamin D we need from supplements? In fact, the model got those estimates on preventing internal cancers with vitamin D from intervention studies involving giving people vitamin D *supplements*, not exposing them to UV rays.[6341] The sun debate is framed as needing to choose between the lesser of two evils: skin cancer or vitamin D deficiency. This framework ignores the fact that there's a third way: vitamin D supplements.

Black Salve Swindle

Skin cancers are usually just excised, but what about using "black salve" instead? Listed as a "fake cancer cure" by the FDA and similarly condemned by the American Academy of Dermatology, black salve is still promoted on the internet as a "natural alternative remedy for skin cancers." I detail how damaging and dangerous it can be in see.nf/salve.

Some cancer patients are duped by disinformation, but many who refuse conventional therapies described their oncologists as "impersonal," "'intimidating,' 'cold,' 'uncaring,' 'unnecessarily harsh,' 'thinking they were God,' and 'not even knowing [their] names,'" and becoming "adversarial" when questioned about recommended treatments. Few believed their doctors had their best interests in mind, and many said they would have been more likely to initially accept conventional treatment had they felt they had "caring physicians" who treated them with respect.[6342]

SUNSCREEN PROVEN TO PREVENT CANCER

As I noted before, there are randomized controlled trials that have shown that regular use of sunscreen can arrest signs of skin aging,[6343] including biopsy-proven reductions in UV-related skin damage.[6344] But, are there interventional trials proving that sunscreen can prevent cancer? Yes.[6345] In fact, it can actually reverse the progression of precancerous skin growths, causing them to spontaneously regress and vanish. I profile the mind-blowing study in see.nf/sunscreenuse. The body can sometimes heal itself once we stop bombarding it with so many cancer-causing rays.[6346]

PROPER SUNSCREEN USE

For maximum effectiveness, sunscreen needs to be applied properly. Several studies have demonstrated that this rarely happens,[6347] with as few as one in twenty-five complying with recommendations.[6348] In the same video (see.nf/sunscreenuse), I detail the proper amount using the "teaspoon rule,"[6349] why SPF 50+ is often recommended[6350] even though SPF 15 should theoretically be enough to prevent cancer,[6351] how cloudy skies can sometimes be even worse,[6352] and timing of application before[6353] and after water[6354] and sand[6355] exposure.

It's Black and White

The average built-in SPF of Black skin (also known in the medical literature as "ethnic skin" or "SOC," skin of color)[6356] is 13, compared with only 3 for white skin.[6357] Though there have been no interventional studies on sunscreen effectiveness for skin cancer prevention in people with darker skin, SPF 13 is not considered sufficient sun protection, so the American Academy of Dermatology recommends regular sunscreen use with an SPF of 30 or higher for people of all skin shades.[6358] Unfortunately, only about 12 percent of non-Hispanic Blacks and 31 percent of Hispanics report regularly using sunscreen, compared to around 44 percent of non-Hispanic whites.[6359] Despite this, the incidence of melanoma, the deadliest skin cancer, is five times lower in Hispanics compared to whites and twenty-five times lower among Blacks. However, the mortality rate if melanoma does develop is higher among Blacks, presumed to be from delayed diagnosis.[6360]

Photoaging in darker skin is less likely to appear as wrinkles and more likely to appear as pigmentation issues, such as uneven skin tone, melasma (dark patches),[6361] and dermatosis papulosa nigra (small dark bumps on the face).[6362] To combat skin aging and cancer risk, transparent chemical sunscreens are often marketed to those with darker skin, since the mineral sunscreens (i.e., titanium dioxide and zinc oxide) often leave a white residue. However, there are now micronized mineral sunscreens that are much less visible after application.

MINERAL RIGHT

What kind of sunscreen should you use? Cream-based is preferable to spray-on, since it's easier to see where you've applied the sunscreen.[6363] To help with adequate coverage, spray-on sunscreens should be rubbed around immediately after spraying.[6364] I don't recommend aerosolized sunscreens. They are flammable and can combust on the skin upon exposure to an open flame even after the sunscreen has dried.[6365] What's more, the safety of breathing in aerosolized sunscreen chemicals has not been adequately studied,[6366] though, frankly, the same thing could be said about rubbing them on your skin.

As I detail in see.nf/safestsunscreen, concerns about the systemic absorption of sunscreen chemicals were underscored by the 2019 FDA bombshell that none of them can be considered generally recognized as safe. Only two active ingredients got the green light, the two nonchemical "mineral" sunscreens titanium dioxide and zinc oxide. The revelation was based on a growing body of evidence that transdermal (through-the-skin) absorption of sunscreen chemicals was greater than we thought, raising "previously unevaluated safety concerns."[6367] Unevaluated, because previously we didn't think so much got into our bloodstreams.

TRIM THE FAT

Other than nicotinamide, how else might we protect against skin cancer from the inside out? Based on studies showing that high-fat diets accelerated skin cancer formation in mice[6368] and population studies showing higher cancer rates tied to higher-fat diets,[6369] the National Cancer Institute and a Veterans Affairs research team published striking results in *The New England Journal of Medicine* showing that randomizing those with a history of skin cancer to a lower-fat diet resulted in a tenfold drop in skin cancer rates.[6370] Details in see.nf/lowfatskin.

VARICOSE VEINS

Varicose veins are not just a cosmetic issue. They can be associated with feelings of pain, heaviness, and itchiness.[6371] Compression stockings were traditionally the standard therapy for management of symptoms,[6372] but over the last decade, the lack of evidence for compression efficacy combined with the development of minimally invasive endovenous ablation techniques has shifted treatment recommendations.[6373] (Details in see.nf/varicose.) However, neither treats the underlying cause.

Topical Vinegar

In see.nf/vein, I profile a study titled "The Effect of External Apple Vinegar Application on Varicosity Symptoms, Pain, and Social Appearance Anxiety: A Randomized Controlled Trial."[6374] Topical vinegar[6375] (not pee)[6376] can help with jellyfish stings, but not eczema.[6377] What about varicose veins? See the video for details, but the potential harms of applying undiluted vinegar[6378] probably outweigh the questionable benefits.[6379]

ANTI-VARICOSITY DIET

In Uganda, a survey found only six cases of varicose veins out of five thousand adults.[6380] Perhaps rural Africans had more than fifty times fewer varicose veins for the same reason that they had fifty times less heart disease, up to fifty times less colon cancer, and up to more than fifty times less of other "pressure diseases," such as diverticulosis, hiatal hernia, and hemorrhoids.[6381] Because their diet was so packed with whole plant foods, rural Africans were among the only known populations ever recorded eating more than 100 g of fiber a day, which is the amount that is considered normal for our species.[6382]

I mention in the Preserving Your Bowel and Bladder Function chapter and detail in see.nf/varicose how straining at stool can push blood flow back into the legs and cause the valves in the veins of our legs to fail.[6383] The root cause of straining is the effort needed to pass unnaturally firm stools, but we can treat that cause by eating enough fiber-containing whole plant foods to create stools so large and soft that you could pass them effortlessly. Given the fiber connection, it's no surprise that Western vegetarians also have lower rates of pressure diseases like diverticulosis,[6384] hemorrhoids, and varicose veins,[6385] but that might not be the only reason. A study of elderly vegetarians found they also have a much lower incidence of varicose veins under the tongue, as well as fewer sublingual bleeding capillaries, a condition known as *caviar tongue*. Given the dilation of veins and thinning of blood vessel walls characteristic of scurvy, the researchers suspect the low rates of varicose veins in vegetarians may also have to do with their greater vitamin C intake.[6386]

NAIL HEALTH

According to the American Academy of Dermatology, nearly everyone will experience some sort of nail disorder during their lifetime. As we age, our nails grow more slowly, become more brittle, and can start to appear pale, dull, or opaque. Starting around age twenty-five, nail growth rates slow by about a half a percentage point a year, perhaps one of the reasons we are more likely to be affected by nail fungus as we get older, the most common of nail disorders.[6387] The prevalence of nail fungus, also known as *onychomycosis*, rises from about 2 percent in our youth to 20 percent over the age of sixty and affects around half of seventy-year-olds.[6388]

TREATING FUNGAL TOENAIL INFECTIONS

Nail fungal infections typically strike the toenails, causing nail discoloration, deformity, detachment, thickening, crumbling, and ridging. They are stubborn to treat, as the fungus can hide deep inside the nail, protected from the blood supply on one side and anything you want to put on topically from the other. So, even if you're able to beat it back, it often recurs due to residual infection.[6389]

Onychomycosis is most commonly treated with oral antifungal drugs[6390] because they are much more effective than topical antifungals, but they carry more side effects and drug interactions.[6391] Terbinafine, sold as Lamisil, is typically the drug of choice for treatment in the elderly.[6392] It can cause a metallic taste in the mouth by the second month of treatment, and skin rashes are common and sometimes severe.[6393] Other common side effects include headache and gastrointestinal symptoms, with rare cases of liver, kidney, and heart failure.[6394] Cure rates in the elderly from oral antifungals are only about 64 percent, but that's a lot better than the topical drugs.[6395]

Oral antifungals are typically given for twelve weeks for toenail infections, whereas topical antifungals may take twelve months. (Fingernail fungus is usually treated in half the time.) Such long treatment courses can limit patient compliance, especially among those who want to use nail polish to cover it up, and, even after a full year of daily application, cure rates for most topical medications are only about 9 percent versus around 1 percent for placebo.[6396] There are some newer topical agents that can be applied once or twice a week that may work better, but, apparently, not significantly so.[6397] Given the poor response rate, topical treatment alone is generally only recommended in mild cases or where oral drugs are con-traindicated.[6398] (For example, terbinafine is not recommended for people with liver disorders.[6399]) To increase the cure rates, oral and topical treatments can be combined.[6400] Based on in vitro data on the antifungal effects of an acidic pH,[6401] some recommend nightly diluted vinegar foot baths of half water and half vinegar before topical antifungal application.[6402]

What about other natural remedies? Diluted tea tree oil appears to help against the fungus that feeds on your scalp to cause dandruff[6403] and the athlete's foot fungus between your toes, so what about topical application for nail fungus?[6404] As I detail in see.nf/teatree, it was pitted head-to-head against the popular anti-fungal medication clotrimazole, sold as Lotrimin, in a double-blind, randomized, controlled trial and was found to be comparable in efficacy of cure, clinical assess-ment, subjective improvement, and even cost.[6405] Even better, though, is to treat the underlying causes.

Preventing and Treating Ingrown Toenails

While fingernails tend to become thinner with age,[6406] toenails can become thicker and harder, making them more difficult to cut.[6407] To prevent toenails from becoming ingrown, when the side or corner of the nail digs into the adjacent flesh, toenails—especially on the big toe—should be trimmed straight across.[6408] Unlike the curve you get trimming your fingernails, the top of your toenails should make a straight line. You can round the corners,[6409] but the nail should always extend beyond the skin on both sides.[6410] Another main cause of ingrown toenails is ill-fitting footwear.[6411] Shoes that are that too tight or small can push the skin of your toe into your nail.

Minor ingrown toenails can be treated at home with cotton packing.[6412] As

(continued)

soon as you feel the corner of your toe getting inflamed, twist off a wisp of cotton from a cotton swab or a cotton ball. Insert it under the corner of your nail, and try to stuff it under and along the lateral edge of the nail to protect the underlying skin.[6413] Although it can be painful to get it in there, you should experience immediate relief when it's in place.[6414] Obviously, if it continues to get worse, see a healthcare professional.

PREVENTING FUNGAL TOENAIL INFECTIONS

First there's the pathogen. The leading culprit is the same fungus that also causes jock itch, ringworm, and athlete's foot.[6415] So, keeping feet clean and dry can help prevent the foot from being a fungal reservoir.[6416] Then, we can prevent fungal penetration of the nail by making sure nail grooming instruments are sanitized. Even sharing nail polish can be risky, as the fungus can live for months in top coat products.[6417] Artificial nails can put fingernails at risk,[6418] presumed to be because the acrylic nails trap dampness that would otherwise evaporate through the nail.[6419] (Due to the low-fat content of nails, they are normally about a thousandfold more permeable to water than skin.[6420])

Then, there's the host. Fungal nail infections may be a manifestation of poor peripheral blood circulation that would normally allow your body's natural defenses to keep the fungus from taking root in the first place. A study of four hundred patients found a greater than 50 percent reduction in blood flow in patients with athlete's foot and nail fungus compared to patients without. So, fungal nail infections may just be a symptom of an underlying process, such as declining immunity or circulation, which can help explain why the eradication of these infections can be "unrealistic." This has led to a fatalistic response: "A more appropriate goal may be the amelioration of symptoms. . . ."[6421] But, if circulation is a problem, why not instead try to improve the circulation?

We've known since the 1950s, from one of the first dietary cardiovascular disease reversal studies ever published, that you can effectively turn peripheral artery disease circulation on and off like a light switch within days just by switching people between a low-fat plant-based diet and the more conventional diet that contributed to the problem in the first place.[6422]

Separation Anxiety

Many over-the-counter products purport to improve nail quality, but little evidence supports these claims and the products can sometimes even make things worse. Cuticles serve a function. They are a barrier to pathogens and should be left in place, not cut or pushed back. The nail surface shouldn't be filed, as the thinning may make the nail prone to split, and sharp objects should not be placed under the nails, as they can breach the onychodermal band, the natural smile line that seals the nail bed against infection, which can increase the risk of onycholysis, the partial separation of the nail from the nail bed.[6423]

Acrylic nails can also be a predisposing factor for onycholysis, as the adhesive can be stronger than the natural bond between the nail and the nail bed.[6424] The accumulation of moisture beneath artificial nails can also make the nail more likely to detach. Nail hardeners are another potential cause because they contain up to 5 percent formaldehyde (also listed as "formalin" or "methylene glycol" on the label),[6425] which can cause inflammation that can lead to nail separation.[6426]

HOW TO PREVENT BRITTLE NAILS

Brittle nails affect about one in five, with women affected about twice as frequently as men.[6427] Reported risk factors include dehydration, certain chemicals, and trauma.[6428] A common trope is that nail hardness depends on nail hydration. Nails become soft when overhydrated and are said to become brittle when they get too dry,[6429] leading to advice to soak brittle nails every day[6430] and apply nail moisturizing creams, oils, or ointments.[6431] When actually put to the test, though, the water content of brittle fingernails didn't seem significantly different than that of normal fingernails. In fact, the brittle nails had slightly more water. What did appear linked to the risk, however—tripling the odds of brittle nails—was professional manicures.[6432]

Rather than manicures leading to brittle nails, might those with brittle nails just be more likely to get manicures?[6433] Nail cosmetics, including nail polish removers, solvents, nail hardeners, cuticle removers, and premixed acrylic gels, as well as procedures such as nail wrapping and nail sculpturing, can weaken the very structure of the nail. You'd think nail hardeners would help, but, again, the formaldehyde in these products may do more harm than good in the long term.

At home, choose non-acetone nail polish removers (like acetate) and try to minimize use to once a week or less,[6434] as they are considered a major cause of brittle nails.[6435] Artificial nails can protect brittle nails, but the problem is that removal is always traumatic for the nail and prolonged use may weaken the nail by reducing oxygen transport.[6436] Finally, prevent trauma by avoiding filing the surface of your nails or subjecting them to repetitive stress, such as from typing.

BIOTIN FOR BRITTLE NAILS?

Biotin supplements for nail growth are popular,[6437] but, as we explored on page 284, the same could be said about biotin for hair growth, and, in that instance, biotin was a total flop. Could the same be said about biotin for nails? We don't have a good sense, since there apparently hasn't been a single placebo-controlled study published on the matter.[6438]

Where did anyone get the idea that biotin might help? Serious biotin deficiency is associated with poor nail quality,[6439] though this tends to only strike those who eat raw egg whites.[6440] Biotin works in ponies, affecting a 15 percent increase in hoof horn growth rate.[6441] (Their hooves are made out of the same stuff as our nails.) So, what about biotin in people?

There have been two uncontrolled before-versus-after studies that suggest 2.5 mg of biotin a day may help.[6442] One trial showed a 25 percent increase in nail thickness after six to fifteen months.[6443] There has only been one controlled trial, though. Once a day for four months, brittle fingernails were treated with a nail lacquer with or without taking daily 10 mg supplements of biotin. Nail appearance improved substantially in 80 percent of the biotin group versus 53 percent in the control group.[6444] Unfortunately, at that dose, biotin may disrupt laboratory measurements.

For scheduled blood tests, like thyroid function or pregnancy, you may want to stop the biotin one to five days before the blood draw, depending on how much you're taking.[6445] The FDA was prompted to put out warnings about biotin after a case where biotin interfered with a test (troponin) that would have revealed a missed heart attack and the patient died.[6446] Those are the kinds of tests you can't foresee.

A survey of dermatology outpatients taking biotin found that only 7 percent had ever heard about the FDA warning,[6447] and a nationwide survey of physicians also showed that there were significant professional knowledge gaps.[6448] A dose of 2.5 mg a day may be too low to interfere with lab results,[6449] so it may be worth a try for brittle nails even though we don't have firm evidence that it will help.[6450]

PRESERVING YOUR TEETH

More than 65 percent of the U.S. population over the age of sixty-five have periodontitis.[6451] The word is derived from the Greek *peri-*, meaning "around," *-odont*, meaning "tooth," and *-itis*, meaning "disease." Periodontal disease is an affliction of the tissue surrounding and supporting our teeth, and a major cause of tooth loss.[6452]

Poor diet quality is associated with oral health problems such as periodontitis and tooth loss, and the relationship may be bidirectional. For example, as a pro-inflammatory food component, saturated fat could be contributing directly to tooth loss. Or, tooth loss could be contributing to eating more fatty foods like processed meat because they're easier to chew. In the same vein, the foods associated with fewer missing teeth—fruits and vegetables—are both anti-inflammatory and may require more chewing.[6453] Is a poor diet leading to poor dentition, poor dentition leading to a poor diet, or both?

LONG IN THE TOOTH

As we grow older, we already tend to eat less—and eat less healthfully. Between the ages of forty and seventy, food intake drops by about a quarter due to a declining appetite. We also start losing our taste buds, and sweet and salty tastes are often the first to slip. This can lead to diets particularly excessive in sugar and salt.[6454] Throw in a shift to preprocessed foods due to poor dentition, and you can imagine how this could kick off a vicious cycle, though longitudinal studies don't present clear evidence that tooth loss indeed leads to a loss in nutritional status.[6455] However, tooth loss is associated with premature death and dementia.

A systematic review and meta-analysis found that both periodontitis and tooth loss are predictors of a shortened lifespan. Not all studies accounted for confounding factors, such as smoking, which could easily increase the risk of both,[6456] but those that did control for these other considerations still found missing teeth to be associated with premature death.[6457] Dentition could just be a surrogate for overall health status or genetic robustness.[6458] For example, centenarians have better oral health than those in the same generation who died forty years previously, and so do the children of centenarians compared to their same-age peers.[6459] There is, however, a potential causal pathway by which peri-odontal disease could cut a life short.

Periodontitis is a chronic inflammatory bacterial disease that leads to the de-struction of tooth-supporting structures, such as the gums and underlying ligaments and bone.[6460] These bacterial pathogens can invade the bloodstream and trigger a systemic inflammatory burden.[6461] This could explain the association between missing even just a few teeth and the elevated risk of heart attacks,[6462] as well as connections between periodontal disease and other signs of vascular inflamma-tion, such as erectile dysfunction.[6463] (By looking in your mouth, your dentist may find out more about you than you realize!) Does that explain the dementia link as well?

INDENTURED CONSERVANT

Systematic reviews and meta-analyses have found that tooth loss or periodontitis is associated with both cognitive impairment[6464] and dementia.[6465] Reverse causation might be an intuitive explanation—dementia leading to a decline in oral hygiene.[6466] But, prospective studies following people over time have found that tooth loss appears to predict future cognitive decline, and the more missing teeth, the higher the associated risk.[6467]

I detail a fascinating series of experiments in see.nf/overdentures, where, for example, in a study subtitled "New Teeth for a Brighter Brain," researchers found that replacing missing molars with crowns affects the size of your pupils, suggesting that a gap in the sensation of teeth pushing against each other adversely affects brain function.[6468] If you think that's wild, check out this one: Ten toothless individuals—nine out of ten of them cognitively impaired, six severely so—were given conventional dentures for a month before being fitted with overdentures, which are snapped onto titanium implants surgically screwed into the jawbone. The conventional dentures, held in place by adhesives and natural suction, did nothing to significantly alter cognitive function, but the ones securely attached to implants in the bone appeared to have a dramatic effect. The overdentures presumably transmitted the same kind of chewing pressure sensations to nerves in the jaw that the natural roots of teeth might. Nine out of ten of the subjects went into the study cognitively impaired, but eight out of ten left the study cognitively intact.[6469] This suggests that well-fitting, secure dental prostheses aren't just about improving self-confidence, social contact, and quality of life, but proper brain functioning as well. Even better, though, is to preserve the teeth you have.

Building a Better Mouthwash

If tooth decay is a bacterial disease, why not just use antibiotics to kill the cavity-causing bugs? Many such attempts have been made. However, undesirable side effects, such as antibiotic resistance, vomiting, diarrhea, and teeth-staining, have precluded their use.[6470] There are antiseptic mouthwashes with chemicals like chlorhexidine, which is considered to be the "gold standard" anti-plaque agent, but as I show in see.nf/mouthwash, there is a cheaper, safer, better option: using green tea as a mouthwash,[6471] with or without added amla.[6472]

DON'T SUGARCOAT IT

Our ancestors who lived more than 10,000 years before the toothbrush was invented had almost no cavities.[6473] Why? Because candy bars hadn't been invented yet, either. Now, dental cavities may be humanity's most prevalent disease,[6474] and, as I show in see.nf/sugar, sugar consumption is considered to be the one and only cause.[6475]

The recommended 3 percent cap on total daily intake of added sugars[6476] wouldn't even allow for a single average serving for young children of any of the top ten breakfast cereals most heavily advertised to them.[6477] Obviously, soda is off the table. One can would be nearly two days' worth of sugar.

The official position of the American Academy of Pediatric Dentistry was that frequent consumption of sugary drinks can be a significant factor in the initiation and progression of dental cavities[6478]—that is, it was the official position before it accepted a million-dollar grant from Coca-Cola.[6479] After the grant, its tune changed to "Scientific evidence is certainly not clear on the exact role that soft drinks play. . . ."[6480] As the Center for Science in the Public Interest's Integrity in Science Project put it, *"What a difference a million dollars makes!"*[6481]

If we were really interested in minimizing disease, the ideal goal would be to drop the intake of added sugars to zero.[6482] Though that may be able to get rid of cavities, wrote a Kellogg's-funded researcher, "this ideal is impractical."[6483] The "dictatorial use of foods 'friendly to the teeth'" might promote "dietary celibacy" not "acceptable to all individuals."[6484]

Rather than recommending "draconian" reductions in sugar intake, the sugar industry responded that "attention would be better focused on fluoride toothpaste."[6485] That's the perfect metaphor for medicine's approach to lifestyle diseases: Why treat the cause when you can just treat the consequences?

Are Dental X-Rays Safe?

Every year, doctors may cause an estimated 29,000 cancers by dosing patients with X-rays during CT scans.[6486] What about dentists? Dental X-rays are the most common artificial source of contact with high-energy radiation,[6487] subjecting tens of millions of Americans a year to exposure.[6488] Don't the lead apron and thyroid (neck) shield protect your vital organs? All your vital organs except for one—your brain!

As I detail in see.nf/dentalxrays, dental X-rays appear to increase the risk of the most common type of brain tumor.[6489] There is little evidence to support

(continued)

irradiating asymptomatic patients in search of problems hiding in their mouths.[6490] Accordingly, dentists should only take X-rays when there is a patient-specific reason to believe there is a reasonable expectation the imaging will offer unique information that will influence diagnosis or treatment.[6491]

TOOTH-PRESERVING DIET

What is the role of diet in periodontal disease? I review the evidence in see.nf /periodontitis, including interventional studies showing that the superior peri-odontal health among vegetarians[6492] may be due to eating fewer pro-inflammatory foods[6493] or more anti-inflammatory components like high-fiber diets.[6494] As I detail in see.nf/chewing, there was even a remarkable trial in which more than a thousand participants were randomized to decades of a healthy dietary intervention practically from birth. Those in the lower saturated fat and cholesterol arm ended up with better saliva flow, which is essential for the maintenance of oral health. This was thought to be a function of greater chewing required of fiber-rich foods.[6495] Similarly, foods requiring more intensive chewing have been found more effective at improving bad breath.[6496]

Brush with Greatness

Surprisingly, as I review in see.nf/flossing, the evidence is limited that adding flossing to a brushing regimen reduces gum inflammation,[6497] but it is still recommended on a daily basis.[6498] Researchers have compared unwaxed to woven to shred-resistant floss, and they all appear to have about the same plaque-removal efficacy.[6499] Should you floss before or after you brush? A randomized controlled trial on flossing sequence was performed to put to rest dueling intuitions. Flossing first won hands down.[6500]

GREENS FOR GUMS

When researchers took advantage of a *Survivor*-type reality TV show in which contestants agreed to live under Stone Age conditions to study the natural progression of dental disease without toothbrushing, they were surprised to find a lack of gingivitis. Normally, as I review in see.nf/plaque, plaque buildup is followed by gum inflammation, but perhaps this is only in the context of eating a lot of processed foods rich in sugar and low in anti-inflammatory, whole plant foods.[6501] Randomized, double-blind, placebo-controlled trials of the amount of lycopene in as little as one tomato a day, equivalent to about a daily tablespoon of tomato paste,[6502] found a significant reduction in gingivitis within just one week,[6503] as well as an improvement in gum bleeding in chronic periodontitis patients.[6504] However, half the dose didn't appear to help, so it looks like you have to go the whole tomato.[6505]

A few plants—namely, greens and beets—have another secret weapon: nitrates. Beyond improving circulation, nitrates may also play an important antimicrobial role in our saliva,[6506] proven in a randomized, double-blind, placebo-controlled clinical trial to alleviate gum inflammation.[6507] Check out see.nf/chewing for the full story.

Oil Pulling My Leg?

Coconut oil is safe to put on your hair or your skin,[6508] but, according to the American Heart Association[6509] and the American College of Cardiology,[6510] you don't want to be eating it. In fact, you may not even want to be in the same kitchen when coconut oil is being heated. I don't know where people got the idea that it's safe to use for cooking. Coconut oil has one of the lowest smoke points and releases a variety of toxic emissions at typical frying temperatures.[6511] What about just swishing coconut oil around in your mouth?[6512]

I have a four-part video series starting with see.nf/oilpulling on a time-honored folk remedy that involves "pulling" oil back and forth between the teeth for minutes before spitting it out for a variety of purported "oral and systemic health benefits." There appear to be no such systemic benefits,[6513] and effects on oral health are mixed (good,[6514] bad,[6515] and neutral[6516]). The reason to avoid it completely is the very real risk of lipoid pneumonia, a potential consequence of aspirating small amounts of any oily substance into the lung.[6517] In fact, the reason some of the dental studies were performed on "a stored collection of human extracted teeth"—sounds like straight out of a horror movie—instead of on real-life subjects is that the researchers considered it "not ethically sound to conduct a human trial of [oil pulling] . . . with the knowledge that there was a chance of inducing lipoid pneumonia in study volunteers."[6518]

DON'T END ON A SOUR NOTE

A meta-analysis of eighteen studies on the oral health implications of vegetarian diets showed that vegetarians have significantly fewer decayed, missing, and filled teeth.[6519] This isn't surprising given that vegetarians eat more antioxidants[6520] and anti-inflammatory[6521] foods. Those eating plant-based also have significantly lower rates of oral cancer in every study to date on the topic,[6522,6523,6524,6525] leading to a review on oral cancer prevention published in *The Journal of the American Dental Association* to conclude: "Evidence supports a recommendation of a diet rich in fresh fruits and vegetables as part of a whole-foods, plant-based diet. . . ."[6526] Vegetarians do appear to have an Achilles' tooth, though: an increased risk of dental enamel erosion,[6527] thought due to their consumption of more acidic fruits and vegetables, such as citrus and tomatoes.[6528]

As I cover in see.nf/sour, the solution is to rinse out your mouth with water after consuming sour foods or beverages[6529] and waiting to brush your teeth for at least thirty, and preferably sixty, minutes after consumption to allow your teeth to first remineralize, so as not to brush them in a softened state.[6530]

Is Fluoride Safe and Effective?

One of the studies that bucked the trend and showed that vegetarians had more cavities blamed the excess decay on the fact that vegetarians were significantly less likely to choose fluoride-containing toothpaste,[6531] which has clearly been shown to reduce tooth decay.[6532] Adding fluoride to drinking water is more controversial. Though characterized by the CDC as one of the top ten public health achievements of the twentieth century,[6533] growing evidence about the adverse effects of fluoride on brain development[6534] led to the National Toxicology Program's draft conclusion that fluoride should now be "presumed to be a cognitive neurodevelopmental hazard to humans."[6535]

Ironically, it was the anti-fluoridationists who were accused of their "anti-scientific" attitudes, but now it's the pro-fluoridationists who may be ignoring evidence that doesn't conform to their beliefs.[6536] How can society get the cavity-preventing benefits of fluoride without the risks? Since the primary risk arises from systemic absorption, yet the primary benefits arise from topical contact with our enamel, we can safely reap the rewards by using fluoride toothpaste and mouthwashes.[6537] For an in-depth look into why I changed my mind on water fluoridation, see my five-part video series starting with see.nf/fluoride.

PRESERVING YOUR VISION

More than a million Americans are legally blind. The good news is that a healthy diet can help prevent all four of the most common causes of vision loss—macular degeneration, diabetic retinopathy, glaucoma, and cataracts.

MACULAR DEGENERATION

Age-related macular degeneration is the leading cause of blindness in the developed world.[6538] The macula is the central bull's-eye of the retina in the back of our eyes and is responsible for high-resolution vision. What makes it degenerate?

The retina, the inner rear lining of our eyeballs, transforms light into vision. This continuous feat requires a massive load of oxygen and energy, making the retina one of the most metabolically active tissues in the body—more so, gram for gram, than even the brain.[6539] The oxidative stress due to this firestorm of activity is compounded by the free radicals created by the sun's rays that are focused like a magnifying glass angling straight back into the macula.[6540] This cumulative oxidative strain is thought to play the central role in age-related macular degeneration.[6541]

Eyes donated to science after death from people with age-related macular degeneration show increased oxidative stress[6542] and more free radical DNA damage than do the eyes from those without the condition.[6543] Even the bloodstream of those with age-related macular degeneration shows higher levels of oxidative damage, suggesting a systemic breach of antioxidant defenses.[6544] The pro-oxidants in cigarette smoke[6545] help explain why smokers have up to quadruple the risk of having the disease.[6546] To slow its progression, macular degeneration sufferers are strongly encouraged to quit cigarettes if they smoke and include in their diet a special mixture of antioxidant pigments that go straight to the macula.[6547]

The technical term for the macula is *macula lutea*, which comes from Latin *macula*, meaning "spot," and *lutea*, meaning "yellow." That's what it looks like when we doctors peer into the back of your eye with that bright light. The color comes from two yellow plant pigments that home onto the macula like a laser beam, achieving a concentration a thousand times higher than other tissues. Even just one or two millimeters off from the dead center of your vision, the pigment concentrations drop a hundredfold. Your body knows just where to put them. The two primary pigments, lutein and zeaxanthin, protect the retina from photo-oxidative damage by absorbing blue light.[6548]

The yellowing of our lenses when we develop cataracts may actually be our body's defense mechanism to protect our retinas. In fact, when cataracts are removed, the risk of blindness from macular degeneration may shoot up because we removed the protection.[6549] Instead of trading one type of vision loss for another, it's better to pigment the back of our eyes through diet instead of pigmenting the front of our eyes with cataracts. The pigment in the back of our eyes is entirely of dietary origin.

YELLOW CORN, GREENS, AND GOJIS

Where in our diet can we get these pigments? In an apparent attempt to distract from the cholesterol content of eggs, the egg industry scrambles to boast that eggs contain the pigments lutein and zeaxanthin that protect the retina from photo-oxidative damage.[6550] And it's true. Eggs can have up to 250 micrograms (μg), but a single serving of collard greens has closer to 18,500 μg and just one serving of kale tops the chart at nearly 44,700.[6551] Though yellow yolks might fool you, the two yellow pigments are found mostly in greens. (During autumn splendor, you can see some of the yellow pigments peek out of green leaves as the chlorophyll fades.)

One spoonful of spinach has as much of the pigments as eight eggs.[6552] For eye protection, the recommendation is to get 10,000 μg a day, which is about a third of a cup of spinach or forty eggs—more than three cartons a day. The plant pigments in eggs come from chickens that got it from pecking at corn or blades of grass. We can cut out the middle-hen and get the pigments straight from corn and greens. All the top ten sources of these critical, eyesight-saving nutrients in the USDA nutrient database are greens. Eggs don't even make the top one hundred. To get to eggs, you have to scroll down a couple of pages, and, according to the USDA, they come in right behind Cap'n Crunch with Crunch Berries (which is presumably on the list due to its yellow corn content).[6553]

This discrepancy pans out when put to the test. When study subjects ate around six high-lutein, free-range, certified organic eggs every week for three months, the pigmentation in their eyes hardly changed.[6554] Instead of getting the plant pigments from eggs that came from chickens that got them from pecking at plants, when researchers went straight to the source by offering these nutrients from plants directly—a cup of corn and a half cup of spinach a day—most individuals saw a dramatic boost in protective macular pigmentation within the first month.[6555]

Three months after the subjects stopped eating the corn and spinach, the levels of these pigments remained relatively high, indicating that once we build up our macular pigment with a healthy diet, our eyeballs really try to hold on to it. So, even if we go on vacation and end up eating more iceberg lettuce than spinach, our eyes will try to hold out until we get back.

Yellow corn has about seventy times more lutein than white corn,[6556] but spinach has sixty times more than yellow corn. Corn beats greens for zeaxanthin, though. The word comes from modern Latin *zea*, meaning "maize," and *xanthin*, "yellow coloring." However, a few food sources can crack corn. Orange bell peppers have eight times more zeaxanthin than corn,[6557] but goji berries reign supreme, with about twelve times more than orange peppers.[6558] In see.nf/gojis, I profile a double-blind, randomized, placebo-controlled study that found that gojis may even help people already suffering from macular degeneration.

Goji berries may cost about twenty dollars per pound in natural foods stores, but they're even cheaper than raisins in Asian supermarkets, where you can buy them as "Lycium" berries. I encourage you to swap out raisins for goji berries—in your breakfast oatmeal, as a snack, in muffins, and anywhere else. As one review concluded, goji berries offer a "'whole food' dietary supplement for the maintenance of retinal health as well as for prevention and/or delay in progression of retinal diseases commonly seen in clinical practice."[6559]

PASS WITH FLYING COLORS

Lutein and zeaxanthin are both fat-soluble, so make sure you pair your greens with nuts, seeds, nut and seed butters, or any other Green Light source of fat. They'll taste better, and you'll maximize absorption of these important macular pigments. So, you can add walnuts to your pesto, whip up a creamy tahini-based salad dressing, top your sautéed kale with sesame seeds, or choose produce that has the fat baked in: avocados.

In see.nf/avocados, I run through all the experiments showing how pairing avocados with salsa or salads can dramatically increase the absorption of the carotenoids in vegetables.[6560] Another way to boost the bioavailability of the macular pigments in greens is to steam them,[6561] but heat isn't the only way to liberate lutein from greens. If you finely chop spinach, you can apparently double the amount of lutein released during digestion. And, if you really blend it up—a green smoothie, pesto, or some kind of pureed spinach dish, for instance—you may triple the bioavailability.[6562]

PLANT PIGMENTS PUT TO THE TEST

The Age-Related Eye Disease Study (AREDS) randomized thousands of men and women who had at least the beginnings of age-related macular degeneration to a combination of antioxidants and zinc versus placebos for more than five years[6563] and was able to decrease the risk of progression to advanced macular degeneration by 25 percent.[6564] The AREDS formulation quickly became the medical standard of care for those suffering from the disease. In see.nf/areds, I detail all the changes in the formula since. Fish oil was tried and flopped, the zinc dose was lowered, and "vegetarian" levels of lutein and zeaxanthin[6565] beat out the original beta-carotene.[6566]

There is a consensus among professional eye health associations and guidelines that these kinds of supplements should be given to people with macular degeneration,[6567] but they have not been found effective for primary prevention. In fact, the Harvard Physicians' Health Study II found that those randomized to a multivitamin (Centrum Silver) developed *higher* rates of macular degeneration compared to placebo.[6568] To prevent the disease in the first place, a diet "high in green leafy vegetables" is recommended instead of supplements.[6569]

To protect your eyes, everyone is recommended to incorporate two to three servings of greens into your daily diet.[6570] Think of this as greens at every lunch or supper with bonus points for sneaking them into breakfast—perhaps in a green smoothie or a savory oatmeal dish. It may be especially important for white people to eat their green leafies, as they have significantly higher rates of age-related macular degeneration. This is likely due to eye color. Blue eyes let through a hundred times more light, so people with blue or gray eyes appear to be significantly more vulnerable to damage compared to those with brown or black eyes. (Green and hazel fall somewhere in the middle.)[6571]

I Can See for (Twenty-Seven) Miles

The macular pigments lutein and zeaxanthin not only protect our eyesight but may also improve it. Their peak light absorbance just so happens to be the wavelength of the color of our planet's sky. By filtering out that blue haze, those fortifying their retinas with a lot of greens are estimated to be able to distinguish distant mountain ridges up to twenty-seven miles farther than those with little macular pigment when standing atop a mountain on a clear day.[6572]

There have been nine randomized controlled trials investigating the effects of macular pigment supplementation on visual function in normal healthy subjects. All have found significant improvements,[6573] including improving visual acuity, contrast sensitivity (important for low-light conditions),[6574] chromatic contrast (the vividness of colors), and photo-stress recovery time (the time needed to recover sight after a bright flash).[6575]

Are there any other foods that can improve vision in healthy people? Given the fact that cocoa powder can acutely boost cerebral blood flow,[6576] researchers compared the effects of eating a Trader Joe's dark chocolate bar (72 percent cocoa) versus a Trader Joe's milk chocolate bar (31 percent cocoa).[6577] Two hours after consumption, contrast sensitivity and visual acuity were significantly improved in the dark chocolate group compared to the milk chocolate group, meaning they were better able to pick out small, low-contrast targets. The researchers suggested it may be due to the enhanced availability of oxygen and nutrients afforded by the improvement in blood flow to the metabolically voracious retina.

The blood flow in the *choriocapillaris*, the massive network of tiny blood vessels that feed our retinas, may actually be the highest in the body.[6578] That may help explain why higher meat intake is associated with a significantly increased risk of developing macular degeneration.[6579] Those with higher cholesterol intake have up to 60 percent higher odds of early age-related macular disease, and higher saturated fat consumption bumps it up to 80 percent.[6580] Drusen, the spots of debris in the back of the eye that are the hallmark of macular degeneration, are actually cholesterol-rich deposits with a composition similar to that of atherosclerotic plaques in arteries.[6581] The level of oxidized cholesterol in drusen is so high that it would be lethal in most cell systems.[6582] Injecting LDL cholesterol into rats for seven days causes retinal changes "quite similar" to that of early-stage age-related macular degeneration in humans,[6583] but the current evidence regarding the use of statin drugs to prevent or treat the disease in people is inconclusive,[6584] which would argue against a strong role of blood cholesterol in macular pathology.

FLOWER POWER

In addition to two to three daily servings of green leafy vegetables, berries are considered a healthy choice for conserving our eyesight.[6585] As I detail in see.nf /saffronvision, there are interventional studies showing that berries can improve various aspects of our vision,[6586,6587] but only one pigmented food has been put to the test for macular degeneration: the spice saffron. I run through all the studies in the video, but basically, a tiny daily pinch of saffron (20 mg) can cause a significant, yet modest, improvement in visual acuity in older adults with mild or moderate age-related macular degeneration.[6588]

Diabetic Retinopathy

Diabetes is another leading cause of blindness, as well as amputations and kidney failure. Thankfully, type 2 diabetes can be prevented and even reversed, as I discuss at length in my chapter on diabetes in *How Not to Die*.

GLAUCOMA

Glaucoma is now the leading cause of irreversible vision loss in the world. It's caused by the deterioration of the optic nerve that connects the eye to the brain. Most commonly, this is due to excessive pressure inside the eyeball. Up to 40 percent of glaucoma patients end up going blind in at least one eye.[6589] To prevent this from occurring, most treatments concentrate on trying to lower the intraocular pressure.[6590]

KALE GRAIL

Might greens be the go-to again? The nitric oxide that is boosted by vegetable nitrate consumption helps to balance pressure in the eyeball by reducing the overproduction of *aqueous humor* (the fluid that fills and inflates the eyeball) and improving outflow of any excess.[6591] The pharmaceutical industry has been working on coming up with Viagra-type drugs to increase the amount of nitric oxide in the eye,[6592] but we already have veggies that can get it up.

Only about one in ten white people eat even a single serving of dark-green leafy vegetables a *month*. To study the relationship between greens and glaucoma, researchers sought a cohort of Black women, of whom nearly nine out of ten regularly eat their greens.[6593] Compared to those eating a single serving of kale or collard greens once a month or less, those eating more than one serving a month had less than half the odds of glaucoma.[6594] It didn't seem to take much at all. At so few servings a month, even studies of white people might be informative, so Boston researchers looked to the Harvard Nurses' Health Study (97 percent white)[6595] and the Harvard Health Professionals Follow-Up Study (only 1 percent Black).[6596] Based on the more than 100,000 men and women followed for decades, higher nitrate intake (mostly from green leafy vegetables) was indeed associated with significantly lower risk of developing glaucoma.[6597]

NO HEAD STANDS

Is there anything else we can do? Aerobic exercise can at least transiently reduce intraocular pressure,[6598] and one study suggested that chronic conditioning can maintain lower pressures over the long term.[6599] However, bungee jumping,[6600] scuba diving,[6601] and inversion (head-down) yoga positions may have the opposite effect.[6602]

A study of nearly 30,000 runners found a dose-dependent effect, with farther distances and faster times associated with a lower incidence of glaucoma.[6603] Of course, such observational data are complicated by the specter of reverse causation. Instead of exercise maintaining people's vision, maybe those who maintain their vision are more likely to exercise. And, indeed, those with glaucoma do tend to exercise less than same-age peers.[6604] There has yet to be a randomized controlled trial to put exercise to the test, but we do have interventional data on berries.

SWIM WITH THE CURRANT

Japanese researchers have shown that black currant pigments can slow down glaucoma vision loss. (Details in see.nf/currants.) This was accompanied by an increase in ocular blood flow, but no change in intraocular pressure, suggesting that berries might also work for "normal tension" glaucoma, the type in which the optic nerve deterioration proceeds despite normal eyeball pressure.[6605] Note that most "currants" sold in the United States are little raisins (*Vitis vinifera*) and not actual currants (*Ribes nigrum*), which were illegal to grow until recently, due to pressure from the lumber industry because they can carry white pine blister rust.[6606]

GINGKO?

As I detail in see.nf/gingkonic, one study found suggestive benefit of *Ginkgo biloba* extracts for open-angle glaucoma,[6607] and one[6608] of two[6609] found a significant benefit for closed-angle glaucoma. If you want to try it despite the underwhelming results, make sure you first discuss it with your healthcare professional due to a possible increase in bleeding risk from the herb.[6610]

NICOTINAMIDE

In the same video, see.nf/gingkonic, I detail a randomized, double-blind, placebo-controlled, crossover trial showing that the B vitamin nicotinamide may cut the risk of further visual field deterioration of glaucoma patients from 12 percent down to 4 percent within a matter of months.[6611] A 2022 study found a significant improvement in visual function compared to placebo with two months of an escalating nicotinamide dose, going from 1 g to 3 g a day, but it is not directly comparable since pyruvate, another important part of energy metabolism, was also added.[6612] See page 585 for my discussion of cost, labeling confusion, and potential side effects of taking nicotinamide.

CATARACTS

Age-related cataract, the clouding of the normally clear natural lens of the eyes, typically starts between the ages of forty-five and fifty. It is the leading cause of blindness in low- and middle-income countries, but only responsible for about 5 percent of blindness in higher-income countries, thanks to the availability of cataract surgery, the current standard of care. These days, high-tech cataract surgery is a relatively quick, safe, and simple procedure, with rapid recovery. It involves the removal of the clouded lens and replacement with an artificial lens usually made out of silicone or acrylic.[6613]

Overall, about half of patients don't recover vision better than 20/40 after cataract surgery, but the most common complaint is *dysphotopsia*, light artifacts manifesting as streaks or flashes that can result from internal reflections within the implanted lenses. Anywhere between 33 and 78 percent of cataract patients are affected,[6614] and it typically doesn't improve without surgical replacement.[6615] The most serious sight-threatening complication is *endophthalmitis*, the introduction of infection into the eye. Though it's extremely rare—less than one in twenty-five hundred surgeries—it's concerning enough that bilateral cataract surgery is done in two separate operations instead of both at the same time to avoid the risk of going completely blind from infections in both eyes.[6616]

GREENS *AGAIN?*

How about preventing the cloudiness in the first place? Cataracts are a direct result of oxidative stress,[6617] free radical damage to the normally transparent crystallin proteins that make up the lenses in our eyes.[6618] The oxidative stress can come from hyperbaric oxygen therapy, the natural UV rays of the sun, artificial UV rays of tanning beds, or other forms of high-energy radiation.[6619] For example, all twenty-one studies of healthcare workers exposed to X-rays, such as those who do angiograms, found higher rates of cataracts, sixteen of which significantly so.[6620]

If cataracts are caused by oxidation, how about eating more antioxidants? The body concentrates vitamin C in the lens at levels fifty times higher than the blood to defend against oxidative attack.[6621] Experiments in which samples of eye fluid were taken during cataract surgery after vitamin C supplementation confirm that changing what goes into our mouth can change what ends up in our eyes,[6622] but does that translate into lower risk?

Those eating diets with a higher total antioxidant content do tend to have lower risk of age-related cataract.[6623] The same could be said for the intake of some individual antioxidants—vitamin C, beta-carotene, and lutein and zeaxanthin—but not others, such as vitamin A, vitamin E, or alpha-carotene.[6624] For vitamin C, both intake and blood levels correlated with lower cataract risk.[6625] Those getting the amount of vitamin C found in about two oranges a day appeared to have approximately 40 percent lower risk.[6626] Researchers concluded that dietary vitamin C intake "should be advocated for the primary prevention of cataract," mirroring similar advice from a meta-analysis on dietary lutein and zeaxanthin and cataract risk: "[O]phthalmologists should counsel individuals to increase consumption of lutein-rich foods, such as dark-green leafy vegetables."[6627] Why not just recommend antioxidant supplements instead?

ANTIOXIDANT SUPPLEMENTS?

Details in see.nf/antioxmulti, but supplements containing vitamin C, vitamin E,[6628] and beta-carotene[6629] with or without[6630] zinc failed to affect the rate of cataract formation. Perhaps there's a threshold effect such that supplementation would only work in the context of dietary deficiency.[6631] For example, consider the case of lutein and zeaxanthin. They are the only carotenoids present in the human lens,[6632] so perhaps it's no surprise that beta-carotene failed to help.[6633] Lutein and zeaxanthin supplementation also failed, but only among those getting enough in their diet. Those with the lowest baseline intake did appear to benefit from supplementation.[6634] Presumably, those with an inadequate baseline intake of greens would also benefit from just eating more greens.

MULTIVITAMIN SUPPLEMENTS?

Taking supplements just as an "insurance policy" is a common sentiment heard in the context of multivitamins, but as I note in see.nf/antioxmulti, the results for cataract prevention are mixed. For example, one study showed that those randomized to Centrum for about a decade had a 34 percent lower risk of developing or worsening one kind of cataracts, but a 100 percent higher risk (a doubled risk) for developing or worsening a different type of cataract. The contrasting effects, concluded the researchers, "prevent us from making recommendations. . . ."[6635]

SEEING CLEARLY

In addition to antioxidant-rich foods,[6636] eating more anti-inflammatory foods is also associated with lower cataract risk.[6637] As well, the aging toxin AGEs (see page 54) may accelerate cataract formation by cross-linking lens proteins.[6638] That may help explain why the consumption of meat (including poultry) has been associated with increased cataract risk.[6639] In contrast, those eating at least about an ounce a day of daily legumes have less than half the odds of posterior cataracts, but the researchers didn't adjust for meat consumption, so it's hard to know if this is just an indirect benefit of eating less meat.[6640]

The European Prospective Investigation into Cancer and Nutrition is a large enough study to get more granular. The study compared the rates of cataract development in "high" meat eaters, "low" meat eaters, and pescatarians versus those eating vegetarian and those eating vegan. The researchers went out of their way to choose health-conscious subjects to help factor out smoking, exercise, and other non-diet variables, so the "high" meat-consuming group was defined as just one serving a day (100 g) or more.[6641] Yet even compared to health-conscious light-meat consumers, those cutting back on meat even further (eating less than 100 g a day) had a 15 percent lower cataract incidence.

Compared to the one-serving-or-more-a-day meat eaters, those cutting out all meat except for fish (the pescatarians) had a 21 percent lower risk, those cutting out *all* meat (the vegetarians) appeared to drop their risk by 30 percent, and those going a step further and also eliminating eggs and dairy (the vegans) had 40 percent less risk of developing cataracts.[6642] Similar stepwise reductions of risk can be seen with other diseases, such as diabetes, hypertension, and obesity, as one's diet gets more and more centered around plants.[6643] A subsequent study out of Taiwan confirmed that those eating no meat were significantly less likely to develop cataracts compared to those eating on average just about a half serving of meat a day.[6644]

Why do vegetarians have higher rates than vegans? It might be the dairy. We've known that galactose, the breakdown product of the milk sugar lactose, can cause cataracts from studies dating back to 1935[6645] with titles like "Cataracts Produced in Rats by Yogurt."[6646] Galactose buildup in the eye causes an injurious swelling of the lens.[6647] Thankfully, human livers have a greater capacity to detoxify galactose than do rat livers.[6648] There are children born with genetic defects who can't handle it as well (and subsequently develop cataracts),[6649] but might a lifetime of consuming dairy increase the risk of cataracts even in those with normal detoxification enzyme activity?[6650] After all, drinking milk into adulthood is an evolutionarily novel behavior.

Across the general population, milk consumption does not appear to increase the risk of cataracts, but some people may be more susceptible.[6651] People are born with different capacities to detoxify galactose. Among those with normal, but lower, levels of the galactose-detoxifying enzyme *galactokinase*, high-lactose intake from milk and other dairy products may quadruple the risk of developing cataracts later in life.[6652] This has been used to help explain why women have higher cataract rates than men, since women tend to have weaker galactokinase activity.[6653]

PRESERVING YOUR DIGNITY

I'm breaking with the alphabetical sequence by placing this section at the end.

HOW TO DIE A GOOD DEATH

We have all sorts of detailed data about dying, but little about the experience of death. For the minority who die while receiving palliative care, death could probably be described as good, but there is a suspicion that the experience is bad for the majority who die in hospitals or nursing homes.[6654] Unfortunately, that's where most people die.[6655]

In spite of widespread preference to die at home, in almost all populations most deaths occur in institutions. Approximately 80 percent of Americans say they would prefer to die at home,[6656] yet fewer than 30 percent do.[6657] Highly medicalized institutional deaths have consequences not just for the patient but for their bereaved caregivers as well. Not only do patients with cancer who die in a hospital tend to experience more physical and emotional distress and worse quality of life at the end of life but their caregivers suffer five times the odds of developing post-traumatic stress disorder and nearly nine times the odds of severe, prolonged, disabling grief. Now, that was from an observational study.[6658] It's not like the patients were randomized to die in different locations, so this doesn't prove cause and effect, but it certainly raises concerns.

When researchers have looked into the care of dying patients in hospitals, it hasn't been pretty. Basic interventions to maintain patients' comfort were often not provided, contact with dying patients was minimal, and the distancing and isolation worsened as death approached. For example, in one heart-wrenching case report, a fifty-two-year-old woman with metastatic cancer that had spread to her liver had gross abdominal distension and was jaundiced, very breathless, but alert. Her eyes were swollen and she shed yellow tears. The patient received *no care* from the nurses delegated to attend to her. Yet in the nursing log, it was recorded that attention had been given to her personal hygiene, pressure areas to prevent bed sores, oral hygiene, and eyes—but it was all a lie. The only attention she got was to receive a commode from a nursing assistant. Contact time totaled six minutes over the four and a half hours the researchers kept track.[6659]

What would a good death look like? It looks like retaining control, dignity, and privacy. Having pain relief, emotional support, and respect for your wishes. Choosing where and how you spend your last days. Being able to say goodbye, and being able to leave when it is time to go and not have life prolonged pointlessly.[6660]

The best bet to ensure that your death is yours is access to hospice care. Palliative care involves comfort measures to relieve symptoms and improve quality of life that can be utilized at any stage of a serious illness, whereas hospice is *just* comfort measures, embodying a shift of focus from curing the disease to improving the quality of one's last days.[6661] About half of Medicare patients receive some hospice care, but for many (28 percent), they are enrolled mere days before death.[6662]

Hospice is often framed as "giving up," but, ironically, when you compare hospice versus nonhospice patient survival, the patients in hospice actually tend to live longer. Patients who choose hospice care live on average about a month longer than similar patients who do not choose hospice.[6663] In one study, people with lung cancer randomized to early palliative care lived two and a half months longer.[6664] That's the kind of survival benefit you might get with a standard chemotherapy regimen.[6665] In fact, that's one of the ways hospice could extend survival in cancer patients: by avoiding the risk of overtreatment with chemo and its related toxicity.[6666]

PHYSICIAN AID IN DYING

There are limits to palliative care. Even under hospice, where one would assume such care to be excellent, there are those who spend their last months in uncontrolled pain.[6667] And this unbearable suffering, despite our best efforts, leads to requests by patients to end their lives prematurely.[6668] Physician-assisted suicide, or perhaps more accurately *physician-assisted dying*[6669] or *medical aid in dying*, allows the terminally ill to end their lives through the voluntary self-administration of a lethal dose of medication expressly prescribed by a physician for that purpose.[6670] As I discuss in <u>see.nf/aid</u>, any physician aid in dying is illegal and punishable by law in forty U.S. states. In contrast, VSED is legal throughout the United States: Voluntarily Stopping Eating and Drinking.[6671]

THE BENEFITS OF VSED

In an ideal world, every patient with a life-limiting illness would receive optimal hospice and palliative care comfort measures such that no one would ever wish to hasten their own death. Unfortunately, the reality is that some with terminal illness continue to suffer despite our best efforts,[6672] leading increasing numbers of patients to explore VSED to escape intolerable suffering.[6673] In Europe, as many as 1 to 2 percent of deaths are attributable to this practice.[6674]

VSED can be defined as a conscious decision to voluntarily and deliberately choose to stop eating and drinking with the primary intention of hastening death because of the persistence of unacceptable suffering.[6675] In <u>see.nf/vsed</u>, I discuss all the benefits: dying at home, no waiting period for approval, it's legal, you can change your mind, and you don't need anyone's permission. Just knowing there's a "way out" can provide relief from feelings of desperation and entrapment, engendering a feeling of control that may itself be therapeutic.[6676] It can also prevent people from contemplating a more violent way out or feeling pressured to end their lives prematurely while they still can.[6677]

WHAT IS VSED LIKE?

What is it like to die from voluntarily stopping to eat and drink? There are a lot of anecdotes floating around describing death from VSED as peaceful, painless, and dignified.[6678] Fortunately, there have been several independent studies to evaluate these claims,[6679] which I explore in <u>see.nf/vsed</u>.

The average time of death after stopping eating and drinking is about seven days, though 8 percent lived for more than two weeks. The last days of life were rated as peaceful, with low levels of pain and suffering, even more so than a physicianassited death.[6680] Most hospice workers said they would consider VSED themselves should they become terminally ill.[6681]

The state of terminal dehydration may even have some analgesic (painkilling) effect,[6682] presumed to be due to the release of endorphins, which act as natural pain blockers.[6683] So, concluded a systematic review published in a palliative care journal, VSED may reflect all twelve principles of a "good death," with an emphasis on retaining dignity and control.[6684]

One of the most famous accounts of VSED is a doctor's description of his own mother's death in the *Journal of the American Medical Association*.[6685] I asked permission from the journal to reprint two particularly poignant paragraphs for you here. It was happy to oblige—for $12,867.28. So, I just put them in my see.nf/vsed video instead. (Make sure to have a box of tissues at hand.)

The Dementia Trap

There are other side benefits to the dehydration process.[6686] There is less worry about incontinence, catheters, or bedpans, and less nausea and vomiting as our digestive secretions dwindle. Fewer respiratory secretions mean less coughing and choking and fewer drowning sensations. Dehydration can also decrease swelling, which can be a problem with end-stage cancer. That can relieve pain by taking pressure off the nerves. Mental awareness may also decline, which can also bring some relief, but it can also present a serious ethical dilemma. What if you become delirious, forget you ever made the decision, and start asking for something to drink? I cover this in my video see.nf/dignity, as well as how to create advance directive documents to specifically address the issue of hand feeding should you want to avoid end-stage dementia.

YOU ARE IN CONTROL

Thanks to the Fourteenth Amendment, everyone in the United States has the right to refuse medical care.[6687] Critics contend that food is different because it's a necessity.[6688] But, if you can refuse to be put on a respirator to save your life, the counterargument goes, then you should be able to refuse food and drink. (After all, nothing is more necessary than breathing!) In see.nf/dignity, I run through other common criticisms and potential pitfalls, including how to manage the associated thirst. The bottom line is that VSED appears to provide most patients with a peaceful and gentle death.

IV. Dr. Greger's Anti-Aging Eight

INTRODUCTION

Anti-aging quackery is an age-old phenomenon, but the convergence of three factors has been blamed for the recent explosion: the seventy-two-million-strong wave of aging baby boomers, online availability and advertising, and the passage of the 1994 Dietary Supplement Health and Education Act (DSHEA).[6689]

ANTI-AGING SCAMS

When surveyed, most people incorrectly believe that supplements must be approved for safety by a government agency such as the FDA before they can be sold to the public or, at the very least, must include a warning on the label about potential side effects. Nearly half even believed supplement manufacturers had to show some sort of effectiveness.[6690] None of that is true, though, thanks to DSHEA. The act removed the burden of proof for quality control, safety, or efficacy from the supplement manufacturers, and the market blew up from a $4 billion industry with 4,000 products before DSHEA's passage to a $40 billion industry with an excess of 50,000 products.[6691] By 2012, sales of dietary supplements in the United States were averaging more than $100 per person per year.[6692]

By law, over-the-counter medications must meet standards for safety, efficacy, and quality control, but dietary supplements are exempt.[6693] Prior to DSHEA, supplements were regulated like food additives, so manufacturers had to show that the products were safe before they were brought to market, but not anymore. What's the harm? Watch my video see.nf/dshea.

Because of the lack of government oversight, there is no guarantee that a supplement bottle even contains what's listed on its label. In one study, only two out of twelve supplement companies were found to have products that were labeled accurately.[6694] FDA inspectors have even found that seven out of ten supplement makers violated Good Manufacturing Practices, which are considered the *minimum* quality standards,[6695] such as ingredient identification and basic sanitation. Not 7 percent, but 70 percent in violation.

The problem isn't limited to fly-by-night phonies lurking in some dark corner of the internet either. The New York State attorney general commissioned DNA testing of seventy-eight bottles of commercial herbal supplements sold by GNC, Walgreens, Target, and Walmart, and four out of five bottles didn't contain *any* of the herbs listed on their labels. Instead, the capsules often contained little more than cheap fillers, such as powdered rice and "houseplants."[6696]

At least you hope it's just houseplants. Some supplements are tainted with pharmaceuticals—sometimes even banned substances that had already been yanked from the market. As I note in see.nf/adulterated, recalled supplements may pop right back on store shelves, sometimes with even *more* banned ingredients.[6697] As a founding fellow of the Institute for Science in Medicine put it, "Fines for violations are small compared to the profits."[6698]

PAYING TO CUT YOUR LIFE SHORT?

A nationally representative sample of thousands of Americans over the age of sixty found that 70 percent reported using dietary supplements.[6699] Perhaps that should be 100 percent, since the Institute of Medicine's official recommendation is for everyone fifty and older to take a B_{12} supplement (or consume foods fortified with B_{12}),[6700] but the most common supplement taken was a multivitamin. What might that do for our lifespan?

As you can see in see.nf/multi, there have been nine randomized controlled trials of multivitamin and multimineral supplements, randomizing more than 50,000 men and women to typically years of such supplements, and no overall benefit to mortality was found.[6701] "[W]e believe that the case is closed," read an editorial published in the *Annals of Internal Medicine* titled "Enough Is Enough: Stop Wasting Money on Vitamin and Mineral Supplements."[6702] Instead of trying to get our nutrients from pills, concluded a 2021 review on vitamin and mineral supplements, we should "move to more plant-based diets, as advised now internationally."[6703]

At least multivitamins appear to be safe.[6704] The fact that they were not associated with mortality was heralded as good news, after results from the Iowa Women's Health Study had found multivitamin use associated with a higher risk of premature death.[6705] However, there are a few supplements for which it appears people are actively paying to live a shorter life. Meta-analyses of randomized controlled trials have found that high-dose vitamin A, beta-carotene,[6706] and extended-release niacin[6707] can all increase mortality risk compared to placebo.

One way that any supplement could harm more than a user's wallet is through a fascinating glitch of human psychology called *self-licensing*.[6708] In see.nf/glitch, I explore why smokers smoke more[6709] and dieters eat more[6710] when randomized to take "supplements" that were actually placebos.

WHAT VITAMIN D CAN AND CANNOT DO

What about those so-called life extension formulas? Researchers fed mice human-equivalent doses of combinations of the highest-quality purported longevity supplements incorporating more than a hundred components, and not a single one extended lifespan. One mixture even cut their lives short. (The researchers suspect it was the fish oil that was at least partially responsible for the reduced lifespan.)[6711]

One supplement was shown in randomized controlled trials to extend human life: vitamin D.[6712] So why isn't it part of my Anti-Aging Eight? Vitamin D has been touted as a veritable cure-all,[6713] but as I note in my video see.nf/dpanacea, when actually put to the test in randomized controlled trials, vitamin D supplementation was found to be ineffective for the prevention and treatment of most conditions against which it's been tested.[6714] It failed to help with cardiovascular disease,[6715] type 2 diabetes,[6716] multiple sclerosis,[6717] obesity,[6718] or prostate cancer.[6719] It's the old story of reverse causation and confounding. Sick people don't tend to go out in the sun, and low vitamin D levels may just be a marker for inactivity.[6720] Just because low vitamin D levels are correlated with high disease rates doesn't mean the low vitamin D levels are *causing* the disease.

There are a few exceptions. Besides the obvious vitamin D–deficiency diseases of softened bone—rickets and osteomalacia[6721]—vitamin D supplements have been found to be effective for preventing exacerbations of asthma[6722] and chronic obstructive pulmonary diseases like emphysema in people with low baseline vitamin D levels.[6723] Although vitamin D was ineffective for preventing depression,[6724] it does appear to be helpful for treating it,[6725] and the converse was true for acute respiratory tract infections—effective for preventing them[6726] but apparently not for treating them.[6727]

VITAMIN D FOR DEFYING DEATH?

The vast majority of observational population studies also show that those who have higher vitamin D levels in their blood have a lower risk of premature death.[6728] Once put to the test, though, will life extension flop, too? Sufficient

D is certainly not necessary for a long life.[6729] A study of centenarians found appallingly low vitamin D levels. In fact, they were mostly undetectable using standard testing.[6730] But might taking vitamin D supplements help our chances at a longer life?

A Mendelian randomization study found that those born with genetically predetermined lifelong low D levels did tend to live shorter lives,[6731] but interventional trials looking at intermediate risk factors for our leading killer, such as artery stiffness[6732] or function, failed to show benefits for vitamin D supplements.[6733] However, what we really want are randomized, double-blind, placebo-controlled studies looking at the endpoint that matters most: premature death. Not to worry—there have been sixty-five of them![6734]

The reason I've made videos telling people to take vitamin D supplements to live longer (see.nf/dlongevity) is a Cochrane review of the first fifty-six such trials published in 2014. But by 2019, seventeen additional randomized controlled trials were published, with some so massive that they were able to tip the balance.[6735] For example, the VITAL study randomized more than 25,000 men and women to five years of vitamin D, fish oil, both, or neither (placebos). Neither vitamin D[6736] nor fish oil[6737] was able to prevent major cardiovascular events or cancer, and neither prevented premature death. Critics argue that only a small percentage (12.7 percent) of the study subjects started out deficient in vitamin D,[6738] and all participants—even those in the placebo group—were allowed to take additional vitamin D on their own. It was not deemed ethical to randomize those who might be deficient to abstain from a vital nutrient of which they might not otherwise get enough. This is a common problem with vitamin D trials.[6739] In the VITAL trial, more participants in the placebo group took their own vitamin D than did those in the actual vitamin D supplementation group, presumably because they tested low.[6740] You can imagine how this would dilute the results.

Adding the results of VITAL to the mix, along with all the large new studies that failed to find a mortality benefit, the updated meta-analysis found that the reduction in mortality risk no longer reached statistical significance.[6741] Taking vitamin D_3 supplements did seem to reduce the risk of dying from cancer, though. The effect was small, such that you'd have to supplement 250 people for a year to prevent a single cancer death.[6742] One could argue that this reduction in the risk of dying from the second most common killer could translate into life extension for those at reduced risk of dying from killer number one, heart disease (or for those at particularly high cancer risk), but there isn't enough evidence to confirm this supposition. At the current rate, as many as a thousand new trials of vitamin D supplementation are set to be reported over the next decade, so things may change.[6743] But, as of the time of this writing, there have been more than five dozen randomized controlled trials, and the latest, largest meta-analysis of such studies shows no statistically significant mortality benefit overall.[6744] So, while I went into this book expecting I'd recommend them for lifespan extension, vitamin D_3 supplements didn't make the list, but there are eight things that do.

NUTS

According to the World Health Organization, the constituents of a healthy diet are vegetables, fruits, legumes like beans, lentils, and chickpeas, nuts, and whole grains, while cutting down on added sugars, salt, and saturated and trans fats, which are found predominantly in junk foods, meat, and dairy.[6745] Meta-analyses of prospective studies have shown reduced overall mortality risk for each of those healthy components. Each additional daily serving of vegetables was associated with a 4 percent lower risk of premature death, with 6 percent lower risk for each additional daily serving of fruits, 8 percent lower risk per serving of whole grains, 10 percent lower risk for a single daily serving of legumes, and 15 percent lower risk for eating even a daily half serving of nuts. The primacy of nuts for mortality risk reduction is underscored by the fact that a half serving of nuts is only about 15 g (0.5 oz), whereas servings of the other four groups were all larger, up to 100 g per serving. Of all the dozen or so defined food groups, nothing beats nuts for reducing the associated risk of dying before one's time.[6746]

HEALTH NUTS

Few foods, concludes a review in a top-rated nutrition journal, have experienced such "vindication" as nuts.[6747] Nut consumption is associated with a lower risk of dying from stroke, heart disease, respiratory disease, infections, diabetes, and even cancer—more than half of our top ten killers.[6748] (One study found that patients with stage 3 colon cancer who ate nuts at least twice a week had more than double the chance of surviving an average of six and a half years compared to those who never partook.[6749]) So, it isn't surprising that eating nuts is associated with a lower risk of dying prematurely across the board. In a study of those aged 84 to 107, eating nuts every day was associated with as much life extension as regular donut consumption was associated with lifespan contraction.[6750] The title of an editorial in the *Journal of the American College of Cardiology* suggested succinctly: "Eat Nuts,

Live Longer."[6751] Nuts are one of the very few foods that, just on their own, may literally add years to your life.[6752]

Based on studies tracking the eating habits and deaths of about a half million people over time,[6753] inadequate nut consumption may be responsible for the premature deaths of millions every year around the world.[6754] What does this mean for us on a personal level? Eating nuts at least twice a week appears to halve mortality risk compared to almost never eating them.[6755] So, two handfuls of nuts a week could be the longevity equivalent of jogging for four hours.[6756] Looking at it another way, not eating nuts may risk doubling our chances of dying prematurely. But there's a difference between relative risk and absolute risk.

A healthy, middle-aged person's risk of dying in the next decade may only be about 2 percent. That's a one-in-fifty chance of dying over the next ten years—but only if they don't eat nuts.[6757] If they do eat them, their risk of dying may fall to just 1 percent. So, it's accurate that risk was cut in half, from 2 percent down to 1 percent, but our absolute risk of dying only fell by a single percentage point. That may not sound as impressive, but to me, dying with so much life left seems like such a tragedy that it would be worth making lifestyle changes to drive down that risk as low as possible, especially when one such strategy is a simple, delicious dietary tweak.

This is all assuming that the link between nut consumption and mortality is cause and effect. There are many potentially confounding factors. People who consume nuts tend to exercise more, smoke less, and eat less meat and more vegetables and fruits, for example. But, after controlling for these factors, the mortality benefits appear to persist.[6758] Randomized controlled trials have certainly shown that nuts can improve some of the key risk factors for some of our leading killers, such as cholesterol[6759] and, in the case of walnuts, artery function.[6760] No other food group was found to lower LDL cholesterol as effectively.[6761] Even then, though, there may be displacement effects. When researchers asked study participants to incorporate hundreds of calories of nuts into their daily diet, the subjects ended up just naturally decreasing their intake of animal protein, saturated fat, and sodium,[6762] which would be expected to help regardless of any benefits from adding nuts.[6763] It's not just that people are eating nuts instead of meat, though. The drop in heart attack risk among more frequent nut eaters is just as strong or even stronger among vegetarians.[6764]

How many nuts should we eat for maximal benefit? Remarkably, most of the survival advantage can apparently be achieved by eating only about three servings of nuts a week, which is just an average of 12 g a day,[6765] and no further reduction of mortality risk was found above a little more than a daily 0.5 oz or 15 to 20 g a day.[6766] So, at most, that's a palmful—for instance, nine hazelnuts (filberts), ten walnut halves, thirteen cashews, seventeen almonds, or twenty-five peanuts.[6767]

How Many Nuts Are Too Much?

Surprisingly, not a single one of dozens of studies adding an average of hundreds of calories of nuts a day for fifteen weeks to people's diets resulted in significant weight gain.[6768] However, there is a limit. Do not regularly eat more than a cup of nuts a day for the same reason we should avoid consuming multiple cups of spinach, beet greens, or Swiss chard, more than a few starfruits,[6769] multiple cups of rhubarb,[6770] or even spoonsful of chaga mushroom powder[6771] a day: oxalates.

Refer to see.nf/oxalaterisk to see who is at particular risk and see.nf/oxalatefood for other risky doses, including sixteen glasses of iced tea a day[6772,6773] and regularly eating in excess of a cup of cashews[6774] or almonds,[6775] or a combination of five handfuls of almonds and six tablespoons of chia seeds a day.[6776] See page 128 for a caveat about getting too much selenium in Brazil nuts.

WHICH NUT IS HEALTHIEST?

What about peanut butter? Details in see.nf/pblongevity, but basically, the longevity benefits associated with nuts (including peanuts) do not appear to extend to peanut butter, perhaps due to the lack of intact cellular structures that deliver a bounty of prebiotic goodness to our friendly gut flora. (See page 548.) The healthiest nut, however, is probably walnuts. Not only do they have some of the highest antioxidant[6777] and omega-3[6778] levels, but walnuts are the only nuts known to significantly improve artery function,[6779] and they beat out others in suppressing cancer cell growth in vitro.[6780]

While nut consumption in general has been associated with lower risk of impaired agility and mobility in older men and lower risk of impaired overall function in older women,[6781] in the Harvard Nurses' Health Study, only walnuts were significantly associated with healthy aging after controlling for confounding factors.[6782] Of all the nuts investigated in the PREDIMED study, the researchers discovered the greatest benefits associated with walnuts, particularly when it came to cancer.[6783] Individuals eating more than three servings a week of walnuts appeared to cut their risk of dying from cancer in half. A review of the available evidence concluded that "the far-reaching positive effects of a plant-based diet that includes walnuts may be the most critical message for the public."[6784]

GREENS

Nuts seem to beat out vegetables in terms of food groups associated with a longer life, but that was compared to vegetables *in general*. Green leafy vegetables can match nuts for potentially decreasing the risk of premature death,[6785] and consumption of greens is also associated with lower risk of heart disease, stroke, and a few types of cancer and may even help prevent some of the leading causes of age-related vision loss.[6786] (See the Preserving Your Vision chapter.) Greens can also boost our immunity, slow our metabolism, and protect our body against the effects of air pollution, one of the leading causes of death worldwide.

BOOSTING GUT DEFENSES WITH BROCCOLI

Our greatest exposure to the outside world is through our gut. When you take into consideration all the little folds in our intestinal lining, its total surface area is about half the size of a badminton court.[6787] Yet the lining is extremely thin, at just fifty-millionths of a meter. In other words, the barrier between our bloodstream and the outside world is many times thinner than a piece of tissue paper. If the lining of our gut were any thicker, it would be difficult for nutrients to pass through. Our skin needs to be waterproof so we don't start leaking, but our intestinal lining must allow for both nutrients and fluids to be absorbed. Since we have such a fragile layer separating our inner core from the outer chaos, we need a good defense mechanism in place to keep out the bad.

Enter our immune system, specifically, our intraepithelial lymphocytes, which are special types of white blood cells that have two functions: serving as our gut's first line of defense against pathogens and conditioning and repairing the thin intestinal lining.[6788] The "Ah receptor" covers these lymphocytes and activates the cells.[6789] This crucial receptor is significantly upregulated in centenarians, whereas its loss leads to premature aging (at least in mice).[6790] For years, scientists were unable to find the key that fit into the Ah receptor lock. If only we could uncover how to activate these cells, we might be able to boost our immunity.[6791] That key, it turns out, is found in broccoli. For more details, go to see.nf/gutdefenses.

The immune boost we get from consuming broccoli and other cruciferous vegetables not only protects us against pathogens found in food but also against pollutants in the environment, like car exhaust or tobacco smoke. Because dioxins and certain other pollutant chemicals exert their toxic effects through the Ah receptor system, cruciferous compounds may block them.[6792] Lest you think concerns over toxic chemicals floating around whiff of overblown hippie paranoia, in reality they are likely the fifth leading cause of death.[6793]

BILLIONS OF YEARS LOST EVERY YEAR

According to the preeminent Global Burden of Disease Study, air pollution is the fifth leading killer of humanity, wiping out about four million people a year[6794] from lung cancer, emphysema, heart disease, stroke, and respiratory infections.[6795] Ironically, one respiratory infection—COVID-19—may have saved lives in some parts of the world. In the early months following the lockdown in China, the decrease in air pollution was so great that as many as 30,000 air pollution fatalities *a month* may have been averted in that country alone. In other words, the air quality in China was so bad that COVID-19 may have ended up *saving* around a thousand lives a day.[6796]

Nine out of ten people live in areas that violate the World Health Organization's air pollution guidelines.[6797] It's estimated that improving air quality to those standards would increase the average global lifespan by more than two years. So, every year, polluted air appears to shave off billions of years of life expectancy.[6798] Traffic-related air pollution exposure has also been associated with premature skin aging[6799] and dementia.[6800] What can we do about it?

In 2014, China declared a "war against pollution," and their pollutant particle levels have since dropped by 29 percent, potentially adding years onto their average life expectancy.[6801] Elsewhere, however, such strict policy actions "might not be politically acceptable" as they "might indirectly affect the comfort of the population."[6802] Until we have better vehicle inspections, public transport, bus lanes, bicycle lanes, and perhaps even urban tolls to fund air cleanup efforts, what can we do to protect ourselves?

Personal strategies to minimize effects of air pollution include limiting physical exertion outdoors on high air pollution days and near heavy traffic areas.[6803] A randomized, crossover trial of older men and women found that walking along busy streets "curtails or even reverses the cardiorespiratory benefits of exercise."[6804] Close-fitting particulate respirators, such as N95 face masks, should even be considered on high pollution days.[6805]

Thanks in part to our changing climate, even if we uproot our families and move out to the countryside, worsening forest fires can bring pollution home, almost no matter where you live and breathe. Home air purifiers are increasingly recommended during fire smoke events,[6806] as numerous studies have shown that they can lower particulate exposure and benefit respiratory and cardiovascular health.[6807] I'd recommend HEPA filter models and avoiding air cleaning technologies that may emit harmful by-products,[6808] such as electrostatic precipitators (ionizers)[6809] and negative ion generators.[6810]

Diet contributes to more than twice as many deaths as air pollution, though.[6811] Fortunately, we may be able to bring the power of diet to combat the effects of polluted air.

DIETARY DETOX

I detailed how cruciferous vegetables can boost the activity of the detoxifying enzymes in our liver (see page 122) such that heavy broccoli eaters have to drink more coffee to get the same caffeine buzz.[6812] We also have detoxification enzymes lining our airways. Studies show that people born with less effective ones have an exaggerated allergic response to diesel exhaust, suggesting that these detox enzymes actively combat the inflammation caused by pollutants in the air.[6813] Might broccoli boost the activity of those enzymes, too?

Given that the cruciferous compound sulforaphane is the "most potent known inducer" of a major class of detox enzymes, researchers tried to see if it could combat the pro-inflammatory impact of pollutants.[6814] Details in see.nf/pollutiondetox, but basically, by squirting both diesel exhaust and flu viruses up people's noses, researchers discovered that eating a cup or two of broccoli could offer the best of both worlds—less inflammation from the pollution[6815] and an improved anti-viral immune response.[6816] Broccoli was also found to cut inflammation levels in smokers[6817] and dramatically accelerate the clearance of carcinogenic pollutants like benzene from the body.[6818]

What About Broccoli Supplements?

What if you don't like the taste of cruciferous veggies but still want their benefits? Researchers put BroccoMax, a leading commercially available broccoli supplement, to the test. Its manufacturer boasts that each capsule of BroccoMax contains the equivalent of half a pound of broccoli. Each day, study participants were given either six capsules or about a cup of broccoli sprouts. In the end, the supplement hardly worked at all, while the sprouts boosted blood levels about eight times higher and about eight times cheaper.[6819] Newer enzyme-treated broccoli sprout extract supplements claim comparable bioavailability, but they, too, were found to pale in comparison to the real thing.[6820]

GREEN IS FOR SLOW

One of the ways caloric restriction may extend the lifespan of animals is by slowing their metabolism.[6821] Like a candle, burning with a smaller flame may allow us to last longer. Thanks to the nitrates in green leafy vegetables, we may be able to achieve a similar metabolic benefit by eating a big salad every day.

The nitrate naturally found in leafy greens and beets improves the efficiency of our mitochondria, the little power plants within our cells, boosting athletic performance by extracting more energy from each breath.[6822] That's why a single shot of beet juice enables free divers to hold their breath for thirty seconds longer than usual, for instance.[6823] See what else vegetable doping can do for athletic performance in see.nf/nitrates. No drug, supplement, steroid, or any other intervention has been shown to do what vegetable nitrates can do.[6824]

Beets barely even reach the top ten list of common nitrate-rich foods, though. Eight of the top ten are greens, and, with four times the nitrate content of beets, arugula comes out on top with a whopping 480 mg of nitrate per 100-g serving.[6825]

Overall, green leafy vegetables contribute to 80 percent of our nitrate intake.[6826] So, if we eat a lot of greens, might we be able to slow our metabolism since our body would be able to function so much more efficiently, effectively drawing more energy from each calorie? Indeed, researchers found that the resting metabolic rates of study participants slowed by an average of about 4 percent after they consumed a dose of nitrate equivalent to a few servings of greens or beets.[6827] That's nearly a hundred calories of slowing a day.[6828] The researchers conjectured that this may be a way our body evolved to use vegetables to help preserve energy during lean times in our ancient past. Either way, slowing our metabolism may have benefits for our longevity[6829] and explain why those who eat more greens tend to live longer than those who eat less.[6830]

Top Ten Common Food Sources of Nitrates

1. Arugula
2. Rhubarb
3. Cilantro
4. Butter Leaf Lettuce
5. Spring Greens (e.g., Mesclun Mix)
6. Basil
7. Beet Greens
8. Oak Leaf Lettuce
9. Swiss Chard
10. Beets

VEGETABLE NITRATES TO COMBAT MUSCLE AGING

Nitrate supplementation can significantly increase exercise tolerance[6831] and performance,[6832] not only because it enables our body to extract more energy from oxygen[6833] but because it helps to dilate our arteries so they can deliver more oxygenated blood to our muscles[6834] and even directly improves muscle function (contractility) through an unknown mechanism.[6835] Nitrate-rich diets have been associated with improved muscle strength and physical function, leading researchers to conclude that "vegetables may be an effective way to limit any age-associated declines in muscle function." Causality, however, can't be inferred due to the cross-sectional nature of the data.[6836]

Catch see.nf/nitrateaging for more, but there have been acute interventional studies, such as one in which older men and women with an average age of seventy-one were given a beet juice supplement equivalent to about a cup of cooked greens.

The participants experienced a significant boost in knee extension (quads) power and velocity. Based on the steady annual rate of muscular decline, the extent of the nitrate enhancement was said to be "functionally equivalent to acutely reversing the effects of several decades of aging."[6837] A similarly aged group consuming a similarly sized dose also significantly improved upper body strength recovery (forearm hand grip).[6838]

VEGETABLE NITRATES TO COMBAT ARTERY AGING

In an editorial titled "Cardiac Aging and the Fountain of Youth," a Mayo Clinic research chair commented on the results of an "impressive array of experiments suggesting that this dream of reversing cardiac aging might not be as mythical as we had once believed."[6839] Spiking the water of old mice with nitrates was able to reverse age-related heart and artery stiffness,[6840] but what about people?

A meta-analysis of a dozen randomized, controlled human trials found that between two-thirds of a cup to two cups of cooked greens' worth of nitrates significantly improved artery function as measured in the arms[6841] or legs,[6842] and, as I detail in see.nf/nitrateaging, this translates into clinical benefit, for example, enabling peripheral artery disease patients to walk 18 percent longer without pain.[6843]

The healthiest way to get your nitrate fix is to eat a big salad every day. People randomized to eat a green leafy salad with arugula and spinach lowered their blood pressures within hours, compared to eating a greens-free salad of cucumber, green beans, and cherry tomatoes.[6844] You could take nitrate- and nitric-oxide-boosting supplements, but they have a questionable record of safety[6845] and efficacy.[6846] What about a juice like V8, which includes beets and spinach juice as ingredients? It must not have much of either, because you'd need to drink nineteen quarts of it a day to reach your daily nitrate intake target.[6847] (Details in see.nf/nitratetarget.)

FEEDING YOUR ORAL MICROBIOME

When all the studies are put together, nitrate-rich vegetables are found to significantly lower blood pressure on average,[6848] but some studies show no benefit whatsoever.[6849] To understand this variability and why eating greens is especially important as we age, you must first understand the nitrate activation step that happens in your mouth, thanks to good bacteria on your tongue. I explain the whole fascinating process in see.nf/scrape, but the bottom line: Foster the growth of nitrate-metabolizing bugs by eating nitrate-rich vegetables regularly,[6850] don't use antiseptic mouthwash,[6851] and clean your tongue daily[6852] (unless you have heart valve problems, a pacemaker, or anything else that puts you at risk for endocarditis).[6853]

HOW TO KEEP NITRATES FROM TURNING INTO NITROSAMINES

Note that the nitrate strategy may only work in the context of a healthy diet.[6854] Adding saturated fat (in the form of meat and dairy) to a vegetable-rich Mediterranean diet was found to raise blood pressure, not lower it.[6855] Furthermore, the nitrate strategy may only be *safe* in the context of a healthy diet.

The activation step that occurs on our tongue is the conversion of nitrates into nitrites. *Nitrites?* Isn't that what's added to cured meats? Why are nitrates and nitrites from vegetables okay, while the very same compounds from meat are linked to cancer?[6856] Because nitrites on their own are not carcinogenic; they *turn into* carcinogens. Nitrites only become harmful when they become nitro*samines* and nitro*samides.* For them to do that, amines and amides must be present, both of which are found in abundance in animal products.

So, adding nitrites to meat leads to the formation of carcinogens. (In the case of "uncured" bacon, you may see "fermented celery juice" or something similar in the ingredients list; that's just a deceptive way to add nitrites without using the word "nitrites.")[6857] The threat from processed meat is so great that the second-largest prospective study ever on cancer and diet determined that reducing consumption of processed meat to less than 20 g a day, a portion smaller than a matchbook, would prevent more than 3 percent of all deaths in Europe.[6858] The largest prospective study of diet and health in U.S. history—the NIH-AARP study of more than half a million Americans—found that the fraction of preventable deaths may be even higher. For instance, suggested the researchers, if the highest consumers of processed meat would reduce their intake to the equivalent of less than half a bacon strip a day, 20 percent of heart disease deaths among U.S. women could be averted.[6859] It's no surprise that the American Institute for Cancer Research recommends that we simply "avoid processed meat such as ham, bacon, salami, hot dogs and sausages."[6860]

So, nitrite-laden processed meats are a no-go, but what if the amines and amides in unprocessed meat mixed with the nitrites from activated vegetable nitrates? Remember, on their own, nitrites aren't carcinogenic; it's only when they're turned into nitrosamines and nitrosamides in the presence of amines and amides. So, for example, what if you eat a big salad, then, two or three hours later, eat unprocessed meat? The swallowed nitrites off your tongue from the salad-nitrate that got pumped back into your mouth could then mix in your stomach with the amides and amines from the meat. Researchers put this possibility to the test by having volunteers drink nitrate-rich water with a daily meal of cod, salmon, pollack, or shrimp. (Seafood is high in amines.) The level of carcinogenic nitrosamines flowing through their bodies shot up during the week they were asked to eat fish and fell back down once they cut out the seafood.[6861] A similar reaction was found in another study, with unprocessed chicken and turkey breast instead of seafood.[6862] This explains why having omnivores drink a single bottle of beet juice can lead to a significant rise in these carcinogenic compounds in their urine within twenty-four hours.[6863]

On the other hand, the vitamin C and other antioxidants naturally found in plant foods help block the formation of these carcinogens in our stomach.[6864] This helps explain why intake of nitrate and nitrite from processed meats has been linked to cancer, but no increased risk has been found for intake of nitrate or nitrite from plants.[6865] It may take more than a side serving, though. In the seafood study, the research subjects ate some vegetables with their fish, but evidently not enough to block carcinogen formation.[6866] So, those wanting to take full advantage of nitrate-rich vegetables may want to center all their meals around whole plant foods.

SALAD DAYS

In 1777, General George Washington issued an order that American troops should forage for wild greens around their camps "as these vegetables are very conducive to health, and tend to prevent . . . all putrid disorders."[6867] Since then, however, most Americans have declared their independence from greens. Today, only about one in twenty-five even reach a dozen servings throughout the course of an entire month,[6868] whereas I advise getting more than a dozen servings a week.

Greens have been suggested as one of the Okinawan secrets for longevity.[6869] Eating greens at least nearly every day may be one of the most powerful steps we can take to extend our lifespan. A study titled "Healthy Lifestyle and Preventable Death" identified six lifestyle factors that were associated with cutting in *half* the risk of dying over a period of twelve years for men and women in their sixties and seventies. Beyond nondietary factors, such as not smoking and walking an hour or more a day, the sole criterion for dietary quality the researchers used was "eating green-leafy vegetables" at least "almost daily."[6870]

Of all the food groups analyzed by a Harvard University research team, greens were associated with the strongest protection against major chronic diseases,[6871] including up to about an associated 20 percent reduction in risk for heart attacks[6872] and strokes[6873] for each additional serving per day.

So no wonder that of all the different types of fruits and vegetables, the best evidence for reducing mortality risk overall is seen with the consumption of green leafy vegetables.[6874] Imagine if there were a pill that could prolong your life and only had good side effects. Everyone would be taking it! It would be making billions of dollars for the lucky drug company that created it. All health plans by law would have to cover it. People from every walk of life and every corner of the globe would be clamoring for it. But when that "pill" is just eat-your-greens, people's eyes just glaze over.

IMPORTANT CAVEAT: Greens and Warfarin

If you are on warfarin (also known as the drug Coumadin), be sure to speak with your physician before you increase your intake of greens. The drug works by hampering the enzyme that recycles vitamin K, which is involved in blood clotting. If your system gets an influx of fresh vitamin K, which is concentrated in greens, you may undermine the effectiveness of the drug.[6875] You should still be able to enjoy your greens, but your doctor will need to titrate the dose of the drug to match your regular greens intake.

BERRIES

For all the national dietary guidelines from around the world, the most common key message is simple: Eat more fruits and vegetables.[6876] But not all fruits and vegetables are the same. Those who think berries are the berry best live longer, but those who are bananas over bananas do not.[6877] I've already talked about the benefits of berries for cognition in the Preserving Your Mind chapter, for immunity in the Preserving Your Immune System chapter, and for eyesight in the Preserving Your Vision chapter. Rarely in research are berries separated out from the generic fruit category,[6878] but combining the three prospective studies on eating berries and overall longevity, it's clear that those with high berry consumption tend to live significantly longer than those with low intake.[6879] Tastes great *and* may help us live longer? That's what plant-based eating is all about.

JAM-PACKED WITH ANTIOXIDANTS

Berries appear to reduce all-cause mortality risk as much as green leafy vegetables.[6880] Greens are the healthiest vegetables, and berries the healthiest fruits—in part due to their respective plant pigments. Leaves contain chlorophyll, the green pigment where the firestorm of photosynthesis takes place, so greens have to be packed with antioxidants to deal with the free radicals that are formed. Meanwhile, berries evolved to have bright, contrasting colors to attract fruit-eating critters to help disperse their seeds, and the same molecular characteristics that give berries such vibrant colors may account for some of their antioxidant abilities.[6881]

Apples and bananas are America's favorite fruits, with antioxidant power of about 60 and 40 units, respectively (in modified FRAP assay daμmol antioxidant units). Mangos are the preferred fruit everywhere else and have much more anti-oxidant punch at around 110 units. (If you think about how much more colorful mangos are on the inside, this makes sense.) But none of these fruits is a match for berries: Per cup, strawberries have about 310 units; blueberries, 380; raspberries, 430; cranberries, 490; and blackberries, a staggering 680 antioxidant units. There are some Dr. Seuss–sounding berries in the Arctic tundra, like red whortleberries, that have even more antioxidant power, but when it comes to what is readily available in the store, it's blackberries for the win. Selecting blackberries over strawberries may give you twice the antioxidant bang for your berry.[6882]

Super-Dupe-Er Fruit

Açaí berries have anti-aging effects in mice,[6883] though they don't prolong the lifespan of *C. elegans*.[6884] Açaí does improve the survival of fruit flies fed a high-fat diet, but what might it offer people?[6885] I profile the disappointing clinical results in see.nf/acai. Even the antioxidant effects are overblown. Those who hawk supplements love to talk about how açaí consumption can "triple antiox-idant capacity" of your blood. If you look at the study they cite, though, you'll find that the antioxidant capacity of participants' blood did actually triple after eating açaí—but the same tripling was achieved in the control group consuming plain applesauce.[6886]

DEAD AND BERRIED

As I noted on page 124, the stomach acts as a bioreactor.[6887] The fat in muscle starts to oxidize (turn rancid) from the moment an animal is slaughtered, but when meat hits the acid bath of the stomach, a burst of free radicals is generated.[6888] Within hours of consumption, oxidized fat by-products like malondialdehyde (MDA) are created and then absorbed into the bloodstream,[6889] where they can damage pro-teins and mutate DNA.[6890] But berries can help.

Polyunsaturated fats are most susceptible to oxidation, which explains why a digested chicken leg results in six times more MDA equivalents than beef or pork and salmon results in fourteen times more. What about high polyunsaturated plant foods like pecans? Add handfuls of pecans to people's diets, and MDA levels go *down*.[6891] Why? Because whole plant foods come prepackaged with antioxidants to protect against oxidation. On average, plant foods have *sixty-four times* more antioxidants than animal foods. Even iceberg lettuce has more antioxidants than meat, and it's 96 percent water.[6892] That's why most of the oxidized fat we get in our diet comes from meat products and fatty processed foods.[6893]

If antioxidants in plants can counter fat oxidation in the stomach, what about just eating plants and meat together? It worked in pigs. When pigs were fed a mixture of oil and beef, they had a fivefold increase in MDA equivalents, but when they were fed the same oily beef with fruits and vegetables (plums, apples, and artichoke hearts), the meal appeared to only double MDA levels.[6894] Researchers in Italy decided to try this in humans by having people eat a McDonald's Big Tasty Bacon and fries with or without one and a half glasses of fermented berry juice (red wine). Within four hours of eating the Big Tasty Bacon and fries without the wine, there was a significant rise in oxidized LDL cholesterol in the blood, but not after the same McDonald's meal was paired with merlot.[6895] The same neutralization of the effects on oxidized fats and cholesterol in the blood was found with two glasses of red wine with a double cheeseburger.[6896]

The one food group with more antioxidant power than berries is spices. Herbs and spices have been used in meat preservation to reduce rancidity for thousands of years.[6897] Researchers prepared a spice mix composed of about a teaspoon of paprika, one and a half teaspoons of oregano, a half teaspoon of garlic powder, a half teaspoon of ginger, and about a quarter teaspoon each of black pepper, cloves, cinnamon, and rosemary to a half pound of ground beef. Compared to the burgers without the spice mix, the spiced burgers cut the MDA flowing through the subjects' systems approximately in half (as measured in their urine).[6898] Just adding about a half teaspoon of turmeric to a half pound of ground beef can cut its MDA content by around 20 percent. Although black pepper alone doesn't seem to help, combining the turmeric with even just an eighth of a teaspoon of black pepper appears to double turmeric's effect.[6899]

Turkey is a tougher challenge. Although red wine could fully quiesce the fat oxidation of a double cheeseburger, it was able to drop MDA blood levels by only 40[6900] to 75 percent after consumption of turkey cutlets. However, if you presoak the cutlets in red wine in addition to drinking it with the meal, you can fully defuse the MDA bump.[6901] The same with a concentrate of cranberries, blackberries, blueberries, raspberries, Chilean guava, and Chilean wineberries. Mixing the berries into ground turkey meat cut the MDA spike from turkey burgers nearly in half, and drinking two cups of the berry combination in beverage form with the meal was able to fully quash the rise in MDA.[6902]

Rather than making berry burgers, what about just eating a side salad? Researchers combined about a quarter pound of turkey breast with a half cup of a Mediterranean-type salad made up of tomato, raw pink onion, black olives, extra-virgin olive oil, and fresh basil into an in vitro digester and were able to reduce the formation of oxidized fats in half. A full cup of salad stopped the oxidation completely. Testing the different salad components separately, the most potent appeared to be the onion and the olive oil.[6903]

Unlike tuna fat or fish oil supplements, which can quintuple the MDA formation from digesting turkey meat, the antioxidants in extra-virgin olive oil can cut it in half.[6904] There can be a paradoxical effect at higher concentrations, though. At a concentration of 2.5 percent, which is about a half teaspoon of oil for a 3-oz serving of turkey breast, extra-virgin olive oil has a powerful antioxidant effect. But at 5 percent (a full teaspoon) or 10 percent, it had a pro-oxidant effect, making MDA formation from digesting turkey even worse.[6905] No such paradoxical effect has ever been reported with whole plant foods. Only about one in five Americans eats salad on a given day, though.[6906] How about just a simple cup of joe?

Given the sad state of the standard American diet, coffee is actually one of the leading sources of antioxidants.[6907] Turkish coffee is like the matcha of the coffee kingdom in that you drink the powdered beans, and a cup of it can cut the MDA levels in your bloodstream caused by a meat meal by more than half, comparable to the effect of red wine. Instant coffee is the least potent. It would take four and a half cups of instant coffee to have the same effect as one cup of Turkish.[6908]

To quantify just how many plant foods it would take to neutralize the free radicals produced in the stomach after consuming animal foods, researchers created the Postprandial Oxidative Stress Index, defined as "the capacity of a plant derived food in grams to completely (100%) inhibit MDA formation from 200 g turkey meat incubated in SGF [simulated gastric (stomach) fluid] for 180 min at 37°C" body temperature. How much tomato would you have to put on that turkey sandwich to not end up with mutagenic oxidized fat in your blood? Thirty-one slices, which is about five tomatoes' worth. Spinach has, gram for gram, six times more free radical–quenching power, but it is so light that you'd need three cups of spinach, which might topple the sandwich but could be doable as a large side salad. Having one large apple would also do it, but berries would be the best. Even just an eighth of a cup of blackberries would sop up the free radicals created by the turkey meal in the stomach, or a quarter cup of blueberries, a half cup of raspberries, or a full cup of strawberries.[6909]

Fatty fish like tuna or salmon would be worse than turkey because of the polyunsaturated fat content in fish, and beef and pork would be better. The worst of the worst would be a combination of poultry (turkey) and fish fat (tuna oil), which creates five times more oxidized fat in the stomach than turkey alone. Still, that's nothing that less than a cup of blackberries couldn't handle.[6910] So, whenever you eat meat or fatty junk food, you should make sure your stomach also has potent plants in it at the same time to deal with the pro-oxidant aftermath.

If you're going to buy bulk vitamin C to make your own DIY facial youth serum (see page 454), why not just sprinkle some on a meal? Because it could make things worse. Straight vitamin C in the stomach can convert the ferric iron (Fe^{3+}) in meat into ferrous iron (Fe^{2+}), which causes toxic hydroxyl radical,[6911] resulting in a net pro-oxidant effect at all vitamin C doses tested when mixed with high-fat beef during digestion.[6912]

No Wild Goose Chase

As a Western-trained physician, I had never heard of amla, which is dried, powdered Indian gooseberry fruit. I was surprised to find more than seven hundred articles on it in the medical literature and even more surprised to find papers with titles like "Amla, a Wonder Berry in the Treatment and Prevention of Cancer." Arguably the most important plant in Ayurvedic medicine, amla is used traditionally for everything from a hair tonic to a snake venom neutralizer.[6913] I eat it because it's apparently the single most antioxidant-packed whole food on Earth.[6914] See what four cents' worth can do to the antioxidant power of a smoothie in see .nf/breakfast.

In the Ayurvedic lexicon, amla is considered "the best medicine to increase the lifespan"[6915] and a "potent aphrodisiac," but the evidence to support these claims derives from fruit flies.[6916] The Elens-Wattiaux mating chamber I detail in see.nf/amla has since been replaced with the "Copulatron." But when you read about aphrodisiac effects, you're probably not thinking *more maggots*. What effects have been documented in people?

A lifespan-extending effect wouldn't be surprising given the cholesterol-lowering benefits of amla[6917] I note in the video. Amla has also been shown to reduce triglycerides,[6918] improve blood fluidity, reduce markers of oxidative DNA damage[6919] and systemic inflammation,[6920] improve blood sugar control in diabetics,[6921] and may decrease the effects of stress on the heart.[6922] As noted in see.nf /dyspepsia, it can also work as well as antacids for calming an upset stomach, in addition to significantly reducing heartburn and regurgitation.[6923] See my Amla section in *How Not to Die* for tips on buying and using it.

CHASE RAINBOWS

Leading health organizations such as the American Heart Association and the American Institute for Cancer Research encourage people to "eat the rainbow," a wide spectrum of naturally colorful foods.[6924] Beyond the fact that 94 percent of Americans don't even reach the minimum recommended number of servings of fruits and vegetables (five to thirteen, depending on gender, age, and activity), there is a "phytonutrient gap." We are missing out on the colors. If the average American should eat about ten servings a day, that could be visualized as two from each color category, yet about eight out of ten Americans fall short of every color. The worst is the purple/blue group, our source of anthocyanin pigments, for which more like nine out of ten are deficient.[6925] Blueberries are the main source in the U.S. diet, yet people average only about a single blueberry a day.[6926]

Anthocyanin comes from the Greek *anthos*, meaning "flower," and *kyanos*, meaning "blue."[6927] The same pigments color red, blue, and purple berries, but their names still hint at their floral origins—for example, the petunidin in blueberries or the peonidin in cranberries.[6928] Able to cross the blood-brain barrier, anthocyanins are thought to be responsible for the cognitive benefits of berries in terms of improving brain perfusion, memory, executive function, processing speed, attention, and overall cognitive performance.[6929] They may also benefit our eyesight.

In the Preserving Your Vision chapter, I talked about their potential for helping with macular degeneration, glaucoma, and cataracts, but berries also can benefit our vision in other ways. Randomized, double-blind, placebo-controlled trials have shown that berry anthocyanins can significantly improve both objective and subjective signs and symptoms of eye strain,[6930] as well as improving light[6931] and dark[6932] adaptation. Anthocyanins appear to be important for regenerating a receptor protein known as "visual purple" in our retina that helps convert light into electrical signals for the brain, speeding up how fast our vision can adjust to changing light levels.[6933]

As discussed in the Inflammation chapter, berries have systemic anti-inflammatory effects throughout the body, though they can also suppress inflammation directly within the gut.[6934] Ninety percent of patients with ulcerative colitis responded to bilberries, with most achieving remissions within six weeks; disease activity surged back, however, once the berries were stopped.[6935] Part of this may derive from the prebiotic effect of anthocyanins on the gut flora. Eating berries increases the number of good bugs and decreases the number of bad ones.[6936] For example, eating blueberries every day increases the number of *Lactobacilli* and *Bifidobacteria*.[6937] Similar effects have been shown for black currants[6938] and tart cherries.[6939]

Anthocyanins have also been found to improve short- and long-term blood sugar control,[6940] in part by improving insulin sensitivity,[6941] so it's no surprise that higher berry intake is associated with a lower risk of developing type 2 diabetes.[6942] A famous pair of Harvard studies chalking up millions of person-years of data found that just two or more servings a week was associated with 23 percent lower risk.[6943]

Berries may also acutely improve artery function,[6944] which could help explain why higher anthocyanin intake is associated with a significantly lower risk of dying from cardiovascular disease[6945] and, by extension, all causes put together.[6946] A bowl of blueberries can even mediate much of the arterial dysfunction induced by smoking a cigarette. Smoke just one, and the ability of your arteries to relax naturally drops by 25 percent within two hours.[6947] But if you eat two cups of blueberries a hundred minutes before smoking, that same cigarette causes less than half the damage. (Of course, all the damage could be prevented by not smoking in the first place.)

We suspect it's largely the anthocyanin component since purified anthocyanins alone can improve artery function,[6948] though not as well as whole berries.[6949] At doses over 300 mg a day, anthocyanins can also lower LDL cholesterol.[6950] That translates into as little as a single daily serving, like a half cup of high-anthocyanin berries such as blueberries.[6951] Even just daily consumption of blueberry tea— powdered blueberries in a teabag steeped for five minutes—can lower cholesterol, though it took three months for the tea to start having a significant effect.[6952]

Anthocyanins are cleared from our bloodstream within about six hours, so, by the afternoon, the berries you had on your oatmeal may have run their course.[6953] In my mind, berries make the perfect dessert for any meal. There are other anthocyanin-containing fruits, like plums, pomegranates, and red or black grapes. Anthocyanins can also be served in your main course, thanks to red onions, blue potatoes, red cabbage, or purple barley. I like to air-pop purple popcorn for a snack or air-fry purple sweet potato fries for a side. For a drink, what do you think makes hibiscus tea as ruby red as Dorothy's slippers? Anthocyanins may also be responsible for the blood-pressure-lowering benefits of hibiscus.[6954] In animal models, the anthocyanins in black rice help ameliorate the accelerated aging induced by galactose in mice,[6955] and those in purple wheat prolong the lifespan of *C. elegans* by about 10 percent.[6956]

CHERRIES, CRANBERRIES, GOJIS, AND GRAPES

For about half a century, we've known that tart cherries are so anti-inflammatory that they may be used to successfully treat gout, a painful type of arthritis, as I mentioned in the Inflammation chapter.[6957] Cherries can also reduce inflammation in healthy people, as indicated by decreasing C-reactive protein levels.[6958] Overall, eleven out of sixteen interventional trials on the consumption of cherries, both tart and sweet ones, found a decrease in inflammation, and a drop in oxidative stress was found in eight out of ten studies, a decrease in exercise-induced muscle soreness and loss of strength in eight out of nine, a drop in blood pressure in five out of seven, improvements in arthritis in five out of five, and improved sleep in four out of four (presumably due to the melatonin content, see.nf/melatoninfoods). Most of these studies were less than two weeks in duration and involved giving people the equivalent of 45 to 270 cherries a day.[6959]

When not in season, tart cherries can be found canned in water and sweet cherries can be found in the freezer section. (I still like to suck on frozen dark cherries like little popsicles—a trick my mom taught me.) In *How Not to Die*, I recommend using the drained liquid from canned cherries in a hibiscus punch recipe and mixing cherries into your morning oatmeal with cocoa powder for a chocolate-covered cherry-like sensation.

As we saw in the Preserving Your Bowel and Bladder Function chapter, cranberries have benefits for urinary health for both men and women. Cranberries can increase the lifespans of flies[6960] and worms[6961] and slow the age-related decline in insulin production in rats,[6962] but they haven't been put to the test for mammalian longevity.

I highlighted goji berries in the Preserving Your Immune System and Preserving Your Vision chapters. Also known as *wolfberries*, goji berries have long been considered a "potent anti-aging agent" in traditional Chinese medicine and have been used to counteract premature hair graying, for example.[6963] There is little scientific evidence to confirm such effects, though. Goji berries do extend the lifespan of *Drosophila*, but fruit being good for fruit flies isn't exactly revelatory.[6964] However, they have at least four times the antioxidant activity of other dried fruits, like raisins or dried cranberries that you might otherwise sprinkle on your oatmeal or add to your trail mix.[6965] Goji berries also have anti-inflammatory effects in vitro (on cells from umbilical cords),[6966] as well as in randomized, double-blind, placebo-controlled trials of whole people,[6967] and may even help with weight loss, as I detail in my Inflammation Quenchers chapter in *How Not to Diet*.

Whatever you now do with raisins, do it with gojis instead. Domesticated more than 6,000 years ago,[6968] the grapevine is now the single largest fruit crop grown in the world.[6969] What can they do for us? A meta-analysis of more than fifty randomized controlled trials involving thousands of study participants found that various grape products can cause a small (five-point) drop in LDL cholesterol, but raisins did not seem to work.[6970] This may be because most raisins are made from "white" grapes, the ubiquitous pale green Thompson grapes. In a head-to-head comparison between red grapes and green ones, eating about three cups a day of red grapes for eight weeks significantly reduced LDL cholesterol, but the same amount of green grapes did not.[6971]

Similarly, raisins were not able to acutely improve artery function,[6972] but a cup and a quarter of various fresh grapes, including red and blue-black ones, can even blunt the arterial dysfunction caused by a McDonald's Sausage McMuffin with Egg meal.[6973] Chronic improvement in artery function was also demonstrated in a randomized, double-blind, placebo-controlled trial (using powdered red grapes).[6974]

Grape Seed Extract Supplements

The McMuffin mediation study included grapes with seeds, which harbor the bulk of the polyphenols in the fruit. Only 1 percent is found in the pulp and 5 percent in the juice. The skins of grapes hold 30 percent of the polyphenols, but the seeds contain the remaining 64 percent.[6975] Unfortunately, it can be hard to find seeded grapes these days. What about just taking grape seed extract supplements? I review the available studies for you in see.nf/gse. The bottom line? Stick to the seeded grapes. I've found the best odds of finding seeded grapes are at Asian markets, where you might be lucky enough to find Concord-like Kyoho grapes (from the Japanese *Kyohō budō*, meaning "giant mountain grape"), dark purple globes with tasty large oval seeds.

XENOHORMESIS AND microRNA MANIPULATION

Xenohormesis and microRNAs represent cross-kingdom communication pathways between plants and animals that we may be able to use to our advantage.

XENOHORMESIS

Hormesis can be thought of as the "that which doesn't kill you makes you stronger" principle.[6976] Physical activity is the classic example:[6977] You put stress on your muscles and heart, and are all the healthier for it, provided there is sufficient recovery time. Mild stresses like exercise can trigger a protective response that leads to strengthened defenses in the long run.[6978]

In the sixteenth century, the Swiss physician Paracelsus, the "father of toxicology," coined the Latin phrase *sola dosis facit venenum*, which is translated as "only the dose makes the poison."[6979] This aphorism is typically summoned to explicate how some of the most helpful or harmless substances (like water) can be toxic at high enough concentrations, and, conversely, how even some of our most poisonous substances (like cyanide) can be harmless at sufficiently infinitesimal doses. The field of toxicology adopted this threshold dose-response model, where at low enough concentrations, there may be no effect, but above that, the hazard is proportional to the dose. Hormesis added a new wrinkle, forcing toxicology to challenge this assumption.[6980]

Hormesis takes the notion "too much of a good thing can be bad" and turns it on its head by suggesting that, sometimes, a little of a bad thing can be good.[6981] Hormesis comes from the Greek term *hormáein*, meaning "to excite."[6982] Rather than a linear model in which there are small effects at small doses and the same but larger effects at larger doses, hormesis describes a biphasic response characterized by one effect at a low dose and the opposite effect at a higher dose. For example, herbicides kill plants, but in tiny doses they can actually boost plant growth, presumably by stressing the plant into rallying its resources to successfully fight back.[6983]

What began as a biological curiosity used in a misguided nineteenth-century attempt to vindicate homeopathy[6984] is now undergoing a resurgence of interest.[6985] In the 1980s, as few as a single study a year were published on hormesis in the scientific literature. Now, on average, more than one paper is published every day.[6986] This is in large part due to interest in the role of hormesis to combat aging.[6987]

BASK IN THE GLOW?

Hormesis was first shown to extend life more than a century ago when low doses of radiation were found to increase the lifespan of beetles[6988] by presumably ramping up DNA repair.[6989] That which didn't kill them made them stronger. I run through the wild ride of a story in see.nf/radiation, including studies suggesting longer lives among atomic bomb survivors[6990] and experiments done more than a mile down into the Earth to counter the cosmic rays bombarding us every second.[6991] "Nothing in life is to be feared," Marie Curie, who won the Nobel Prize for pioneering work in radioactivity, is quoted as saying, "it is only to be understood."[6992] Of course, this is coming from a woman who died of bone marrow failure from radiation exposure,[6993] such that her remains had to be interred in a lead-lined coffin.[6994] Watch the video, but the bottom line is that we don't know enough about low-level radiation to exploit any hormetic effects without potentially being exposed to unacceptable risks. There are, however, salutary ways to harness hormesis for health and longevity.

NO PAIN, NO GAIN

We all know that exercise is ultimately good for us, but, nonetheless, it places inseparable stress on the body.[6995] Ultramarathon runners generate so many free radicals during a race that they can damage the DNA of a significant percentage of their cells.[6996] But, within a week, they don't just go back to the baseline level of DNA damage; they have significantly *less* damage, presumably because they had revved up their antioxidant defenses.[6997] So, exercise-induced oxidative damage may ultimately be beneficial. In other words, classic hormesis, where low levels of damage can upregulate protective mechanisms and ultimately leave you better off. For those interested in how not to undermine the benefits of athletic recovery, check out see.nf/exercisehormesis.

WHAT DOESN'T KILL PLANTS MAY MAKE US STRONGER

Hormesis may be why dietary restriction can lead to lifespan extension.[6998] The mild stress placed upon the body by not eating enough may activate a wide variety of protective pathways, ramping up anti-inflammatory and antioxidant defenses.[6999] Your body is preparing itself for the coming famine it thinks is about to occur.

In the Caloric Restriction chapter, I'll explore ways to exploit the benefits of dietary restriction to extend life and prevent disease, but chronically restricting food intake is not a realistic health strategy for many. Given the powerful evolutionary drive to eat, it's hard for most people to cut food intake by even 10 or 20 percent.[7000] A more feasible alternative may be to activate dietary restriction–induced stress response pathways by other means. One such possibility is *xenohormesis*, derived from the Greek *xenos*, meaning "stranger," "foreigner," or "other." Xenohormesis refers to the bestowal of stress resistance from stressed plants to the animals who eat them.[7001] In other words, instead of exposing ourselves to the stressor to trigger our body's defenses and shore up protection against future stressors, why not let plants take the hit?[7002]

Couch potatoes don't have anything on real potatoes. Plants live the ultimate sedentary lifestyle. Because they can't move, they've had to evolve a whole other way to respond to threats, and they do so biochemically. They manufacture—from scratch—a dizzying array of compounds to deal with whatever's coming their way.[7003] For example, if we get too hot, we can move into the shade, but if plants get too hot, they're stuck. They *are* the shade!

Plants have had nearly a billion years to create a whole chemistry set of protective substances, some of which can play a similar role in us. After all, where do most vitamins come from? Plants make them for their own needs, and we hijack them for broadly analogous cellular roles in our own body.[7004] There is also a shared set of "vitagenes" conserved through evolution to encode an array of repair and maintenance processes, such as heat-shock proteins that confer fitness and survival benefits.[7005] Nature programs marvel how closely we're related to chimps, but we share about a fifth of our genes with a banana[7006] even though it's been more than a billion years since we had a shared ancestor—before the human and the banana split.[7007] Nature didn't reinvent the wheel for critical cellular processes, such as basic metabolism and preserving DNA integrity. Plants and animals even share some of the same stresses.

We get attacked by bacteria, and so do plants and fungi.[7008] When bacteria muscle in on a particular fungus, it creates a molecule called penicillin—provided free for us—and when a fungus muscles in on a particular bacterium, it produces rapamycin as an antifungal to slow its growth, inhibiting the target of rapamycin (TOR) pathway conserved in fungi, plants, and animals, including us.[7009] Remember, that's the same "engine of aging" enzyme pathway that can be tweaked to extend lifespans. (See page 102.)

When plants get infected, they produce the compound in aspirin, which can come in handy when we get infected ourselves. Plants heal wounds, and so do we, using similar signaling systems.[7010] Plants have DNA they need to protect from free radical damage, so they cook up complex antioxidants that we can use for ourselves instead of reinventing the wheel. In a sense, the crispers in our fridges are like nature's medicine cabinet.

We can just let the plants get stressed because, incredibly, the stress response molecules in plants may activate the same protective responses in us.[7011] The majority of known health benefits of edible plants may be attributable to the pharmacologically active substances of plants' sophisticated stress responses, off which we can then piggyback. For example, I've often mentioned polyphenols, a class of phytonutrients for which there's a huge medical literature on health-promoting effects.[7012] Plants produce polyphenols to protect themselves,[7013] and we may be able to expropriate and commandeer them for our own similar purpose.[7014]

Xenohormesis explains how environmentally stressed plants produce bioactive compounds that can confer survival benefits to those of us who consume them. Drought-stressed strawberries, for example, have more antioxidants and other phytonutrients. Have you ever eaten a wild strawberry? The taste is incomparable to the flat flavor facade of the cultivated kind. The healthiest grapes often grow in relatively dry, sun-exposed, infertile soil.[7015] Studies show that commonly consumed fruits and vegetables can be nutritionally enhanced by light, water, nutrient deficits, cold stress, or being nibbled on by bugs.[7016] That may help explain why the levels of phytonutrients are estimated to be 10 to 50 percent higher in organic vegetables compared with conventionally grown ones.[7017] Organic grape juice, for instance, contains more polyphenols and resveratrol than conventional grape juice.[7018] Similarly, soups prepared from organically grown vegetables contain levels of salicylic acid that are nearly six times higher than soups prepared from nonorganic ingredients.[7019]

If you starve plants, they do the same thing mammals do: activate preservation pathways. So, let the plants face the adversity to create the molecules that trigger cell stress resistance, alter metabolism, and improve disease resistance. Then, we can just capture them for the same uses in our own body. The fact that many phytonutrients act as "dietary restriction mimetics," in that they mimic the physiological effects of dietary restriction, may be no coincidence. The plants produce these compounds to save their own green butts from scarcity. So, instead of having to starve, thanks to xenohormesis, we may be able to let plants bear the brunt and enable us to harness their hardships as a means to promote our own health.

PLANT POKES

The flip side of xenohormesis is that plant compounds themselves can act as a source of hormetic stress that ends up bolstering us. If you remember from the Oxidation chapter, green tea's rallying of antioxidant and DNA repair defenses appears to be a consequence of its mild *pro*-oxidant qualities.[7020] It ends up doing a lot of good by being a little bad. The constant small jabs with every sip rev up our defenses to better protect us when a more serious insult comes along. It's like minor irritations that build up calluses on our hands to fortify our resilience. The end result? Interventional studies on rodents show that green tea extends their lifespan,[7021] and observational studies on human populations show that tea drinkers may average lives that are years longer.[7022,7023]

Remember the broccoli story from the same chapter?[7024] How the cruciferous compound sulforaphane is the most potent natural inducer of Nrf2, a "guardian of healthspan and gatekeeper of species longevity"? Our body wouldn't ramp up the detoxification enzymes in our liver every time we ate broccoli if it didn't consider broccoli to be a threat at some level. It's like how applying the hot pepper compound capsaicin on our skin can trigger heat receptors and fool our body into sweating and flushing its way to actually bring down our internal body temperature.[7025] Our body seems to picture each floret of broccoli as a miniature medieval mace and responds by battening down the hatches. We may then reap the rewards of this veggie vigilance and enjoy a longer life as a result.

It's no surprise that our body is finely tuned to react defensively to so many compounds in plants. After all, plants don't want to be eaten. Sulforaphane is thought to be created in plants to dissuade nibblers with its bitterness. Allicin, the garlicky compound in garlic, is presumably made for the same purpose. At petri dish concentrations exceeding that which could be achieved by even garlic-lover levels of consumption, certain garlic compounds can be toxic to mammalian cells (obtained from human foreskin,[7026] so no applying raw crushed garlic to your skin),[7027] but at culinary levels our body evolved to handle, subtoxic dosing in pasta sauce can induce the adaptive stress responses thought responsible for garlic's health benefits.[7028] Whether some of our healthiest plants are actually mildly toxic[7029] or our body merely treats them as such, the end result is the same: health through hormesis.

POWER PLANTS

There are thousands of phytonutrients that will never make it onto the side of a cereal box, yet may play a role in reducing the risk of chronic diseases—and those are just the ones we know about.[7030] The terms *phytonutrient* and *phytochemical* refer to natural compounds found in plants that can affect our health. (*Phyto-* comes from the Greek *phyton*, meaning "plant.") They are not considered "essential" nutrients like vitamins, as we can technically survive without them. Instead, they have been called "lifespan essential," meaning they're necessary for the longest possible life.[7031] In this way, they are like dietary fiber—critical for optimal health and longevity, but not technically essential, as coma patients can survive for years on an intravenous mixture of sugar water, electrolytes, amino acids, vitamins, and a few essential fats and trace minerals.

How many people are dying these days of vitamin deficiencies, like scurvy, compared to the number dying from phytonutrient deficiencies? An estimated 7.8 million premature deaths are attributed annually to the inadequate consumption of fruits and vegetables, not getting at least eight servings a day.[7032] Millions of lives hang in the balance, the balance being the scales that hang in the produce aisle.

In the United States alone, if you add up all the fatal cancers, strokes, heart attacks, and other deaths that could have been averted by simply eating more fruits and vegetables, it comes out to about 450,000 deaths every year.[7033] There is a phytonutrient deficiency pandemic that could be wiped out with a few more daily servings of plants. Yet, the pandemic is getting worse, not better. Over the last few decades, dietary quality has continued to deteriorate. Consumption of both fruits and vegetables (excluding potatoes) has dropped by more than half,[7034] and intake of legumes, also an important source of phytonutrients,[7035] has dropped by about 40 percent. At the same time, saturated fat consumption is on the rise. Only about 1 in 250 people even meet 80 percent of the American Heart Association's recommendations for a healthy diet.[7036]

Perhaps people just don't understand the power of plants. Consider the first phytochemical, isolated in 1804 from the poppy plant: morphine.[7037] In the fourth century, the first handbook of emergency medicine was published in China and recommended wormwood for malaria.[7038] Seventeen hundred years later, this discovery was immortalized in a Nobel Prize in medicine for the phytochemical *artemisinin*, now included in the most effective combination therapies against the scourge of malaria.[7039] In my video see.nf/herbs2drugs, I dive into other powerful examples.

POLYAMORY

Polyphenols are among the front-runners in developing dietary approaches to fight age-associated diseases. More than 8,000 different polyphenols have been identified, but only a small proportion have had their health effects cataloged.[7040] Still, there is such a critical mass of data in favor of the protective benefits[7041] of these "lifespan essentials" that recommended daily intakes of polyphenols have been proposed.[7042] I review what they can do and why in see.nf/polyphenols, where I also note the one source of flavonoids associated with an *increased* mortality: grapefruit, chalked up in part to grapefruit's suppression of a set of detoxification enzymes in our intestines.[7043]

NATURAL GEROPROTECTORS

Geroprotectors are substances that increase longevity and/or have other anti-aging properties.[7044] More than two hundred have been found. (See geroprotectors.org.) Some of the most powerful ones that even beat out synthetic compounds are natural plant extracts of simple herbs and spices, like celery seed.[7045] There are phytonutrients that can increase the maximum lifespan of animals by as much as 78 percent.[7046]

Plant extracts that have been shown to increase the lifespan of lower organisms include açaí, apples[7047] (including boring Red Delicious),[7048] asparagus, blueberries, cinnamon, cocoa, corn,[7049] fenugreek seeds, grape skins, holy basil leaf,[7050] peach, pomegranate, rose, and turmeric.[7051] Fewer improve the lifespan of mammals like mice, and those that do—like lemon—are tested on inbred strains chosen for their rapid aging.[7052]

Many of the "superfoods" that can extend the lives of enfeebled mice have no significant effect on robust, long-living ones, and those that do may be a result of inadvertent dietary restriction.[7053] For example, mice fed a turmeric compound lived longer than control group mice, but they weighed about 3 percent less, suggesting they were eating less.[7054] (Maybe they weren't curry fans.) The dietary restriction alone could potentially account for the longevity. When researchers subsequently fed mice iso-calorically instead of ad libitum, effectively forcing those groups of mice to eat the same amount, the turmeric benefit appeared to vanish.[7055]

Speaking of dietary restriction–induced life extension, might the hormetic or xenohormetic benefits of phytonutrients undermine the longevity dividends of the stress of caloric restriction? A mixture of synthetic antioxidants completely blunted the life extension from a 20 percent diet restriction in mice,[7056] but if you give polyphenols from blueberries, pomegranates, and green tea to intermittently fasted mice, they live even longer than had they just fasted intermittently.[7057] The longevity benefit was potentiated by phytonutrients. The researchers suggest that although alternate-day fasting in mice may have a net beneficial effect on lifespan, it also may entail harmful stresses that can be successfully countered by polyphenol intake.

PLANTS, NOT PILLS

If phytonutrients can be so healthful, why not just take plant extract supplements rather than go to all the trouble of eating the plants themselves? Besides the misidentification, contamination, and adulteration issues rife within the poorly regulated supplement market[7058] we've discussed, there is a question of dose. Taking polyphenol supplements can result in blood levels nearly an order of magnitude higher than that of a polyphenol-rich diet.[7059] When it comes to hormesis, less may be more.

For a series of examples of how isolated phytochemicals and plant extracts can be life-extending at one dose but life-shortening at a higher one, check out see .nf/dosing. After all, many flavonoids function as "nature's pesticides," protecting plants from predators like us.[7060] We coevolved to counter these defenses, and thanks to hormesis, a smidgen of toxin can actually be beneficial, but a profusion of toxin can be toxic. To paraphrase a quote from a review on the anti-aging effects of polyphenols: It's easier to overdose on supplements than on salad.[7061]

SYNERGY WITHIN PLANTS

Some phytonutrients are so potent that functional doses can be encapsulated in a capsule, allowing for placebo-controlled trials of whole foods. For example, the sesame seed phytonutrient sesamin extends the lives of *C. elegans*[7062] and fruit flies.[7063] To see if it might have clinical effects, researchers pitted 2.5 g a day of ground black sesame seeds stuffed into capsules against placebo. Within one month, less than a teaspoon of sesame seeds a day drove down systolic blood pressures by eight points in middle-aged men and women. If sustained, that alone would decrease the risk of stroke by more than 25 percent.[7064]

The downside of whole-food studies is you're never quite certain which component—or components—may be responsible. Was it the sesamin or other sesame phytonutrients, such as sesamol, sesamolin,[7065] or anthrasesamones A, B, C, D, E, or F?[7066] In a certain sense, who knows, but who cares, as long as it works. It's hard to patent produce, which is perishable and relatively unprofitable, so Big Pharma and supplement companies (which are often one and the same) use a reductionist approach to try to uncover the "magic bullet" active ingredient(s) of foods. But this ignores the concept of synergy. Sometimes, the whole food is greater than the sum of its parts.

For example, check out what happens when you pit various fractions of pomegranate polyphenols against prostate cancer cells in vitro. One subfraction reduced cancer cell growth by 30 percent compared to control, and another subfraction didn't help at all; the cancer grew as if it wasn't even there. So, mixing both together, you might expect the effect to land somewhere between the two, maybe 15 percent inhibition with the ineffectual fraction washing out the better one? But, no. Put them together, and you get *70 percent* lower cancer growth.[7067] Thirty percent + 0 percent = 70 percent. That's synergy, where 1 + 1 is greater than 2. A pomegranate extract supplement that includes only one of the fractions would miss out on most or all of the benefit.

When cranberry fractions were pitted against colon cancer cells, the discrepancy was even more extreme.[7068] Separately, two polyphenol fractions only suppressed cancer cell growth by 15 percent at most, but, when they were combined into the total polyphenol complement of cranberries, colon cancer growth was suppressed by as much as 90 percent. Similar synergistic effects against human cancer cells in vitro have been found in components of ginger root,[7069] grape skins,[7070] rosemary leaf,[7071] and tomatoes.

In see.nf/tomatosynergy, I give a remarkable account of synergy in action. Basically, supplements of the red tomato pigment lycopene have repeatedly failed to successfully prevent[7072] or treat[7073] prostate cancer, but tomato sauce seemed to help.[7074] This makes sense, given studies showing how tomato components that are noneffective[7075] or worse[7076] *individually* can suddenly show anticancer effects when combined. For phytonutrients, plants are better than pills. To quote a past president of the American College of Lifestyle Medicine, "The active ingredient in broccoli is broccoli."[7077]

SYNERGY BETWEEN PLANTS

Each plant not only has thousands of different phytonutrients, but very different phytonutrient profiles.[7078] So, there may be synergistic effects when eating different foods together, too.[7079] The reason it's better to get vitamin C in citrus form than pill form is that you won't miss out on all those citrus phytonutrients, like lemonin, limonol, or tangeretin, that may interact, work together, and complement one another. But you'd also miss out on them if you instead ate an apple. Comparing apples and oranges is like, well, comparing apples and oranges.

At least all fruits are fruits, whereas vegetables can be any other part of the plant. Roots harbor different phytonutrients than shoots. Carrots are roots, celery is a stem, dark green leafies are leaves, peas are pods, and cauliflower is true to its name, a collection of flower buds. Combining foods across different categories appears to increase the likelihood of synergy.[7080] The combined antioxidant power of raspberries and adzuki beans together, for example, is greater than just the sum of one plus the other. Neither soy phytonutrients nor green or black tea components alone decreased the tumor load or metastasis of human prostate cancer implants in mice, but soy and tea together did.[7081] Hot pepper extracts alone appeared to have little effect on the growth of cervical or breast cancer cells, but mixed with green tea, the cancer killer power rose tenfold in the case of cervical cancer and a hundredfold for breast cancer over green tea alone.[7082]

These are interesting proof-of-principle studies, but they have limited human relevance if the cancer-stopping concentrations used in the petri dishes couldn't be achieved in the bloodstream through normal dietary consumption. To resolve this issue, researchers exposed breast cancer cells from different patients to six different plant compounds individually, then all together at the level you might find in your bloodstream after eating foods like broccoli, grapes, soybeans, and turmeric. While individual plant compounds had little or no effect on their own, in combination, dietary blood levels significantly suppressed breast cancer cell proliferation by more than 80 percent, inhibited cancer cell migration and invasion, stopped the cancer cells in their tracks, and eventually killed them all off. All the while, this "phytochemical super-cocktail" had no deleterious effects on the normal, noncancerous cells used as control.[7083]

A 10 percent tomato diet reduced the prostate cancer tumor burden of rats by 33 percent, and a 10 percent broccoli diet reduced the amount of tumors by 42 percent.[7084] Put them together, though, and a diet enhanced with both tomato and broccoli cut tumor levels by more than half. A spouse wrote to the editor of the *Harvard Men's Health Watch*, saying their husband, having heard about lycopene, wants to have pizza for his prostate but they don't think it's a healthy food. The doctor replied with the suggestion of a "cheese-free pizza (with broccoli instead of pepperoni, please)."[7085]

GARDEN VARIETY

Though there are generic plant compounds like vitamin C that are found scattered throughout the plant kingdom, there are also specific phytonutrients produced by specific plants to perform specific functions—both in their organs and in ours.[7086] We miss out on these if we're stuck in a fruit and vegetable rut, even if we're eating many servings a day.

Airline pilots experience high rates of DNA damage due to being bombarded with radiation from the galaxy without the protection of the full atmosphere. A study found that pilots eating a greater mixture of phytonutrients had less chromosomal damage, but the researchers didn't control for total fruit and vegetable intake.[7087] Maybe the greater variety was just a proxy for greater quantity. Those randomized to eat fourteen servings of fruits and vegetables a day for even just two weeks show a reduction in oxidative DNA damage compared to those randomized to eat only four servings a day,[7088] but what about a study in which the number of servings is held constant and you just increase the diversity of the produce? That's exactly what a group of researchers in Colorado did.

Both diets had the same number of daily servings (eight to ten), but the high botanical diversity diet included fruits and vegetables from eighteen different families versus emphasizing just five in the low diversity diet. Only those randomized to the high diversity diet experienced a significant reduction in DNA damage.[7089] The researchers concluded that "smaller amounts of many phytochemicals may have greater potential to exert beneficial effects than larger amounts of fewer phytochemicals." Observational studies have also found that fruit and vegetable variety is associated with lower inflammation[7090] and better cognition[7091]—again, independent of quantity. Does this mixing and matching of a variety of plant foods actually translate into a concrete difference for patients?

Check out see.nf/foodcombining for a wild experiment involving secretly giving cancer patients a combination of a fruit, a vegetable, a spice, and a leaf—about one one-hundredth of a pomegranate, less than one floret of broccoli, less than an eighth of a teaspoon of turmeric, and about a sixth of a tea bag's worth of green tea a day, hidden in capsules and randomized against placebo. Surely such tiny amounts couldn't affect the progression of cancer, right? Wrong.[7092] As I show in the video, the cancer was significantly slowed down.

Based on an update of the most extensive report on diet and cancer ever published, the foundation of cancer prevention is a diet centered around plants—whole grains, vegetables, fruits, and beans—while cutting down on alcohol, soda, meat, and processed junk.[7093] As I documented in How Not to Die, a completely plant-based diet may even shrink the tumor, not just slow down its growth, but there's no reason we can't do both with a plant-based diet chock full of particularly powerful plants.[7094]

microRNAS

If you thought the interspecies communication between the plant and animal kingdoms with xenohormesis was interesting, hold on to your hat. The "Central Dogma" of molecular biology has been challenged by a revolutionary twenty-first-century discovery: microRNAs.[7095]

Allow me to transport you back to high school biology. If you remember, our genetic code is stored in our DNA. Those are the instructions for creating and maintaining our body. There's no point in just having a set of blueprints if they can't be communicated to the builders to become manifest in the real world. RNA is that messenger. Messenger RNA transcribes a stretch of DNA code (called a gene) and has it translated into the finished product, a structural protein or an enzyme. The Central Dogma describes this flow of information as one gene to one messenger RNA to one protein. Then along came a shocking discovery from the Human Genome Project.

Only about 2 percent of our DNA actually codes for proteins. So, what does the other 98 percent do? When I was in medical school, the more than one billion letters of seemingly purposeless DNA[7096] were dismissed as "noise," "garbage sequences,"[7097] or "junk DNA," perhaps just accumulated genetic schmutz from throughout our evolutionary past.[7098] That would seem a little wasteful, though. A parallel from astrophysics was drawn to this mystery: dark matter,[7099] the apparent fact that we can't account for about 85 percent of the matter in the universe.[7100] The mystery of the dark matter of our genome was solved in 2001:[7101] Most of our DNA violates the Central Dogma by being actively transcribed into *noncoding* RNA—that is, RNA that doesn't code for proteins.[7102] Then what does it do?

We now know that there are more than a hundred types of noncoding RNAs, but let's focus on the OG: microRNA.[7103] It takes a stretch of DNA thousands of letters long to encode the average messenger RNA.[7104] In contrast, microRNAs are only about twenty letters long. For example, the first microRNA ever discovered was twenty-two letters long in the four-letter RNA alphabet: UUCCCUGAGAC-CUCAAGUGUGA.[7105] What exactly do microRNAs do? They are generally created to glom on to messenger RNAs to prevent them from being translated into proteins.[7106]

If DNA is the blueprint and messenger RNAs are the construction workers translating those instructions into building parts of a house, microRNAs are like regulatory bureaucrats who intercede and keep particular workers from carrying out their duty. This is a good thing. Without building inspectors, minimum safety standards could be flouted. And different elements need to be timed properly. It makes sense to hold off the roofers until well after the foundation is poured.

Understanding microRNA regulation is particularly insightful[7107] because a single microRNA can block more than a thousand different messenger RNAs.[7108] So, one microRNA can effectively silence more than a thousand different genes. In my building analogy, one simple instruction can put all the second-floor workers on hold until the first-floor workers finish construction. Then, there are regulators who regulate the regulators, other noncoding RNAs that stop the microRNAs from stopping the messenger RNAs,[7109] but let's not even go there.

Just when the complexity seemed overwhelming, researchers realized that even though there are a trillion possible microRNA twenty-letters-long combinations made from the four-letter RNA alphabet, only a few thousand microRNAs seem to be active in the human body.[7110] And, in any given cell, the five most abundant microRNAs average half the overall microRNA pool in the cell.[7111] However, in 2007 things got a lot more interesting.

MicroRNAs have been found circulating in at least twelve different human bodily fluids.[7112] (When I read that, I had to stop and think, *Wait. Can I even name a dozen bodily fluids?*) We didn't think this possible since we have enzymes that chop up any floating RNA outside our cells (as a precaution against viruses, which often come bearing RNA). It turns out they're being transported in *exosomes*, tiny bubble-like vessels that pinch off from cells. We used to think these budding blebs were just a waste disposal device for the cells.[7113] (Why do scientists seem to just jump to junk when they don't understand something?) But, in 2007, we discovered that they were packed with microRNA.[7114] Our cells were communicating with each other! In this way, a liver cell could send out microRNAs to regulate the genes in a lung cell, which could then regulate a brain cell, or vice versa. They could even talk to the next generation by depositing their microRNA load into a sperm or egg cell.[7115]

What's the upshot of all this? It is now safe to say that microRNAs probably regulate virtually every biological process, playing essential roles in virtually every aspect of health.[7116] Mice genetically engineered to be unable to make microRNAs never even make it past the embryo stage.[7117] Diseases of all shapes and sizes have been linked to the dysregulation of microRNAs.[7118] But the good news is that there is something we can do about it. MicroRNA expression can be modified through diet.[7119]

microRNAS AND AGING

What does this have to do with aging? As a major regulator of all cellular pathways,[7120] it would make sense for microRNAs to play a role, but the connection has special salience. The very first microRNA was discovered in the humble roundworm *C. elegans*.[7121] Guess what it did? Regulated its lifespan. Reducing the activity of the simple microRNA reduces lifespan and accelerates tissue aging, whereas overexpressing it significantly extends life. It turns out that the target of the microRNA was a DAF-16 suppressor gene.[7122] DAF-16 is the worm equivalent of the FOXO gene, which can confer immortality to certain primitive animals[7123] and is one of the most important genetic determinants of extreme longevity in humans.[7124] By blocking the repression of this longevity gene, the microRNA had a lifespan-extending effect. Knowing the expression patterns of just a few micro-RNAs in *C. elegans* can effectively predict the longevity of individual animals.[7125]

To study the effects of microRNAs on mammalian lifespan, a series of lifestyle interventions were set up in mice. One group of mice was put on a high-fat diet, and they lived for 101 weeks. A second group was put on a high-fat diet with added voluntary exercise, and they lived for 114 weeks. The next group was put on a low-fat diet, which brought them up to 127 weeks. A fourth group was put on a low-fat diet plus exercise and lived for 131 weeks. Group five was put on caloric restriction on a high-fat diet and lived for 137 weeks. And, finally, mice were put on caloric restriction on a low-fat diet and lived for 153 weeks, a lifespan more than 50 percent longer than those in the regular high-fat group. Using this approach, the researchers found that ninety-two microRNAs were correlated with lifespan, including eighty-four in an inverse manner. In other words, the microRNAs generally appeared to be suppressing longevity genes, so certain microRNA levels were up to 90 percent lower in the longest-living group.[7126] However, there are exceptions.

For example, miR-17 (short for microRNA-17) directly extends the lifespans of mice. Transgenic mice created to overexpress miR-17 live longer and healthier lives, proving that microRNA isn't just correlated with a longer life but directly causes it (in part by repressing mTOR, which I explored starting on page 101).[7127] Such "longevi-miRNAs" may account for the parabiosis findings.[7128] Remember the mad scientist experiments (see page 40) of rejuvenating old animals by sewing them to younger cagemates and hooking together their circulations? That effectively proved that there are blood-borne determinants of aging. Perhaps microRNAs fit the bill.

In humans, dozens of circulating microRNAs are upregulated as we age, and dozens are downregulated.[7129] The blood levels of seven microRNAs may be able to differentiate Alzheimer's patients from healthy controls with up to 95 percent accuracy.[7130] If these dynamics are all just genetic, then microRNA levels could still be useful as biomarkers or diagnostics, but they might be harder to tweak to control our fate. But, no, a study on identical twins who died about a decade apart found they had highly discordant microRNA levels, suggesting that nongenetic factors, such as diet and lifestyle, are pivotal in microRNAs related to life expectancy.[7131]

EXERCISE POWER OVER microRNAS?

More than 6,000 patents have been filed on the potential use of synthetic microRNA mimics and inhibitors to fight aging and disease,[7132] but, to date, no such drugs have been approved.[7133] Is there anything we can do naturally?

MicroRNAs may be one of the reasons randomized controlled trials have shown that exercise can prevent cognitive decline in older adults[7134] and improve cognition for those already suffering from Alzheimer's disease.[7135] There are microRNAs that are reduced in Alzheimer's (like miR-132[7136] and miR-338[7137]) but boosted by exercise,[7138,7139] and, conversely, there are microRNAs that are overexpressed in Alzheimer's (like miR-7[7140] and miR-766[7141]) but reduced by exercise.[7142,7143] The picture isn't completely clear, though. MiR-146a has consistently been found to be elevated in the blood,[7144] brain,[7145] and cerebrospinal fluid[7146] of Alzheimer's disease patients. And, although acute resistance training[7147] and chronic basketball training[7148] were found to reduce circulating levels of the microRNA, rowing training[7149] and marathon running[7150] were found to increase them. So, we still have much to tease out about the possible role that microRNAs play in the way physical activity can improve mental activity.[7151]

MODULATING microRNAS WITH MEALS

MicroRNAs may also be a mediator of the benefits of polyphenols.[7152] A dozen different phytonutrients have been shown to change the expression of dozens of microRNAs in vitro.[7153] As we know, one problem with petri dish studies is that sometimes concentrations are used that far exceed that which can be achieved through regular dietary consumption, but a few foods have been put to the test. For example, a study showing that extra-virgin olive oil with a high polyphenol content has a different microRNA impact than lower-polyphenol olive oil suggests that the polyphenols may be playing an active role.[7154] Nuts—either one to two handfuls of walnuts a day for a year[7155] or a single handful of a combination of almonds and walnuts for eight weeks—also change the levels of an array of microRNAs in the bloodstream.[7156] But to what end?

There are well-known inflammiRs, inflammatory microRNAs like miR-155, that are suppressed by a variety of flavonoids—genistein in soy, quercetin in apples and onions, allyl isothiocyanate in onion family vegetables, curcumin in turmeric, and apigenin in parsley, celery, and chamomile tea.[7157] MiR-155 also plays a role in cancer. For example, miR-155 is implicated in the development of acute myeloid lymphoma, the deadliest form of leukemia and the most common acute leukemia among adults. In a study titled "Alleviating the Progression of Acute Myeloid Leukemia (AML) by Sulforaphane Through Controlling miR-155 Levels," not only could miR-155 levels be dropped by about 80 percent by the cruciferous vegetable compound in vitro, but this led to a significant drop in cancer cell viability.[7158] Unfortunately, broccoli sprouts, the most concentrated source of sulforaphane, have yet to be tested on AML patients to assess clinical outcomes.

Flavonoids have been found to suppress the proliferation of tumor cells by both suppressing oncogenic (cancer-causing) microRNAs and boosting tumor suppressor microRNAs.[7159] Long-term soy consumption in breast cancer patients had this effect,[7160] perhaps helping to explain why soy consumption appears to help prevent the development of breast cancer in pre- and postmenopausal women,[7161] as well as improve survival in breast cancer patients and reduce the chances of the cancer coming back.[7162] This may also help explain the upregulation of tumor suppression microRNAs in vegetarians and vegans compared to omnivores,[7163] and the subsequent lower cancer risk,[7164] though meat consumption can affect microRNAs, too.

Rectal biopsies taken before and after a month of eating three daily servings of beef or lamb found significant upregulation of oncogenic microRNA clusters in rectal tissue. Adding resistant starch to the diet was able to reduce, but not completely eliminate, this effect.[7165] Similarly, the cooked meat carcinogen PhIP, found particularly in grilled, broiled, fried, and barbecued chicken, causes estrogen-like effects on microRNAs implicated in the initiation and progression of breast cancer.[7166] MicroRNA modulation has also been used to explain why saturated fat increases insulin resistance, though, so far, this has only been demonstrated in rat muscle.[7167]

Beyond potentially contributing to the lower cancer[7168] and diabetes[7169] rates among those eating plant-based, diet-induced microRNA changes may also contribute directly to life extension. A study on circulating microRNA expression in the Loma Linda blue zone, where healthy Adventist vegetarians live about a decade longer than their fellow Californians, found half a dozen microRNAs related to aging differentially expressed between vegetarians and nonvegetarians that potentially provide mechanisms for the longer plant-based life expectancy. Interestingly, for one of the anti-aging measures, semi-vegetarians and vegans both beat out ovo-lacto vegetarians, those who eschew meat but eat eggs and dairy. Semi-vegetarians were defined as eating meat at least once a month, but no more than once a week. The researchers suggest that they might have ended up eating fewer animal products overall than the vegetarians who more regularly ate eggs and dairy.[7170]

XENO-microRNAS

Intercellular microRNA communication is conserved throughout the evolutionary tree of life, raising the possibility of cross-kingdom gene regulation. In the eighteenth century, life was classified as belonging to either the plant kingdom or the animal kingdom.[7171] In the nineteenth century, single-celled organisms like amoebas got their own kingdom,[7172] and with further improvements in microscopy, bacteria got one as well. (These days we're up to seven kingdoms—algae and fungi each got their own, as did bacteria-like organisms originally described as extremophiles, living in previously thought uninhabitable zones like hot springs.[7173])

With a common language of microRNAs, might inhabitants of different kingdoms communicate with one another? In 2011, we learned that microbiome microRNAs could modulate the gene expression of their host.[7174] For example, there are gum disease bacteria that secrete vesicles filled with microRNA shown to penetrate host cells, apparently to suppress our immune response.[7175] Sneaky! Then, in 2016, we learned that we have our own microRNA counterinsurgency program. Fecal microRNAs produced by our intestinal lining cells infiltrate our gut bacteria, regulate their gene expression and growth, and may be essential for the maintenance of a healthy microbiome.[7176] If there is microRNA manipulation happening between the simplest and most complex organisms on Earth, what about cross-talk with an intermediate—the plant kingdom?

The nerd's cartoonist, Randall Munroe at xkcd.com, used a comic captioned "Really, *every* gathering is a family reunion" to remind us that ultimately, we're all related. If you go far enough back, each of us can trace back to a common ancestor, all the way back to the very first *Homo sapiens* to whom we're all related. So, the cartoon shows a party scene with stick figures labeled "me," "2nd cousin," "14th cousin," and "35th cousin," and also a pet cat, labeled "17,000,000th cousin." Yes, if you go back far enough, you and Fluffy actually had a real flesh-and-blood common ancestor. The cartoon also has a houseplant labeled "50,000,000,000th cousin."[7177] Using molecular clock–dating techniques on shared DNA deviation, it's estimated that plants and animals diverged 1.576 billion years ago, give or take 88 million years.[7178] So, even you, Fluffy, and the ficus shared an ancestor. Family reunion indeed.

Recognition of the ubiquitous presence and activity of microRNAs in plants followed soon after their discovery in animals.[7179] Cotton plants, for example, use microRNAs to silence the virulence genes of a pathogenic fungus.[7180] What influence might plant microRNAs be having in another cross-kingdom interaction—with us? Just like we share many microRNAs with other animals, some microRNA sequences in plants have such close overlap with animal microRNAs that scientists suspect they're actually the same microRNA, conserved through 1.5 billion years of evolution.[7181] Regardless, matching up the sequences of plant microRNA to human messenger RNA, there appear to be at least a thousand different human genes that plant microRNAs could target.[7182]

Plant-based diets contain thousands of biologically active microRNAs.[7183] While the scientific community has historically chalked up the benefits of fruits, vegetables, and herbal medicines to the presence of phytonutrients, it may be their microRNAs playing a role.[7184] Isolated phytonutrients have often failed to fully replicate the effects of the whole foods from which they were extracted. This failure has been attributed to the synergistic symphony of interactions between the various components working together. As we've seen, one way that phytonutrients like polyphenols affect our physiology is by manipulating our microRNA expression, but perhaps plant microRNAs are silencing our genes directly.[7185]

The exploration of the potential for cross-kingdom gene regulation with "xeno-microRNAs"[7186] from plants is currently considered among the most exciting topics in all of science.[7187] Broadly, the concept of cross-kingdom genetic manipulation is nothing new. After all, RNA and DNA from viruses have been hijacking human cells since time immemorial. But, if food-derived microRNAs are altering our gene expression, that certainly offers new meaning to the phrase "you are what you eat."[7188]

DIETARY microRNAS

Dietary microRNAs would mean that food may provide information as well as nutrition—information that could effectively switch our genes on or off.[7189] Some researchers have conceptualized dietary microRNAs as "dark nutrients," in another nod to dark matter, claiming that they play a "significant role in human health."[7190] Yes, plant microRNAs have been shown to enter human cells and alter our gene expression,[7191] but let's take a step back. Would microRNAs in our diet even survive cooking or digestion?

Some processed plant products, such as olive oil and beer, seem to have lost their microRNAs in the production process.[7192] What about microRNA loss on the stove? We used to think cooking destroyed genetic material, but more recent experiments show that some plant microRNAs can take the heat.[7193] Some, such as miR-159 in broccoli, remain stable after cooking,[7194] while those like artichoke microRNA-319 are partially destroyed.[7195] And the levels of other microRNAs, like those found in cooked beans and brown rice, rise even higher after cooking, presumably by being liberated into the cooking water.[7196] Mammalian and avian microRNAs in meat, dairy, and eggs survive cooking and processing, based on studies of pork and poultry sausages,[7197] ham,[7198] salami, hard-boiled eggs, cheese, and pasteurized milk. There was little change in microRNA levels between raw beef and beef roasted until well done;[7199] however, they would still have to survive the acid bath of the stomach.

Again, the conventional wisdom was that microRNAs would be destroyed during digestion,[7200] but if you dunk them in acidic gastric fluid, the majority of plant and microRNAs appear to survive for at least six hours.[7201] In the small intestine, though, there are RNases, enzymes that chew up naked RNA. How might they survive that gauntlet? They may not have to. A study in mice found that the stomach itself appears to be the primary site of dietary microRNA absorption into the bloodstream.[7202] Alternately, microRNAs may travel wrapped in protective exosomes.

From plants, exosome-like vesicles have become known as "edible nanoparticles," and they can be filled with microRNAs.[7203] A pound of fruit can contain 1 g of these little delivery vehicles.[7204] This packaging has been proposed as a solution to the microRNA bioavailability problem.[7205] In that form, they could be absorbed by our intestinal lining, repackaged into exosomes, then released into our circulation.[7206] The proof is in the pudding, though. When we eat microRNAs, do they show up in our bloodstream?

Unlike typical animal microRNAs, the tips of plant microRNAs are tagged with a methyl group.[7207] (See page 46.) This not only makes them more resistant to digestion but it allows researchers to differentiate them from preexisting microRNAs circulating in animals.[7208] Feed mice some cruciferous vegetables, and cruciferous vegetable microRNAs peak in their bloodstream within six hours and can be picked up in multiple organs.[7209] Corn microRNAs peak in the bloodstream of pigs fed fresh corn between six and twelve hours after consumption.[7210] Most plant microRNAs are carried in exosomes,[7211] which can even transport RNA into the brain.[7212] The cruciferous microRNAs were found circulating for more than thirty-six hours.[7213] What about in people?

Researchers found that as many as 5 percent of all detectable microRNAs circulating in people's bodies may be from plants. The first report of plant microRNAs circulating in humans was published in 2012, the consistent finding of rice microRNAs in bloodstreams of Chinese consumers.[7214] Just as fish-eating seals have circulating fish microRNAs and cows have plant microRNAs from foraged crops and grasses, most of the plant microRNAs in us are from fruit and vegetable species.[7215] Plant microRNAs have been found throughout the human body, including the brain, breasts, kidneys, liver, and lungs, as well as in breast milk, amniotic fluid, and umbilical cord blood.[7216] Are these just incidental findings, or are dietary microRNAs doing anything to us or for us?

FRUIT AND VEGETABLE microRNAS

Hundreds of different microRNAs have been found in the edible nanoparticles of common fruits and vegetables.[7217] In a proof-of-principle study, edible nanoparticles from grapes were fed to mice. They were taken up into intestinal cells, changed gene expression, and protected the mice from gut inflammation.[7218] Similar experiments with carrot, ginger, and grapefruit nanoparticles found a range of beneficial regulatory effects, but how do we know it was necessarily the microRNAs?[7219]

MicroRNAs are such simple molecules that we can make them from scratch. So, researchers synthetically made strawberry microRNA-156, rice microRNA-168, and cabbage microRNA-874 to isolate out microRNA-specific effects. And, indeed, they were found to have anti-inflammatory effects on human cells. RNA extracts of blueberries, raspberries, and apple peels had a similar effect. To make sure this was not a generic RNA effect, an RNA extract from beef was tested and it failed to dampen inflammation.[7220]

One plant microRNA found circulating in people is microRNA-156a. Decreased levels were found in the blood and blood vessels of patients with cardiovascular disease, suggesting it might have a protective effect. But where is microRNA-156a concentrated? In green vegetables. Give people a salad, and you can see a bump in 156a within an hour. Might lower levels of 156a in heart disease patients just be a proxy for low levels of greens intake? To find out if it was actually cause and effect, researchers exposed human artery endothelial cells to pure (synthesized) microRNA-156a and showed that it targets a sticky protein called *junctional adhesion molecule-A* that abets in the attraction of inflammatory immune cells into the artery wall to trigger atherosclerotic plaques. And indeed, boosting microRNA-156a reduced the attachment of inflammatory cells to artery lining cells.[7221] So, the protective effect of green vegetables on cardiovascular disease[7222] may be more than just a nitrate effect.

A similar story was found with breast cancer and microRNA-159a, which is found in abundance in broccoli.[7223] Lower blood levels correlated with higher breast cancer incidence and tumor progression. MicroRNA-159a wasn't just a broccoli biomarker, though, but an active player, targeting a cancer-promoting gene called transcription factor 7. When mice implanted with human breast tumors were fed straight microRNA-159a, they experienced a dramatic decrease in tumor weight and growth. So, the protective effects of cruciferous vegetables on breast cancer[7224] may be more than just a sulforaphane effect.

HERBAL microRNAS

Might some of the effects of herbal medicines also be ascribed to plant microRNAs? In see.nf/herbalmirnas, I review the evidence on microRNAs in ginseng,[7225] licorice,[7226] red sage (*danshen*),[7227,7228] and another traditional Chinese herb, honeysuckle, which appeared to have remarkable efficacy in hospitalized COVID patients.[7229] Unfortunately, as I explain in the video, like so many impromptu pandemic trials, the study left a lot to be desired. The bottom line is that microRNAs may shed some light on how plants can be so powerful (including why some poisonous plants are so poisonous![7230]).

APPLE OF DISCORD

The concept that dietary miRNAs could be therapeutic has been called "compelling, fresh, and revolutionary."[7231] However, the first reports were met with suitable skepticism,[7232] which have since evolved into a fierce controversy.[7233] Many subsequent attempts at replication failed to unambiguously confirm the initial findings,[7234] leaving the medical literature littered with editorials with titles like "Diet-Derived MicroRNAs: Unicorn or Silver Bullet?"[7235] and "Dietary Non-Coding RNAs from Plants: Fairy Tale or Treasure?"[7236] I run through the tug-of-war controversy in see .nf/discord. Though it continues to be an exciting area, the biological role of dietary plant microRNAs remains far from being firmly established.[7237]

EATING ANIMAL microRNAS

What about eating or drinking animal microRNAs present in meat, milk, and eggs?[7238] Animal-derived microRNAs can sometimes be absorbed in much more significant amounts than plant microRNAs.[7239] The problem is it's much more difficult experimentally to distinguish between dietary animal microRNAs and the ones our own animal body makes, since they can be nearly or completely identical.[7240]

One way researchers have tried to solve this conundrum is to genetically engineer "knockout" mice, in which the gene for a particular microRNA is "knocked out," inactivated or deleted. For example, researchers made microRNA-451 knockout mice drink the blood of wild mice, chickens, and pigs. When they then found microRNA-451 circulating in their bloodstreams and carrying out its regulatory function, they knew that ingested animal microRNAs could indeed affect physiology.[7241]

Vampiric mice aside, how could confirmatory experiments be carried out in people? This is an important question since there are a number of pro-inflammaging and cancer-promoting microRNAs in animal products that are a 100 percent match with the same microRNAs in humans.[7242] Even if you couldn't differentiate meat microRNA from me microRNA, you could at least test to see if you get a rise in blood levels after consumption. Tracking three shared cow microRNAs in people after eating beef failed to show a bloodstream bump,[7243] though, if you remember, that rectal biopsy study did at least show microRNA changes down in the colon after red meat consumption.[7244] Chicken microRNAs from egg consumption, however, can be detected in the human bloodstream after intake.

In the USDA-funded study published as "MicroRNAs in Chicken Eggs Are Bioavailable in Healthy Adults and Can Modulate mRNA Expression in Peripheral Blood Mononuclear Cells," volunteers were fed hard-boiled eggs. Within nine hours, blood levels of microRNA-181a and microRNA-181b rose to about 150 percent and 300 percent above baseline, respectively, reflecting their relative abundance in eggs. This was accompanied by a suppression of the validated gene target of miR-181b in their white blood cells. To verify that chicken microRNAs actually make it into the human bloodstream after egg consumption and don't just indirectly bump up endogenous microRNA levels, the researchers were able to track the entry of a chicken-specific microRNA into their circulation.[7245]

DRINKING ANIMAL microRNAS

The greatest evidence for the potential for cross-kingdom gene regulation comes from the dairy literature. Of all body fluids tested, milk contains the largest load of microRNAs.[7246] Milk is a secretory product of mammary gland epithelial cells, which discharge miRNA-packed exosomes into the milk.[7247] Based on the human breast milk literature, most are immune-modulatory,[7248] especially during the first six months of lactation.[7249] We've long known that breast milk contains antibodies and other protective agents missing from baby formula to provide passive immunity and help with immune system development, but microRNAs may add additional urgency to the entreaty that breast is best.[7250]

Babies aren't just breastfed but breast-programmed.[7251] Milk is no longer perceived just as food for infants but rather as a highly sophisticated communication system orchestrating early development.[7252] For example, we've known for more than a decade that something in milk prevents allergies. Rat milk, but not rat formula, prevents allergies in rat pups.[7253] MicroRNAs may help explain why breast-feeding seems to protect against childhood asthma[7254] and pediatric infections and results in higher intelligence compared to formula feeding.[7255] If milk microRNAs can so manipulate an infant's physiology, what happens if we drink milk after weaning as an adult, or even drink milk from another species?

The milk of pandas and pigs, humans, and cows and water buffalo share a few common highly expressed microRNAs,[7256] but cow's milk also contains large quantities of hundreds more,[7257] as many as 1,500 different microRNAs.[7258] Because most milk microRNAs are encapsulated in exosomes, they are resistant to heat. While most exosomes and their cargo are destroyed by boiling or ultra-high-temperature processing (used to make shelf-stable creamers), commercial pasteurization leaves a significant proportion of milk microRNAs intact.[7259] Most then survive conditions of digestion in adults.[7260]

To prove that milk microRNAs from one species can make it into the circulation of another species who drinks it, milk microRNAs were tagged with a fluorescent label as a tracker. Loaded into cow's milk, the microRNAs ended up distributing and accumulating in the spleens, livers, hearts, and brains of mice. In vitro, human cells take them up and have multiple genes upregulated and downregulated as a result.[7261] Of course, mice suckling from cows is ludicrous. Primates, on the other hand . . .

MADE FOR EACH UDDER

Government-funded researchers at the University of Nebraska had men and women drink different quantities of dairy milk—one, two, or four cups. Considerable amounts of milk microRNAs appeared in their blood in a dose-dependent manner, peaking within four hours after consumption and affecting target gene expression. The bovine microRNAs tested were identical to human microRNAs, though. How do we know that drinking milk doesn't somehow boost the endogenous production of our own microRNAs instead of crossing over from the digestion tract into our bloodstream? The levels of a control microRNA not found in milk were unaffected,[7262] but more robust evidence came from subsequent studies using highly sensitive PCR techniques that could detect tiny differences between bovine and human microRNAs. And indeed, blood concentrations of bovine-specific microRNAs end up circulating throughout our body within hours of milk consumption,[7263] providing compelling evidence that dairy milk exosomes from commercial pasteurized milk right off store shelves can end up in the tissues of human consumers.[7264] What consequences may this have?

The most abundant microRNA in milk is microRNA-148a, and it's a key inhibitor of crucial suppressors to the engine-of-aging enzyme mTOR that I talked about in the Aging Pathways section.[7265] After all, what does an infant need more than accelerated aging? This may be even more apparent in dairy cows, whose newborns double their birthweight in forty days, more than four times faster than our infants.[7266] Cows have been selectively bred for lactation performance, which incidentally appears to have exaggerated microRNA-148a expression.[7267]

The species-specific growth stimulation programmed by milk microRNAs was meant to be confined to infancy. The concern is that continuous exposure to growth-promoting exosomes of pasteurized milk may confer substantial risk for the development of chronic diseases—from acne and obesity to diabetes and cancer.[7268] MicroRNA-148a, for instance, directly stimulates prostate cancer growth in vitro,[7269] which may help explain why dripping milk on human prostate cancer cells boosts their growth rate by more than 30 percent.[7270] Maybe that's why a systematic review of observational studies reported that an overwhelming majority of them—nineteen out of twenty—found a link between milk consumption and increased risk of developing prostate cancer.[7271] MicroRNA-21, one of the earliest identified cancer-promoting "oncomiRs,"[7272] is also a signature microRNA of dairy milk.[7273]

MicroRNAs may also help explain the difference in associated mortality between fresh milk and fermented milk in two large Swedish studies. Significant increases in mortality risk in men and women were associated with the consumption of fresh milk, but not soured milk.[7274] Bacteria fermentation of milk can lead to exosome and microRNA breakdown,[7275] though this did not appear to affect prostate cancer risk, which seemed to be elevated by both milk and yogurt consumption.[7276]

A recent review titled "Cow's Milk May Be Delivering Potentially Harmful Undetected Cargoes to Humans" suggested that dairy recommendations need to be reconsidered in light of the fact that an estimated thirty-five trillion bovine exosomes are floating around in each glass of milk.[7277] Given the role of exosomes in pasteurized milk to boost mTOR activity, some researchers have concluded that "milk exosomes should not reach the human food chain,"[7278] as milk "is not a suitable food for adults."[7279] In other words, milk is for babies.

PREBIOTICS AND POSTBIOTICS

The human colon may represent the most biodense ecosystem in the world.[7280] Though many may believe that our stool is primarily made up of undigested food, about 75 percent is pure bacteria[7281]—trillions and trillions, in fact, about half a trillion bacteria per teaspoon.[7282] As Neil deGrasse Tyson put it, "More bacteria live and work in one linear centimeter of your lower colon than all the humans who have ever lived."[7283]

Do we get anything from these trillions of tenants taking up residence in our colon, or are they just squatting? They pay rent by boosting our immune system, making vitamins for us, improving our digestion, and balancing our hormones. We house and feed them, and they maintain and protect their house, our body. Prebiotics are what feed good bacteria. Probiotics are the good bacteria themselves. And postbiotics are what our bacteria make.

Our gut bacteria are known as a "forgotten organ,"[7284] as metabolically active as our liver and weighing as much as one of our kidneys.[7285] They may control as many as one in ten metabolites in our bloodstream.[7286] Each one of us has about 23,000 genes,[7287] but our gut bacteria, collectively, have about three *million*.[7288] About half the cells in our body are not human.[7289] We are, in effect, a superorganism—a kind of "human-microbe hybrid."[7290]

What we eat plays the dominant role in determining our gut microbiome, based on studying stool samples from around the world, those who eat different habitual diets, and what comes out of fraternal versus identical twins.[7291] Change your diet, change your gut flora, within days or weeks, for good or for ill.

THE GOOD, THE BAD, AND THE BUGLY

Having coevolved with us and our ancestors for millions of years,[7292] the relationship we have with our gut flora is so tightly knit as to affect most of our physiological functions.[7293] Yet our microbiome is probably the most adaptable component of our body. Gut bugs like *Escherichia coli* (*E. coli*) can divide every twenty minutes.[7294]

The more than ten trillion bugs we churn out every day can therefore rapidly respond to changing life conditions.[7295] Every meal, we have the opportunity to nudge them in the right direction.

Thousands of years ago, Hippocrates is attributed as saying that all diseases begin in the gut[7296] or, more ominously, "death sits in the bowels."[7297] Of course, he also thought women were hysterical because of their "wandering uterus."[7298] ("Hysteria" comes from the Greek *husterikos* for "of the womb.") So much for ancient medical wisdom. The pendulum then swung to the point of incredulity when the medical community refused to accept the role of one gut bug, *Helicobacter pylori*, as the cause of stomach and intestinal ulcers.[7299] Out of frustration, one of the pioneers chugged a brew of the bugs from one of his ulcer patients to prove the point, before finally being vindicated with the Nobel Prize in 2005 for his discovery.[7300]

In some ways, the pendulum has swung back, with overstated causal claims about the microbiome's role in a wide range of disparate diseases that are casually bandied about.[7301] Perhaps the boldest such claim dates back more than a century to Élie Metchnikoff, who argued that senility and the disabilities of old age were caused by "putrefactive bacterial autotoxins" leaking from the colon. He was the first to emphasize the importance of the gut microbiome to aging.[7302] He attributed healthy aging to gut bacteria that fermented carbohydrates into beneficial metabolic end products like lactic acid and associated unhealthy aging with putrefaction, the process in which bacteria degrade protein into noxious metabolites as waste products.[7303]

There is no shortage throughout history of old-timey crackpots with quack medical theories, but Metchnikoff was no slouch. He was appointed Louis Pasteur's successor,[7304] coined the terms "gerontology"[7305] and "probiotics,"[7306] and won the Nobel Prize in medicine to become the founding "father of cellular immunology."[7307] More than a century later, some aspects of his theories on aging and the gut are now being vindicated.[7308]

YOUNG AT GUT

Full-term, vaginally delivered, breastfed babies are said to start out with the gold standard for a healthy microbiome, which then starts to diverge as we age.[7309] The microbiomes of children, adults, the elderly, and centenarians tend to cluster together,[7310] such that a "microbiomic clock" can be devised.[7311] Dozens of different classes of bacteria in our gut so reliably shift as we age[7312] that our age can be guessed based on a stool sample within about a six-year margin of error.[7313] If these changes turn out to play a causal role in the aging process, then, hypothetically, our future high-tech toilet may one day be able predict our lifespan as well.[7314]

The transition from adulthood into old age is accompanied by pronounced changes to the microbiome.[7315] Given large interpersonal differences, there is no "typical" microbiome of the elderly,[7316] but the trends are in the very direction Metchnikoff described: a shift from the fermentation of fiber to the putrefaction of protein.[7317] This deviation from good bugs to bad is accompanied by an increase in gut leakiness, the spillage of bacterial toxins into the bloodstream, and a cascade of inflammatory effects. This has led to the proposal that this microbiome shift is a "primary cause of aging-associated pathologies and consequent premature death of elderly people."[7318]

As profound a change in microbiome composition from early adulthood into old age, there's an even bigger divergence between the elderly and centenarians.[7319] When researchers analyzed centenarian poop, they found a maintenance of short-chain fatty acid production from fiber fermentation.[7320] For example, in the Bama County longevity region in the Guangxi province of China, fecal sample analyses found that centenarians were churning out more than twice as much butyrate as those in their eighties or nineties living in the same region. If you recall, butyrate is an anti-inflammatory short-chain fatty acid critical for the maintenance of gut barrier integrity. At the same time, there were significantly fewer products of putrefaction, such as ammonia and uremic toxins like p-cresol. The researchers concluded that an increase of dietary fiber intake may therefore be a path toward longevity.[7321] An abundance of fiber feeders also distinguished healthy individuals ninety years and older from unhealthy nonagenarians.[7322]

CENTENARIAN SCAT

Interestingly, the microbiomes of Chinese centenarians shared some common features with Italian centenarians, suggesting that there could be certain universal signatures of a longevity-promoting microbiome.[7323] For example, centenarians have up to about a fifteenfold increase in butyrate producers.[7324]

A study of dozens of semi-supercentenarians (those aged 105 to 109) found higher levels of health-associated bacteria, such as *Bifidobacteria* and *Akkermansia*.[7325] In vaginally delivered, breastfed infants, *Bifidobacteria* make up 90 percent of colon bacteria, but the level may slip down to less than 5 percent in adult colons and even less in the elderly and those with inflammatory bowel disease.[7326] But centenarians carry more of the good bacteria in their gut.[7327]

Bifidobacteria are often used as probiotics, but anti-aging properties may exist in their *postbiotics*. *Bifidobacteria* are one of the many bacteria that secrete "exopolysaccharides," a science-y word for slime.[7328] That's what dental plaque is, the biofilm created by bacteria on our teeth.[7329] Exopolysaccharides produced from a strain of *Bifidobacteria* isolated from centenarian poop were found to have anti-aging properties in mice, reducing the accumulation of age pigment in their brains and boosting the antioxidant capacity of their blood and livers.[7330]

Akkermansia muciniphila is named after the late Dutch microbiologist Antoon Akkermans[7331] and from Latin and Greek for "mucus-lover." The species is the dominant colonizer of the protective mucus layer in our gut that is secreted by our intestinal lining.[7332] Unfortunately, that mucus layer thins as we age,[7333] a problem exacerbated by low-fiber diets. When we eat a fiber-depleted diet, we starve our microbial selves. Our famished flora, the microbes in our gut, have to then compete for limited resources and may consume our own mucus barrier as an alternative energy source, thereby undermining our defenses.[7334,7335] Mucus erosion from bacterial overgrazing can be switched on and off on a day-to-day basis in mice supplanted with human microbiomes with fiber-rich and fiber-free diets.[7336] You can even show it in a petri dish. Researchers successfully re-created layers of human intestinal cells and showed that dripping fiber (from plantains and broccoli) onto the cells at dietary doses could "markedly reduce" the number of *E. coli* bacteria breaching the barrier.[7337] Aside from eating fiber-rich foods, *A. muciniphila* helps to directly restore the protective layer by stimulating mucus secretion.[7338]

A. muciniphila is a likely candidate for a healthy aging biomarker,[7339] as its abundance is enriched in centenarians[7340] and it is particularly scarce in elders suffering from frailty.[7341] A comparative study was undertaken of the microbiomes of people in their seventies and eighties experiencing "healthy" versus "non-healthy" aging, defined as the absence or presence of cancer, diabetes, or heart, lung, or brain disease. *Akkermansia*, the species most associated with healthier aging, were three times more abundant in the fecal samples of the healthy versus non-healthy aging cohort. Among centenarians, a drop in *A. muciniphila* is one of the microbiome changes that seems to occur about seven months before death, despite no apparent changes in the physical status, food intake, or appetite at the time.[7342] To prove a causal role in aging, researchers showed that feeding *A. muciniphila* to aging-accelerated mice significantly extended their lifespans.[7343]

CAUSE, CONSEQUENCE, OR CONFOUNDING?

A recurring recommendation from centenarian poop studies is the promotion of high-fiber diets,[7344,7345,7346] one of the most consistently cited pieces of lifestyle advice in general for extreme longevity and health.[7347] An alternative proposal is a fecal transplant, from a cocktail of centenarian stool. Both approaches assume a cause-and-effect relationship between fiber-fueled feces and long lives, but there remains much controversy over whether age-related microbiome changes are cause, consequence, or confounding.[7348]

Aging is accompanied by *dysbiosis*, an unhealthy imbalance of gut flora characterized by a loss of fiber-fed species.[7349] Rather than a changing microbiome contributing to the aging process, it's easier to imagine how aging could instead be contributing to a changing microbiome. Loss of taste, smell, and teeth with age could lead to decreased consumption of fiber-rich foods, replaced by salted, sweetened, easier-to-chew processed foods.[7350] The drop in the quantity and diversity of whole plant foods—the only naturally abundant source of fiber—could result in a dysbiosis[7351] that leads to early death and disability. Or, the decline in diet quality could directly dispose to disease, with the dysbiosis just an incidental marker of an unhealthy diet.

There are also ways aging can be connected to dysbiosis independent of diet. While the rates of antibiotic prescriptions in childhood and through middle age have dropped in recent years, prescription rates among the elderly have shot up.[7352] Even non-antibiotic pharmaceuticals can muck with our microbiome. A study pitting more than a thousand FDA-approved drugs against forty representative strains of gut bacteria found that 24 percent of marketed drugs inhibited the growth of at least one strain.[7353] Reduced physical activity could also contribute to sluggish, stagnant bowels that could leave our gut bugs no other choice but to turn to protein for putrefaction once preferred prebiotics are used up.[7354] Nursing home residents are often fed the kind of low-fiber diet that can contribute to the "decimation" of a healthy microbiome.[7355] So, while researchers have interpreted the link between dysbiosis and frailty as a poor diet leading to poor gut flora leading to poor health,[7356] the arrows of causality could potentially go in every which direction. Maybe there's even a chicken-or-the-egg feedback loop in play.[7357] With so many interrelated factors, you can imagine how hard it is to tease out the causal chain of events.

These questions crop up all the time in microbiome research. For example, the microbiomes of centenarians aren't just better at digesting fiber. They're better at detoxifying industrial pollutants, such as petrochemicals; food preservatives like benzoate and naphthalene, used in petroleum refinement; and haloalkanes, widely used commercially as flame retardants, refrigerants, propellants, and solvents. None of these detoxification pathways was found in the microbiomes of the Hadza, one of the last hunter-gatherer tribes in Africa.[7358] Did the enhanced detoxification in centenarian guts (compared to younger individuals) contribute to their longevity, or did their longevity contribute to their enhanced detoxification (given their longer lifetime exposure and accumulation of chemicals)?[7359]

The microbiomes of centenarians and semi-supercentenarians are better able to metabolize plant fats than animal fats, but maybe that's just due to their eating more plant-based diets.[7360] The Bama County longevity region centenarians who had such an abundance of fiber feeders were eating more than 70 percent more fiber (38 g versus only 22 g per 2,000 calories) compared to those aged eighty through ninety-nine living in the same region.[7361] The only way to know if their longer lives eating more healthfully just led to a better microbiome or if their better microbiome actually contributed to their living longer is to put it to the test.

FECAL TRANSPLANT EXPERIMENTS

Longevity researchers have good reason to suspect a causal, rather than bystander, role for age-related microbiome changes, given fecal transplant studies I detail in see.nf/transplant, showing that the lives of old animals can be extended by receiving gut bugs from younger animals.[7362] Centenarian stool has anti-aging effects when fed to mice. Researchers fed mice fecal matter from a 70-year-old individual that contained *Bilophila wadsworthia*,[7363] a pro-inflammatory bacteria enriched by a diet high in animal products,[7364] versus feces from a 101-year-old containing more fiber feeders. Mice transplanted with the centenarian microbiome ended up displaying a range of youthful physiological indicators, including less age pigment in their brains. This raises the possibility that we will one day be using centenarian fecal matter to promote healthy aging.[7365] Why bathe in the blood of virgins when you can dine on the dung of the venerable?

DYSBIOSIS

An unhealthy imbalance of gut bacteria can result from a deficiency of fiber or an excess of antibiotic exposure, salt, protein, and certain food additives.

PLUGGING LEAKS WITH FIBER

One of the mechanisms by which intestinal dysbiosis may accelerate aging is a leaky gut. Watch see.nf/leaky for details, but basically, across animal species, intestinal barrier integrity has been shown to decline with age.[7366] This can lead to tiny bits of undigested food, microbes, and toxins slipping through our gut lining and entering uninvited into our bloodstream, triggering chronic systemic inflammation.[7367] Thankfully, there's something we can do about it.

To avoid gut dysbiosis, inflammation, and leakiness, plants should be preferred. The reason vegetarians tend to have a better intestinal microbiome balance, a high bacterial biodiversity, and enhanced integrity of the intestinal barrier,[7368] and also produce markedly less uremic toxins in the gut,[7369] is likely that fiber is the primary food for a healthy gut microbiome.[7370] Cause and effect was established in a randomized, double-blind, crossover study of pasta with or without added fiber.[7371]

Other ways to heal a leaky gut, detailed in see.nf/sealthegut, is to stop alcohol consumption,[7372] avoid NSAIDs, like aspirin, ibuprofen, and naproxen,[7373] which can cause gastrointestinal lining damage within five minutes,[7374] and (from see.nf /leaky) get the amount of daily zinc found in about a cup of cooked lentils.[7375]

DYSBIOSIS INFLAMMATION IMMUNOSUPPRESSION

The most important role a healthy microbiome has for preserving health as we age is thought to be the prevention of systemic inflammation.[7376] Inflammaging is a strong risk factor not only for premature death.[7377] Those with higher-than-average levels of inflammatory markers in their blood for their age are more likely to be hospitalized,[7378] frail,[7379] and less independent,[7380] and suffer from a variety of diseases, including common infections.[7381]

In Japan, for example, more than 40 percent of all centenarian deaths are due to pneumonia and other infectious diseases.[7382] In one of the largest studies, involving nearly 36,000 British centenarians, pneumonia was the leading identifiable cause of death.[7383] Inflammaging has not only been shown to increase susceptibility to coming down with the leading cause of bacterial pneumonia[7384] but older adults with more inflammation also tend to suffer increased severity[7385] and decreased survival.[7386]

As we age, our immune system macrophages (from the Greek for "big eaters") start to lose their ability to engulf and destroy bacteria.[7387] The same happens in regular mice. But mice raised microbe-free don't suffer from the leaking gut, subsequent inflammation, and loss of macrophage function. To connect the dots between the inflammation and loss of function, researchers found that the macrophage impairment could be induced in microbe-free mice by infusing them with an inflammatory mediator, which, when dripped on macrophages in a petri dish, could directly interfere with their ability to kill pneumonia bacteria.[7388] Because our immune system is also responsible for cancer defense, immune dysfunction caused by the inflammation resulting from dysbiosis may also help explain why cancer incidence increases so steeply as we age (and why microbe-free mice have fewer tumors and live longer).[7389]

AVOIDING DIETARY ANTIBIOTICS

Other than getting enough fiber, what else can we do to prevent dysbiosis in the first place? There are a number of factors that contribute to microbiome imbalance. For example, on any given day, an average of about two and a half doses of antibiotics are consumed for every one hundred people in Western countries.[7390] The havoc this can play on our microbiome may explain why antibiotic use predicts an increased risk of cancer, though confounding factors, such as smoking, that are associated with both, could also potentially explain this link.[7391]

Up to three-quarters of antibiotic use is of questionable therapeutic value.[7392] Avoiding unnecessary use of antibiotics and using targeted, narrow-spectrum agents whenever possible can help protect our gut flora,[7393] but most people may not realize they're consuming antibiotic residues every day in the meat, dairy, and eggs they eat. As much as 80 percent of the antibiotics used in the United States doesn't go to treat sick people but rather is fed to farm animals[7394] in part as a crutch to compensate for the squalid conditions that now characterize much of modern agribusiness.[7395] But do enough antibiotics make it onto our plates to make a difference?

Infections with multidrug-resistant bacteria are on target to become the world's leading cause of disease and death by the year 2050, poised to surpass even cancer and heart disease. Excessive antibiotic use can result in our guts becoming colonized with these superbugs,[7396] so researchers set out to calculate how many animal products one would need to eat to achieve antibiotic concentrations in our colon to give resistant bugs an advantage. Single servings of beef, chicken, or pork were found to contain enough tetracycline, ciprofloxacin, tilmicosin, tylosin, sarafloxacin, and erythromycin to favor the growth of resistant bacteria. One and a half servings of fish (150 g) exceeded minimum selective concentrations of ciprofloxacin and erythromycin. Two cups of milk could tip the scales for tetracycline, ciprofloxacin, tilmicosin, tylosin, and lincomycin. And, legal levels of erythromycin and oxytetracycline in two eggs could also exceed safe levels.[7397]

Most resistant bacteria have mobile genetic elements like plasmids, little circles of DNA that carry the resistance genes that they can pass on to other bacteria, including those in our own gut.[7398] In an intestinal model, the transfer of an antibiotic-resistance plasmid from an *E. coli* bacterium originating from a chicken into human gut bugs occurred within two hours. This explains why the antibiotic-resistance gene loads in those eating strictly plant-based diets are significantly lower than in omnivores or ovo-lacto vegetarians. A higher incidence of resistance genes to even vancomycin was found in consumers of eggs, poultry, and fish.[7399] Vancomycin is one of our antibiotics of last resort, used to treat serious life-threatening strep and staph infections, including MRSA.

We need to stop squandering lifesaving miracle drugs just to speed the growth of farm animals reared in unhygienic conditions, and we also need to stop the reckless overuse in medicine. But, sometimes, you have to take antibiotics. To reduce the collateral damage to your friendly flora, a series of mouse studies suggest that you can make your microbiome more resilient by eating healthfully—for example, by consuming more fiber and less sugar.[7400] Prebiotics protect mice from colonization by the bad bug *Clostridium difficile* during antibiotic treatment,[7401] and higher-fiber, lower-fat diets can even protect mice from dying from sepsis after surgery due to antibiotic microbiome disruption.[7402]

FOOD ADDITIVES TO AVOID

The ultraprocessed foods that make up the majority of our diet[7403] aren't just deficient in fiber but include additives that have been shown to muck with our microbes. Even something as simple as salt can affect our microbiome. Approximately doubling sodium intake by adding a teaspoon of salt to people's diets not only increases their blood pressure and boosts pro-inflammatory cells[7404] implicated in autoimmune disease[7405] but it rapidly depletes the gut of the good bacteria *Lactobacillus*. Nine out of ten study subjects who started out with *Lactobacillus* in their gut had it completely wiped out by the added salt within just two weeks.[7406]

Check out see.nf/notsosweet to learn about the adverse microbiome effects of artificial sweeteners. The good news is that after stopping them, the original balance of gut bacteria may be restored within weeks.[7407] It's more difficult to avoid the ingestion of emulsifiers, the most widely used food additives.[7408] Details in see .nf/emulsifiers, but the bottom line is that out of twenty different commonly used emulsifiers, most appeared to have detrimental effects, including carboxymethyl-cellulose and polysorbate 80, but two emulsifiers seemed to be okay: soy lecithin and mono- and diglycerides.[7409]

PROTEIN PUTREFACTION

Have you heard the takeoff of the industry slogan "Beef: It's What's for Dinner"? "Beef: It's What's Rotting in Your Colon." I saw this on a shirt once when I was with some friends and was such a party pooper—no pun intended—that I explained to everyone that meat is fully digested in the small intestine and never makes it down into the colon. (It's no fun hanging out with biology geeks.) But I was wrong! (About meat in the colon, not about being the occasional science-based buzzkill.)

On a typical Western diet, it's been estimated that up to 12 g of protein can escape digestion, and, when it reaches the colon, it can be turned into toxic substances like ammonia.[7410] This degradation of undigested protein in the colon is called putrefaction. So, a little meat *can* actually end up putrefying in our colon. The problem is that some of the by-products of this putrefaction process can be toxic.[7411]

As I explain in see.nf/sulfide, animal proteins tend to have more sulfur-containing amino acids like methionine, which can be turned into hydrogen sulfide in our colon. This may help explain[7412] why those who eat meat appear to be at higher risk of both inflammatory bowel disease[7413] (see.nf/hsibd) and colon cancer[7414] (see.nf/hscancer). Sulfur preservatives (sulfites and sulfur dioxide) in nonorganic wine and dried fruit may also be an issue,[7415] but the sulfur-containing compounds in cabbage-family vegetables don't seem to be a problem.[7416]

Silent, but Deadly

There's a reason hydrogen sulfide is called "rotten egg gas." It's thought to be responsible for the "malodorous rectal flatus" associated with a low-carb diet.[7417] One of the strongest predictors of fecal odor when comparing fresh stool samples was found to be whether or not someone eats meat.[7418] To shrink the stink, the *Harvard Health Letter* offers the recommendation to cut back on meat and eggs.[7419] Randomize people to different quantities of meat, and a clear correlation with fecal sulfide concentrations can be found.[7420] Compared to those eating plant-based diets, individuals who regularly eat meat were found to generate up to fifteen times as much.[7421]

HOW TO REDUCE TMAO EXPOSURE

Prebiotics, like fiber and resistant starch, can feed our probiotic good bacteria, like *Lactobacillus* and *Bifidobacteria*, to make beneficial postbiotics, like butyrate and acetate. However, feeding the wrong foods can foster the growth of bad bacteria that create toxic postbiotics, like TMAO.

Short for *trimethylamine oxide*, TMAO is considered the "smoking gun" of microbiome-disease interactions.[7422] It was identified when researchers compared the blood of patients who had had a stroke or heart attack against the blood of those who hadn't.[7423] (View the full story in see.nf/tmaodiscovery.) Whether young or old, male or female, smoker or nonsmoker, with high blood pressure or low blood pressure, high cholesterol or low, having high levels of TMAO is associated with a significantly higher risk of having a heart attack or stroke, or dying prematurely in general.[7424]

In mice, TMAO promotes atherosclerosis by promoting the accumulation of cholesterol and inflammatory cells within artery walls.[7425] Two other mechanisms for the role of TMAO in cardiovascular disease have been directly demonstrated in human interventional trials. One of the reasons high TMAO levels appear to increase the odds of stroke by 68 percent[7426] and quadruple the odds of dying from it[7427] is that it effectively makes our blood-clotting platelets stickier, the opposite effect of aspirin.[7428] This results in a prothrombotic (clot-promoting) state, whereas the reason TMAO impairs artery function appears to be due to oxidative stress, as an IV infusion of vitamin C can restore TMAO-impaired function in middle-aged and older adults.[7429]

We used to think the toxic effects of TMAO were limited to cardiovascular disease,[7430] but, more recently, it has been associated with everything from psoriatic arthritis[7431] to polycystic ovary syndrome (PCOS),[7432] including eight of our ten leading causes of death: cancer (ovarian,[7433] colorectal,[7434] and breast[7435]), COPD,[7436] dementia,[7437] diabetes,[7438] pneumonia,[7439] and kidney failure.[7440] See details in see.nf/tmaorisk. Based on twenty studies following more than 30,000 people for an average of about five years, a systematic review and meta-analysis found that higher TMAO was associated with a nearly 50 percent increase in all-cause mortality risk.[7441]

Where does TMAO originate? From bad bacteria in our gut when we eat a lot of choline, which is concentrated in eggs and lecithin supplements, or carnitine, which is found in abundance in meat and some energy drinks. Within hours of eating eggs[7442] or meat,[7443] TMAO levels get bumped up—unless antibiotics had recently been taken, wiping out our gut flora. (It can take weeks for bad bacteria to grow back.) Instead of taking drugs, why not prevent the growth of these bad bacteria by not feeding them to begin with? Researchers found that even after a vegan ate steak, virtually no TMAO was produced, presumably because the growth of steak-eating bacteria had not been fostered on a meat-free diet.[7444]

Remarkably, even if you give plant-based eaters the equivalent of an 18-oz steak[7445,7446] every day for two months, only about half of them start ramping up production, showing how far their gut flora had changed.[7447] But it's not all or nothing. As I explore in see.nf/swap, even just exchanging two servings a day of regular meat for plant-based meat can lower TMAO levels within a matter of weeks.

Even plant foods that are relatively rich in choline don't seem to cause the same problem. For example, pistachios[7448] and brussels sprouts[7449] can even make TMAO levels go down. I explore the mixed effects of different plant foods and the pros and cons of carnitine supplements in aging in my video see.nf/tmaoupdate. In short, the best strategy to reduce TMAO exposure is probably to prevent the bloom of bad bacteria in the first place. As one endocrinology journal editorial put it, maybe TMAO should stand for "Time to Minimize intake of Animal prOducts."[7450]

PROBIOTICS

It's been said that the only thing that stops a bad microbiome is a good microbiome.[7451] The question is how to establish that healthy gut flora. There is a multibillion-dollar industry pushing probiotic supplements,[7452] but despite thousands of clinical trials, we, like our microbiome, are left largely in the dark. When researchers analyzed the first 150 results that Google pulled up on probiotics, commercial sites were the most common, which provided, on average, the least reliable information. Most of the claimed benefits were found to be supported by little or no scientific evidence.[7453]

SAFETY AND EFFICACY OF PROBIOTIC SUPPLEMENTS

As I explore in see.nf/probiotics, a recent systematic review of randomized controlled trials of probiotic supplements for healthy older adults found that there was insufficient evidence for the improvement of health outcomes,[7454] and an analysis of hundreds of trials found harms reporting was often missing, insufficient, or inadequate, which undermines our confidence in the safety of these supplements.[7455] For example, there are concerns about antibiotic resistance.

Probiotics are often intentionally selected to be antibiotic-resistant so they can be coadministered with antibiotics to reduce diarrhea rates,[7456] but they may transfer that resistance to pathogens in the gut.[7457] The irony is that probiotics can actually interfere with microbiome recovery after taking antibiotics rather than facilitate it, so just as it may be wise to bank your own blood before an elective procedure should you need a transfusion, those saving their own stool before the course of antibiotics were able restore their microbiomes back to normal within a matter of days.[7458]

MISLABELING AND CONTAMINATION OF PROBIOTIC SUPPLEMENTS

Even if a particular probiotic is proven to be beneficial, there's no guarantee that what's listed on the supplement label is present in the product. No probiotic formulation has been approved by the FDA, so they are sold under the lax regulatory rubric of the dietary supplement industry.[7459] There are products on the market containing microorganisms like *Bacillus licheniformis* not known to even inhabit the human digestive tract.[7460] (It's a soil microbe used to degrade chicken feathers for use in animal feed.[7461]) What about just choosing a probiotic generally considered safe and effective, like *Bifidobacteria*? Good luck. A survey of sixteen commercial *Bifidobacteria* supplements found that only one matched the contents claimed on its label. Even within the same brand, the contents sometimes changed from lot to lot or even sometimes from pill to pill within the same bottle.[7462]

An analysis of commercial probiotics in the United States found that many major brands, including GNC, Walgreens, Procter & Gamble, NaturesPlus, Nature's Bounty, and New Chapter Organics, failed to live up to their label content claims. Most were also contaminated with microorganisms not listed on the label, including, in the case of a GNC product, mold.[7463] Most foods making probiotic claims were also inaccurate.[7464] For example, as few as two in twenty-five "probi-otic" dairy products tested, like yogurt, matched their labeling.[7465] Unfortunately, no improvement in the quality of probiotic products has been found.[7466] A review titled "The Unregulated Probiotic Market" explained the simple reason why: With such poor regulation, there's just no incentive for producers to accurately represent their products.[7467]

The probiotic data are said to be so tainted by personal and commercial biases and so inapplicable due to insufficient regulation that they "make objective inter-pretation close to impossible."[7468] Even if you could get the right dose of the right strain of the right probiotic, they don't appear to actually colonize our gut.[7469] Presumably, if the conditions within your gut were amenable to the growth of good bugs, they would be there already. Without a change in diet to change the gut eco-system, probiotics don't take root, so you'd have to keep taking them forever.[7470] Stool transplants and probiotics may only be temporary fixes if we keep using the wrong fuel. If we don't change our diets, it may be a waste of money to go shop-ping for vegan poop on the black market. (Brown market?) On the other hand, by eating foods rich in *prebiotics*, in other words, increasing "whole plant food con-sumption,"[7471] we may select for *and* foster the growth of our own good bacteria.

What About Fermented Foods?

If commercial probiotics are unreliable, how about the ones that occur naturally in fermented foods? I talked about the potential benefits of souring milk to elimi-nate some of the galactose, branched-chain amino acids, or microRNAs (see page 107). Beyond the aging implications, fermented dairy would be less distressing to those who are lactose-intolerant (which includes the majority of humanity).[7472] Although no significant differences were noted for abdominal pain or diarrhea after the consumption of milk versus kefir, a fermented milk product, the kefir caused fewer farts—seven over the subsequent eight hours versus thirteen after the milk.[7473]

A randomized, double-blind, placebo-controlled trial of kefir found no benefit for preventing antibiotic-associated diarrhea compared to a heat-killed matching placebo with no live microbes.[7474] Similarly, a randomized controlled trial found no benefit of live versus dead (pasteurized) sauerkraut for irritable bowel syn-drome.[7475] In Japan and Korea, pickled vegetable consumption is associated with higher risk of stomach cancer (whereas consumption of fresh vegetables is linked to lower risk).[7476] This is suspected to be due to the salt added to fermenting vegetables to keep unwanted microbes from growing.[7477] However, in Japan, pickled vegetable consumption is associated with lower all-cause mortality, though no more than fresh vegetables.[7478]

Bacillus subtilis, the bacterium used to make a fermented slimy soy food called natto, was found to extend the lifespan of *C. elegans*.[7479] In people, greater natto consumption is associated with living longer, but not necessarily when adjusting for other dietary and lifestyle traits, suggesting that it may be more of a marker of a traditional Japanese eating pattern rather than the natto itself.[7480]

PREBIOTICS AND POSTBIOTICS

If you look at the most frequently cited articles in the scientific nutrition literature, the original glycemic index paper comes in at number ten, cited more than a thousand times.[7481] But, in the top five, cited more than two thousand times, is "Dietary Modulation of the Human Colonic Microbiota: Introducing the Concept of Prebiotics." As I've discussed, prebiotics are the food components that feed and nourish the good bacteria in the gut, like fiber and resistant starch.[7482] For every 1 g of fiber we eat, we can get an increase of nearly 2 g of stool because we are boosting bacterial growth.[7483] Though probiotic pills have been positioned as the next big source of Big Pharma billions,[7484] why take a pill when you can grow your own at home? A meta-analysis of more than five dozen randomized controlled trials of prebiotics found that they boosted the abundance of common probiotics, such as *Bifidobacteria* and *Lactobacillus*.[7485]

Prebiotics don't just boost growth of preexisting *probiotics*. They are used by our friendly flora to create *postbiotics*, those by-products of microbiome metabolism that can be beneficial. Our good bugs eat prebiotics like fiber and make short-chain fatty acids (SCFAs) that are then absorbed into our bloodstream from our colon, circulate throughout our body, and even make their way to our brain.[7486] These far-reaching fiber-sourced SCFAs may have wide-ranging effects on everything from inflammation and immune function[7487] to mental health.[7488]

Remember from page 332 how just one high-fiber meal can improve lung function in asthmatics within a matter of hours? SCFA postbiotics may explain why higher fiber intake is associated with a lower risk of developing osteoarthritis[7489] and worsening knee pain over time.[7490] To give you an idea how protective fiber-rich foods can be, those randomized to eat more whole plant foods during radiation therapy for cancer not only experienced reduced toxicity during the treatments but suffered fewer long-term side effects a full year later.[7491]

Hormones are defined as signaling messengers produced in one organ that circulate throughout the bloodstream and have a regulatory effect on another organ. So, SCFAs could be considered to be hormones—it's just that the organ producing them is the community of bacteria in our gut. But just like our thyroid gland can't make its hormones unless we eat iodine, our microbiome can't make SCFAs unless we eat fiber.

PREBIOTICS FOR FRAILTY

The anti-inflammatory effects alone can help explain why those who eat more fiber tend to live longer and healthier lives. A systematic review and meta-analysis based on more than a hundred million person-years of data found that, compared with those who consumed the least fiber, those who consumed the most had about a 15 to 30 percent decrease in the risk of dying prematurely from all causes put together, including the risk of getting and dying from heart disease, stroke, and cancer.[7492] Fiber intake is also associated with significantly greater likelihood of "successful aging," which is defined as the absence of disability, cognitive impairment, depression, respiratory symptoms, or chronic disease.[7493]

Prebiotics[7494] and postbiotics[7495] can be shown to extend the lives of model animals, but interventional trials in humans are largely limited to risk factors. For example, a meta-analysis of more than fifty randomized controlled trials showed that prebiotics like fiber can significantly improve blood sugar, blood pressure, weight, and cholesterol control.[7496] However, as I note in see.nf/frailtyprebiotics, there was a randomized, double-blind, placebo-controlled trial of prebiotics for frailty, showing significant improvements in both exhaustion and muscle strength.[7497]

When we eat fiber-rich foods, we get a double benefit: the formation of short-chain fatty acids and the selective cultivation of the bugs that make them. The contents of the colons of people eating more plant-based have nearly three times the capacity to form short-chain fatty acids, ounce for ounce.[7498] We get not only more raw materials for SCFA production when we eat healthfully but also improved microbial machinery to create even more of them. In contrast, short-chain fatty acid production can be slashed by up to 75 percent on a low-carb diet.[7499]

PROMOTING *PREVOTELLA*

In my Microbiome-Friendly chapter in *How Not to Diet*, I detail how all of humanity basically clusters in one of two *enterotypes*, those who eat healthier diets and grow mostly *Prevotella* species and those who eat westernized diets and grow mostly *Bacteroides*.[7500] If that sounds curious—thousands of bacteria species but only two enterotypes—think of our guts as ecosystems.[7501] On our planet, there are millions of different species of animals, but they aren't distributed randomly. There are jungle species in the jungle and desert species in the desert. Each ecosystem has its own collection of unique selective pressures, like temperature, humidity, or rainfall. It seems that there are two types of colon ecosystems, so we can be divvied up into groups whose guts grow a lot of *Prevotella*-type bacteria and those whose guts are better homes for *Bacteroides* species.

As fiber-feeders, *Prevotella* churn out more short-chain fatty acids,[7502] helping to explain why African Americans (who typically have a *Bacteroides* enterotype) have fifty times more colon cancer than native Africans (who typically harbor *Prevotella*).[7503] Within days, though, by switching between plant- and animal-based diets, you can flip your gut flora from one to the other.[7504]

Prevotella also tend to be anti-inflammatory, which could explain why lower levels of that bacteria are also something you see in autoimmune conditions, such as Hashimoto's thyroiditis, multiple sclerosis, and type 1 diabetes.[7505] That may be one reason why autoimmune disorders were rare or virtually unknown among those in rural sub-Saharan Africa eating diets composed nearly entirely of plant foods.[7506] Most studies reported that vegetarians harbor higher numbers of *Prevotella*,[7507] but when researchers put them on a diet of meat, eggs, and dairy, their levels were driven down within as few as four days.[7508]

Plant-based diets have been recommended for maintaining beneficial gut microbiota for healthy aging.[7509] Vegetarians tend to harbor a greater abundance of potential probiotic (good) bacteria, whereas omnivores teem with more potential pathobiont (bad) bacteria.[7510] Plant protein intake is associated with more *Bifidobacteria* and *Lactobacillus*, greater short-chain fatty acid production, decreased inflammation, and an improved gut barrier, whereas animal protein intake fosters the growth of bacteria like *Bilophila* and leads to a drop in short-chain fatty acid production and a rise in toxic metabolites like TMAO.[7511]

A comparison of the stool samples of vegans, vegetarians, and omnivores found a continuum of inflammatory markers, with a significant increase from the most to the least plant-based[7512]—inflammation that can be doused by switching to a completely plant-based diet.[7513] This may have more to do with protective effects of plants, though, than any adverse effects of animal products.[7514] An in-depth study of the microbiomes and habitual diets of more than a thousand people found that the dietary factor that most shaped gut flora was the quantity and diversity of healthy plant foods. The microbiomes of those eating fiber-depleted processed foods, such as soda and refined grain products, clustered with those eating more animal foods.[7515] So a junk-food vegan may not be doing their good bugs many favors.

It needn't be all or nothing. People following a Mediterranean-type diet brimming with beans, fruits, and vegetables, while avoiding meat (including fish), eggs, or dairy on a day-to-day basis, had short-chain fatty acid levels that were comparable to vegans, despite not being totally plant-based all the time.[7516]

WITH EVERY FIBER OF YOUR BEAN

The benefits of short-chain fatty acids rely on us eating fiber *and* having fiber-feeding bugs, just like the detrimental effects from TMAO need us to not only eat eggs, dairy, or meat but also carry the egg-, dairy-, or meat-munching bugs. Remember the steak-scarfing vegan? Their gut didn't harbor the bad bugs that make TMAO, and it could take months of eating steaks to ramp up production. Similarly, it may take months for those eating less healthy diets to realize the full potential of increased fiber consumption as their microbiome of fiber-eating organisms grows.[7517]

As I detail in see.nf/cultivate, the benefits of eating more fiber plateaus when our available fiber-feeders are maxed out, but the sky's the limit for those who have habitually been cultivating the growth of fiber-feeders like *Prevotella*.[7518] The U.S. federal recommendation for fiber intake is at least 14 g per 1,000 calories, which comes out to about 25 g a day for women and 38 g a day for men.[7519] Even though that's a far cry from the 100 g our body was designed to get (based on the diets of isolated modern-day hunter-gatherer tribes[7520] and analyzing coprolites, human fossilized feces[7521]), fewer than 3 percent of Americans even reach the minimal minimum recommendation.

We know that fiber is only found in plants by definition,[7522] with typically little found in processed foods and none at all in any animal foods. Since fruits and vegetables are mostly water, the fiber-rich superstars of the plant kingdom are the whole grains and legumes.[7523] A cup of fruit may only have about 3 g of dietary fiber and a cup of vegetables 5 g, but a cup of beans or a cup of intact whole grains, like barley groats, may have 15 g.

50-FOOD CHALLENGE

The Yanomami tribe in the Amazon jungle have the richest microbiomes ever recorded. They had had no prior contact with the modern world,[7524] which makes me wonder how that conversation went: *We come in peace. Can we have your poop?*

Today's low-fiber diet is thought to be a key culprit in microbiome depletion.[7525] In its profound and potentially catastrophic upheaval of the microbiome ecosystem, the loss of dietary fiber in the modern diet has been compared to the Chicxulub impactor, the meteor that killed off the dinosaurs.[7526] Why can't we just take a fiber supplement? There are literally thousands of types of fiber in plant foods, and each may support different communities of bacteria in our gut.[7527] Unlike whole foods, like brown rice or whole-grain barley, fiber supplements don't seem to work to improve the richness of the microbiome.[7528] What's more, a combination of brown rice and barley synergistically works better than either alone.[7529] That's the reasoning behind recommendations that people take a "50-food challenge," eating at least fifty different plant foods a week to achieve a diet diverse enough to feed a vast spectrum of bacteria.[7530]

No wonder fiber supplements are a poor substitute. Some, like psyllium (sold as Metamucil), don't appear to be utilized by our microbiome at all.[7531] The hubris reminds me of probiotic supplements. There are thousands of different species of bacteria in our guts[7532] that all potentially interact with one another, yet we're surprised a half dozen out of thousands stuffed into a pill don't have more of an impact? No microbe is an island.[7533] Major starch munchers like *Bifidobacteria* produce acetate, which feeds some of the major butyrate producers, and lactate, which acidifies the gut. This further stimulates the growth of butyrate producers, as well as suppressing the growth of bad bugs,[7534] in the same way sauerkraut does. The best way to support this symphony of interaction is to eat plants—not pills or powders.

RESISTANT STARCH

Fiber isn't the only prebiotic. For example, about 30 percent of the caloric content of human breast milk is made of "indigestible" oligosaccharides.[7535] Though we may not be able to digest them, guess who can? *Bifidobacterium infantis*, good bacteria in the guts of infants. That's how important the human-bacteria relationship is. We were designed to be a symbiotic species.

Inulin, concentrated in such vegetables as onion and garlic, can have a "huge" bifidogenic effect.[7536] Ironically, some people with irritable bowel syndrome actively avoid inulin because it is a type of FODMAP, or fermentable oligo-, di-, and monosaccharides and polyols. Individuals following FODMAP-restricted diets tend to end up with depleted levels of *Bifidobacteria*, so it's been theorized that such eating patterns could actually impair long-term gut health.[7537]

There is "resistant starch"—starches resistant to digestion in our small intestines so they make their way to our colon, where they can act as prebiotics to feed our good bacteria, just as fiber does. I mentioned the trick of cooling cooked starches on page 63, but the best source of resistant starch are legumes.[7538] Two daily servings of cooked chickpeas can reduce the colonization of pathogenic and putrefactive gut bacteria within three weeks. Study participants had about a 50 percent reduction in the presence of a highly ammonia-producing bug.[7539] Perhaps this explains why a single serving of legumes a day is associated with about a 20 percent lower risk of colorectal cancer.[7540] In rats, feeding them black beans cuts down by 75 percent the incidence of colon cancer caused by a carcinogen.[7541]

As with fiber, you need to eat the prebiotics *and* have prebiotic-eating bugs to benefit. Those carrying starch scarfers like *Ruminococcus* can ferment nearly all the resistant starch they eat, whereas those who don't are only able to take advantage of 20 to 30 percent.[7542] How do you foster the growth of more of these good bugs? Eat more foods containing resistant starch! Within just ten days of being randomized to a diet high in resistant starch, the abundance of starch eaters like *Ruminococcus* can be quadrupled.[7543]

SURVIVING INTACT

The preferred prebiotic of *Bifidobacteria* is starch, so how can we ferry more starch to our colon?[7544] Wrap it in fiber. That is, within intact grains and legumes. I allude to this on page 90 and do a deep dive in my Wall Off Your Calories chapter in *How Not to Diet*. When we chew and our stomach churns, anything we eat gets reduced down to smaller than two millimeters or so, about one-sixteenth of an inch, before entering our intestines.[7545] That may sound tiny, but a two-millimeter piece of wheat may contain about 10,000 plant cells filled with starch and only approximately 3,800 of them would be ruptured open on their surface,[7546] leaving 62 percent of the starch in that particle of grain protected inside indigestible plant cell walls, which leads to ample leftovers to feed our microbiome.[7547]

Compare that to even whole *milled* grains. Ground flour particles can be a hundred times smaller—even smaller than the cells themselves—so nearly every one may be ruptured open, spilling their contents early and leaving our gut flora in the lurch.[7548] That's why we should try to de-flour our diets. Whole grains are good, but intact whole grains (groats) are better. It's the same reason why eating nuts can alter our microbiome for the better, boosting the growth of good bugs that produce short-chain fatty acids, but there appears to be no prebiotic influence when we eat the same amount of nut butter.[7549]

Remember acarbose from page 60, the drug that effectively turns regular starch into resistant starch? The average and maximum lifespan extension in mice from acarbose may be from the release of a hormone called GLP-1[7550] from specialized *L cells* that line our colons.[7551] That's the same hormone mimicked by the expensive new class of injectable weight-loss drugs like Wegovy.[7552] This same effect can be obtained in a drug-free manner with prebiotics. Researchers have achieved this in a petri dish[7553] or in a person, by infusing their rectum with an SCFA enema[7554] or just having them eat fiber[7555] or, even better, fiber-rich foods.[7556]

POLYPHENOL PREBIOTICS

Another major class of prebiotics are the polyphenols concentrated in fruits and vegetables.[7557] Those who discount the power of polyphenols often refer to studies showing their low bioavailability. Up to 85 percent of the polyphenol pigments that make blueberries blue do not get absorbed and end up in our colons, for example,[7558] but more advanced detection methods have recently shown that the majority of polyphenols may be absorbed after all.[7559] And our colon may be exactly where some of the magic happens.

When blueberry polyphenols[7560] are mixed with a culture of fecal bacteria, beneficial bugs like *Bifidobacteria* and *Lactobacillus* grow within a matter of hours.[7561] If you randomize people to a cup or so of wild blueberries,[7562] they get a significant bump in *Bifidobacteria* in their stools.[7563] How can we know that the polyphenols caused it and not the fiber? Well, apples also boost *Bifidobacteria*,[7564] but the isolated apple fiber pectin on its own does not.[7565] Bananas and berries have a similar fiber content, but bananas have fewer polyphenols. Eating bananas does not significantly boost *Bifidobacteria*,[7566] which is more evidence that polyphenols may be playing a special role.

An interventional trial in which older individuals were randomized to swap out some low-polyphenol snacks for foods like berries and dark chocolate experienced a significant increase in good (butyrate-producing) bacteria and a bolstering of the gut barrier.[7567] However, polyphenol-rich beverages probably provide the best proof. Tea leaves and coffee beans have a lot of polyphenols that end up in the brew, whereas the fiber is completely left behind. Both green tea[7568] and coffee[7569] are bifidogenic. Three cups of coffee a day can raise *Bifidobacteria* levels in the gut significantly within three weeks.[7570]

Isn't tea antimicrobial? It's used in mouthwash to kill plaque bacteria,[7571] in acne creams to kill pimple bugs,[7572] and in foot baths to help control athlete's foot fungus.[7573] That indeed may be one of the ways it helps increase the proportion of good bugs like *Bifidobacteria*—by inhibiting the growth of the bad,[7574] though polyphenols from green, black, and oolong tea also boost *Bifidobacteria* and short-chain fatty acid production.[7575]

In a gut simulator, ginger extracts also promote *Bifidobacteria* growth in fecal samples. Fresh ginger extracts have been shown to ameliorate antibiotic-associated diarrhea in rats and accelerate microbiome recovery, but clinical studies are still lacking.[7576]

Microbiome Manipulation for Dementia

In see.nf/gutbrain, I profile a remarkable case report titled "Rapid Improvement in Alzheimer's Disease Symptoms Following Fecal Microbiota Transplantation"[7577] and review the inconsistent results of dozens of randomized controlled trials of prebiotics, probiotics, and fermented foods for cognition.[7578] Unfortunately, some of the most promising findings are plagued by concerns of data integrity,[7579] including oligomannate,[7580] a prebiotic conditionally approved in China in 2019 to treat mild to moderate Alzheimer's disease.[7581]

POLYPHENOL POSTBIOTICS

Just as the benefits of fiber result from both the prebiotic fueling of good bacteria and the resulting postbiotic metabolites (short-chain fatty acids), polyphenols can act as prebiotics and also result in beneficial postbiotics. For example, there is an immediate bump of blueberry pigments in our blood within an hour of consumption, but a day later, new blueberry-derived compounds continue to appear in our bloodstream as our bacteria churn out new goodies from them.[7582] In this way, berry polyphenols can be the gift that keeps on giving.

As I detail in see.nf/urolithins, one class of postbiotics important to aging are urolithins, which are created in our large intestine by our friendly flora from ellagic acid, which is formed in our small intestine when we eat ellagitannins,[7583] the most common form of tannin,[7584] characteristically astringent-tasting natural compounds found in many of our ancestral foods, including berries, nuts, acorns, and tree leaves.[7585] Since tannins aren't bioavailable, they have been neglected in the field of nutrition or even considered as "antinutrients," a view that has "changed dramatically" once it was recognized that they could be metabolized by the microbiome into urolithins, now thought responsible for some of the benefits of berries, nuts, and pomegranates.[7586]

In *C. elegans*, urolithins extend lifespan by inducing mitophagy, mitochondria autophagy, the prevention of the accumulation of dysfunctional mitochondria with age.[7587] A decline in mitophagy has been linked to low muscle mass and poor physical function (slower walking speed) in the elderly.[7588] Urolithins have been found to counter age-related muscle function decline by improving the exercise capacity of older rodents[7589] and, in people, induced a molecular signature of improved mitochondrial health and biogenesis in muscle biopsies, similar to what one might see after an aerobic exercise regimen.[7590] This then translates into improved muscle endurance even in the absence of any exercise training.[7591] Like any postbiotic, though, it depends on having the requisite microbial machinery. Studies show that some people are poor urolithin producers and some people's microbiomes can't make it at all.[7592]

Give people a pomegranate extract, and producers of urolithins experienced a significant reduction in LDL cholesterol, but the nonproducers did not. After a few weeks of supplementation, though, there were a few conversions—nonproducers turned into producers.[7593] This may explain why vegetarians tend to have a higher abundance of urolithin-producing microbes, their greater intake of plants.[7594] However, some plants have more than others. Among berries and nuts, the highest levels of ellagitannins are found in boysenberries, marionberries, yellow raspberries, pomegranates, and walnuts.[7595]

CALORIC RESTRICTION

Three meals a day (plus snacks!) is an evolutionarily novel behavior. In see.nf /fasting, I review how the story of life on Earth is a story of starvation.[7596] If our physiology is so well tuned to periodic scarcity, maybe it would be beneficial to cut back? Beyond just freeing up all the resources that would normally be used for nutrient digestion and storage, during fasting, our cells switch over to a protective mode[7597] that results in a reduction of free radical damage and inflammation.[7598] It's the hormesis concept of that-which-doesn't-kill-us-makes-us-stronger.[7599] This was perhaps most starkly demonstrated in a set of cringe-worthy experiments in which mice were blasted with Hiroshima-level gamma radiation sufficient to kill 50 percent within two weeks. But, of the mice that had been intermittently fasted for six weeks before the radiation blast, not a single one died.[7600]

A TIME TO FAST

Benjamin Franklin said, "To lengthen thy life, lessen thy meals."[7601] Might this hormetic bolstering of defenses result in a longer life? Using caloric restriction to slow aging became a topic of interest during the Great Depression in the 1930s when, contrary to expectations, average lifespan appeared to increase.[7602] The same was noted earlier during World War I in Denmark, when blockaded food supplies were accompanied by a 34 percent reduction in death rates, and later in Norway during World War II, when a 20 percent drop in calories was accompanied by a 30 percent drop in death rates.[7603] The quality of the diets changed as well, though, complicating the picture, with the switch to eating feed crops like barley rather than the livestock to which they were being fed.[7604]

In the lab, caloric restriction without malnutrition is one of the most powerful non-pharmacological interventions for extending healthspan and lifespan across a multitude of species,[7605] considered perhaps "the most important discovery in the biology of aging to date."[7606] Simply reducing food intake can double or triple the lifespans of yeast, fruit flies, and worms, and prolong the average and maximum lifespans of rats and mice by up to 50 percent.[7607] The experiments can be as simple as feeding some flies to some spiders (cutely named *bowl and doily spiders*): One fly a week and they live an average of eighty-one days, three flies a week and they only live sixty-four days, and at five flies a week, only forty-two days.[7608]

The animals in some of these experiments live not just longer lives but healthier lives. The apparent slowing of the aging process conserved up through primates is accompanied by resistance to a range of age-related diseases, preventing or delaying autoimmune diseases, cancer, cardiovascular disease, glaucoma, kidney disease, and neurodegeneration.[7609] In Part I, I covered many of the theoretical underpinnings to the longevity benefits of caloric restriction, from boosting AMPK to "cleaning out the cupboards" autophagy—clearing out misfolded proteins, damaged cell structures, and senescent cells.[7610] As one review on the mechanisms by which intermittent fasting benefits cardiometabolic disease was subtitled, "The Janitor Is the Undercover Boss."[7611]

THE CANDLE THAT BURNS TWICE AS BRIGHT BURNS HALF AS LONG

Another potential mechanism may be the slowing of our metabolism. Because of our millions of years of evolution hard-wiring us to survive scarcity,[7612] when we start losing weight, in addition to unconsciously starting to move less as a behavioral adaptation to conserve energy,[7613] there are metabolic adaptations as well.[7614] Every pound of weight loss may reduce our resting metabolic rates by seven calories a day.[7615] Though a bane for dieters (see.nf/biggestloser), a slower metabolism may actually be a good thing.

Caloric restriction can increase the lifespans of animals,[7616] and the metabolic slowdown may be the mechanism.[7617] That may be why the tortoise lives ten times longer than the hare.[7618] (Harriet, a tortoise evidently collected from the Galápagos by Charles Darwin in the 1830s, lived until 2006.[7619]) Slow and steady may indeed win the race.

One of the ways our body lowers our resting metabolic rate is by creating cleaner-burning, more efficient mitochondria, the power plants that fuel our cells.[7620] It's like our body passes its own fuel-efficiency standards. These new mitochondria appear to create the same energy with less oxygen and produce less free-radical "exhaust." After all, our body is afraid that famine is afoot, so it tries to conserve as much energy as it can.

The largest caloric-restriction trial to date found both metabolic slowing and a reduction in free radical–induced oxidative stress, both of which may slow the rate of aging.[7621] The metabolic slowing from eating nitrate-rich vegetables (see page 494) may be why eating leafy greens has been found to be among the six most powerful things we can do to potentially live longer.[7622] Whether restricting calories will translate into greater human longevity is an unanswered question. Caloric restriction has been said to extend the lifespan of "every species studied,"[7623] but this isn't even true of all strains within a single species.[7624]

STRAIN FOR EFFECT

If rodent results could be replicated in humans, what kind of life extension might people expect? Well, a 50 percent lifespan increase would extend the current U.S. life expectancy from 77 years[7625] to around 115, but that's based on experiments that restricted food intakes between 40 and 60 percent, starting immediately after weaning.[7626] See a full chart in see.nf/extrapolate, but even cutting down one's intake from 2,500 calories a day to 1,750 calories, a 30 percent drop, for a few decades starting in one's forties could potentially add a few years to your life. Same for reducing caloric intake just to 2,125 starting in one's thirties. Again, though, this is assuming we can extrapolate from rodents to humans.[7627]

A study of more than forty strains of mice found that caloric restriction *shortened* the lifespans of three times as many strains as it extended. Cutting food intake by 40 percent, one of the most common experimental regimens, extended the lifespans of five strains of mice, shortened it in fifteen, and had no significant effect on the majority. In one strain, the longevity of female mice was increased while that of male mice was decreased.[7628] If we can't even extrapolate the effects of caloric restriction from one strain of mouse to another, how can we extrapolate from mice to men or women? I explore other problems with generalizing results to humans in see.nf/extrapolate.

CALORIE RESTRICTION OR JUST OBESITY RESTRICTION?

One important critique of the entire field is that even the most successful studies more likely illustrate the life-shortening effects of obesity rather than the life-extending effects of caloric restriction.[7629] The control group animals in most caloric restriction experiments are allowed to eat ad libitum, meaning as much as they want.[7630] So maybe any benefits researchers find are less about restricting and more about just not overeating.

As anyone with pets knows, if you allow them to eat as much as they want, they can get fat.[7631] Middle-aged Labrador retrievers given unlimited food access in their youth end up with more than twenty pounds of body fat and only live about eleven years.[7632] If you pair litter puppies and restrict one to 75 percent of what their sibling eats ad libitum during that period, they put on less than ten pounds of fat and live an average of thirteen years. Nine out of twenty-four of the diet-restricted dogs (37.5 percent) survived past the time all their unrestricted siblings had died. Is that evidence that caloric restriction is good, or just evidence that obesity is bad?

Ironically, this aspect of the experiments may make them more generalizable to the human populace. Nearly three-quarters (73.6 percent) of the U.S. adult population is overweight or obese.[7633] So, using ad libitum controls may be the appropriate comparator. Those who are very obese (BMI ≥ 35) throughout their adult lives lose at least seven years of life and nineteen years of healthy life.[7634] Obviously, caloric restriction would be good for them, but most of the restriction experiments don't offer insight into whether someone who is already at a healthy weight would benefit from restricting further. Control group considerations play heavily into the interpretation of conflicting results found in a famous pair of long-term caloric restriction monkey experiments.

MONKEYING AROUND WITH DIETARY RESTRICTION

There have been four investigations of caloric restriction and lifespan in nonhuman primates.[7635, 7636, 7637, 7638] The particulars are worth exploring, as I do in detail in see.nf/primatecr, but bottom line, if I had to sum up what we've learned from the primate data in one sentence, it would be: If you're overweight or living off junk food, eating less is a good idea.

CRONIE CATABOLISM

What about human data? Lifelong randomized controlled trials aren't going to happen,[7639] but there have been shorter-term ones, studies of those who calorically restrict voluntarily, as well as a variety of creative approaches to answer the question: *Does eating less help you live more?* For example, do those suffering from anorexia live longer? Far from it. Anorexia nervosa is one of the deadliest mental disorders. Anorexics die at a rate about ten times that of the general population,[7640] suffering from a range of electrolyte abnormalities, anemia, osteoporotic bone fractures, and cardiac arrhythmias.[7641] Researchers found that developing chronic anorexia from age fifteen would be expected to shave twenty-five years off a woman's lifespan.[7642]

Anorexia is an example of extreme caloric restriction. As many as nearly one-third of those diagnosed with the disease who seek treatment have a BMI under 15,[7643] about half the weight of the average American woman.[7644] Unlike laboratory protocols that dictate caloric restriction without malnutrition, those with anorexia can suffer from starvation-related nutrient deficiencies so severe that they can go blind.[7645] Their contracted lives may therefore not bear direct relevance to the question at hand, not to mention that one in five anorexia victims die by suicide.[7646]

The only long-term human study of extreme caloric restriction was the (in)famous Minnesota Starvation Experiment that used conscientious objectors as guinea pigs during World War II. Unlike caloric restriction experiments designed to meet recommended daily allowances of essential nutrients, the Minnesota Starvation Experiment was deficient on purpose. The malnourished study subjects suffered from chronic weakness, painful leg swelling, and severe emotional distress. Interestingly, though, half the study participants went on to celebrate their eightieth birthdays, living at least eight years longer than expected for men in their generation,[7647] though other factors peculiar to a pacifist cohort could have played a role.

Speaking of unusual groups, self-styled CRONies (for *calorie restriction with optimal nutrition*) are active members of the Calorie Restriction Society, started by caloric restriction researcher and practitioner Roy Walford. He attempted to popularize the practice in the 1980s with his book *The 120 Year Diet*. Sadly, Walford himself died well short of the promised 120 at age 79 (of ALS).[7648] I review all the research on CRONies in see.nf/cronies. All in all, long-term practitioners of calorie restriction appear to be in excellent health, but they're a rather unique, self-selected bunch of individuals.[7649] As always, you don't really know until you put it to the test. Enter CALERIE, the Comprehensive Assessment of Long-Term Effects of Reducing Intake of Energy, the first large, long-term, clinical trial to test the effects of caloric restriction.[7650]

THE CALERIE TRIAL

Although the standard caloric restriction diet used in rodent studies is 40 percent less than the quantity consumed by ad libitum controls, even a 10 percent reduction can extend the lifespan of rats.[7651] Caloric restriction that modest would be amenable to a randomized controlled trial.

In the CALERIE trial, hundreds of nonobese men and women were randomized to two years of caloric restriction. (Details in see.nf/calerie.) As I mentioned, the study participants in the Minnesota Starvation Experiment suffered both physically and psychologically.[7652] However, the subjects started out lean and had their caloric intakes cut in half. The CALERIE study ended up being four times less restrictive, at only about 12 percent below baseline caloric intake, and enrolled normal-weight individuals, which in the United States these days means overweight on average. As such, the CALERIE subjects experienced nothing but positive quality-of-life benefits, with significant improvements in mood, general health, sex drive, and sleep.[7653] They also wiped out more than half of their visceral abdominal fat,[7654] which translated into significant improvements in blood pressure, insulin sensitivity, triglycerides, and cholesterol levels.[7655] During the final year, they were eating only about 300 fewer calories than they had been at baseline,[7656] so they got all those benefits after cutting only about a snack-sized bag of chips' worth of calories from their daily diets.

What happened at the end of the trial, though? In both the Minnesota Starvation

Experiment[7657] and experiments on U.S. Army Rangers,[7658] as soon as subjects were released from restriction, they tended to rapidly regain the weight—and sometimes more. The leaner they started out, the more their bodies seemed to drive them to overeat to pack back on extra body fat. In contrast, after the completion of the CALERIE study, even though their metabolisms were slowed by about a hundred calories a day,[7659] they retained about 50 percent of the weight loss two years after the trial ended.[7660] They must have acquired new eating attitudes and behaviors that allowed them to keep their weight down and did so without any signs of increased susceptibility to eating disorders.[7661] Indeed, after extended caloric restriction, cravings for sugary and fatty foods can go down.[7662]

The slowed metabolism, presented as "a reduction in the rate of living," would be expected to contribute to longevity[7663] and may explain part of the reduction in whole body oxidative stress within the first year of caloric restriction.[7664] However, even just culturing cells in the blood of those practicing caloric restriction makes them significantly more resistant to free radical damage, perhaps due to a doubling of antioxidant enzyme activity within cells bathed in calorically restricted blood.[7665] Furthermore, two different biomarker algorithms used to calculate "biological age" found that the caloric restriction intervention appeared to slow the rate of aging, and this appeared to be independent of the degree of weight loss. By one estimate, the ad libitum control group appeared to be aging at an average rate of 0.7 "years" per year, whereas the caloric restriction group averaged only 0.1. Based on that algorithm (the Klemera-Doubal Method), the caloric restriction group hardly appeared to be aging much at all.[7666]

The multitude of physiological, psychological, and aging benefits attributed to this sustained, moderate (11.9 percent) caloric restriction must be interpreted with the proviso that the composition of the diet changed along with the quantity. Much of the caloric restriction was achieved through a reduction in fat intake.[7667] The type of fat was not specified, but given that the leading sources of fat in the American diet have typically been meat and dairy, followed by desserts like donuts, cookies, and cake, this may have been accompanied by an improvement in diet quality that could account for some of the measured effects.[7668] That caveat aside, the CALERIE trial does suggest that even "normal weight" individuals should eat less to improve their health and longevity.[7669]

Thinking Outside the Icebox

Studies following more than five million men and women found that abdominal obesity was associated with an increased likelihood of developing cognitive impairment and dementia in men and women older than sixty-five.[7670] Caloric restriction has been deemed one of the most effective dietary interventions to improve the cognitive performance of rodents.[7671] What about in people? There don't appear to be any human caloric restriction trials for dementia,[7672] but there have been about a dozen randomized controlled trials on cognitive effects on those who are cognitively intact or mildly impaired.[7673]

Although hardly any of the individual studies were able to show significant improvements, when all the studies were compiled together, there did appear to be cognitive benefit to cutting down calories. Most of the thousand or so study subjects were obese, so the benefit may have derived more from the weight loss than the caloric restriction per se.[7674] It doesn't take much, though. When overweight, borderline obese elderly men and women (BMI of 29.9) were advised to reduce their calories by 30 percent for three months, they only achieved about a 12 percent reduction in caloric intake, losing about five pounds, but nonetheless experienced a significant improvement in verbal memory performance.[7675]

A 12 percent reduction is what the CALERIE intervention group participants averaged. At the end of the two years, they had better working (short-term) memory than those randomized to the control group. Interestingly, the cognitive improvement was related mostly to lower protein intake.[7676] This was directly tested in a study titled "Dietary Effects on Cognition and Pilots' Flight Performance." Commercial airline pilots were randomly rotated through four-day high-carbohydrate, high-protein, high-fat, or control diets, then had their flying performance evaluated using a full-motion flight simulator. Compared to being on any of the other three diets, when the pilots were on the high-protein diet, their flight performance suffered.[7677]

More extreme fasting appears to have rather equivocal effects on cognition in the short term.[7678] Those randomized to eat nothing for a day subjectively feel greater "mental fatigue" than those given about 500 calories of food throughout the day, but they perform just as well on objective tests of cognitive performance.[7679] Given the potential for psychological influence, there was actually a randomized, double-blind, placebo-controlled trial of forty-eight hours of caloric deprivation. How can you blind someone to whether they eat or not? They were fed indistinguishable gels, either nearly calorie-free or providing thousands of calories a day. Surprisingly, two days of near-total caloric deprivation didn't affect the cognitive performance, activity, sleep, or mood of healthy young adults. This makes sense from an evolutionary point of view. Remaining sharp during a downturn in food availability would presumably offer a survival advantage.[7680]

POTENTIAL DOWNSIDES OF CALORIC RESTRICTION

Caloric restriction has been heralded as a fountain of youth.[7681] The near-universal benefits seen in the CALERIE trial support the potential health and longevity benefits of mild caloric restriction without the downsides seen with more extreme restriction: loss of libido, strength, and bone mass; menstrual irregularities; infertility; cold sensitivity; slower wound healing; blood pressure dropping too low; and psychological conditions such as depression, emotional deadening, and irritability[7682] (not to mention walking around starving all the time).

Two of the most potentially serious pitfalls—impaired wound healing and recovery from infection—could possibly be restored sufficiently by temporarily resuming a full diet in the event of injury or illness. Full wound healing capacity was reestablished in calorically restricted rats[7683] and mice[7684] within days or weeks of full feeding, but the refeeding was done *before* the wounds were inflicted. This could be useful in the case of scheduled surgery but may have limited relevance to spontaneous injury.

One might presume that immune suppression could result from steroid stress hormones released in an underfed state, but, although total fasting can dramatically increase cortisol levels—as much as doubling them within five days[7685]—less severe caloric restriction does not.[7686] Though many indicators of immune function improve during caloric restriction,[7687] this doesn't necessarily translate into improved survival from infection.[7688] Despite an apparent rejuvenation in immune system parameters, when actually put to the test, feeding rodents 20 to 40 percent less than ad libitum intake has been found to have detrimental impacts in fighting bacterial,[7689] viral,[7690] fungal,[7691] and parasitic[7692] infections. Refeeding calorie-restricted mice two weeks before influenza infection improved survival back toward the level of normal-fed mice.[7693] For those without crystal balls, the researchers suggest unrestricting caloric intake before, or perhaps throughout, the flu season.[7694]

One of the most consistent benefits of caloric restriction is improvement in blood pressure in as short as one or two weeks.[7695] Unfortunately, this can work a little too well and cause orthostatic intolerance,[7696] manifesting as light-headedness or dizziness upon standing, which, in severe cases, can cause fainting. Staying hydrated can help.[7697]

What about loss of muscle mass? Unintuitively, caloric restriction appears to actually delay age-related muscle loss in rats and monkeys. Details in see.nf/restrictionpitfalls, but in the CALERIE trial, participants generally got stronger. There was also a small increase in aerobic capacity in the restricted group compared to control.[7698] Increased protein intakes are commonly suggested to preserve more lean mass, but most studies fail to show a beneficial effect on preserving muscle strength or function, whether young or old, active or sedentary,[7699] and high-protein intake during weight loss has been found to have "profound" negative metabolic effects, undermining the benefits of weight loss on insulin sensitivity. Lose twenty pounds, and you can dramatically improve your body's ability to handle blood sugars, compared to a control group who maintained their weight. Lose the exact same amount of weight but while on a high-protein diet (getting about an extra 30 g a day), and, from a blood sugar control standpoint, it's like you never lost any weight at all.[7700]

Though you can always bulk back up afterward, the best way to preserve muscle mass during weight loss is exercise. Resistance training even just three times a week can prevent more than 90 percent of lean body mass loss during caloric restriction.[7701] The same may be true of bone loss. Lose weight through caloric restriction alone, and you experience a decline in bone mineral density in fracture-risk sites like the hip and spine. However, in the same study, those randomized to lose weight with exercise didn't suffer any bone loss.[7702] It's hard to argue with calls for increased physical activity, but even without an exercise regimen, the "very small" drop in bone mineral density in the CALERIE study might only increase the ten-year risk of osteoporotic fracture by about 0.2 percent.[7703] A high-resolution MRI study of the bones of CRONies found a reduction in bone quantity but not bone quality. The honeycomb-like microarchitectural structure within the bone appeared to be preserved despite the reduction in bone mass.[7704]

Chipping Away at Pollutants?

Body fat may play a protective role by sequestering toxic pollutants, such as PCBs and DDT, which come spilling out when we lose weight.[7705] That's one of the reasons health authorities recommend that women don't try to slim down during breastfeeding.[7706] I cover the ways in which we can protect our vital organs in see.nf/fastingdetox. Eating Pringles made with the fake fat olestra doesn't seem to help,[7707] but fiber can bind to these pollutants and potentially flush them out of the body.[7708] See see.nf/eatlow for ways to prevent the buildup of industrial toxins in the first place.

MORE FOOD, LESS CALORIES

The bottom line is that the benefits of mild caloric restriction revealed by the CALERIE trial—improved blood pressure, cholesterol, mood, libido, and sleep—would seem to far outweigh any potential risks. The fact that a reduction in calories seemed to have such wide-ranging positive effects led commentators in the American Medical Association's internal medicine journal to write: "The findings of this well-designed study suggest that intake of excess calories is not only a burden to our physical homeostasis but also on our psychological well-being."[7709] This is all the more remarkable given how little they were actually restricting.

By the end of the twenty-four months of the CALERIE trial, the caloric restriction group was eating just one hundred fewer calories a day than the ad libitum control group, a slip in compliance from the two hundred or so fewer calories a day at the end of the first year.[7710] A common refrain from commentators is that all of this benefit can be yours by skipping your daily latte or cutting your muffin du jour in half,[7711] but by switching to healthier foods, you can achieve the same caloric reduction while eating *more* food, not less.

The reason obesity rates among vegans may run as low as 2 to 3 percent[7712] is that those eating more plant-based eat as many as 464 fewer calories a day while eating the same amount of food[7713]—or even more.[7714] That's the beauty of foods with low calorie density: more food, less weight. For an in-depth discussion of caloric density, please see my book *How Not to Diet*.

The founding director of Harvard's center on aging research, David Sinclair, wrote: "After twenty-five years of researching aging and having read thousands of scientific papers, if there is one piece of advice I can offer, one surefire way to stay healthy longer, one thing you can do to maximize your lifespan right now, it's this: eat less."[7715] Eating fewer calories, however, doesn't necessarily mean you need to cut portions. For example, part of Okinawans' longevity may be because they were only eating about 1,800 calories a day. However, because whole plant foods are so calorically dilute, they were actually eating a greater quantity of food.[7716]

INTERMITTENT FASTING

Rather than cutting calories day in and day out, what if, instead, you just ate as much as you wanted every other day? Or for only a few hours a day? Or what if you fasted two days a week or five days a month? These are all examples of intermittent fasting regimens, and they may even be the way we were built to eat. For millennia, our ancestors often may have consumed only one large meal a day or went several days at a time without food.[7717]

Might intermittent fasting stress our body in a good way, like exercise, through hormesis? Mark Twain thought so: "A little starvation can really do more for the average sick man than can the best medicines and the best doctors. I do not mean a restricted diet; I mean *total abstention from food for one or two days*."[7718] But Twain also said, "Many a small thing has been made large by the right kind of advertising."[7719] Is the craze over intermittent fasting just hype?

I cover all the important studies on alternate-day fasting in see.nf/altdayfasting and 5:2 fasting (eating five days a week) in see.nf/52fmd. The bottom line: There do not appear to be any advantages over chronic daily restriction.[7720] And, as I discuss in see.nf/altdaysafety, the largest and longest trial of alternate-day fasting disturbingly found a significant increase in LDL cholesterol.[7721] One study of post-menopausal women also found that intermittent caloric restriction led to twice the loss of lean body mass compared to weight loss from chronic restriction.[7722] I also caution diabetics[7723] and those on medications,[7724] though concerns about mood, cognition, and eating disorders have been eased. Symptoms of irritability and in-ability to concentrate on fasting days may wane over time.[7725] And, of eleven inter-ventional studies, although four showed an increase in binge eating, two showed no change and the other five showed decreases in bingeing.[7726]

INTERMITTENT FASTING AND LONGEVITY

Most intermittent fasting studies focus on weight loss. What about life extension? Mormon teachings call for a once-monthly fast when adherents are expected to skip two consecutive meals (thereby fasting about twenty-four hours). Could this play a role in Utah routinely having among the lowest rates of death due to heart disease[7727] and help explain why men active in the Mormon church have tended to live about seven years longer than the U.S. average?[7728]

In a study of a cardiac patient population with a preponderance of Mormons, routine fasters were found to have lower rates of diabetes and severe heart dis-ease.[7729] Does this translate into living longer? About two thousand patients in a medical center in Salt Lake City were followed for four years after cardiac catheter-ization. About four hundred were routine fasters, adhering to the monthly practice for an average of forty-two consecutive years, about two-thirds of their lives. Did they do better than their nonfasting colleagues? Yes, they had a 46 percent lower risk of dying in the subsequent years of follow-up.[7730]

The obvious confounding would be other tenets of religious observation. Those following Mormon teachings on fasting to the letter might be more likely to follow other doctrines of the church, and indeed routine fasters were significantly less likely to smoke and significantly more likely to be teetotalers. However, both of these factors were taken into account, and the survival benefit remained.[7731] What they didn't control for, though, is diet composition. In addition to monthly fasting, the Mormon church recommends consumption of whole grains, fruits, and vege-tables,[7732] with meat only to be eaten "sparingly."[7733] Hence, it's not clear how much of the survival advantage among the fasters was due to the quality of their diets rather than the periodic dips in quantity. The only way to prove cause and effect is to put intermittent fasting to the test, which it was, remarkably, in the 1950s.

Inspired by the data being published on life extension with caloric restriction on lab rats, researchers split 120 residents of a senior home in Madrid into two groups. Sixty residents continued to eat their regular diets, and the other sixty were put on an alternate-day modified fast for three years. Details on the study and its outcomes are in see.nf/fastinglongevity, but basically, it's held up as evidence that caloric restriction may improve one's healthspan and potentially even one's lifespan, given that there were approximately twice as many deaths and hospitalization days in the control group.[7734] But, as I explain in the video, serious caveats are in order.[7735]

FASTING-MIMICKING DIET

Instead of 5:2, what about 25:5, spending five days a month on a "fasting-mimicking diet"? Longevity researcher Valter Longo designed a five-day meal plan to try to simulate the metabolic effects of fasting by being low in proteins, sugars, and calories with zero animal protein or animal fat. By making it plant-based, he was hoping to lower the level of the cancer-promoting growth hormone IGF-1, related to animal protein consumption, which he accomplished, along with a drop in markers of inflammation, after three cycles of his five-days-a-month program.[7736] Check out see.nf/52fmd for the pros and cons.

Dr. Longo created a company to commercially market his meal plan but says, to his credit, that he donates the profits to his nonprofit research foundation.[7737] The whole diet ("ProLon") appears to be mostly a few dehydrated soup mixes of vegetables, mushrooms, and tomatoes, herbal teas like hibiscus and chamomile, kale chips, nut-based energy bars, an algae-based DHA supplement, and a multivitamin dusted with vegetable powder.[7738] I figure, why spend fifty dollars a day on a few processed snacks when you could instead just eat a few hundred calories a day of real vegetables?

TIME-RESTRICTED EATING AND LONGEVITY

What about fasting a little bit every day? The reason many blood tests are taken after an overnight fast is that meals can tip our systems out of balance, bumping up certain biomarkers for disease, such as blood sugars, insulin, cholesterol, and triglycerides, yet fewer than one in ten Americans may even make it twelve hours a day without eating.[7739] Might it be beneficial to give our body a bigger break?

Time-restricted eating is defined as fasting for periods of at least twelve hours but less than twenty-four.[7740] In see.nf/tre, I present evidence that early time-restricted eating, a narrow eating window shifted toward the morning, carried a variety of metabolic benefits. For example, as I profile in see.nf/earlytre, those randomized to stick to a six-hour eating window ending before 3:00 p.m. experienced a drop in blood pressures, oxidative stress, and insulin resistance even when all the study subjects were maintained at the same weight. The average drop in blood pressures was extraordinary, from 123 over 82 down to 112 over 72 in just five weeks, comparable to the effectiveness of potent blood pressure drugs.[7741]

As I note in see.nf/earlytre, studies suggest that prolonged nightly fasting with reduced evening food intake may decrease cancer risk and recurrence.[7742] It may even play a role in the health of perhaps the longest-living population in the world, the Seventh-day Adventists in California. Slim, vegetarian, nut-eating, exercising, nonsmoking Adventists live about a decade longer than the general population.[7743] Their greater life expectancy has been ascribed to these healthy lifestyle behaviors, but there's one lesser-known component that may be playing a role. Historically, eating two large meals a day, breakfast and lunch, with a prolonged overnight fast was a part of Adventist teachings. Today, only about one in ten Adventists surveyed was eating just two daily meals, but most (63 percent) reported breakfast or lunch was their largest meal of the day.

A study of older Italians found that those who had a food window that was narrower than ten hours a day had 72 percent lower odds of suffering from cognitive impairment. However, this was limited to those practicing early time-restricted feeding (i.e., not skipping breakfast). In general, shifting food intake toward the morning—eating breakfast like a king, lunch like a prince, and dinner like a pauper or skipped entirely—has beneficial cardiometabolic effects, whereas the same eating window pushed toward the evening (skipping breakfast) can have null or negative effects.[7744]

DON'T TRY THIS AT HOME

What about periodic longer fasts? Proponents speak of fasting as a cleansing process, but some of what they are purging from their body are essential vitamins and minerals.[7745] In see.nf/fastingsafety, I cover the very real risks of prolonged fasts. Contrary to the popular notion that the heart muscle is specially spared during fasting, the heart appears to experience similar muscle wasting.[7746] Breaking the fast appears to be the most dangerous part.[7747] After World War II, as many as one in five starved Japanese prisoners of war tragically died following liberation.[7748] Now known as "refeeding syndrome," multiorgan system failure can result from resuming a regular diet too quickly.[7749]

Medically supervised fasting has gotten much safer now that there are proper refeeding protocols, we know what warning signs to look for, and we know who shouldn't be fasting in the first place,[7750] such as those with advanced liver or kidney failure, porphyria, uncontrolled hyperthyroidism, and pregnant and breastfeeding women.[7751] Fasting for longer than twenty-four hours and particularly for three or more days should only be done under the supervision of a physician and preferably in a live-in clinic. This is not just legalistic mumbo jumbo. For example, your kidneys normally dive into sodium conservation mode during fasting, but should that response break down, you could rapidly develop an electrolyte abnormality that may only manifest with nonspecific symptoms, like fatigue or dizziness, which could be easily dismissed until it's too late.[7752]

Fasting for Cancer Treatment

Short-term fasting before and immediately after cancer treatment can minimize side effects while, at the same time, may actually make cancer cells more susceptible.[7753] I review the preclinical studies in see.nf/fastingcancer, including experiments showing how fasting can mean the difference between 100 percent of animals dying versus 100 percent surviving.[7754]

In see.nf/fastingchemo, I run through the clinical trials. Water-only fasting for a total of seventy-two hours before and after chemo appeared to reduce the toxicity of treatment[7755] without detectable harm.[7756] Fasting-mimicking diets have also been tested.

In the DIRECT trial (DIetary REstriction as an Adjunct to Neoadjuvant Chemo-Therapy), more than one hundred breast cancer patients were randomized to the same sort of plant-based, low-calorie, low-protein, and low-carbohydrate fasting-mimicking diet (FMD) of mostly soup, teas, and broth for three days before, and the day of, each chemotherapy cycle. Unfortunately, there was no difference in quality of life or chemo side effects between those randomized to the FMD or those in the regular diet control group. However, a per-protocol analysis did find benefits, meaning that if you took compliance into account and only counted those who actually followed the instructions and stuck to the FMD, they did significantly better across a range of emotional and physical function scores. Isn't that what we care about—what happens when you actually do it? The problem with per-protocol analyses is that we lose the bias-busting power of randomization. For example, maybe people who felt better in the first place were more likely to stick to the program.[7757]

Quality of life aside, did the FMD make the chemo work any better? Fasting-mimicking diets appear to help control cancer in mice, and a series of promising human case reports have been published,[7758] but what happened in the DIRECT trial where it was actually put to the test? There was no significant difference in the most important measure: complete response rate, the disappearance of all signs of cancer from the body. (That occurred in about 11 percent of cases in the FMD group versus 13 percent in the control group.) There was, however, three times the rate of radiological evidence of tumor shrinkage on MRI or ultrasound in the FMD group,[7759] though the impact of this on long-term outcomes is uncertain.[7760] In the per-protocol analysis, there was also an improvement in pathological response (the disappearance of cancer cells in surgical specimens), though, as with any per-protocol analysis, this carries the potential for selection bias.[7761] The lack of more robust evidence of benefit has been blamed on the lack of compliance with the FMD regimen, which was attributed mainly to the dislike of certain prepackaged components. A suggestion was made that future trials consider incorporating fresh foods.[7762]

LOWERING IGF-1 WITH DIETARY RESTRICTION

Is there anything we can tweak in our diet to get similar benefits without having to fast? As I elaborate in see.nf/fmdcancer, one of the ways fasting works is by reducing the levels of the cancer-promoting growth hormone insulin-like growth factor 1[7763] (see the IGF-1 chapter). Reduced levels of IGF-1 appear to mediate the differential protection of normal versus cancer cells in response to fasting because restoration of IGF-1 can be sufficient to reverse the protective effects.[7764] Add chemo to various types of cancer in a petri dish, and half or more of the cancer cells can be wiped out.[7765] Under starvation conditions, the same dose of chemo can wipe out about twice as many cancer cells in a petri dish, but this effect vanishes when IGF-1 is added back to the mix.

The downregulation of IGF-1 through fasting is conceptualized as a way of "turning anti-ageing genes against cancer."[7766] If you remember, the lowering of IGF-1 levels, genetically or otherwise, can lead to a significantly longer lifespan. But fasting isn't the only way to drop IGF-1. Yes, a few days of fasting can cut levels in half,[7767] but that's largely because you're cutting your protein intake. Protein intake is considered a key determinant of circulating IGF-1 levels in humans, suggesting that some of the anticancer and anti-aging benefits of eating less food could be captured by just eating less protein.[7768]

In rodents, caloric restriction alone can reduce IGF-1, but in people, just cutting down on food in general isn't enough.[7769] For example, in the CALERIE trial, two years of caloric restriction didn't lower IGF-1 compared to the control group. This isn't surprising, since there was no concomitant drop in protein intake.[7770] Even severe caloric restriction doesn't decrease IGF-1 levels unless protein intake is also reduced.[7771]

CRONies practicing about a 30 percent caloric restriction for an average of six years had IGF-1 levels similar to those eating a full standard American diet. Again, no surprise, as the CRONies were eating 1.7 g per kg of protein a day, twice the recommended dietary allowance (RDA) of 0.8 g/kg. In contrast, a group of vegans eating right around the RDA for protein had about 25 percent lower IGF-1 levels in their blood. This was assumed to be due to the protein difference, since interventional trials show increasing protein intake increases IGF-1,[7772] but how can we be sure it's not some other factor? By putting it to the test. And indeed, when CRONies eating 1.7 g/kg of protein dropped their intake to 1 g/kg or less, within three weeks their IGF-1 dropped by 25 percent, on par with the vegans.[7773]

PROTEIN RESTRICTION

Reducing protein intake would seem to be a more feasible lifelong strategy than serious long-term caloric restriction,[7774] but the relative contribution of protein restriction to the overall longevity benefits of caloric restriction is controversial. In insects, the life extension from restricting overall food intake appears to be wholly a protein reduction phenomenon,[7775] but in mammals, the data appear to be mixed. There is a body of evidence that suggests that protein restriction alone accounts for approximately half of the life-extending effects of caloric restriction—a 20 percent average increase in maximum lifespan of rodents compared to about 40 percent with caloric restriction.[7776] At the same time, there are rodent studies showing lifespan extension with dietary restriction that appears independent of protein intake—nearly identical longevity from cutting food intake by 40 percent whether or not protein intake is held steady.[7777] More recently, the pendulum has swung in the other direction, suggesting that all the lifespan benefits of caloric restriction derive from the drop in protein intake.[7778] In this chapter, I'll explore how can we account for these discrepancies and what implications this has for human longevity.

FGF21

In the year 2000, a new human hormone was discovered. It was the twenty-first documented fibroblast growth factor, so it was named FGF21.[7779] Since its discovery, it has emerged as a key agent for promotion of metabolic and artery health, leanness, and longevity.[7780] Inject FGF21 into fat monkeys, and they lose body weight without reducing food intake, and not just a little—a 27 percent drop in body fat eating the same amount.[7781] In mice, it increases their lifespan by

30 to 40 percent, comparable to lifelong caloric restriction, but achieved without decreasing food intake.[7782] FGF21 appears to act through multiple aging pathways, boosting AMPK and sirtuin activity,[7783] while inhibiting IGF-1 and mTOR signaling. The thought that FGF21 could potentially be used as a hormone therapy to extend lifespan got Big Pharma salivating,[7784] raising the question, "Can aging be 'drugged'?"[7785]

The idea that one drug could treat obesity, diabetes, and hypertension, all the while slowing aging, might have seemed impossible but suddenly became a tantalizing prospect.[7786] The reason you can't just give people straight FGF21 is that it gets rapidly broken down in the body, so you'd have to get injections every hour or two around the clock.[7787] So, drug companies started to patent a variety of longer-acting FGF21 look-alikes.[7788] And indeed, give people some PF-05231023, and they can lose about ten pounds in twenty-five days, along with dramatic drops in triglycerides and cholesterol.[7789] But then the side effects of these newfangled drugs start cropping up.[7790] What about packaging the FGF21 gene into a virus, then injecting the virus and having it stitch extra FGF21 genes into your DNA?[7791] Or you can just lace up your running shoes.[7792]

EXERCISE AND FASTING TO BOOST FGF21

Exercise boosts FGF21 levels, which may in fact be one of the reasons it's so good for us.[7793] Circulating FGF21 rises immediately after a bout of exercise, peaking an hour afterward and returning to baseline within three hours.[7794] Which works better, though? Aerobic exercise (eight weeks of running training) or resistance exercise (eight weeks of lifting weights)? The answer is both, but the resistance exercise edged out the running, a 42 percent increase in FGF21 versus a 25 percent increase, respectively.[7795]

What can we do with diet? Rather than gene editing or injections, wouldn't it be easier to just stimulate our own endogenous, natural production through diet?[7796] One way is through no diet at all.[7797] FGF21 is known both as the "prolongevity hormone" and the "starvation hormone."[7798] Fasting induces FGF21, but not just a day or two without food.[7799] Unlike mice, which show an increase after only six hours of fasting, humans don't get a notable surge in FGF21 until after a week. Fasting can quadruple FGF21, but that takes ten days of fasting, which is the very poster child of an unsustainable eating pattern.[7800]

HOW TO BOOST FGF21 WITH DIET

How can we get the benefits of fasting without the starvation? Might a ketogenic diet be able to mimic the fast?[7801] In rodents, keto diets raise FGF21 levels,[7802] but in people, they don't work.[7803] In fact, FGF21 levels may drop by 40 percent after one[7804] to three[7805] months on a ketogenic diet. High-fat diets may even interfere with the boost you get from exercise, as demonstrated in a twelve-week study of high-intensity interval training.[7806] Thankfully, the starvation hormone, characterized as a "systemic enhancer of longevity," can be raised by less drastic measures than a prolonged fast:[7807] by eating more carbs and less protein.[7808]

Even without reducing protein intake, FGF21 levels shoot up when people are fed lots of starchy foods.[7809] The healthiest sources would likely be legumes and intact whole grains.[7810] FGF21 is bumped up by butyrate, the short-chain fatty acid our good gut flora make from fiber,[7811] as well as the starch-blocking drug acarbose (at least in mice).[7812] This suggests slow-digesting starches, such as pasta, beans, and intact grains, could have a similar "pro-longevity" effect.[7813]

Circulating FGF21 levels are also "rapidly and robustly" induced by dietary protein restriction. Researchers saw a more than 150 percent increase in FGF21 within four weeks, even in the context of overeating calories.[7814] And the "protein restriction" was just restricting protein intake from the typical excess that most Americans get down close to the recommended amount.

The recommended dietary allowance for protein is around 50 g a day (46 g for women, 56 g for men).[7815] The researchers took men who were averaging twice that—112 g, which is about the average of what many American men get[7816]—and randomized them down to 64 g of protein a day. So, the "protein-restricted" group was still getting more than enough protein. Do that, and you can essentially double FGF21 levels in the blood within about six weeks.[7817] That may help explain why, despite them getting significantly more calories,[7818] they lost more body fat.[7819] How can you eat hundreds more calories a day and still lose two more pounds of straight body fat? By just bringing your protein levels down to recommended levels. Who hasn't fantasized about a diet that allows ingestion of excess calories that are burned off effortlessly by ramping up fat burning?[7820] The researchers concluded that "even a quite modest PR [protein restriction] regimen may have significant clinical benefits."[7821]

A similar study found that even less protein restriction, taking men down to 73 g a day, resulted in a sixfold increase in FGF21 within a single week, accompanied by a significant increase in insulin sensitivity. The researchers concluded that "dietary protein dilution" promotes metabolic health in humans.[7822] Switching men and women from a high-protein diet of 138 g per day down to a more than adequate 67 g[7823] also multiplied FGF21 levels in the blood sixfold, but within just four days.[7824]

FGF21 may help explain the mounting evidence suggesting that a lower protein intake is associated with increased health and survival.[7825] Interestingly, both studies were feeding people about 9 percent of calories from protein, which is what the

Okinawans were getting when they were among the longest-living populations in the world.[7826] However, not all proteins are the same.

ANIMAL PROTEIN VS. PLANT PROTEIN

Some proteins may be more important to restrict than others. FGF21 is considered to be the most important mediator of the metabolic health benefits of restricting the amino acid methionine.[7827] As we know, amino acids are the building blocks of proteins. There are about twenty different kinds of them,[7828] similar to the number of letters in the alphabet. Just as different sentences can be made from different combinations of letters, different proteins are made from stringing together different sequences of the various amino acids. Since methionine is one such amino acid, found predominantly in animal proteins,[7829] we could potentially boost FGF21 levels by lowering methionine intake even without changing overall protein consumption just by switching from animal to plant sources. Legumes (beans, split peas, chickpeas, and lentils) deliver as much as five to ten times less methionine than meat.[7830] (See the chart on page 577.)

FGF21 has been proposed as an explanation for the protection from cancer, autoimmune diseases, obesity, and diabetes afforded by vegan diets.[7831] Maybe that's one of the reasons plant-based interventions have yielded such extraordinary results. Take Dr. Esselstyn's work, for example, suggesting that heart disease, our number one killer, can largely be halted or reversed, and risk for heart attack almost eliminated, with the help of a whole food, low-fat, plant-based diet. This benefit cannot be attributed solely to cholesterol reduction, as we now have powerful drugs that can force cholesterol levels as low as healthy eating can, but the pills appear to have far less effect. So, maybe it's not just the fat and cholesterol but the quantity and quality of protein playing a role.[7832]

Harvard School of Public Health researchers proposed the "protein package" explanation for why plant protein sources are preferable to animal protein sources.[7833] Food is, after all, a package deal, so why get your protein prepackaged with saturated fat and cholesterol when you can get it with fiber and phytonutrients instead? But FGF21 presents a reason why the plant protein itself may be healthier. The theory was first proposed in 2015,[7834] but the first testing of vegan FGF21 levels wasn't published until 2019.[7835]

FGF21 levels were found to be markedly higher in those eating plant-based.[7836] To prove cause and effect, omnivores were switched to a vegetarian diet and the FGF21 levels in their blood shot up by more than 200 percent after just four days free of meat. The bottom line? A major review out of NIH's National Institute on Aging and the USC Longevity Institute published on the clinical applications of fasting concluded that "various fasting approaches are likely to have limited efficacy, particularly on aging and conditions other than obesity, unless combined with high-nourishment diets such as the moderate calorie intake and mostly plant-based Mediterranean or Okinawa low-protein diets. . . ." The researchers specified that by "low protein" they meant 0.8 g of protein per kg of body weight, which is, rather, the recommended daily intake.[7837]

HOW TO LOWER IGF-1 WITH DIET

In mice, protein restriction not only increases lifespan but reduces frailty and improves physical performance later in life. FGF21 is suspected to mediate these benefits because all the anti-aging effects of protein restriction disappear in mice engineered to be unable to express FGF21.[7838] In people, other aging pathways may be involved. Diets with excess protein may be associated with increased oxidative stress[7839] and inflammation, as well as lower levels of NAD^+, which is critical for sirtuin function.[7840] Reducing protein intake can also reduce blood levels of IGF-1.

Low IGF-1 levels predict survival in people with exceptional longevity.[7841] Remember from page 70 how age-related pathologies like cancer were practically absent in those born with lifelong low IGF-1?[7842] IGF-1 appears to mediate the benefits of fasting for cancer,[7843] and its reduction with fasting is what causes the differential protection of normal cells and cancer cells, improving chemo's ability to kill cancer but spare normal cells. We know this because restoration of IGF-1 was sufficient to reverse fasting's protective effects.[7844] Starved cancer cells are more vulnerable to chemo in vitro, but this effect vanishes if the diminished IGF-1 is added back to the petri dish.[7845]

A few days of fasting can cut IGF-1 levels in half,[7846] but that's largely because you're cutting your protein intake.[7847] A key determinant of circulating IGF-1 levels in humans is protein, particularly animal protein. Women[7848] and men[7849] eating strictly plant-based diets have significantly lower IGF-1 levels compared to those eating typical diets, including those who are comparatively slim (long-distance endurance runners).[7850] It's not because they're eating fewer calories, because, when it comes to lower IGF-1 levels, those eating plant-based also beat out CRONies, the members of the Calorie Restriction Society intentionally eating even fewer calories in an attempt to live longer whom I mentioned earlier.

In mice, caloric restriction alone lowers IGF-1,[7851] but people require protein reduction. The IGF-1 levels of practitioners of serious, long-term caloric restriction remain elevated. As I noted before, the reason we suspect it's the protein is, if you take such practitioners and have them cut their protein intake from 1.67 g/kg down to 0.95 g/kg a day, IGF-1 levels drop more than 20 percent within three weeks. IGF-1 is presented as the reason reduced protein intake may represent an important component of anti-aging and anticancer diets.[7852]

Potential Downside of IGF-1 Lowering

For at least twenty years, whole food, plant-based diets have been advocated for slowing the human aging process by way of lowering IGF-1.[7853] IGF-1 also appears causally linked to cancer,[7854] heart disease, diabetes,[7855] and osteoarthritis, so it may help account for a panoply of plant-based perks.[7856] Those born with lower lifetime IGF-1 also have enhanced cognitive performance.[7857] However, as I detail in see.nf/igf1bp, there may be a downside of IGF-1 lowering among those with high blood pressure.[7858] So, those cutting down on animal protein should be particularly mindful of their blood pressure by reducing processed foods and added salt, while ensuring an ample supply of potassium-rich foods, such as beans, sweet potatoes, and dark green leafy vegetables.[7859]

PROTEIN RESTRICTION

Evidence that protein restriction extends lifespan[7860] actually predates the evidence from studies using caloric restriction.[7861] Data on the relative importance of protein versus caloric restriction are mixed,[7862] but a comprehensive comparative meta-analysis of dietary restriction of more than a hundred studies across dozens of species found that when it comes to life extension, protein reduction was more important.[7863] Sometimes it's hard to tease out, though. For example, when studies find that mice restricted to 70 percent of what they'd normally eat live longer, this may be chalked up to caloric restriction, even though protein was cut by the same amount. On the other hand, "protein restriction" studies in which mice are given all-they-can-eat low-protein chow may fail to show benefits because the mice eat more food to compensate, so they don't end up cutting their protein after all.[7864]

The most impressive study to date tried to control for these factors by randomizing nearly a thousand mice to one of twenty-five different diets systematically differing in protein, carbohydrate, fat, and calorie content. They found that the diets with the lowest protein-to-carbohydrate ratios yielded the longest maximum lifespans independent of calories.[7865] Markers of late-life health, including improved blood pressure, cholesterol, mitochondrial function, insulin sensitivity,[7866] and immune function were also best on the low-protein diets and worst on the high-protein or high-fat diets.[7867] Low-protein, high-carbohydrate diets are able to generate the metabolic[7868] and immunity[7869] benefits of up to a 40 percent caloric restriction without restricting calories at all. As the protein levels dropped, average lifespan increased from about 95 weeks to 125 weeks, an approximate 30 percent increase in lifespan even at the same caloric intake.[7870]

The restriction of protein, not calories, was found to be driving the survival effect.[7871] In fact, researchers discovered that only restricting calories appeared to *shorten* lifespans.[7872] How can we square that with past studies with the same mouse strain that found the opposite?[7873] The new twenty-five-diets mega-study used a novel method for restricting calories. The researchers designed all the diets ad libitum. How can you restrict calories if the animals can eat all they want? The calorie-restriction diet was bulked up with indigestible cellulose (basically sawdust) such that even when the mice gorged themselves, they would still be left with a 30 percent calorie deficit.[7874] Yet, despite the caloric restriction, they lived shorter, not longer, lives.[7875]

How do we explain same calories, different effects? Maybe the customary caloric restriction effect is really more of an intermittent fasting effect.[7876] Unlike the cellulose dilution diet where the mice can eat anytime they want, if you just underfeed mice by giving them a fraction of what they'd normally eat, then once they finish their daily ration, they are effectively fasting until the next day. Might the conventional benefits instead be due to hunger signal pathways in the brain you might get from dietary restriction but perhaps not from dietary dilution?[7877] Or maybe traditional caloric restriction cuts protein, too, and that's the real driver of longevity.[7878]

One potential caveat that arose from these series of experiments involves the "protein leverage" effect. On low-protein diets, the mice tended to overeat to try to compensate, so they were in effect eating more calories and still living longer.[7879] Obesity was prevented by feeding them high-fiber diets,[7880] but you can imagine how you wouldn't be doing your body any favors if your idea of a low-protein diet is one filled with ultraprocessed junk like SnackWell's cookies. Indeed, low-protein longevity is undercut in mice fed diets high in refined carbs.[7881] In humans, any negative effects of protein leverage[7882] may be countered by eating whole plant-based foods.[7883]

ANIMAL PROTEIN VS. PLANT PROTEIN

The optimum ratio of protein to carbohydrates across species for lifespan appears to be about one to ten,[7884] which is remarkably similar to the Okinawan ratio.[7885] The traditional Okinawan diet was 9 percent protein and 85 percent carbohydrates (mostly from sweet potatoes, if you recall).[7886] Before they westernized their diets, they had among the highest numbers of centenarians in the world, with 80 percent lower rates of common cancers[7887] and five times lower mortality rates from a variety of age-related diseases in general.[7888] Some have suggested this was due to their relative caloric restriction, consuming about 20 percent fewer net calories than Americans,[7889] but they were also consuming about 50 percent less protein.[7890]

In animal studies, the shortest lifespans were among those fed high-protein diets.[7891] This is consistent with a meta-analysis of prospective human cohort studies showing that higher total protein intake is associated with higher all-cause mortality rates.[7892] But that's because most protein eaten in the Western world comes from animal sources.[7893] The higher the animal protein intake, the higher the mortality rates, whereas the higher the plant protein intake, the lower the mortality rates.[7894]

There is some evidence that those over age sixty-five could benefit from slightly higher protein intakes[7895]—for example, 1.0 g per kg of body weight instead of 0.8 g/kg,[7896] which is still less than what most older Americans get.[7897] However, longevity experts suggest that this should be from plant-based sources to prevent excess IGF-1 activation.[7898] As I mentioned, the NIH-AARP study, based on more than six million person-years of observation, found that swapping just 3 percent of calories from animal protein to plant protein was associated with 10 percent decreased overall mortality in both men and women.[7899] Not all such studies showed this effect,[7900] but a meta-analysis of thirty-two such prospective cohort studies following people for up to thirty-two years found that, overall, as little as a 3 percent increase in plant protein was associated with significantly lower risk of dying from all causes put together.[7901]

Significant improvements in healthspan appear to be achievable by even just a 1 percent animal-to-plant swap. A study of unhealthy aging used a "deficit accumulation index," tracking more than fifty different functional impairments, measures of self-reported health and vitality, mental health indicators, chronic diseases, and needs of health services. Those who increased their plant protein by even 1 percent at the expense of animal protein (a swap of only about 5 g a day) accumulated significantly fewer deficits over a period of eight years.[7902] In the Women's Health Initiative, which followed 100,000 older women for eighteen years, a 5 percent animal-to-plant protein swap was associated with about a 20 percent drop in the risk of dying from perhaps the biggest deficit of all, dementia.[7903] One study even found that swapping out a single serving *a week* of unhealthy protein sources, like eggs, for a healthy source like nuts or whole grains, would hypothetically extend your lifespan.[7904] A 2022 meta-analysis on plant versus animal protein substitutions concluded their findings suggested "introducing plant protein-rich sources to replace animal proteins to prevent aging-related diseases, and promote longevity and healthy aging."[7905]

Even more distinct than the caloric or protein restriction in the Okinawan Japanese was the skew toward plant sources. Animal products constituted less than 1 percent of their traditional diet, the equivalent of one serving of fish a week, other meats once a month, one egg about every two months, and practically no dairy.[7906] As we've discussed, the only formally studied population with a longer life expectancy didn't eat a 99 percent meat-free diet, but rather 100 percent meat-free, the California Adventist vegetarians,[7907] even though they were eating 30 percent over the RDA for protein.[7908] As a review on the impact of protein intake on longevity concluded, the protein source may be more important than the overall level of protein intake,[7909] though, at high enough protein intake, IGF-1 levels may not drop even with a switch to mostly plant-based sources.[7910]

What about randomizing people to a switch from animal to plant sources of protein and also a drop in overall protein intake? Sixteen weeks later, the lower-protein plant-based group lost about ten pounds of straight body fat, including hundreds of cubic centimeters of visceral fat, the dangerous deep belly fat, and experienced a significant decrease in insulin resistance.[7911] In *Ageing Research Reviews*, this study was characterized as suggesting that a decrease in animal protein "may be pivotal in improving metabolic health and aging," but given the concordant drop in animal fat as well, it's hard to tease out the primary driver of metabolic improvements.[7912]

Cancer Restriction via Protein Restriction

T. Colin Campbell and colleagues showed nearly a half century ago that rats on a 5 percent casein (milk protein) diet developed 75 percent fewer precancerous lesions in response to a carcinogen compared to rats fed a 20 percent casein diet.[7913] Protein reduction can extend the lifespans of mice by about 30 percent,[7914] but cancer accounts for more than 90 percent of deaths of common inbred strains of laboratory mice. Given the outsized impact of protein reduction on cancer, we wouldn't expect the same life extension in people, who die more often from heart disease.[7915]

Human cancers show a similar response when transplanted into mice fed different diets. Human breast and prostate tumors show a 56 to 70 percent reduction in cancer growth rates in mice switched from 21 percent of calories from protein down to 7 percent. Even at the higher protein intake, just switching from animal protein to plant protein can decrease tumor weights by 37 percent, though, at the low protein intake, source didn't seem to matter.[7916]

The decrease in tumor size from protein reduction was presumed to be due to a drop in cancer growth fueled by IGF-1,[7917] but low-protein diets were also found to stimulate the targeted killing of cancer cells by the immune system, increasing tumor infiltration by lymphocytes[7918] and enhancing the "tumoricidal capacity" of macrophages.[7919] Low-protein diets can also cause shrinkage of tumors in immune-deficient mice, suggesting it's a combination of factors.[7920] Even just limiting a single amino acid, methionine, can also slow the growth of cancerous tumors.[7921]

METHIONINE RESTRICTION

Just as many of the benefits of dietary restriction can be replicated simply by restricting protein,[7922] most of the benefits of protein restriction may be due to the reduction of just a few of the amino acids that make up proteins, for example, methionine.[7923] Methionine is the only amino acid that strongly correlates with maximum lifespan across mammals, such that the more methionine in body tissues, the shorter the animal lives. ($r = -0.96$ for the stat nerds out there.) The hearts of guinea pigs have about 40 percent more methionine than the hearts of rabbits, which can live about 40 percent longer.[7924] Mice have threefold higher methionine levels than naked mole rats,[7925] which can live seven times longer.[7926] To prove cause and effect, you'd have to show that lowering methionine levels actually prolongs lifespan, and indeed methionine restriction does just that.

Simply restricting that one amino acid can increase the maximum lifespan of rats by up to 44 percent,[7927] more than one tends to see with caloric restriction.[7928] Methionine restriction also prolongs the maximum lifespan of mice, as well as improving stress resistance,[7929] decreasing visceral fat,[7930] and slowing aging of the eyes and immune system.[7931] The exact mechanisms by which reducing dietary methionine leads to slower aging are not known,[7932] but methionine restriction boosts FGF21,[7933] induces autophagy,[7934] and reduces inflammation[7935] and IGF-1.[7936] The IGF-1 pathway may be critical, as mice with growth hormone signaling defects don't respond to methionine restriction,[7937] but there are other possibilities.

In studies in which animals are fed excess amounts of different amino acids, methionine has consistently been found to be the single most toxic one.[7938] This may be because methionine has a pro-oxidant effect.[7939] Supplementing rodent diets with extra methionine results in a spike in oxidative stress markers in their blood[7940] and a depletion of tissue antioxidants.[7941] Conversely, reducing methionine intake profoundly reduces mitochondrial free radical generation and oxidative damage to mitochondrial DNA,[7942] consistent with the mitochondrial theory of aging (see page 109), the only amino acid ever shown to do so. Even restricting every other amino acid except for methionine fails to reproduce this effect.[7943]

Of all the amino acids, methionine is also one of the most vulnerable to oxidation.[7944] When it becomes oxidized while incorporated into a protein, that may lead to the loss of protein function.[7945] Thankfully, there's an enzyme—*methionine sulfoxide reductase*—that repairs this damage to protect cells against methionine-related oxidative damage.[7946] Genetically engineering animals to overexpress just this methionine detox enzyme alone was shown to markedly extend longevity.[7947]

Mild restriction of protein synthesis has been shown to rejuvenate senescent cells, enabling "zombie" cells to start growing again. This was demonstrated in vitro using a drug called cycloheximide, which blocks a final translation step of protein formation. The researchers conclude, "It is desirable to find a substitute for cycloheximide . . . to exert a holistic health promoting effect, to reduce excess or unnecessary protein synthesis. . . ."[7948] This same effect may be had by methionine restriction, because methionine acts as the starting code for the translation of most proteins.[7949] Indeed, reducing the methionine concentration in a cell culture medium can result in a 60[7950] to 75 percent[7951] increase in the replicative lifespan of human cells (the Hayflick limit, the number of times a cell can double before becoming senescent—see page 38). Methionine-restricted cells are also significantly better at robustly resisting various stressors, including heat, radiation, carcinogens, and free radicals.[7952]

HOW TO LOWER METHIONINE INTAKE

Pharmaceutical companies are fighting to be the first to come out with a drug that decreases methionine levels[7953]—methionine-munching enzymes to give to patients with advanced cancer, for example.[7954] But, since methionine is sourced mainly from food, a better strategy may be to lower methionine levels by lowering methionine intake.[7955] There are three ways to accomplish this. The first is caloric restriction—by decreasing your intake of food in general, you reduce your intake of methionine. The purported pro-longevity benefits of alternate-day fasting,[7956] for instance, have been ascribed to the periodic depletion of the "pro-aging amino-acid methionine."[7957] Second, since methionine is in protein, instead of reducing food intake across the board, you could just cut down on protein. Simply reducing protein intake from present excessive levels down to the recommended intake is expected to offer a large potential for health benefit.[7958] Third, even keeping portions and protein consumption the same, methionine restriction could be accomplished by switching from animal to plant protein sources, which tend to be relatively low in methionine. To achieve methionine restriction, a review on the impact of dietary protein intake on health and longevity concluded that individuals may need to "eat less animal-based food."[7959]

Termed the Hoffman effect, one of the universal hallmarks of cancer is "methionine addiction."[7960] The methionine dependency of cancer cells has led to attempts to feed cancer patients a methionine-free "amino acid–modified medical food powder." Made mostly out of corn syrup, oil, and all the other amino acids, it is meant to crowd out methionine sources in the daily diet.[7961] The problem is that it's considered "not palatable," so few people stick with it.[7962] Failed compliance with these oily corn syrup concoctions has led researchers to conclude it is "necessary to develop palatable foods in which methionine has been selectively removed." We already have them. They're called fruits and vegetables.

WHERE IS METHIONINE FOUND?

Plant-based diets may "make methionine restriction feasible as a life extension strategy."[7963] Here's a graph comparing bioavailable methionine levels in common representative plant and animal foods:[7964,7965,7966]

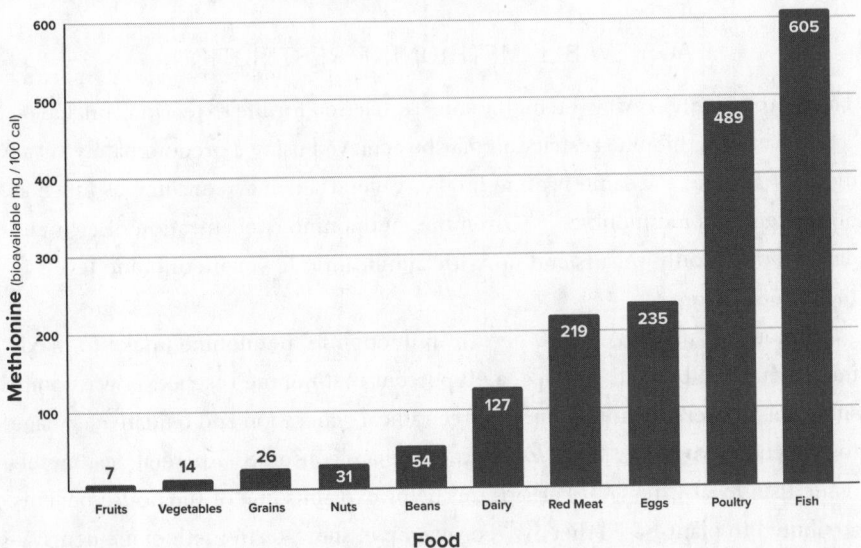

Methionine Content of Foods

As you can see, fish and poultry tend to have the highest levels of methionine. I used canned tuna as the representative fish, but a hundred calories of fish such as haddock, halibut, or roughy can deliver even worse levels, up to 709 mg. The lowest seafood levels are found in oysters, with levels as low as 92. For poultry, I graphed grilled chicken breast, though roasted chicken breast can reach 587.

Dairy, red meat, and eggs have less. I used hard-boiled eggs, but a whites-only omelet could top the charts at 714. I used ground beef as the representative red meat, but pork and lamb can go as high as 509 and 564, respectively (though blood sausage dips as low as 49). I used milk for dairy in the graph, though a dairy product like butter has nearly none, since it's almost all fat. In contrast, high-protein dairy foods like low-fat cottage cheese can go as high as 482.

The lowest methionine foods tend to be fruits, nuts, veggies, grains, and beans. I used canned chickpeas, but all the other beans have similar amounts, even the "methionine-rich" legume,[7967] the kidney bean, at 65. Only when plant protein is concentrated into a food like tofu can you get up around 114. For grains, I used whole-wheat bread, but teff, the most methionine-rich grain, has 99, followed by quinoa with 64. For nuts, I used mixed nuts. Most nuts are similar, with the exception of Brazil nuts at 136. Hemp seeds are also high (135). For vegetables, I used carrots. Spinach is surprisingly high at 184, but it's so low-calorie that you'd have to eat about fifteen cups to get a hundred calories. Kale is lower, at 66 for fourteen cups. I used bananas for fruit, but even oranges, the common fruit highest in methionine, average only 34.

ACHIEVABLE METHIONINE RESTRICTION

The bottom line: A review on methionine restriction for life extension concluded, "In humans, methionine restriction may be achieved using a predominately vegan diet."[7968] Even at the same protein intake, vegetarians may consume as much as 36 percent less methionine.[7969] Given the methionine concentration of eggs and dairy, though, only vegans end up with significantly lower methionine levels in their bloodstream.[7970]

Although it may take an 80 percent reduction in methionine intake to maximize metabolic benefits in mice, a 40 percent methionine restriction was found sufficient to decrease mitochondrial free radical generation and oxidative damage to mitochondrial DNA.[7971,7972] On average, vegans consume 47 percent less methionine than meat eaters.[7973] Perhaps this helps explain some of the health benefits attributed to plant-based diets.[7974] For example, short-term methionine deprivation can slim 60 percent of the fat mass off obese mice within two weeks, despite increased caloric intake and decreased physical activity[7975] (by apparently activating a "futile cycle" of simultaneous fat formation and consumption[7976]).

So, maybe methionine reduction helps explain why vegans are forty pounds lighter on average than those who eat conventional diets.[7977] Even vegans at the same weight as typical omnivores appear to have less than half the risk of diabetes,[7978] consistent with a 2022 analysis that followed about 15,000 U.S. adults for seventeen years and found that those who ate the most methionine had more than twice the risk of dying from diabetes.[7979]

On average, American women effectively consume twice as much methionine as they need and American men three times as much.[7980] Given the cardiometabolic risk associated with higher intake, public health researchers suggest that the optimum intake may be down around the recommended intake.[7981] So, just as I'm not advocating for a low-protein diet but rather a diet with the recommended amount, one need not eat a low-methionine diet but rather just one without *excess* methionine. Given what we now know, simply decreasing intake to recommended levels "has a great potential to lower tissue oxidative stress and to increase healthy life span in humans. . . ."[7982]

Cysteine and Glycine

Much of the methionine we eat is converted into another amino acid within the body, called *cysteine*.[7983] Given that the provision of extra cysteine to methionine-restricted animals reverses some of the benefit, cysteine might be responsible for some of methionine's dirty work.[7984] While cysteine may be a partner in crime, the amino acid *glycine* is used by the body to aid in clearance of methionine from the system.[7985] I go into detail on both in see.nf/cysteineglycine. The bottom line is that you get more glycine in your bloodstream the same way you get less methionine and cysteine: by eating more plant-based.[7986,7987]

BRANCHED-CHAIN AMINO ACIDS

The effects of protein restriction can't be completely replicated with methionine restriction alone, since the dietary restriction of all amino acids except methionine continues to have a range of beneficial effects, such as a reduction in free radical production and oxidative DNA damage.[7988] Also to blame may be the three branched-chain amino acids (BCAA)—isoleucine, leucine, and valine.

In the twenty-five-diets mega-study, health and longevity consequences negatively correlated with BCAA levels in the blood, such that the lowest amounts were associated with the longest, healthiest lives.[7989] Interventional studies show that high-BCAA diets shorten mouse lifespans,[7990] whereas BCAA restriction increases the lifespan and delays age-related frailty in fruit flies[7991] and mice.[7992] The researchers suggest "limiting dietary levels of BCAAs may be a key to a long and healthy life."[7993]

This makes sense since BCAAs are potent activators of the engine-of-aging enzyme mTOR,[7994] which I explored in Part I. Reducing mTOR signaling is considered "critical for improved health and lifespan,"[7995] as mTOR suppression is a "robust molecular transducer of diet-induced antiaging signals."[7996] Lower BCAA intake may help explain not only Okinawan longevity but why a disease like acne was rare or even nonexistent,[7997] as pimples are considered a visual manifestation of elevated mTOR activity.[7998] Insight into potential cognitive effects comes from maple syrup urine disease.

The irreversible breakdown of branched-chain amino acids is tightly regulated within the body.[7999] Babies born with a rare congenital defect in detoxifying BCAAs develop sweet-smelling urine and can go on to suffer encephalopathy, brain swelling, and death. The disease clearly shows that large excesses of BCAAs are hazardous to the brain, raising the question of whether milder elevations might also be neurotoxic.[8000] In a mouse model of Alzheimer's disease, high-BCAA diets made cognitive performance worse, whereas low-BCAA diets made it better.[8001] This is consistent with a Mendelian randomization analysis that found that people born with a genetic predisposition to higher isoleucine levels were significantly more likely to develop Alzheimer's disease,[8002] but a meta-analysis of eight cohort studies found that higher levels of BCAAs (including isoleucine) were associated with a *lower* risk of dementia.[8003]

The BCAA literature seems surprisingly rife with this kind of contradictory evidence, with studies suggesting that BCAAs have harmful, harmless, or helpful effects on aging and age-related conditions.[8004] For example, there was an observational study that found that higher BCAA intakes were associated with a significantly lower all-cause mortality.[8005] With "such levels of complexity," concluded a recent review on BCAAs and aging, "there is unlikely to be any unifying conclusion about overall benefits or harms of BCAAs in older people."[8006] However, at least when it comes to metabolic effects, we have human interventional trials to prove harms or benefits one way or another.

BCAAs AND INSULIN RESISTANCE

Insulin resistance is the cause of prediabetes and type 2 diabetes.[8007] Even in nondiabetics, insulin resistance[8008] and the elevated blood sugars that can result[8009] are associated with premature death, based on meta-analyses of prospective cohort studies. (For a backgrounder on what insulin resistance is and what it does, see my Low Insulin Index chapter in *How Not to Diet*.) Insulin resistance, the inability of our body to sufficiently respond to the blood sugar–lowering hormone insulin, can be caused by the intake of saturated fat (see.nf/insulin), as well as the intake of branched-chain amino acids.[8010] It turns out a BCAA breakdown product appears to stimulate fat uptake and accumulation inside the muscle cells,[8011] which interferes with insulin signaling.[8012]

Reducing BCAA intake in obese mice reduced insulin resistance, caused dramatic fat loss even without a reduction of calories, and restored metabolic health,[8013] whereas a high-BCAA diet induces mouse obesity.[8014] In people, an "overwhelming" number of studies[8015] have consistently shown that blood and urine levels of branched-chain amino acids are tied to insulin resistance. In fact, increased BCAA in the blood, dubbed the "BCAA signature," is a hallmark of obesity and diabetes.[8016] This doesn't necessarily mean that decreasing intake of BCAAs will help, though, since there are other factors that influence levels in the blood.[8017]

Yes, BCAAs can cause insulin resistance,[8018] but insulin resistance also seems to cause an increase in BCAA levels[8019] due to a reduction in BCAA breakdown, potentially leading to a positive feedback loop that can spiral out of control.[8020]

The epidemiology is contradictory, though.[8021] The microbiome has even been thrown into the mix by a study of twin pairs showing that a fecal transplant from a heavier twin increases blood BCAA levels in mice more than a fecal transplant from the thinner twin.[8022] The proof is in the pudding, though. Just like you can make someone insulin-resistant by infusing fat into their bloodstreams,[8023] you can do the same by infusing BCAAs.[8024] Just as a single dose of butter can cause insulin resistance within hours, so can downing a protein drink of straight whey and water.[8025,8026]

This may help explain the results of the study I detailed in the FGF21 section above (see page 565), in which protein intakes were dropped from typical American diet levels down to recommended levels. Not only did FGF21 double within about six weeks compared to the control group, but the drop in BCAA levels in the participants' blood was accompanied by a significant drop in blood sugars and pounds of fat loss despite averaging hundreds more calories a day.[8027] Given the restoration of metabolic health demonstrated by decreasing consumption of branched-chain amino acids, leaders in the field have suggested the invention of pharmaceuticals to block BCAA absorption to "promote metabolic health and treat diabetes and obesity without reducing caloric intake."[8028] Or, we can just try to not eat so many branched-chain amino acids in the first place.

BCAA Supplements

Branched-chain amino acid supplements are a multimillion-dollar business, marketed for the widely believed claim that BCAAs can boost muscle mass by stimulating muscle protein synthesis,[8029] a belief based on rat studies going back more than forty years.[8030] Yet, the only two human studies showed that BCAAs actually cause a *reduction* in muscle protein synthesis.[8031,8032] I review the somewhat mixed research on BCAA supplementation in older adults in see.nf/bcaas, but basically, we're left with the bottom line of a recent review in a journal of exercise metabolism: "In conclusion, the proposed benefits of BCAA used in the marketing of supplements appear to be at odds with the overall state of the current literature, which does not support the efficacy of supplementation on muscle strength and hypertrophy [size]."[8033]

HOW TO LOWER BCAA INTAKE

Since BCAAs are mostly found in meat, including chicken and fish, dairy products, and eggs,[8034] this may explain why animal protein intake intensifies insulin resistance[8035] and is associated with higher diabetes risk,[8036] whereas plant foods tend to have the opposite effect. Substituting in even just 5 percent of plant protein for animal protein may decrease diabetes risk by more than 20 percent.[8037] Although fasting blood levels of BCAAs taken in the morning don't necessarily correlate with dietary intake,[8038] meals high in animal protein can quadruple levels in the bloodstream, which can remain elevated for seven to eight hours.[8039]

A crossover clinical trial found that those randomized to replace just two servings of meat for lentils, chickpeas, split peas, or beans a few days a week can significantly improve fasting blood sugars and insulin levels, beyond just the improvements you'd expect, like lower cholesterol and triglycerides.[8040] Based on more than a dozen randomized controlled trials, even just swapping a third or so of protein from animal to plant sources can significantly improve blood sugar control.[8041]

Like methionine, branched-chain amino acid intake is lower among vegetarians compared to omnivores, but only vegans achieve significantly lower fasting levels in their blood, consuming 30 percent less compared to only about 15 percent less among vegetarians.[8042] Randomizing people to a strictly plant-based diet for a month can significantly drop fasting levels of all three BCAAs, which correlated with anti-inflammatory effects of the switch.[8043]

BCAAs may explain why those randomized to a plant-based diet eliminate significantly more of the deeper, more dangerous fat, even when taking in the same number of calories.[8044] Those eating plant-based also had lower levels of fat stuck inside individual muscle fibers themselves, which may help explain why vegans in particular are often found to have the lowest odds of diabetes.[8045,8046] It's not only because they're slimmer. Even if you match subjects pound for pound, significantly less fat has been found inside the muscle cells of vegans compared to omnivores, as measured in one of their calf muscles.[8047] It is therefore no wonder why those eating plant-based diets average significantly lower insulin levels and have less insulin resistance, even compared to nonvegetarians at the same body weight.[8048,8049]

Those who eat meat have up to 50 percent higher insulin levels in their bloodstreams.[8050,8051] Compared to a control group who made no dietary changes, people randomized to a plant-based diet experienced a significant drop in insulin resistance, fasting blood sugars, and insulin levels.[8052] But add some egg whites to a plant-based diet, and you can cause a "dramatic"[8053] rise in insulin output—by as much as 60 percent within just four days.[8054] Add tuna to mashed potatoes, and the insulin reaction is about 50 percent higher than eating the mashed potatoes alone.[8055] Adding broccoli instead, however, results in the insulin response being cut by about 40 percent within the first thirty minutes after consumption.[8056] This didn't appear to be a fiber effect, either, since giving the equivalent amount of isolated broccoli fiber provided no significant benefit. The differential effect of plant versus animal protein has been attributed to their contrasting amino acid profiles.[8057]

The reason branched-chain amino acids are suspected is, if you give some vegans straight BCAA supplements, you can make them as insulin-resistant as omnivores, in effect proving that BCAAs can have a direct negative impact on insulin sensitivity.[8058] Conversely, take some omnivores and put them through even just a "48-hour vegan diet challenge," and you can produce significant improvements in metabolic health.[8059] After two days on a healthy plant-based diet, not only did cholesterol and triglycerides drop but so did insulin and insulin resistance, presumed to be due in part to the "strong modulatory effect" on circulating BCAA levels. This has been suggested to explain some of the lifespan benefits of plant-based diets,[8060] but because the benefits appeared so rapidly, the researchers suggested metabolic benefits could be gotten from an "intermittent vegan diet" or even the "flexitarian approach" of alternating between animal and plant protein choices.[8061]

Turning It Up to Eleven

Note that protein restriction is the only intervention in the chart on page 148 that blocks every one of the eleven aging pathways, yet the prevailing dogma in our society is to eat more protein.[8062] A survey of U.S. adults suggests that about 65 percent are trying to do just that.[8063] Although high-protein diets can help with compliance in weight-loss interventions,[8064] they do not align with the protein reduction recommended in anti-aging diets.[8065] The best available balance of evidence supports the advice of longevity experts like Drs. Valter Longo[8066] and Luigi Fontana to advise cutting down on protein to live longer: "Eating more protein than what is needed . . . will not increase muscle mass but will accelerate aging and increase the risk of developing many chronic diseases."[8067]

NAD⁺

Our understanding of *nicotinamide adenine dinucleotide* (NAD⁺) arose from humble beginnings as a factor noted to enhance yeast fermentation in a 1906 paper unassumingly titled "The Alcoholic Ferment of Yeast-Juice."[8068] Little did the authors know that waves of NAD-related discoveries would go on to yield, thus far, a total of four Nobel Prizes.[8069] NAD⁺ is now known as an essential molecule for all living organisms,[8070] required for the function of about five hundred enzymatic reactions,[8071] including, notably, the extraction of metabolic energy from food.[8072] The twenty-first century has produced yet another scientific renaissance for NAD⁺ with the realization that it was critical for the activity of sirtuins,[8073] those "guardians of mammalian healthspan"[8074] I detail in Part I.

NAD$^+$ is one of the most abundant molecules in our body. Once considered relatively stable, it is now known to be in a constant state of synthesis, recycling, and breakdown.[8075] Our pool of NAD$^+$ is turned over as often as several times a day.[8076] To maintain cellular vitality in the face of this turnover, an adequate supply of NAD$^+$ precursors and sufficiently high NAD$^+$-synthesizing enzyme activity is critical.[8077] The importance of NAD$^+$ is exemplified by the devastating consequences of a deficiency of its precursors like niacin (vitamin B$_3$).[8078] The deficiency syndrome, called *pellagra*, is characterized by the four Ds: dermatitis, dementia, diarrhea, and, eventually, death.[8079]

Thankfully, since life as we know it can't exist without it,[8080] NAD$^+$ and its precursors are found in everything we eat—plant, animal, or fungi.[8081] The niacin in corn is tightly bound up but can be released by presoaking in alkaline limewater. Sadly, when maize was exported from Latin America to become a dietary staple elsewhere without the requisite knowledge about traditional processing techniques, an epidemic of pellagra ensued.[8082] An estimated 100,000 Americans died from pellagra in the first few decades of the twentieth century before bread started to be fortified with niacin in 1938.[8083]

DO NAD$^+$ LEVELS DECLINE WITH AGE?

The pitch for NAD$^+$ boosting as an anti-aging strategy is as follows: All species, including humans, naturally experience a decline in NAD$^+$ levels over time, and this decline is in fact one of the major reasons organisms age.[8084] By restoring youthful levels, the argument goes, these age-related disorders can be delayed or even reversed.[8085] Two leaders in the field, one from Harvard and the other from MIT, have said, respectively, that NAD$^+$ boosters may "hold the promise of increasing the body's resilience, not just to one disease, but to many, thereby extending healthy human lifespan"[8086] and that sirtuin activation by NAD$^+$ repletion "may be the most actionable item to emerge from aging research."[8087] Of course, both of them have been involved with multimillion-dollar dietary supplement companies.[8088,8089]

The first premise, that NAD$^+$ levels decline with age, has been called into question. For example, a 2022 review titled "Age-Dependent Decline of NAD$^+$— Universal Truth or Confounded Consensus?" concluded that, despite systemic claims to the contrary, the evidence supporting the premise is very limited.[8090] Indeed, the most comprehensive study to date found significant changes in NAD$^+$ levels in only about half of tested tissues in old versus young mice.[8091] The human data, which I review in see.nf/nadecline, are similarly inconsistent.

The bottom line is that, given the conflicting findings from the remarkably few studies on the subject, it is misleading to say NAD^+ universally decreases with age.[8092] Regardless, the proof is in the pudding. What about the second premise, that boosting levels late in life can improve health and longevity?

INCREASED HEALTHSPAN AND LIFESPAN IN RODENTS

The effects of NAD^+ boosters on aged rodents have been described in the medical literature as "dramatic" and "remarkable."[8093] Treated mice had increased physical activity[8094] and endurance, improved vision, and strengthened bones,[8095] while delaying, preventing, or reversing muscle atrophy,[8096] hearing loss,[8097] ovarian aging,[8098] and cognitive decline.[8099] Benefits to nearly every organ system have been documented,[8100] including improved functions of the arteries,[8101] brain,[8102] heart,[8103] immune system,[8104] kidneys,[8105] liver,[8106] and muscles. For example, a single week of a NAD^+ booster was sufficient to restore key markers of muscle health in a twenty-two-month-old mouse to levels similar to those of a six-month-old mouse.[8107] That's roughly the equivalent of reverting those of a seventy-year-old person back to age twenty.[8108]

NAD^+ boosters can also extend the lifespans of other animals, presumed to be due to the elevation of NAD^+-dependent sirtuin activity.[8109] This longevity effect was first demonstrated more than twenty years ago in yeast cells. An overexpression of the genes involved in NAD^+ synthesis extended replicative lifespans by up to 60 percent.[8110] In the microscopic worm *C. elegans*, NAD^+-boosting compounds have been shown to extend lifespans by up to 16 percent.[8111] In mice, one NAD^+ booster was able to extend lifespan by a more modest 5 percent, but this was accomplished even when supplementation was started late in life, which is unusual for longevity treatments.[8112]

No wonder people are excited about all manner of NAD^+-boosting supplements. The big question is whether any of these healthspan or lifespan effects translate to humans.[8113]

NAD+-BOOSTING SUPPLEMENTS

There are four major NAD^+-boosting supplements on the market these days: nicotinic acid (NA), also known as niacin, nicotinamide (NAM), also known as niacinamide, nicotinamide riboside (NR), and nicotinamide mononucleotide (NMN). NAD^+ can also be given directly, as can the hydrogenated form NADH. There are also hydrogenated forms of NMN (NMNH) and NR (NRH). So, there is quite the alphabet soup: NAD, NA, NAM, NR, NMN, NADH, NMNH, and NRH. Our body can also make NAD^+ from scratch from the amino acid tryptophan. Given the critical nature of NAD$^+$, it is perhaps unsurprising that the body has so many different pathways utilizing a panoply of precursors.[8114]

Converting tryptophan to NAD$^+$ requires eight steps, whereas NA, NAM, and NR can be turned into NAD$^+$ in only two or three steps.[8115] NMN is a direct precursor of NAD$^+$, but when NMN or NR is taken orally, it appears to just turn into NA or NAM via rapid degradation in the bloodstream[8116] or active conversion in the liver or by the microbiome.[8117] So, why take the more expensive NMN or NR if it's just going to end up as NA or NAM? Bought in bulk, NA or NAM would cost just pennies a day versus more like a dollar a day for NR or NMN. That would add up to hundreds of dollars a year for NR or NMN compared to closer to five bucks for NA or NAM. But is it worth taking any of them?

NICOTINIC ACID (NA)

The name nicotinic acid was changed to niacin in the 1940s to avoid any confusion with nicotine.[8118] Either name has to be better than the original moniker, though: vitamin PP (for *pellagra preventing*).[8119]

In the 1950s, NA became the world's first cholesterol-lowering drug.[8120] This led to about two dozen trials involving tens of thousands of individuals taking high-dose NA for up to five years,[8121] resulting in by far the most robust safety data we have on any of the NAD$^+$ precursors. The most striking benefit was found in the Coronary Drug Project, a trial carried out in the pre–statin drug era of the 1960s and 1970s. The fifteen-year follow-up found that those who had been randomized to years of high-dose NA ended up with a 6.2 percent drop in absolute mortality (52 percent had died in the NA group versus 58.2 percent in the placebo group).[8122] This sparked major clinical trials that, sadly, failed so spectacularly that one was even stopped prematurely.[8123, 8124]

All in all, a Cochrane meta-analysis concluded that "no evidence of benefits from niacin therapy" was found.[8125] One possible explanation for the contrasting results is that the promising early trials used immediate-release niacin, and the newer failed trials used slow-release formulations (also known as extended or sustained release).[8126] At high doses, regular niacin commonly causes an intense flushing redness and prickly heat sensation, similar to a menopausal hot flash. A slow-release version was developed to reduce the flushing reaction, catapulting it into a billion-dollar blockbuster drug,[8127] but it simply doesn't work as well to reduce cholesterol.[8128]

The major clinical trial failures led to the withdrawal of the drug in Europe[8129] and its removal from U.S. clinical guidelines for cardiovascular disease prevention.[8130] There still may be a role for niacin preparations in the treatment of heart disease among patients who cannot tolerate statin drugs,[8131] but what about use for the general public as an NAD^+ booster?

There is a series of rare genetic defects that can lead to a condition called *mitochondrial myopathy* that's characterized by low NAD^+ levels in the blood and muscles. In 2020, researchers demonstrated that these levels could be repleted with 750 to 1,000 mg a day of NA, which led to a significant improvement in their muscle strength.[8132] This was the first and only study to show muscle NAD^+ levels and performance improving with any sort of NAD^+ booster.[8133] In a control group of individuals without the genetic defect, blood levels of NAD^+ were raised by NA, but not muscle levels, suggesting that in normal healthy muscles, NAD^+ levels are already "topped off."[8134] As you'll see, this is a recurring theme among NAD^+ boosters.

We know that large doses of NA can boost NAD^+ levels in human blood,[8135] but a corresponding increase in sirtuin activity has yet to be demonstrated.[8136] Why not give it a try? Because of the side effects unearthed in the cholesterol-lowering trials. NA raises blood sugars[8137] and may increase your risk of developing diabetes. Based on studies of tens of thousands of individuals on high-dose NA followed for years, one would expect that one in forty-three people taking NA for five years would develop diabetes who otherwise wouldn't have.[8138] It's unclear if this risk is only limited to slow-release formulations.[8139]

The safety buffer, the ratio between the tolerable upper limit and the RDA, is the lowest for NA compared to a half dozen other common vitamins.[8140] However, the upper limit is based on the flushing reaction,[8141] which, although uncomfortable, is considered harmless and tends to dissipate over time.[8142] Long-term use can have other adverse consequences, though, including stomach ulcers, vomiting, abdominal pain, diarrhea, jaundice, and other signs of liver damage (particularly with slow-release formulations).[8143] There is also a theoretical concern that excessive NA intake may contribute to the development of Parkinson's disease.[8144] Due to the unpleasant flushing and risk of more serious side effects, interest has moved toward other NAD^+ precursors.[8145]

NICOTINAMIDE (NAM)

Ever since nicotinamide (NAM) was also shown to cure pellagra,[8146] both NA and NAM have been collectively referred to as niacin or vitamin B_3, though they are distinct compounds.[8147] For example, NAM is not plagued by the same kind of hot flash reaction. (Facial flushing attributed to niacinamide in some older studies was likely due to a less purified form contaminated with residual NA.[8148])

The relative capacity of NA versus NAM to generate NAD^+ is unclear.[8149]

Neither has been demonstrated to boost sirtuin activity,[8150] but both do extend the lifespan of *C. elegans*.[8151] I couldn't find any longevity trials for NA in rodents; however, NAM was put to the test and failed to prolong the lives of mice.[8152] What clinical effects might we expect in people?

I explored the proven anti-aging effects for topical nicotinamide on the skin and the remarkable ability of oral nicotinamide to help prevent skin cancer (see page 456). It failed to prevent type 1 diabetes, despite promising mouse data,[8153] though it may help preserve residual function in people newly diagnosed with type 1 diabetes, but apparently not enough to affect blood sugar control.[8154] What about its use as a NAD$^+$ booster?

In those with mitochondrial myopathy, NA had raised muscle NAD$^+$ levels and improved mitochondrial and muscle function, but in healthy individuals, muscle NAD$^+$ levels didn't budge. However, the average age of the control group individuals was fifty. What about in older adults whose muscle NAD$^+$ levels might potentially be lower? Four NAD$^+$ precursors were tested in older adults: tryptophan, NA, NAM, and NR. They all failed to improve muscle strength or function, affect mitochondrial function, and even nudge NAD$^+$ levels in their muscles.[8155,8156] Why not give it a try? Again, side effects.

Like NA, high-dose NAM can cause gastrointestinal disturbances and signs of liver toxicity.[8157] However, NAM may result in more issues involving methylation.[8158] The primary first step in breaking down excess NAM is to transfer a methyl group to it, forming MeNAM. MeNAM can cross the blood-brain barrier[8159] and has been shown to be toxic to nerve cells in vitro.[8160] This may explain why NAM can cause Parkinson's-like symptoms in rats[8161] and why Parkinson's patients may have higher levels of the NAM-methylating enzyme in their brains.[8162] Excess NAM may also deplete the body's pool of methyl groups.

If you remember from the Epigenetics chapter, DNA methylation is critical for the regulation of gene expression. Epigenetic changes caused by NAM-induced methyl depletion[8163] have been blamed as the reason why rats fed megadoses of NAM suffer from fatty livers and swollen kidneys,[8164] but that was at a human-equivalent dose far exceeding what people might take.[8165] Is there any evidence that more modest NAM supplementation might affect methylation humans? Yes, even with a single dose as low as 100 mg.

Methylation also plays a key role in breaking down fight-or-flight hormones like noradrenaline and neurotransmitters like serotonin and histamine. Within hours of a single 100-mg NAM dose, blood levels of all three become elevated, suggesting that their metabolism had been impaired by the shunting of methyl groups to deal with the excess NAM.[8166] Also noted was a significant rise in homocysteine,[8167] a by-product of methylation reactions and a risk factor for cardiovascular disease and dementia.[8168] (See, for example, page 386.)

Another potential problem with NAM is that it's a sirtuin inhibitor.[8169] Wasn't the whole purpose of taking NAD^+ precursors to *boost* sirtuin activity? Sirtuin enzymes use up NAD^+ and spit out NAM. This allows the body to recycle the NAM back into NAD^+ for further sirtuin use. But this also means that the body can use NAM as part of a negative feedback loop. Like a thermostat in the winter that shuts down the furnace when there's too much heat, the body shuts down NAD^+ use by sirtuins when it detects too much NAM. There was no such thing as NAM pills when our body evolved. So, in the wake of a sudden wave of NAM, the body must think sirtuins are churning out too much and dials them back. Perhaps this explains why NAM failed to prolong the lifespans of mice.[8170] When the sirtuin-suppressing effects of NAM were first reported twenty years ago, the researchers cautioned that this could potentially lead to "deleterious consequences of long-term nicotinamide therapy in humans."[8171]

NICOTINAMIDE RIBOSIDE (NR)

NR and NMN seem to be more promising NAD^+ precursors than NA or NAM, since they don't cause flushing or directly inhibit sirtuins.[8172] In mice, NR and NMN both raise liver NAD^+ levels, but only NR raises NAD^+ in the muscles.[8173] Also, NR is so far the only NAD^+ booster shown to prolong the lifespan of mice.[8174]

There have been at least ten clinical trials of NR showing that it can boost human blood levels of NAD^+ up to 168 percent. Note, though, that most of the doses used exceeded 300 mg, the daily dose approved as safe by the FDA and the European Food Safety Authority.[8175] At the approved dose, blood NAD^+ is boosted more on the order of 50 to 60 percent,[8176] but no dose was found to affect NAD^+ levels in human muscle (compared to placebo).[8177,8178,8179,8180]

The greater preponderance of human bioavailability and safety data for NR compared to NMN has led some to proclaim NR as the preferred NAD^+ precursor. And, by some, I mean employees of a chemical company that produces NR for supplements.[8181] The question after all these human NR trials is, *have any of them shown clinical benefit?* Sadly, no.[8182]

After accounting for the sheer number of variables tested, randomized, double-blind, placebo-controlled trials of NR in young, middle-aged, and older adults failed to find any significant benefit over placebo for artery function, artery stiffness, balance,[8183,8184] BAT activation (see page 221), blood pressure, blood sugar control,[8185,8186] body weight,[8187] cardiac energy or ejection fraction,[8188] fat burning,[8189,8190] fatty liver,[8191] exercise capacity, fatigue, insulin sensitivity,[8192,8193] metabolic flexibility,[8194] metabolic health, metabolic rate,[8195,8196] mitochondrial function[8197] or biogenesis,[8198] muscle blood flow,[8199] upper or lower body muscle strength,[8200,8201] pancreatic function or the release of metabolic hormones,[8202] treatment of Parkinson's disease symptoms,[8203] or physical performance.[8204,8205] NR company stockholders can claim that NR is anti-inflammatory,[8206] but in their own study, only three out of ten markers of inflammation were affected[8207] and a subsequent independent study at the same dose that ran for twice as long found that *zero* markers out of twelve were affected.[8208]

Remarkably, the opposite was found for many of these outcomes in rats and mice. In rodents, NR does raise NAD^+ levels in muscle, improving mitochondrial biogenesis and function, fat burning, insulin sensitivity, metabolic health, and on down much of the list.[8209] Why does NR work in rodents but appear to almost entirely flop in people? Some have suggested inadequate dosing.[8210] The typical dose used in mouse studies was about twice that used in many human studies, but a double dose has been tried in people to no avail.[8211]

Another possibility is sirtuin inhibition by NAM, the main degradation product of NR.[8212] Based on mouse studies, NR may metabolize to NAM or NA in the gut before it even makes it into the bloodstream.[8213] Either way, unlike in mice, NR can't seem to elevate NAD^+ in human muscle, so it's no wonder that no alteration of human sirtuin activity was found in muscle biopsies.[8214] That may explain the disparate results. In fact, the key NAD^+-synthesizing enzyme in human muscle biopsies was actually suppressed by NR supplementation. This doesn't happen in mice, but it does in us. Presumably, this downregulation is an adaptive response to the unnaturally large flood of NR coming into the system.[8215]

In mice, not only may their microbiome affect NR, but the NR may affect their microbiome. Some of the benefits of NR can be transferred between mice via fecal transplants. So, at least in mice, some of the benefits of NR may be due to modulating their microbiome. The distinct differences between the gut flora of humans and rodents may offer another explanation as to why NR works in them but not us.[8216]

Unlike NAM, supplementation with NR did not increase homocysteine levels,[8217] but one study of a combination of NR plus a resveratrol analogue called pterostilbene raised LDL cholesterol[8218] high enough to potentially kill as many as one in forty long-term consumers.[8219] However, this effect is presumed to be due to the pterostilbene,[8220] as NR alone hasn't been shown to raise LDL,[8221,8222] whereas pterostilbene has.[8223]

One study did find that NR seemed to cause a small reduction in hemoglobin, hematocrit, and platelet count in people within a week of starting.[8224] This shift toward a more anemic state was suggested to account for impaired exercise performance seen in rats given NR.[8225] However, the 35 percent drop in performance did not reach statistical significance.[8226] NR did cause a significant increase in systemic oxidative stress,[8227] and another rodent study found a worsening of inflammation and deterioration of metabolic health,[8228] but if positive effects in rodents don't translate to people, perhaps we should expect the same from negative ones.

Regulatory authorities from Australia, Canada, Europe, and the United States have all authorized NR as safe,[8229] at least up to 300 mg a day (230 mg in pregnant and lactating women).[8230] But the lack of demonstrable clinical benefit would seem to preclude NR supplementation.[8231]

NICOTINAMIDE MONONUCLEOTIDE (NMN)

Both NR and NMN have been shown to have beneficial effects in rodents, though they haven't been tested side by side.[8232] Both precursors raise blood levels of NAD^+ in people, but similarly haven't been pitted head-to-head against each other.[8233,8234] One potential advantage of NMN over NR is that it may be more stable in the bloodstream. In mouse blood at least, within an hour, most NR is converted into NAM, whereas NMN levels remain steady. You could also argue that NMN is better because it's a direct precursor of NAD^+, whereas NR has to first be converted to NMN, so we might as well just take NMN.[8235] Ironically, the exact opposite argument can also be made based on the inability of NMN to pass through cell membranes.

Structurally, NMN is just NR with a phosphate group on it. The phosphate charge prevents NMN from passing in and out of cells, so to get inside one, it first has to be converted into NR. Then, once inside, the NR can turn back into NMN and make NAD^+. So, if NMN has to be converted to NR for cell entry, the argument goes, maybe you might as well take NR in the first place.[8236] However, an NMN transporter was controversially[8237] recently identified (at least in mouse intestines), so maybe NMN is able to skip the NR step and pass directly into cells to make NAD^+ after all.[8238]

NMN boasts a long list of rodent healthspan benefits,[8239] but, unlike NR,[8240] it has yet to demonstrate an extension of mammalian lifespan.[8241] What about specifically in people? There have only been a few human NMN studies published to date. One small study of healthy middle-aged men found various single doses had no apparent effect on any of the measured variables, including retinal (eye) function, sleep quality, heart rate, blood pressure oxygenation, or body temperature.[8242] A twelve-week study of daily NMN supplementation in middle-aged men and women similarly found no significant effects on any outcome, including lean mass, muscle mass, body fat, blood sugars, cholesterol, or insulin sensitivity. NMN did boost blood NAD^+ levels, though they peaked after the first month and then trended down for months two and three, so there may have been an adaptive drop in NAD^+ synthesis, as was suspected with NR.[8243] Like NR, NMN also fails to raise NAD^+ in muscle tissue.[8244]

One study, evocatively titled "Nicotinamide Mononucleotide Supplementation Enhances Aerobic Capacity in Amateur Runners," tested three different doses of NMN versus placebo for six weeks among young and middle-aged recreational runners. Aerobic capacity was increased at one ventilatory threshold but not the other. No overall benefit for aerobic capacity, peak power, or any of ten other measures of cardiopulmonary function was found. If you measure enough things, though, statistical outliers—both positive and negative—can pop up as flukes. For example, the researchers noted a significantly improved single-leg stance test result, but NMN had no effect on any of the other physical function tests, including grip strength, push-ups, and sit-and-reach flexibility. And, upon closer inspection, the single-leg stance balance benefit was only found in the middle-dose group compared to the high-dose group and not for any of the doses compared to placebo. (The high-dose group ended up doing slightly worse compared to baseline.[8245])

A similar issue can be found in a twelve-week study of NMN supplementation in older adults. The NMN company–funded authors concluded that NMN "improved lower limb function and reduced drowsiness in older adults," but it failed to significantly affect sixteen other measures, including other tests of lower limb function and fatigue.[8246] There are so few NMN studies that this kind of shotgun approach is understandable, casting the widest possible net for effects to be further tested, but it can't on its own be presented as convincing proof of efficacy.

All of the above NMN studies were on healthy individuals. What about testing NMN on those who are already metabolically compromised? Overweight or obese postmenopausal women with prediabetes were randomized to NMN or placebo for ten weeks. NMN didn't seem to affect body weight or composition, liver fat, blood pressure, or a dozen other metabolic variables, but it did improve muscle insulin sensitivity, though not enough to affect insulin levels or short- or long-term blood sugar control.[8247] This may be because insulin sensitivity in the liver and body fat remained unchanged.[8248] NMN also appeared to have no effect on mitochondrial function, muscle strength, fatigability, or recovery.[8249]

In terms of safety, NMN shills[8250] speak of it as being found naturally in fruits and vegetables,[8251] but even the most concentrated sources (edamame, avocado, and broccoli) have more than a hundred times less per serving than the typical NMN supplement dose.[8252] The same could be said for NR in milk (human and otherwise).[8253] There are safety evaluations for NMN on rats[8254] and dogs,[8255] but unlike NR, supplemental doses of NMN have yet to be proven safe for human consumption.[8256] As of early 2023 as I write this, the sale of NMN as a dietary supplement remains in legal limbo.[8257]

There are rodent studies showing that NMN can have negative metabolic consequences,[8258] but the most serious concern regards nerve degeneration. The accumulation of NMN in nerve cells is toxic.[8259] Since NR is converted to NMN, this is a concern for NR supplementation as well.[8260] The type of nerve damage (axon degeneration) is a major contributor to a variety of neurodegenerative disorders,[8261] including glaucoma.[8262] Blocking an NMN-synthesizing enzyme appeared to help damaged neurons in vitro, protection that's reversed by adding back NMN,[8263] and adding an enzyme that chews up NMN was also found to be protective.[8264] However, clinical effects remain theoretical as these adverse effects have only been demonstrated in fish, mice, and petri dishes.[8265]

NMN supplements may not even have NMN in the first place. ChromaDex, which sells a rival supplement, Tru Niagen (a form of NR), claims to have tested the twenty-two NMN brands with the highest market share on Amazon.com and found that most had NMN levels below the limit of detection, so virtually none at all.[8266] Ironically, many of the apparently fake NMN products displayed a "certificate of analysis" and carried hundreds or even thousands of positive reviews.[8267] Evidently, only three out of twenty-two were found to contain as much NMN as advertised on their labels. Of course, ChromaDex isn't above being shady itself; it's been accused of making hyped false claims for Tru Niagen by both the FDA[8268] and the Better Business Bureau.[8269] In short, NR has been demonstrated to be relatively safe but not effective, and neither safety nor efficacy has been established for NMN.

OTHER NAD⁺-BOOSTING SUPPLEMENTS

What about tryptophan, NAD^+, NADH, NMNH, and NRH? I detail them all in see .nf/othernad. In short, if anything, tryptophan *restriction* may be beneficial,[8270,8271] taking NAD^+ directly largely isn't practical because of instability and poor bioavailability,[8272,8273] and, though NMNH[8274] and NRH[8275] have superior potency, this isn't necessarily a good thing as NRH can promote inflammation[8276] and oxidation,[8277] deleterious effects presumed to be shared by NMNH (since it has to be converted to NRH to enter cells).[8278]

POTENTIAL ADVERSE EFFECTS ON
INFLAMMATION AND CANCER

Most of the reported side effects for NAD^+ precursors like NAM, NR, and NMN are relatively rare and minor—for example, diarrhea, nausea, rashes, hot flashes, and leg cramps.[8279] Both NR and NMN raise NAM levels,[8280] so they may share in the same concerns regarding sirtuin inhibition, methyl depletion, and potential adverse effects of NAM breakdown products.[8281] I go into detail in see.nf/nadprecautions, but basically, particular caution should be used for NAD^+-boosting supplements by those with cancer, a personal or strong family history of cancer,[8282] and perhaps also those with inflammatory disorders[8283] and active *Haemophilus* infections.[8284]

WHICH BOOSTER IS BEST?

There's no clear standout in NAD^+-boosting supplements,[8285] as hardly any of the preclinical effects found in the lab have translated into evidence of human clinical benefit. Perhaps this failure is to be expected given the complexity of NAD^+ physiology, with its juggling of multiple precursors, production pathways, recycling routes, and myriad consuming enzymes.[8286] It's just too early to say if NAD^+ booster supplementation will ever live up to even a fraction of the hype.[8287] Many more, larger, and longer-term studies are necessary to establish safety and efficacy.[8288]

The problem is that because NA, NAM, NR, and NMN are all natural products, they can't be patented, so the money for well-designed clinical trials is not as available.[8289] The reason there have been comparatively more trials done on NR than NMN is that patents were originally issued for NR before it was deemed unpatentable in 2021.[8290]

Perhaps blindly overloading the system with NAD^+ precursors is not the best way to go about NAD^+ restoration.[8291] The body seems too smart to allow such a blunt incursion to affect tissue levels. Maybe these supplements are just profit-making distractions from more natural approaches.

NATURAL APPROACHES TO BOOSTING NAD⁺

There are broadly three main approaches for increasing NAD^+ levels. Increasing the supply of NAD^+ precursors is just the first. The other two means are having the body make more by activating NAD^+-synthesizing enzymes and having the body use less via an inhibition of excess NAD^+ degradation.[8292]

AMPING NAMPT

The primary determinant of NAD^+ synthesis is the enzyme *NAMPT*,[8293] and its abundance tends to decrease with age in human muscle, dropping steadily by about 40 percent between the ages of twenty and eighty.[8294] In our liver, it drops by half.[8295] However, age-related diseases, such as atherosclerosis, cancer, diabetes, and rheumatoid arthritis, have been found to exacerbate NAMPT decline, raising a chicken-or-the-egg question.[8296] This is where interventional trials come in.

Similar NAMPT declines have been noted in aging rats[8297] and mice.[8298] Does boosting this enzyme help? Increasing NAMPT or its species equivalent increases the lifespans of yeast,[8299] fruit flies,[8300] and rodents.[8301] An NAMPT boost also increases aerobic capacity[8302] and exercise endurance in mice in addition to helping them live longer.[8303]

Enhanced expression of NAMPT increases the NAD$^+$ levels in the muscles in mice comparably to feeding them dietary NAD$^+$ precursors, but if you remember, NAD$^+$ precursors don't seem to be able to affect NAD$^+$ muscle levels in most people.[8304] In fact, such supplements can actually suppress NAMPT,[8305] while boosting that methylating enzyme to rid the body of the excess. In addition to methyl depletion, chronic administration of these supplements could then potentially leave people worse off should they ever stop taking them.[8306] There is, however, a way we may naturally boost our NAMPT and NAD$^+$ levels without any supplements: exercise.

Athletes have about twice the NAMPT expression in their musculature compared to sedentary individuals. To prove cause and effect, sedentary men and women started a stationary bike exercise protocol, and, within three weeks, NAMPT levels increased by 127 percent.[8307] Resistance training can also increase NAMPT, and this can translate into a 127 percent increase in muscle NAD$^+$ levels and a rise in sirtuin activity.[8308] In other words, exercise can do what NAD$^+$-boosting supplements can't.

PRESERVING NAD$^+$ BY TAMPING PARP-1 AND CD38

The third way to maintain levels of NAD$^+$ is to conserve it. Besides sirtuins, the major consumers of NAD$^+$ are *PARP-1* and *CD38*. PARP-1 is an enzyme that uses NAD$^+$ to repair DNA. The more oxidative DNA damage, the more single- and double-stranded DNA breaks, the more enzymes like PARP-1 need to be activated to come to the rescue.[8309] This uses up a lot of NAD$^+$. As DNA damage accumulates with age, the rising need for repair enzymes like PARP-1 causes a major drain on NAD$^+$ levels.[8310,8311] This has led to the search for PARP-1 blockers to preserve NAD$^+$ levels,[8312] but rather than blocking DNA repair, why not work to prevent so much damage in the first place? See the Oxidation chapter for how to do just that.

CD38 is the other major guzzler of NAD$^+$. It's an enzyme that uses NAD$^+$ to make a type of cellular messenger.[8313] Found concentrated on the surfaces of immune cells, CD38 is robustly induced in the context of inflammation.[8314] The rise of CD38 activity with age[8315] has been blamed on persistent "inflammaging" activation[8316] and may be a major culprit for falling NAD$^+$ levels.[8317] For example, blocking CD38 has been found to raise NAD$^+$ levels in older mice comparable to that of younger mice.[8318] In addition to my chapter on reducing inflammation, my video see.nf/conservingnad dives into a number of natural CD38 inhibitors found in foods.

Conclusion

In the anti-aging journal *Rejuvenation Research*, a commentary was published titled "Finally, a Regimen to Extend Human Life Expectancy."[8319] I was all ears (or rather, eyes). Was it some new exotic gene therapy or stem cell treatment? No, it was a reference to a Harvard analysis titled "Impact of Healthy Lifestyle Factors on Life Expectancies in the US Population." More than 100,000 men and women were followed for thirty-four years, and just a few basic lifestyle behaviors appeared to translate into about thirteen years of extra lifespan for the average fifty-year-old. Even from age seventy, there are still about ten extra years on the table.[8320] Extending that back, earlier than age fifty, a Canadian study found that nearly eighteen years were up for grabs based on simple, commonsense health behaviors.[8321]

That's the kind of life extension we'd expect extrapolating from some of the advances made in laboratory animal longevity,[8322] but after decades of research and hundreds of millions of dollars spent, efforts to translate those results into humans have largely been in vain.[8323] Yet, here we are with *human* data suggesting that dramatic life extension is available to all of us right here, right now. We already have that trillion-dollar pill that anti-aging biotech has been promising us. It just may have to be effectively administered in the produce aisle or the gym. As presciently written in a textbook of geriatric medicine more than sixty-five years ago, "A more promising approach toward prolonging life in the latter years seems to be the prevention of degenerative diseases by good nutrition."[8324]

Might the wide disparity in lifespan arise from a lifelong pattern of behavior? To make sure it's not too late to turn back the clock, researchers tracked what happened to men and women trying to clean up their bad habits starting in middle age. A midlife switch between the ages of forty-five and sixty-four to even just the barest of minimums—at least five daily servings fruits and vegetables, walking about twenty minutes a day, maintaining a healthy weight, and not smoking—resulted in a substantial reduction in mortality even in the immediate future. We're talking a 40 percent lower risk of dying in the subsequent four years. The research-ers conclude that their findings emphasize that "making the necessary changes to adhere to a healthy lifestyle is extremely worthwhile, and middle-age is certainly not too late to act."[8325]

And that's just the beginning. That doesn't include the dozens of other recom-mendations I put forth in Part I of this book, the healthiest of healthy foods and eat-ing patterns in the Optimal Anti-Aging Regimen in Part II, the death-defying tips on circulation and immunity in Part III, or necessarily any of my Anti-Aging Eight. There is so much we can do to extend our lifespan and our healthspan. A recent remarkable study of more than half a million participants, for example, found that those who salted their food at the table (in addition to whatever salt was used in cooking) appeared to have a two-year lower life expectancy at age fifty compared to those who didn't.[8326] So, just swapping out the salt shaker for some savory salt-free seasoning could potentially add years to your life.

All this just from tiny tweaks of the bare basics without getting really serious about diet. What we eat is considered "probably the most powerful and pliable tool that we have to attain a chronic and systemic modulation of [the] ageing pro-cess. . . ."[8327] The apparent benefits are so extreme that they've been used to cast aspersions on the whole field of nutritional epidemiology. Meta-analyses suggesting that you could add years to your life just by avoiding eggs or bacon, or by eating nuts every day or certain fruit? It just seems too good to be true.[8328] Regardless of the absolute magnitude of the effect, diet is understood to be the number one determinant of how long we live.[8329] We are what we eat.

LIFESPAN REGRESSION

Martin Luther King Jr. warned that "human progress is neither automatic nor in-evitable,"[8330] and the same may be true of the human lifespan.[8331] In 1850, life expectancy in the United States was less than forty years,[8332] but it has steadily increased over the last two centuries,[8333] gaining about two years per decade—until recently, that is. Longevity gains have faltered and then, in 2015, started to reverse.[8334] Thanks in large part to the obesity epidemic, we may now be raising the first American generation to live shorter lives than their parents.[8335] And that was before COVID-19 knocked two years off the U.S. life expectancy, a decline not experienced since 1943, the deadliest year of World War II.[8336]

As we get older, the reserve capacity of our organs is diminished,[8337] making it even more important to eat and live healthfully. We can't continue to get away with the fast-food lifestyle we may have led with teen abandon. Unfortunately, most have not gotten the memo. The American Heart Association has tracked diet and lifestyle trends in the United States for decades. In its 2012 report, it noted that most Americans were already not smoking and nearly half achieved their "ideal" goal for exercise (at least twenty minutes or so a day of moderate intensity activity). But when it came to healthy diet score, only about 1 percent scored a four or five out of its zero-to-five diet quality scale. And, "ideal" criteria just included things like drinking less than four and a half cups of soda a week.[8338]

The American Heart Association set what it called an "aggressive" goal of improving these stats by 20 percent by 2020. Did it achieve its objective of bumping up that 1 percent to 1.2 percent? By the 2022 update, we had slipped even farther, from 1 percent down to 0.2 percent.[8339] Today, only one in five hundred Americans even gets close to a modestly healthy diet.

No wonder, in terms of life expectancy, the United States ranked down around twenty-seven or twenty-eight out of the thirty-four top free-market democracies. People in Slovenia live longer than we do.[8340] That was in 2010, down from ranking twentieth in 1990. More recently, U.S. life expectancy dipped to forty-third in the world and is expected to drop to sixty-fourth by 2040,[8341] despite spending trillions on healthcare a year, more than anyone else around the globe.[8342]

The problem isn't healthcare access. The Mayo Clinic estimates that nearly 70 percent of Americans are on prescription drugs.[8343] The problem is that those trillions in healthcare spending aren't addressing the root cause. The leading risk factor for death in the United States is what we eat.[8344] It's the food. The standard American diet is just to die for. Literally. It's almost as if we're eating as though our future doesn't matter. There are actually data to back that up, from a study I profile in see.nf/usa titled "Death Row Nutrition."[8345] The upshot was that there wasn't much difference between the final food requests of death row inmates and what Americans normally eat. If we continue to eat as though we are having our last meals, eventually, they will be.

COALITION CONSENSUS

On the flip side, the good news is how huge the opportunity is for improvement. One of the most beautiful graphs in all of public health is that of the lung cancer death curves. It took decades to finally turn the corner, but with dropping smoking rates, the rates of lung cancer deaths have come tumbling down.[8346] I look forward to the day when we see the same with diet.

Yes, approximately 80 percent of chronic disease and premature death could be prevented by not smoking, being physically active, and "adhering to a healthful dietary pattern," but what exactly is meant by a healthy diet?[8347] Unfortunately, what we hear in the media about nutrition is often inconsistent and confusing. There's a pressure within today's competitive journalism market for sensationalism. Media analysts suggest that there may even be a purposeful disincentive to present the facts in context to sell more copies.[8348] (The analysis was published before the lure of clickbait headlines, which presumably makes matters even worse.)

There's a quote from the 1940s by a leader in the field that seems all the more relevant now, more than three-quarters of a century later: "It is unfortunate that the subject of nutrition seems to have a special appeal to the credulous, the social zealot, and, in the commercial field, the unscrupulous . . . [a combination] calculated to strike despair in the hearts of the sober, objective scientist."[8349]

Arguably, the most important healthcare problem we face may be our poor lifestyle choices based on misinformation.[8350] It reminds me of climate change denial, how healthy dietary advice can be overshadowed by industry interests, ideologues, and a misguided media. What we've needed is an IPCC of nutrition, and I'm proud to have contributed to just such an undertaking. The True Health Initiative is a nonprofit coalition of hundreds of experts from dozens of countries agreeing to a consensus statement as to the basics of healthy living,[8351] "fighting fake facts and combating false doubts to create a world free of preventable diseases, using the time-honored, evidence-based fundamentals of lifestyle as medicine."[8352] Spoiler alert: The healthiest diet is one that is generally comprised mostly of minimally processed plants.[8353]

AS NATURE INTENDED

Perhaps that is not surprising, since it is what we ate from about twenty million years ago when we split with our last common primate ancestor up until we started making tools about two million years ago.[8354] We know that, for the first 90 percent of our evolution, when our nutrient requirements and digestive physiology were being established, we were eating what the rest of the great apes ended up eating, a diet centered around whole plant foods. Even the most carnivorous of apes—chimpanzees—eat a diet that is more than 98 percent plant-based.[8355] You can feed natural omnivores like dogs[8356] five hundred eggs' worth of cholesterol, and they just wag their tail, whereas a fraction of that can clog the arteries of more naturally plant-based species within a matter of months.[8357] Some animals are used to eating and ridding themselves of excess cholesterol. Our body can't handle it, as evidenced by atherosclerotic heart disease being our leading cause of death.

During the Stone Age, there was little selection pressure to protect people from their expanding diet since most prehistoric people didn't live long enough to get heart attacks. When the average life expectancy is twenty-five years,[8358] the genes that get passed along are from those who can live to reproductive age by any means necessary—

and that means not dying of starvation. The more calories in food, the better. Eating lots of bone marrow and brains, human or otherwise, would have a selective advantage (as would discovering a time-machine stash of Twinkies, for that matter). If we only have to live long enough to get our kids to puberty to pass along our genes, then we don't have to evolve any protections against the ravages of chronic disease.

To find a population nearly free of chronic disease in old age, we don't have to go back millions of years. As I detailed in *How Not to Die*, in the twentieth century, networks of missionary hospitals in rural Africa found coronary artery disease to be virtually absent and the same for other leading killers, like high blood pressure, stroke, diabetes, common cancers, and more.[8359] In a sense, populations in rural China and Africa were eating the type of diet we've been eating for 90 percent of the last twenty million years, a diet almost exclusively comprised of plant foods. How do we know it was their diet and not something else? Because of the pioneering research from Pritikin, Ornish, and Esselstyn that showed that plant-based diets could help arrest or even reverse the progression of heart disease in the majority of patients when formally put to the test. Indeed, it's the only diet that ever has.[8360]

Is a healthy diet and lifestyle all you need to fight the ravages of aging? This would have been a much thinner book if it were so. As you've read in these pages, there are a plethora of pills and procedures and salves, supplements, and specific foods that can help reduce wrinkles, grow hair, shrink prostates, and enhance vision, dentition, erection, cognition, and so on. But the foundation is diet and lifestyle, which is good news, because you hold the power.

References

For a full list of searchable citations, point your phone camera at the QR code below or go to nutritionfacts.org/book/how-not-to-age/citations. Each cited source is hyperlinked so you can read the original studies themselves.

Scan for cited sources:

Or visit:

nutritionfacts.org/book/how-not-to-age/citations

Acknowledgments

Primary appreciation goes to the researchers whose enlightenment of the natural world forms the foundation of all my work. There is no evidence-based nutrition without evidence.

Then, first and foremost, I want to thank editing extraordinaire Miyun Park, who expertly coordinated this whole massive project, with sweet potato dreams to her precious Ollie. Then gratitude for everyone every step of the way. We're so fortunate to have a veritable army of volunteer article retrievers, but standout source sleuths include Jolene Bowers, Gregory Butler, Devra O'Gara, Laura McClanathan, Julie Van Horn, and Kevin Wise. Thanks to Marie Townsley and Chrissy Liptrot for annotation compilation, Dawn Chang for citation formatting, Caroline Garriott for the figures, editors Lee Oglesby and Laura Greger (the latter of whom also did the favor of birthing the author), Christi Richards for wrangling all the citations online, Abie Rohrig for helping with promotion, and, finally, fearless fact-checking savant Alissa Finley, who regularly reminds me just how remarkably wrong I can be. (What's five orders of magnitude between friends?) Also deep appreciation to Katie Schloer for keeping NutritionFacts.org running so smoothly, Richard Pine and Bob Miller for negotiating such a great book deal in the midst of pandemic uncertainty, and the amazing charities to which that money is going to help make the world a healthier place.

Index

Page numbers in *italics* refer to charts and figures.

AARP, 379
abdominal fat, 49, 83, 555, 556–57
Academy of Nutrition and Dietetics, 210, 401–2
açai berries, 500, 513
acarbose, 60–61, 90–91, 548, 568
acetaldehyde, 20–21, 52, 169, 170–71
acetaminophen (Tylenol), 342–43
acetic acid, 20–22, 169, 539
acetone, 62
acetylcholine, 361
acid-base balance, 234, 238, 412–14, *413*
acid reflux, 27–28, 234
AcipHex, 234
acne, 19, 106, 107
acromegaly, 74
acrylamide, 25, 38
acupuncture, 346
acute myeloid lymphoma (AML), 521–22
adrenal hormones, 159, 271, 295, 402, 412
aducanumab (Aduhelm), 361–62
aerobic exercise, 24, 38, 142, 178, 215, 218,
        244, 249, 263, 266, 282, 316, 348, 433,
        476, 567
Africa, 254, 290, 601
African Americans, 137, 166, 253, 476
Age-Related Eye Disease Study (AREDS), 473–74
AGEs (advanced glycation end products, or
        glycotoxins), 54–60, 62, 65–66, 81, 100,
        135–36, 305, 402, 479
age spots, 440–41
Ah receptor, 492
air pollution, 49, 115, 123, 141, 372, 373, 441,
        492–94
Akkermansia muciniphila, 532–33
alaria (*Alaria esculenta*), 77

alcohol, 20–21, 25, 52, 94, 115, 120, 124, 141,
        144, 164, 168–72, 225, 229, 234, 239–40,
        266, 279, 316–17, 356, 372–73, 401, 445,
        517, 536
algae, 397, 399, 400, 523
alkaline-forming foods, 238
alkylamines, 331
allergies, 202
allicin, 511
almond milk, 27, 95
almonds, 117, 184, 240, 491
alopecia areata, 287
alpha-carotene, 118, 478
alpha hydroxy acids, 454
alpha-lipoic acid, 127
ALS Parkinsonism dementia complex, 399–400
alternate-day fasting, 560–61, 576
aluminum, 368
Alzheimer's, 39, 40, 42, 48, 55, 59, 80, 125,
        132, 135, 137, 141, 156, 167, 173, 219,
        357–76, 379, 381–85, 388–89, 392–404,
        520–21, 549, 579–80
Alzheimer's Disease Cooperative Study, 386
Alzheimer's Foundation of America, 359
Ambien, 226
American Academy of Anti-Aging Medicine, 2–3
American Academy of Dermatology, 451, 458, 460
American Academy of Family Physicians, 299
American Academy of Orthopaedic Surgeons,
        346
American Academy of Pediatric Dentistry, 467
American Academy of Sleep Medicine, 226
American Association of Clinical Endocrinology,
        310
American Association of Retired Persons, 155

American Cancer Society, 253, 315
American College of Cardiology, 269, 469
American College of Family Physicians, 314
American College of Lifestyle Medicine, 212, 515
American College of Obstetricians and
    Gynecologists, 299–300, 428
American College of Physicians, 253, 315
American College of Preventive Medicine, 314
American College of Rheumatology, 356
American Egg Board, 154, 409
American Geriatrics Society, 299, 343, 361
American Heart Association, 95, 159, 262, 269,
    273, 277, 299, 406, 469, 504, 512, 598–99
American Indians, 166
American Institute for Cancer Research, 497, 504
American Medical Association, 161, 427, 559
American Psychological Association, 229
American Urological Association, 315–16, 434,
    437
Ames, Bruce, 191
amino acids, 29, 73–74, 105, 110, 228, 331,
    410–11, 538
aminoglycoside antibiotics, 291
amla, 44, 118, 274, 466, 503
ammonia, 412
AMPK (AMP-activated protein kinase), 14–25,
    38, 104, 105, 131, 133, 136, *148*, 149,
    169, 201, 552, 567
amyloid beta, 361–63, 369–70, 373–74, 378
amyloid cascade hypothesis, 362
anal fissure, 247
androgenic alopecia, 280
andropause, 308
anemia, 58
anesthesia, 391
angiogenesis, 39
angiogram, 272, 293
angioplasty, 272
animal fats, 72, 88, 92, 184, 502
animal foods, 34, 57, 71–72, 84, 89, 152, *153*,
    208, 272, 388
animal microRNAs, 527–39
animal protein, 25, 72–75, 77, 88, 105, 111–12,
    201, 203–4, 277–78, 292, 490, 562,
    569–70, 572–74, 581–82
animal-to-plant protein swap, 573–74, 576, 582
ankle-brachial index, 177
anorexia, 104, 554
antagonistic pleiotropy, 102, 137, 200–201
anthocyanins, 93, 94, 101, 188, 189, 367, 389,
    390, 504–5

anti-aging industry, 1–3, 6, 485–86
antibiotics, 79, 253, 395, 536–38, 540, 541
antidepressants, 215, 438–39
antifungal drugs, 102, 460–61
anti-glycation foods, 447
anti-inflammaging, 91–92
anti-inflammatories, 43, 89–101, 184, 187, 218,
    252, 330, 332, 350, 371, 389, 406, 447,
    469, 479, 504, 506, 532, 544, 545
antioxidants, 26, 43, 51, 57, 65, 93–94, 109,
    110, 112–30, 133, 141, 147, 167, 184,
    187, 191, 195–96, 218, 239, 279, 350–52,
    367, 384, 389, 411–12, 444–45, 447,
    452–53, 469, 471, 473, 478–79, 491, 498,
    500–503, 506, 510–11, 516, 533
antiperspirants, 368
anxiety, 84, 208, 229, 308, 414
apigenin, 521
APOE ε4, 102, 366–67
appetite suppression, 19–20
apple juice, 173
apples, 31, 33, 41–42, 44, 58, 89, 117, 118,
    133–34, 136, 331, 423, 444, 500, 513,
    516, 521, 526, 549
APPROACH (Animal and Plant PROtein And
    Cardiovascular Health) trial, 273
arachidonic acid, 349
arame, 191
arginine, 29, 438
Aristotle, 16, 162
aromatherapy, 381–82, 426
artemisinin, 513
arteries, 19, 21, 31, 42, 58–60, 85, 103, 119,
    167, 172–73, 176–77, 182–83, 193, 223,
    262, 272, 275–76, 307, 363–65, 431–32,
    437, 490–91, 496, 505, 507, 526, 600
arthritis, 5, 48, 55, 89, 94, 113, 137
arthroscopic surgery, 344–45
artichokes, 524
artificial sweeteners, 62, 168, 538
arugula, *495*, 496
ashwagandha, 426
Asians, 166, 290
asparagus, 35, 54, 513
aspartame, 62
aspirin, 98–99, 291, 510, 536
asthma, 20, 89, 332, 487, 528, 543
astragalus, 146
atherosclerosis, 124–25, 169, 177, 182–83, 193,
    217, 263–68, 273–74, 292–93, 356, 360,
    363, 422, 424, 475, 526, 539, 594, 600

athletes, 142, 163, 217–19, 330, 348, 495
athlete's foot, 461–62, 494
Atkins diet, 62, 84, 210, 437
atrial fibrillation, 184
Australia, 175, 455
autism, 107, 340
autoimmune diseases, 88, 330, 338, 538, 545,
    552, 569
autoimmune inflammation, 81, 109
autologous platelet-rich plasma therapy, 284
autophagy, 15, 22–38, 81–83, 100, 102, 111,
    133, *148*, 188, 215, 414, 552, 575
avocado, 87, 99, 182, 221, 393, 473
Ayurvedic medicine, 147, 503

Bacillus licheniformis, 541
Bacillus subtilis, 543
bacon, 66, 144, 155–56, 497
bacteria, 29, 86, 90–91, 510, 523, 530–40,
    544–47. *See also* microbiome
Bacteroides, 544–45
baking powder, 368
baking soda, 414
balance, 140, 215, 244
balding, 280–84
Baltimore Longitudinal Study of Aging, 156–57
Bama County, 532, 535
bananas, 95, 324, 499–500, 510, 549, 578
barberries, 19, 22–23
bariatric surgery, 83, 220, 320
barley, 90, 505
basal cell carcinoma, 446
basil, 99, *495*, 502, 513
bathing, 227, 245
BCAA supplements, 581, 583
B cells, 328, 335
BDNF, 377–78
beans, 37, 51, 53, 61, 89, 90, 92, 111, 152, 165,
    175–79, 189, 241, 388, 411, 413, 546,
    568, 577, 582
beef, 57, 125, 126, 272, 370, 413, 441, 501,
    503, 522, 524, 537, 538
beer, 115, 154–55, 162, 307, 317, 524
beets, 99, 438, 469, 494–96, *495*
bell peppers, 89, 472
benign prostatic hyperplasia (BPH), 258–62
berberine supplements, 19
berries, 27, 64, 93–94, 101, 115, 116, 124, 130,
    167, 263, 304, 324–26, 351–52, 389–91,
    475, 499–507, 550
beta-carboline alkaloids, 418

beta-carotene, 49, 93, 95–96, 112, 118, 126,
    145, 478, 487
beta-glucans, 92, 330–31
beverages, 120, 154, 162–73, *164*, 350–51
bicycle helmets, 372
Bifidobacteria, 36–37, 53, 91, 189, 378–79, 504,
    532–33, 539, 541, 543, 545, 547–49
bilberries, 504
Bilophila wadsworthia, 535
bioflavonoids, 94
biogerontology, 3
bioidentical hormones, 300
biological age, 49–50, 556
biological clock, 138–39
biotin, 284–85, 464
birth defects, 53
blackberries, 500–503
Blackburn, Elizabeth, 141
black cohosh, 307
black cumin, 19–20, 22–23, 44, 308
black currants, 121, 476–77, 504
black-eyed peas, 35
black pepper, 501
black rice, 188, 505
black salve, 457
black tea, 34, 41, 44, 65, 89, 120, 166–67, 394,
    516
bladder, 252–62
bladder cancer, 84
blood, young vs. old, 40
blood-brain barrier, 370–71, 378
blood clots, 163, 240–41, 297–99, 329, 345,
    359, 499, 539–40
blood orange juice, 118, 173
blood pressure, 20, 31, 42, 89, 104, 119, 169,
    176, 189, 194, 220, 231, 264–66, 269,
    275, 292, 307, 328, 349, 354, 364–65,
    496, 505, 506, 514, 544, 555, 558–59,
    562–63, 571. *See also* high blood pressure;
    low blood pressure
blood rheology, 276
blood sugar, 19, 20, 21, 36, 54, 59–61, 63–65,
    127, 130, 132, 176, 178, 194, 208, 218,
    220, 224, 251, 264, 275, 281, 292, 317,
    328, 503–5, 544, 559, 562, 581, 582
blood tests, 464, 562
blood thinning, 329
blood vessels, 262–63. *See also* arteries; veins
blueberries, 43, 95, 117–18, 292, 325, 352,
    367, 389–91, 414, 500–505, 513, 526,
    549–50

blue-green algae supplements, 400
Blue Mountains Hearing Study, 293
blue zones, 112, 174–75, 179–80, 198
BMAA, 399–400
BMPEA, 436
body fat, 39, 82–83, 208, 219–22, 281, 568
body mass index (BMI), ideal, 197, 219, 222–23
body odor, 419–21
Bogalusa Heart Study, 139
Bolivia, 259, 267
bone density, 130, 233, 235–36, 239, 241–44, 281, 305, 307, 312, 558
bone fractures, 215, 237–38, 243–44, 299
bone loss, 104, 215, 239
bones, 12, 132, 154, 233–45
Boseman, Chadwick, 253
Botox, 284, 442, 447
bovine microRNAs, 107
bovine spongiform encephalopathy (mad cow disease), 450
bowel movements, 245–52
BPA, 432–33
brain, 10, 29–30, 39, 58, 125, 154, 169, 192, 218, 219, 362–404, 424, 504
brain-derived neurotrophic factor (BDNF), 375–78
branched-chain amino acids (BCAA), 105, 107, 111, 579–83
Brazil nuts, 128, 491, 578
BRCA mutation, 71
bread, 33, 63–64, 377–78, 413
breakfast cereals, 62–64
breast cancer, 21, 47, 55, 69–70, 74, 76, 84, 104, 106, 125, 169, 184, 201, 208, 240, 241, 297–303, 306–7, 322, 368, 425, 516, 522, 526, 564, 574
breast milk, 56, 209, 328, 407, 528, 547
breast self-exams, 300–301
breastfeeding, 19, 44, 163, 308, 532, 559, 563
broccoli, 54, 96, 107, 117, 119, 121–23, 327, 352–53, 392, 447, 492, 494, 511, 515–17, 524, 526, 582
Broccoli Osteoarthritis (BRIO) study, 353
broccoli sprouts, 96, 122–23, 327, 494, 522
bronchitis, 333
brown adipose tissue (BAT), 221–22, 589
brown rice, 207
Brown-Séquard, Charles-Édouard, 309
brussels sprouts, 118, 122, 540
Buchinger fasting, 131
Buck v. Bell, 200

buckwheat, 99
Buettner, Dan, 174
burgers, 85–87, 155, 272, 370
Burkitt, Denis, 247
butter, 18, 85, 182, 184, 221, 230, 263, 273, 577
butyrate, 89–91, 92, 350, 378–79, 532, 539, 547, 549, 568
B vitamins, 51, 106, 146, 210–11, 385–86. *See also specific types*

cabbage, 34, 122, 123, 392, 505
cadmium, 399
caffeine, 28–29, 123, 145, 225, 256, 282, 286, 415, 494
calcified aortic valve disease, 274
calcium, 154, 165, 211, 235–38, 242, 385, 410
CALERIE (Comprehensive Assessment of Long-Term Effects of Reducing Intake of Energy) trial, 49, 555–60, 565
California Dried Plum Board, 252
California Teachers Study, 302–3
caloric density, 560
caloric dilution, 134
caloric restriction, 15, 24–25, 40, 49, 53, 59, 71, 81, 83, 103–4, 131, 197, 201, 376–77, 494, 509, 514, 520, 551–66, 572, 576
Calorie Restriction Society, 24, 59, 555, 570
Campbell, T. Colin, 206–7, 278, 348–49, 574
Canada, 166, 237
cancer, 5, 6, 18, 20–21, 37, 38, 53, 55, 68–71, 74–78, 83–84, 88, 95–96, 105, 113, 115, 123–25, 130, 132, 139–40, 147, 155–56, 162, 169, 171, 179–80, 189, 201, 203, 208, 213, 237, 241, 250, 254, 262, 276, 279–80, 320–21, 329, 333–34, 337, 406, 410, 435, 481, 483, 488–89, 491–92, 512, 516–17, 521–22, 536, 540, 552, 563–65, 569–70, 574, 576, 594, 601
cannabidiol (CBD) oil, 356
cannabis, 234, 356, 433
canola oil, 186
capers, 41, 44
capsaicin, 511
caramelization, 57
carbohydrates, 25, 57, 60
carboxymethyl-cellulose, 538
cardamom, 134–36, 196, 325
cardiovascular disease, 18, 31, 53, 58, 80, 84, 95–96, 123–24, 132, 154, 176, 180, 186, 189, 203, 234, 237, 262–78, 298, 302,

313, 318, 339–40, 343, 431–32, 462, 487, 526, 539–40, 552, 589

carnitine, 411, 540

carob powder, 118

carotenoids, 49, 124, 145, 209, 393, 443, 445, 479

carotid arteries, 169, 275, 293

carpal tunnel syndrome, 354

carrot juice, 118, 326

carrots, 118, 516, 525, 578

cartilage, 58, 349–51

casein, 27

cashews, 491

Castelli, Bill, 278

castration, 200, 280, 310, 312–14, 319

catalase, 121–22, 195–96

cataracts, 55–56, 113, 125, 470–71, 477–80, 504

cauliflower, 122, 392, 516

caviar tongue, 460

cavities, 467, 470

cayenne pepper, 180

CD38, 595–96

celecoxib (Celebrex), 343

celery, 89, 117, 447–48, 516, 521

celery seed, 513

cell growth, 29, 69–70

cell phone radiation, 291

cellular senescence, 38–44, *148*

Centella asiatica, 147

centenarians, 4–5, 11, 13, 43, 67–68, 70, 91–92, 113, 127, 139–40, 173–76, 187, 200, 220, 488, 492, 532–36, 572

Center for Alzheimer's Disease Research, 362–63

Center for Menopause, Hormonal Disorders and Women's Health, 283

Center for Science in the Public Interest, 188, 467

Centers for Disease Control and Prevention (CDC), 283, 338–39

Central America, 179

Centrum Silver, 384, 474, 479

cereals, 207

cervical cancer, 334, 516

chamomile tea, 64–65, 89, 98, 101, 167, 228, 521

cheese, 18, 34, 85, 88, 125, 351, 368, 370, 413, 524

chemical peel, 443

chemotherapy, 39, 113, 122, 140, 302, 342, 564–65

cherries, 94, 116, 391, 504–6

cherry juice, 120, 351, 391, 504

chia seeds, 491

chicken, 34, 57–58, 60, 72, 85, 87–88, 95, 115, 124–26, 154, 158, 272–73, 349–50, 370, 498, 501, 537, 577, 581

chicken pox, 80, 341

chickpeas, 32–33, 61, 89, 92, 112, 154, 175–78, 547, 577, 582

childbirth, 255, 281

children, 9–10, 28

chili peppers, 99, 179–80, 222, 285, 516

China, 188, 193, 194, 259, 493, 513, 532, 549, 601

China-Cornell-Oxford Project (China Study), 348–49

Chinese medicine, 146, 147, 286–87, 506

chlorella, 328–29

chlorination, 164, 211

chlorogenic acid, 26–28, 38

chlorophyll, 96, 127, 420–21, 499–500

chocolate, 27, 119, 167, 390, 423, 474, 549

cholesterol, 2, 5, 20–21, 36, 42, 43, 82–84, 125, 129–30, 176, 184, 186, 189, 193–94, 208, 213, 217–18, 220, 256, 263–75, 293, 328, 349, 363–64, 366–70, 395, 422–23, 431, 468, 475, 490, 503, 544, 555, 559, 562, 571, 582, 583, 600. *See also* HDL cholesterol; LDL cholesterol

cholesterol-lowering drugs, 127, 268–71, 586

cholesterol oxidation products (COPs), 125–26

choline, 540

cholinesterase inhibitors, 360–61

chondroitin, 356–57

choriocapillaris, 475

Christensenellaceae, 43

ChromaDex, 593

chromosomes, 48, 136

chronic diseases, 6, 7, 213–14, 601

Cialis, 435

cilantro, *495*

cinnamon, 98, 101, 118–19, 130, 501, 513

cinnamon tea, 64

circadian rhythm, 65

circulation, 12, 262–78, 292, 356, 462

citrinin, 270

citrulline, 438

citrus, 94, 447–48, 470, 515–16

Cleveland Clinic, 186

clitoris, 422

clones, 45–46, 50

Clostridium difficile, 538

cloves, 98, 119, 130, 501

Coca-Cola, 6, 165, 467

Cochrane review, 273, 380, 488, 586

cocoa, 98–99, 101, 118–19, 135, 415, 423, 446, 474, 506, 513

coconut milk, 27

coconut oil, 273, 355, 469

coenzyme Q10 (CoQ10), 127, 269, 453

coffee, 25–29, 38, 57, 107, 120, 145, 148, 162, *164*, 165, 167, 240, 256, 282, 317, 390, 394, 414–15, 445, 494, 502, 549

cognition, 43, 184, 215, 305, 517, 521

cognitive decline or impairment, 43, 48, 59, 84, 103, 113, 132, 135, 184, 288–89, 364–65, 369, 371–72, 375–76, 379–81, 466, 556–57

cognitive stimulation, 387

colds, 137, 322, 324, 329, 331–32, 337

cold sensitivity, 104, 558

colectomies, 248

collagen, 55, 73, 357, 411, 439–40, 447–50

collard greens, 96, 122, 392, 476

colon, 22, 530, 532, 538, 548–49

colon cancer, 77, 187, 213, 254, 459, 489, 515, 539

colonoscopies, 253–54

colorectal cancer, 69, 84, 99, 156, 165, 169, 246, 252–55, 547

colorectal polyps, 53

Complete Health Improvement Program (CHIP), 199, 228

compression stockings, 459

constipation, 245–52

Consumer Product Safety Commission, 425

cooking, 56–59, 65–66, 123, 125, 167–68, 524

COPD (chronic obstructive pulmonary disease), 90, 327, 540. *See also* emphysema

copper, 369

corn, 34, 179, 472, 513, 525, 584

coronary artery disease, 202, 266–67, 274, 278, 292, 293, 356, 601

coronary calcium scores, 169, 269

Coronary Drug Project, 586

corticosteroids, 97, 344

cortisol levels, 321, 402, 412, 558

cosmetic surgery, 440, 442

Costa Rica, 176, 179

Coumadin (warfarin), 499

COVID-19, 3, 5, 43, 270, 282, 288, 320, 328, 329, 334, 359, 493, 526, 598

CPAP machines, 225

cranberries, 196, 261–62, 391, 501, 504–6, 515

cranberry juice, 120

cranberry powder, 256, 262

C-reactive protein (CRP), 20, 79–84, 87, 92, 94–95, 100–101, 239, 269, 275, 307, 351, 353, 406, 424, 505

cream, 85

creatine, 59, 235, 408, 415–17

Crete, 180–81

Crohn's disease, 92, 330

CRONies, 555, 559, 565–66, 570

CrossFit, 217, 407

cruciferous vegetables, 96, 107, 122–24, 129, 146, 148, 327, 352–53, 392, 492, 494, 511, 521–22, 525–26

cryostimulation, 387

CT scans, 467

cucumber, 35, 496

cumin, 99, 118, 195

curcumin, 97, 134, 383, 521

Curie, Marie, 2, 508

cuticles, 463

cyanide, 19, 325, 508

cyanocobalamin, 211

cycling, 433–34

cycloastragenol (TA-65), 146–47

cycloheximide, 575–76

cyclosporin, 192

cysteine, 579

cytokine storm, 320

cytomegalovirus (CMV), 81

DAF-16 suppressor gene, 520

dairy, 18, 59, 72, 75–77, 86, 100, 120, 147, *153*, 154, 161, 165–66, 175, 187, 237, 259, 272, 274, 296, 304, 351, 522, 524, 528, 545, 546, 577, 578, 581

dandelion tea, 167

dark green leafy vegetables, 52, 95, 242, 292, 386–87, 391–94, 441, 516

DASH diet, 401

dates, 99, 196

Dawkins, Richard, 432

DDE, 371

DDT, 49, 201, 209, 371–72, 559

death, good, 480–83

deferoxamine, 368–69

dehydration, 163, 445, 483

dementia, 5, 30, 75, 141, 202, 219, 299, 312, 358–75, 380–404, 465, 466, 483, 540, 549, 557, 580, 589

Denmark, 551

dental cavities, 292

dental enamel erosion, 470

dental plaque, 532

dental X-rays, 467–68

dentition, 465

dentures, 466

depression, 84, 104, 144, 208, 215, 218, 228, 250, 258, 305, 308, 382, 414, 431, 438, 487, 551, 558

dermatosis papulosa nigra, 458

desserts, 85, 88

detoxification, 122–23, 494, 513, 534, 559

DHA, 154, 277, 397, 398, 399

DHEA (dehydroepiandrosterone), 295, 425, 428–29

diabetes, 54, 61, 77, 80, 95, 96, 128, 132, 137, 171, 178, 184, 202, 213–15, 250, 265, 275, 292, 320, 351, 419, 480, 489, 503, 522, 540, 561, 569, 582, 594, 601

type 1, 545

type 2, 17, 26, 59, 61, 64–65, 77, 132, 154, 218, 270, 414, 475, 487, 505, 580

Diabetes Prevention Program, 18

diabetic retinopathy, 184, 470, 475

dialysis, 6–7

diarrhea, 90, 542, 587

diclofenac sodium gel (Voltaren), 354

diet, optimal, 151–62, 599–601. See also specific types

dietary fiber hypothesis, 250–51

Dietary Guidelines for Americans, 274

Dietary Inflammatory Index, 83–84, 89–90, 93, 97, 100, 144, 406

dietary quality index, 208

dietary restriction mimetics, 15, 511

Dietary Supplement Health and Education Act (DSHEA), 193, 485

diet soda, 168, 256–57

dignity, 12, 480–84

dill, 32–33, 98, 101

DIM, 107

dioxins, 209–10, 372, 492

DIRECT trial, 564–65

diuretic drugs, 162

diverticulosis, 202, 247, 459

DNA, 29, 35, 40, 44, 46–47, 109–10, 112–13, 120–21, 130, 136, 195, 325, 518, 575, 578

DNA damage, 117–18, 124, 128, 215, 241, 444, 500, 503, 509, 517, 595

DNA methylation, 46, 48–54, 588

DNA repair, 112–13, 118, 120, 122, 130, 140, 215, 447, 509, 511, 595

Dog Aging Project, 103

dogs, as pets, 231, 245

Dolly (cloned sheep), 45–46

donepezil (Aricept), 360–61

Dramamine, 194

Dr. Greger's Daily Dozen app, 52

DrugAge database, 37

drusen, 475

dry eye syndrome, 445

dulse, 191

durian fruit, 33

DXA (DEXA) scanning, 244

dypepsia, 503

dysbiosis, 534–36

dysphoria, 382

earwax, 289–90

Easter Island, 101–2, 290

echinacea, 324–25

E. coli, 86, 530, 533, 537

edamame, 54, 241

EGCG (epigallocatechin gallate), 107, 166, 286, 445

egg cell, human, 45–46, 139

eggs, 27, 34, 57, 75, 77, 115, 125, 153, 154–55, 175, 187, 204, 230, 259, 272–74, 277, 293, 349–50, 377, 393, 409, 413, 472, 522, 524, 527, 537, 539–40, 545–46, 577–78, 581, 600

egg whites, 95

ejaculatory disorders, 258

elastin, 55, 439–40, 447

elderberry, 324–25

electrolytes, 163

ellagitannins, 550

emphysema, 6, 327, 487, 493. See also COPD

emulsifiers, 538

endocarditis, 340, 497

Endocrine Society, 310, 316

endometrial cancer, 84, 297, 428

endophthalmitis, 478

endorphins, 419, 483

endothelial function, 37, 223

endothelial progenitor cells (EPCs), 263

endotoxins, 86–88, 100, 372, 421

endurance training, 16, 217

Enfamil, 56

Ensure, 408

enterotypes, 544

EPA, 154, 277, 397–98

Epic of Gilgamesh, 9

epigenetics, 44–54, *148*, 219

epilepsy, 28, 238

Epsom salts, 249

Epstein-Barr virus, 81, 327

equol producers, 395

erectile dysfunction (ED), 55, 215, 258, 311, 313, 315–16, 356, 423, 431–39, 465

ergothioneine, 12, 191–92

esophageal cancer, 84, 165

Esselstyn, Caldwell, 186, 569, 601

essential amino acids, 73–74, 410–11

essential tremor, 417–18

estrogen-dependent disease, 335

estrogenic products, 125, 132

estrogen-like chemicals, 28

estrogens, 240–41, 297, 303, 428

estrogen therapy, 257, 297–300, 428, 430

ethylamine, 331

eugenics, 200, 280, 319

eunuchs, 200, 280, 313, 319

European ancestry, 137, 166

European Association of Urology, 310, 316, 437

European Food Safety Authority, 589

European Prospective Investigation into Cancer and Nutrition (EPIC) study, 479

exercise, 12, 16, 24, 40, 49–50, 65, 85, 94–95, 110, 120–21, 124, 129, 131, 133, 142, 155, 210, 213–19, 225, 229, 241–44, 249, 282, 316, 321–22, 348, 375–76, 405–6, 419, 495, 507, 509, 520–21, 559–60, 567–68, 595, 599

exercise-induced oxidative stress paradox, 120–21

exopolysaccharides, 532–33

exosomes, 519, 524–25, 528–30

eye color, 474. *See also* vision

face-lifts, 442

facial masks, 454

facial moisturizers, 450–51

facial youth serum, 503

falls, 215, 236, 243–45, 404, 417

fasting, 24, 71, 131, 377, 514, 551, 563–65, 567, 569–70

fasting blood sugar, 60

fasting-mimicking diet, 71, 562, 564–65

fat, dietary, 58, 123–24, 220–21, 234, 556. *See also* body fat; saturated fats; *and specific types*

fat cells, 39, 82–83

fat oxidation, 123–24, 501–2

fat storage, 14–15

fecal impaction, 247

fecal incontinence, 316

fecal transplants, 285, 533, 535

female androgen deficiency, 425

female sexual function, 421–30

femur fractures, 235

fennel creams, 429–30

fennel seeds, 308, 429–30

fenugreek, 308, 317, 430, 513

fermented foods, 107, 190, 542–43

fertility, 199–201, 296

fetal ductus arteriosus, 98

FGF21 (fibroblast growth factor 21), 222, 566–70, 575, 581

fiber, 21–23, 37, 53, 60, 84, 88–92, 101, 114, 124, 141, 145, 148, 176, 178–79, 190, 206, 210, 228, 234, 246–51, 254, 266, 303, 332–33, 350, 372, 378, 387–88, 395, 412, 447, 460, 512, 532–36, 538–39, 543–47, 559, 568, 582

fibrocystic lumps, 208

50-food challenge, 546–47

figitumumab, 71

figs, 252

fillers, 442, 448

finasteride (Propecia, Proscar), 283, 258

FINGER (Finnish Geriatric Intervention Study), 400–401

fingernails, artificial, 462–63

Finland, 230

Finnish Mental Hospital Study, 293–94

fisetin, 43–44

fish, 93, 120, 125, 144, *153*, 154, 175, 181, 187, 228, 273, 277, 283, 304, 396–401, 413, 450, 479, 498, 502–3, 537, 577, 581

fish oil, 93, 144, 146, 154, 277, 356, 391, 396–97, 399, 473, 488, 502

5:2 fasting, 560

flatulence, 178–79

flavones, 89

flavonoids, 43, 107, 377, 415, 423, 513, 514, 521, 522

flavonols, 41

flaxseed, 36, 77, 95, 97, 101, 154, 196, 251, 260–61, 274, 304, 307, 318, 354–55, 397

flexitarians, 583

flibanserin (Addyi), 422

Flomax, 260

flossing, 468

flour, 548

flu, 5, 319, 323–24, 328, 331, 332, 338–39

fluid restriction, 256, 261

fluoride, 470

flu vaccine, 80, 320–22, 325, 328, 333, 337–40

FODMAP, 547

folate, 51–54, 176, 211, 385, 386–87

folic acid, 51–53, 292, 385, 386–87

follicular unit transplanting, 284

Fontana, Luigi, 11, 75, 583

Food and Drug Administration (FDA), 159, 193,
    284, 288, 299–300, 310, 361, 368, 380,
    403, 422, 425, 428–29, 436, 450, 457–58,
    464, 485–86, 541, 589

food chain, eating low on, 209–10

food color, 117, 188

foods, best and worst, 12, 151–60

footbaths, 227

forest bathing, 224, 321–22

FOXO gene, 520

frailty, 43, 48, 58, 84, 113, 132, 135, 404–6,
    408, 412, 544

Framingham Heart Study, 278

Framingham Risk Score, 269, 423

Franklin, Rosalind, 46

Freedom of Information Act, 171

free radicals, 88, 93, 109–13, 119, 121–25, 129,
    187, 195–96, 241, 279, 350, 393, 452,
    471, 500, 502, 509, 551, 556, 575, 578–79

french fries, 25, 38, 143

French paradox, 172

fruit and vegetable dose-response longevity
    study, 209

fruit juice, 129, 172–73

fruits, 49, 50, 56–57, 61, 87, 89–90, 94, 114,
    116, 120–21, 129, 141, 147, 151–52,
    153, 156–57, 172–75, 179, 181, 207, 209,
    213–14, 238, 254, 304, 323, 326, 388–89,
    413, 443–45, 447, 512, 517, 525–26, 546,
    577, 597

fucoxanthin, 190

Fugh-Berman, Adriane, 298, 422

Fuhrman, Joel, 95

fungal infections, 331

fungal meningitis, 373

fungi, 102, 510, 523

furocoumarins, 447–48

furosemide (Lasix), 291

galactagogue, 308

galactokinase, 480

galactose, 107, 237, 308, 480, 542

gallbladder disease, 299

Game Changers (documentary), 218, 439

gamma-delta T cells, 331

gargling, 332

garlic, 33, 89, 97, 101, 119, 130, 193–94, 259,
    262, 329, 394, 414, 447, 511–12, 547

garlic powder, 98, 193–94, 501

garlic supplements, 329

gastritis, 190

gastrocolic reflex, 249

gastrointestinal system, 343

gelatin, 357, 411

GEMINAL study, 47

gene expression, 46–47, 588

genetics, 11, 13–14, 216, 244, 279, 366–67

genistein, 240, 521

genitourinary syndrome of menopause (GSM),
    426–29

genotoxic chemotherapy, 113

Germany, 455

germ theory of disease, 79

Gerontological Society of America, 1

gerontology, 2–3, 10, 531

gerontotoxins, 65

geroprotectors, 513

ghee, 126

ginger, 89, 97–98, 101, 118, 119, 130, 193–95,
    222, 286, 353, 447, 501, 515, 525, 549

ginger tea, 64

gingivitis, 468

gingko, 380, 384, 477

ginseng, 127–28, 335, 380, 426, 436, 526

glaucoma, 28, 435, 475–77, 504, 552

Global BMI Mortality Collaboration, 222

Global Burden of Disease Study, 151–52, 157,
    171–72, 175, 493

GLP-1, 317, 548

glucosamine, 356–57

glutamine, 238, 412

glutathione, 122

glycation, 54–66, 81, *148*, 371, 447

glycemic index, 543

glycemic load, 59–66, 292

glycine, 579

GNC, 486, 542

goji berries, 325, 472–73, 505–6

gonorrhea, 332

Good Manufacturing Practices, 486

gooseberry, 503

gotu kola, 147

gout, 94, 351, 414

grains, 91, 147, 413, 577. *See also* whole grains

grapefruit, 444, 513, 525

grape juice, 120, 172–73, 262, 510–11

grape polyphenols, 172

grapes, 505–7, 510, 516, 525

grape seed extract supplements, 507

grape skins, 131, 513, 515

graying hair, 113, 138, 278–80

great apes, 113–14, 157, 211

Great Protein Fiasco, 407

Greece, 175, 180, 193

green beans, 96, 496

green leafy vegetables, 117, 146, 174, 187, 212, 304, 474, 475, 492, 494–99

green peas, 33, 38, 99, 516

greens, 51, 53, 101, 165, 212, 388, 392, 438, 441, 444, 468–69, 472, 474, 476, 478, 492–99, 526. *See also* dark green leafy vegetables; green leafy vegetables

green tea, 34, 41, 44, 64–65, 77, 89, 98, 101, 107, 118, 120–22, 129, 145–46, 166–67, 240, 263, 286, 287, 330–32, 350, 394, 445–46, 466, 511, 516, 517, 549

green tea lotion, 107, 446

grip strength, 137, 241, 404

groats, 548

guava, 501

Guillain-Barré syndrome, 338–39

Guinness Book of World Records, The, 173

gums, 468–69

gut, 29, 36–37, 43, 61, 90, 91, 97, 241, 251, 252, 379, 492, 504, 523, 525, 530–50, 568

gut leakiness, 532, 535–36

gut permeability, 83, 86

gynecomastia, 258, 307, 318

Hadza tribe, 534

hair, 12, 30, 278–87

hair dyes, 279–80

hair loss, 41, 281, 283–87

hair plugs, 283–84

haloalkanes, 534

ham, 144, 497, 524

hand pain, 342

Harvard Health Professionals Follow-Up Study, 182, 432, 476

Harvard Medical School Center of Excellence in Women's Health, 305

Harvard Nurses' Health Study, 21, 69, 93, 182, 302–3, 392, 402, 428, 476, 491

Harvard Nurses' Health Study II, 322

Harvard Physicians' Health Study II, 474

Harvard School of Public Health, 410, 569

Harvard University, 498, 560

Harvard Women's Health Study, 369

Hashimoto's thyroiditis, 20, 545

Hayflick limit, 38–39, 136, 140, 576

hazelnuts, 117, 184, 491

HbA1c, 54, 132, 251

HDL cholesterol, 169–70, 217

headaches, chronic, 190

head injuries, 372

healthspan, 7, 48, 130–31, 585, 598

Healthy Lifestyle and Preventable Death study, 498

Healthy Man Study, 309

hearing, 12, 103, 287–94

hearing aids, 287–89

heart, 30, 140, 154, 218, 496–97, 503

heart attacks, 4, 5, 21, 31, 138, 163, 171, 176, 183, 184, 186, 213, 230, 236, 272, 274, 298–99, 320, 339, 341, 343, 430, 465, 490, 512, 569

heartburn, 27, 503

heart disease, 5, 42, 55, 77, 83, 88, 99, 124, 126, 137, 141, 144, 151, 157, 165, 169–71, 178–82, 187, 189, 201, 203, 208, 250, 262, 265–78, 294, 340, 459, 488–89, 492–93, 561, 569, 574

heart failure, 6, 127, 159, 171, 274

heart fibrosis, 59

heart rate, 177–79, 231

heavy metals, 122, 399

Hegsted, Mark, 83

height, 68–69

Helicobacter pylori, 531

hematocrit, 590

hemoglobin, 54–55, 590

hemorrhagic colitis, 47

hemorrhagic stroke, 276

hemorrhoids, 202, 247, 459

hemp seeds, 578

hepatitis A vaccine, 322

hepatitis B vaccine, 322, 337

hepatitis C, 328

herbal hair loss treatments, 286–87

herbal medicines, 526

herbal sleep aids, 228

herbal supplements, 486

herbal teas, 121, 167

herbs, 89, 99, 116, 118–19, 130, 158, 239, 285, 308, 380, 501, 513 herniated discs, 39

herniation, 355

herpes (HSV), 328, 374

heterocyclic amines, 59, 124

hiatal hernias, 246–47, 459

hibiscus, 20, 22, 23, 167, 418, 505–6

hidradenitis suppurativa, 92, 330

high blood pressure (hypertension), 55, 157–59, 169, 178, 190, 193, 202, 208, 213–14, 265, 267, 281, 290, 335, 364–65, 414, 423, 480, 601

high botanical diversity diet, 517

high-fat diet, 50, 58–59, 61, 85, 120, 317, 459, 520

high-intensity interval training (HIIT), 24, 142, 217, 568

high-nutrient density, 95

high-protein diet, 317–18, 557–59, 571, 573, 583

hip fractures, 233, 234, 236–45

hip or spine T-scores, 234

hip pain, 342

Hippocrates, 193, 217, 433, 531

hip protectors, 245

Hispanics, 166, 179, 458

HIV, 328, 342

HMB, 415

Hoffman effect, 576

homeopathy, 508

homocysteine, 106, 385–87, 448, 588, 590

honeybees, 47

honeybush, 446

honeysuckle, 526

hops, 307

hormesis, 121, 507–9, 511, 514, 551, 560

hormone replacement therapy, 240–41, 257, 297–300, 304–5

hormones, 294–319, 543–44

hospice care, 481–82

hospitals, 481

hot dogs, 58, 66, 144, 155, 497

hot flashes, 297, 299–300, 303–8, 427–29

How Not to Age Cookbook, The (Greger), 196, 260

How Not to Die (Greger), 3, 9, 12, 33, 36, 88, 99, 109, 123, 127, 162, 168, 182, 190, 191, 253, 254, 329, 357, 366, 417, 431, 475, 503, 506, 517, 601

How Not to Diet (Greger), 3, 5, 14, 19, 20, 21, 60, 62, 65, 179–80, 193, 199, 219, 221, 222, 226, 332, 506, 544, 548, 560, 580

How to Survive a Pandemic (Greger), 5

HPV (human papilloma virus), 334

human ancestors, 22, 113–15, 157, 523

Human Genome Project, 518

human growth hormone (HGH), 294–95

Hunza Valley, 173

hyaluronic acid, 344, 346, 439–40

hydration, 162, 445–46, 463

hydrogen sulfide, 538–39

hyperfiltration, 88

hypertension. *See* high blood pressure

hyperthyroidism, 335, 563

hypogonadism, 310, 313

hypomethylation, 50–52

hypothyroidism, 20, 279, 281

hysterectomies, 202

ibuprofen (Advil), 97, 291, 343, 353, 536

IGF-1 (insulin-like growth factor 1), 11, 66–78, 105, *148*, 201, 276, 306, 562, 565–67, 570–75

Ikaria, Greece, 174, 180

illicit drugs, 229

Imitrex, 98

immune cells, 30, 595

immune suppression, 318–19, 558

immune system, 12, 30, 39, 79–80, 90, 137, 190, 193, 319–42, 373, 492, 494, 499, 536, 558, 571

immune thrombocytopenic purpura, 338

immunoglobulin A (IgA), 328–30

immunosenescence, 79–80

India, 99, 126, 176, 194, 207, 366

indole-3-carbinol, 107

Indo-Mediterranean Trial, 185

indoxyl sulfate, 412

infant formula, 56

infections, 79, 319, 489, 558

infertility, 104, 558

inflammaging, 79–83, 536, 596

inflammation, 18, 20, 39, 42–43, 55, 59, 65, 78–101, 123, 127, 130, 132, 135, 138, 141, 144–45, 147, *148*, 176, 184, 188, 194, 215, 218, 220, 239, 241, 269, 292, 304, 320, 329, 343, 367, 371, 378–79, 402, 406–7, 432–34, 443, 494, 503, 505–6, 517, 535–36, 545, 551, 562, 570, 575, 595–96

inflammatory bowel disease, 246, 539

inflammatory microRNAs, 521

insomnia, 224–26, 228–29

Institute for Biomedical Aging Research, 2

Institute for Science in Medicine, 486

Institute for the Medical Humanities, 160
Institute of Medicine, 163, 274
insulin, 176, 297, 506, 547, 562, 580, 582
insulin resistance, 18, 19, 59, 62, 241, 270, 562,
      574, 580–83
insulin secretion, 270
insulin sensitivity, 218, 505, 555, 559, 571, 583
interleukin 6 (IL-6), 80, 85, 87, 92, 96, 100,
      172, 252
interleukin 10 (IL-10), 92
interleukin 18, 424
intermittent fasting, 552, 560–63
intermittent vegan diet, 583
International Osteoporosis Foundation, 237
International Society of Sports Nutrition, 416
interval training, 316
intraocular pressure, 476–77
in vitro fertilization, 295
iodine, 191
Iowa Women's Health Study, 486
Iran, 383
iron, 175, 211, 284, 369, 503
irradiation of food, 126
irritable bowel syndrome, 542
isoflavones, 189, 259, 305, 429
isoleucine, 105, 579–80
Italy, 30, 181, 563

Japan, 175, 190, 305, 306, 322, 327–28, 395,
      405, 420, 445, 476, 536, 542–43
jaundice, 246, 587
J curve, 169–72
Jenkins, David, 240
Jews, 68–70, 166, 199
joints, 12, 97, 234, 342–57
Jumpstart program, 275
Junctional adhesion molecule-A, 526
junk food, 59, 115, 124, 143, 206–8, 272–73,
      545
JUST Egg, 409
Justice Department, 126

Kaiser Permanente, 205
kale, 41, 44, 96, 122, 146, 392–93, 443–44,
      476, 578
Kame Project, 173
kanamycin, 291
Kaposi sarcoma, 103
kefir, 542
Kegel exercises, 257
Kenyon, Cynthia, 66–67

ketogenic diet, 61–62, 221, 228, 238, 276, 407,
      567–68
Keys, Ancel, 180–81, 184
kidney cancer, 84
kidney disease, 26, 43, 58, 80, 84, 88, 124, 159,
      269, 552
kidney failure, 37, 125, 137, 234, 414, 540, 563
kidney fibrosis, 59
kidneys, 39, 140, 160, 162–63, 190, 238, 255,
      270, 343, 408, 412–13, 413
kidney stones, 20, 129, 336, 414
kimchi, 190
King, Martin Luther, Jr., 598
kiwifruit, 118, 324, 411
knees, 90, 97, 243, 342, 344–46, 348, 350–55,
      496
Kraft Foods, 76
Kremezin, 66
Kyolic aged garlic extract, 193

lactic acid, 21
Lactobacillus, 21, 91, 189, 252, 378–79, 504,
      538–39, 543, 545, 549
lactose, 165–66, 237, 542
lactucin, 229
lactulose, 251
lacunar infarcts, 365
lamb, 522, 577
Laron syndrome, 70
L-ascorbic acid, 453–54
laser skin resurfacing, 443
lavender, 307–8, 381, 382, 426
laxatives, 162, 248–52
L cells, 548
LDL cholesterol, 19, 65, 124, 169, 172–73,
      182, 186, 189, 206, 207, 217, 241, 251,
      263–77, 307, 317, 367, 475, 501, 505–7,
      550, 561, 590
lead, 87
lecanemab (Lequembi), 361
lecithin supplements, 540
Leeuwenhoek, Antonie van, 29
legumes, 21, 52, 61, 89, 92, 101, 111–12, 141,
      153, 161, 174, 175–79, 189, 207, 259,
      292, 337, 387, 388, 394–95, 411, 479,
      489, 512, 546, 547, 548, 568, 569, 577
lemon balm, 119, 381, 382
lemon-infused water, 118
lemon juice, 64, 123
lemons, 117, 513
lemon verbena tea, 20, 23, 121, 228

lentils, 54, 61, 89, 92, 99, 112, 175–78, 189, 582

lettuce, 34, 41, 228–29, 408–9, *495*, 501

leucine, 105–8, 579

leukemia, 28, 521

Levitra, 435

libido, 104, 201, 313, 317, 421–22, 425, 558–59

licorice, 526

LIFE (Low Inflammatory Foods Every Day) Diet, 95–96

lifestyle, 47–48, 174, 212–14, 233, 320–23, 372–78, 498

light therapy, 224

lignans, 307

lima beans, 189

Lipitor, 42, 268

lipofuscin, 440

lipoid pneumonia, 469

lipoprotein(a) [Lp(a)], 269, 274–75, 307

liposuction, 220

liver, 18–19, 25–26, 30, 49, 53, 73, 84, 122, 140, 146, 189, 343, 408, 426, 480, 587, 588

liver cancer, 84

liver disease, 18, 25–26, 132, 135, 168

liver failure, 137, 563

lobster, 93

Loma Linda University, 210, 388–89

Longo, Valter, 11, 75, 78, 562, 583

Lotrimin (clotrimazole), 461

lovastatin, 192

low back pain, 355–56

low blood pressure, 104, 558

low-carb diet, 59, 61–62, 75, 114, 210, 228, 276–77, 539

low-fat diet, 58, 182, 221, 304, 459, 462, 520

low-glycemic diet, 60–61

low-level laser therapy (LLLT), 284

low-protein diet, 75, 571, 574. *See also* protein restriction

low T syndrome, 309–10, 318

lumbar disc, 355

lung cancer, 19, 69, 76, 152, 156, 165, 267, 299, 493, 599

lungs, 6, 84, 90, 95, 97, 137

lupus, 89, 318

lutein, 393, 471–74, 478–79

lycium berries, 473

lycopene, 77, 468–69, 515, 516

lymphocytes, 492

Lyon Diet Heart Study, 185–86

Mabaan tribe, 290–93

maca, 426

MacArthur Study of Successful Aging, 139

macrophages, 82, 83, 536

macula, 393, 471

macular degeneration, 113, 470–75, 504

magnesium, 211, 415

Maillard reaction, 54, 56, 57

malaria, 513

male hormones, 280–81

male sexual function, 430–39

malondialdehyde (MDA), 500–502

mammograms, 300–302

MAMPs (microbe-associated molecular patterns), 330–31

mangos, 33, 35, 94, 118, 252, 447, 500

manicures, 463

manual labor, 216

marathon runners, 120, 142, 509

marjoram, 119, 130

Mars520 space flight, 89

matcha, 167, 196–97

Mayo Clinic, 41, 257, 322, 496, 599

meat, 18, 34–35, 49, 50, 56, 58, 59, 82–83, 86–89, 75, 92, 100, 113–14, 124–26, 154, 155, 161, 174–76, 181, 202–4, 210, 221, 228, 230, 259, 272–74, 292, 304, 371–72, 377, 416, 421, 441, 475, 479–80, 497–501, 517, 522, 524, 539–40, 545–46, 581. *See also specific types*

Medicare, 342, 481

medications, 205, 213, 342–43, 358. *See also* prescription drugs; *and specific types*

meditation, 49

Mediterranean diet, 32, 120, 145, 180–87, 198, 204–6, 277, 401, 419, 497, 545, 570

melanoma, 137, 435, 455–56, 458

melasma, 458

melatonin, 227–28, 374–75, 506

memantine (Namenda), 360–61

memory, 84, 305, 357, 363, 369, 380–82, 399, 557

MeNAM, 588

meningitis, 340, 398

meniscus damage, 243

menopause, 77, 132, 143, 234, 240–41, 296–308, 425–28, 561

menstruation, 36, 98, 104, 201, 558

mental health, 84, 154, 421

Merck, 258

mercury, 283, 399

messenger RNA, 518–19

meta-analysis, defined, 152–53

metabolic acidosis, 238

metabolic disease, 18

metabolic syndrome, 132, 208, 269, 281

metabolism, 61, 110, 180, 218–19, 492, 494–95, 552, 556, 571

metalloestrogen, 368

Metamucil, 22, 90, 250, 252, 547

metastases, 69–70

Metchnikoff, Élie, 531–32

metformin, 17–19, 21–22, 131, 149

methionine, 105–6, 110–12, 228, 387, 410, 538–39, 569, 574, 577

methionine restriction, 10, 111–12, 129, 575–79

methionine sulfoxide reductase, 575

methylation, 46–48, 50–52, 588–89

methylglyoxal, 62

Mexican Americans, 179

microbiome, 36, 53, 83, 212, 251, 378–79, 440, 447, 496–97, 523, 530–50, 581, 590

microbiome and, 378–79

microlife, 154

microRNAs, 46, 507, 518–30, 542

migraine, 98, 127, 132, 194

milk, 27, 33–34, 56, 72, 76, 95, 106–7, 119, 125, 145, 148, 154, 162, *164*, 165–67, 191, 236–37, 306, 328, 351, 390, 407, 480, 524, 528–30, 537, 542, 577

millet, 63

Million Women Study, 297–98

MIND diet, 401–2

ministrokes, 281, 359, 365

Minnesota Green Tea Trial, 146, 240

Minnesota Starvation Study, 104, 201, 554–56

minoxidil (Rogaine), 283, 286–87

mint, 119, 425

Miocene era, 157

misfolded proteins, 23, 34

miso soup, 187, 190

mitochondria, 16–20, 109–12, 129, 133, 494–95, 550, 552, 571, 575, 578

mitochondrial myopathy, 587–88

MMR vaccine, 332–33, 338, 340

model organisms, 14, 26

Moderate Alcohol and Cardiovascular Health Trial, 171

moles, suspicious, 455

monk fruit, 62

monounsaturated oils, 182, 221

Mormons, 561

morphine, 512

mosquitos, 194

mouthwash, 466, 470, 496

MRSA, 537

MTHFR, 52

mTOR (mechanistic target of rapamycin), 11, 24–26, 38, 101–8, 133, *148*, 149, 201, 409–10, 520, 529–30, 567, 579

Multidomain Alzheimer Preventive Trial, 397

multidrug-resistant bacteria, 537

multiple sclerosis, 89, 318–19, 487, 545

multivitamins, 335–36, 384, 474, 479, 486–87

Munroe, Randall, 523

muscles, 12, 39, 55, 74, 80, 94, 107–8, 113, 137, 215, 241, 404–18, 495–96, 506, 558–59, 581

mushrooms, 30, 32–33, 38, 96, 191–93, 329–31, 394, 420

music, 316, 387, 425

mussels, 35

MyPlate campaign, 175

N-acetylcysteine (NAc), 128

NADH, 585

NAD+ (nicotinamide adenine dinucleotide), 131, 136, *148*, 169, 188, 570, 583–96

nails, 460–64

NAMPT enzyme, 594–95

naproxen (Aleve), 291, 343, 536

National Academy of Medicine, 287, 312

National Cancer Institute, 459

National Cattlemen's Beef Association, 407, 409

National Chicken Council, 154

National Dairy Council, 165, 407

National Football League, 372

National Geographic, 173

National Institute on Aging, 102–3, 569

National Institutes of Health, 155, 171, 311–12, 349

National Osteoporosis Foundation, 235, 237

National Sleep Foundation, 225

National Toxicology Program, 470

natto, 543

natural killer cells, 321, 325–30, 333–35, 419

Natural Science Foundation of China, 286

naturopaths, 295

neomycin, 291

neroli oil (bitter orange), 426

nerves, 50, 361, 381, 593

Nestle, Marion, 115

neu5Gc, 88–89, 100

neuridine, 29

Neurobiology of Aging, 363

neurodegeneration, 18, 552

neurons, 360, 362

neurotransmitters, 361

neurotrophins, 375–76

New Zealand, 309–10, 383

Nexium, 234

NF-κB, 96

niacin (nicotinic acid, NA), 487, 585–88. *See also* Vitamin B₃

nicotinamide (niacinamide, NAM), 452, 456, 459, 477, 585–89, 593–94

nicotinamide cream, 452–53, 588

nicotine, 19, 165, 225

Nicoya Peninsula, 174

Nigerian paradox, 366–67

night sweats, 297, 303–5, 308

NIH-AARP Diet and Health Study, 155, 203, 497, 573

nitrates, 391–92, 469, 476, 494–98, *495*

nitric oxide, 327, 392, 438, 476

nitrites, 497

nitrosamines, 497–98

NMDA blockers, 361

NMN (nicotinamide mononucleotides), 585–86, 589, 591–94

nocturia, 261

noise exposure, 291–92

non-arteritic ischemic optic neuropathy (NAION), 434

noncoding RNA, 518–19

non-Hodgkin's lymphoma, 84

nonmitochondiral DNA, 112

nori, 191, 328

normal pressure hydrocephalus, 358

North American Menopause Society, 426

Norway, 230, 551

NR (nicotinamide riboside), 588–94

Nrf2, 122–23, 129, 511

NSAIDS (nonsteroidal anti-inflammatory drugs), 291, 343–46, 349–50, 353–55, 536

nutritional yeast, 92, 330

NutritionFacts.org, 210, 222, 224

nuts, 35, 66, 75, 87, 90, 93, 97, 99, 117, 119, 141, 146, 152, 157, 161, 175, 182–84, 221, 240, 337, 396, 437–39, 447, 473, 489–91, 521, 548, 550, 577–78

oatmeal, 62, 119, 506

oat milk, 27

oats, 101

obesity, 49, 82–83, 144, 154, 164, 168, 178, 208, 213–14, 219–20, 222, 242, 250, 255, 275, 292, 316, 318, 320–21, 323, 372, 375, 433, 480, 487, 553–54, 569–70, 598

Okinawan diet, 74, 105, 174, 187–98, 498, 560, 569, 570, 572–73, 579

oleic acid, 221

oligosaccharides, 547

olive oil, 18, 145–46, 182–86, 221, 304, 355, 396, 502, 521, 524

olives, 182, 502

omega-3 fatty acids, 93, 144, 154, 186, 277, 304, 396–98, 415, 491

omega-6 fats, 349

omega-7 fats, 420

oncogenes, 47

onions, 41–42, 44, 64, 239, 259, 263, 423, 502, 505, 521, 547

ONTRAC (Oral Nicotinamide to Reduce Actinic Cancer), 456

onychomycosis, 460, 463

opioids, 343

optic nerve, 50, 435, 477

oral cancer, 469, 470

oral contraceptives, 281

orange juice, 27, 118, 120, 173, 445

oranges, 89, 118, 516, 578

oregano, 99, 119, 501

organic foods, 99–100, 210, 326, 432, 510–11

organ transplants, 103

orgasm, 424, 431

Ornish, Dean, 47, 76, 141–44, 147, 210, 403–4, 601

orthopedic surgery, 344–45

oseltamivir (Tamiflu), 324

Osler, Sir William, 340

ospemifene, 429

osteoarthritis, 39, 43, 58, 77, 90, 94, 97, 132, 194, 342–57

osteonecrosis of the jaw, 235

osteoporosis, 5, 39, 43, 55, 58, 125, 137, 140, 233–39, 242, 243–44, 299, 414, 559

ovarian cancer, 69, 84, 162

ovarian hormones, 271

ovaries, 45, 139, 296, 425

overdentures, 466

Over-the-Counter Hearing Aid Act, 288

overweight, 168, 355–56, 375. *See also* obesity

oxalates, 491

Oxford Vegetarian Study, 197

oxidation, 44, 109–30, *148*, 367–68, 500–502, 511

oxidative stress, 59, 88, 109, 111, 113, 117, 119–21, 124–25, 127–28, 135, 141, 147, 172, 184, 194, 196, 218–19, 239, 279, 304, 372–73, 384, 402, 440, 445, 471, 478, 506, 509, 540, 552, 556, 562, 570, 575, 591

oxidized cholesterol, 125–26, 364, 371

oxygen, 82, 441, 495

oxylipins, 97

oxysterols, 125

oysters, 35, 337, 577

PAHs (polycyclic aromatic hydrocarbons), 441

Paleo diet, 113–14, 157, 217–18, 407

palliative care, 481–83

palmitic acid, 18, 86, 106, 221, 238

palm kernel oil, 273

palm oil, 18, 182, 273, 371

PAMPs (pathogen-associated molecular patterns), 330

pancreas, 270

pancreatic cancer, 69, 84

pancreatitis, 324

paprika, 99, 195, 501

parabiotic studies, 40

Parkinson's disease, 5, 26, 34, 39, 48, 80, 165, 358, 417–18, 587–88

PARP-1, 595

parsley, 89, 239, 447, 448, 521

parsnips, 447–48

pasta, 63, 177, 413, 568

Pasteur, Louis, 531

pasteurization, 72

Pauling, Linus, 336

Paxil, 439

PCBs, 209, 372, 399, 441, 559

PCSK9 gene, 267, 270–71

peaches, 513

peanut butter, 491

peanuts, 35, 491

pears, 31, 33

pecans, 18

pectin, 134

pellagra, 584, 586–87

pelvic arteries, 356, 422

pelvic floor exercises, 257

penicillin, 102, 192, 340

penile arteries, 55

penile implants, 434–35

perimenopause, 283

periodontal bone, 103

periodontitis, 132, 464–65, 468

peripheral artery disease, 55, 177, 184, 274, 356, 422, 462

permethrin clothing treatments, 194

persimmons, 117

pesticides, 49, 99–100, 115, 209, 325–26, 371, 432

pesto, 473

pets, 231

Pew Charitable Trusts, 380

pharmaceutical industry, 6, 16, 17, 126, 147, 160, 270, 297, 298, 309, 318, 379, 408, 421, 476, 534

pH balance, 234, 238, 412–14, *413*

Philip, Prince, Duke of Edinburgh, 294

Philip Morris, 76

PhIP, 522

phloridzin, 133–34

photosynthesis, 114, 500

phototherapy, 447–48

phthalates, 424–25

physical activity, 83, 85, 142, 174, 215, 249, 258, 372

physician-assisted dying, 482

phytochemicals, 383, 512–13, 516–17

phytoestrogens, 189, 200, 240–41, 304, 307, 318

phytoncides, 321

phytonutrients, *27*, 41, 49, 84, 99–100, 116, 118, 124, 133, 176, 184, 209, 423, 504, 510–17, 523–24

pickled vegetables, 152, 542

pinene, 224, 321

pine nuts, 35

pippali (piperlongumine), 43–44

pistachios, 437–38, 540

pituitary gland, 69

placebo effect, 345–47

plantains, 259

plant-based diet, 5, 51, 57, 71, 76, 78, 84, 92, 94, 95, 99–100, 105–6, 111–16, 124–26, 129, 145, 147, 152, *153*, 156–57, 165–66, 174–75, 180, 187, 197, 199–212, 217–19, 221, 242, 246–47, 249–50, 260, 265, 270, 275–78, 303–5, 334, 348–50, 366, 387, 403–4, 413, 423–25, 432, 439, 448, 462, 469–70, 517, 545, 582, 601

plant protein, 72–74, 88, 111–12, 277–78, 410–12, 569–74

plasmids, 537

plastics, 432–33
platelet count, 590
Plato, 346–47
plums, 505
pneumococcal disease, 340–41
pneumonia, 79–80, 163, 234, 319, 322, 328, 333, 337, 536, 540
pneumonia vaccine, 321, 323, 340–41
polio vaccine, 338
pollutants and toxins, 83, 93, 115, 184, 209–10, 276–77, 371–72, 398–400, 492, 494, 534, 559. See also air pollution
polycystic ovary syndrome (PCOS), 132, 540
polyethylene glycol, 248
polygonum multiflorum, 286–87
polyphenol chlorogenic acid, 26
polyphenols, 173, 367, 369, 388–90, 394, 507, 511–15, 521, 548–49
polysorbate, 80, 538
polyunsaturated fat, 50, 182, 500–503
pomegranate juice, 173, 438
pomegranates, 94, 120, 351, 505, 513, 515, 517, 550
popcorn, 34, 505
pork, 85, 125, 126, 272, 370, 413, 441, 503, 537, 577
porphyran, 190
porphyria, 563
postbiotics, 530, 539, 543–44
postherpetic neuralgia, 341
potassium, 159, 176
potassium bicarbonate supplements, 412
potassium chloride, 159–60
potato chips, 25, 38
potatoes, 33, 35, 58, 63–64, 96, 505
poultry, 57, 125, 144, 153, 228, 259, 278, 350, 413, 425, 503, 537, 577
prebiotics, 21, 37, 89, 179, 252, 333, 412, 530, 538–39, 543–50
prediabetes, 59, 580
PREDIMED study, 183–84, 204, 396, 491
prednisolone, 97
pregnancy, 19, 28, 53, 98, 163, 169, 464, 563
Premarin, 298, 300
premenstrual syndrome, 194
PremPro, 298
prescription drugs, 98–99, 346, 403, 534, 599. See also medications; and specific types
Prevacid, 234
Prevagen, 379–80
Prevotella, 91, 544–46

Prilosec, 234
Pritikin, Nathan, 177, 601
probiotics, 36, 37, 333, 378–79, 412, 530–31, 539–43, 545
processed foods, 84, 143, 158, 161, 206–8, 304, 368, 371, 388, 413, 517, 534, 538, 545
processed meats, 141, 144–45, 147, 153, 155–56, 497–98
progeria, 14
progesterone cream, 241
progesterone therapy, 297–98
Program to Reduce Incontinence by Diet and Exercise (PRIDE), 255–56
ProLon diet, 562
pro-oxidants, 115, 120–21, 123–24, 129–30
Proscar, 258, 260
prostate cancer, 47, 53, 69, 72, 74, 76–77, 84, 106–7, 141, 162, 165, 241, 258–60, 312, 314–16, 322, 487, 516, 529, 574
prostate enlargement, 258–62, 281
prostate surgery, 258–59
protein, 54–57, 71–75, 78, 175, 261, 407–11, 448–49, 538–39, 562. See also animal protein; plant protein
protein restriction, 78, 104–6, 108, 111, 407, 565–83
Protonix, 234
proton pump inhibitor (PPI) drugs, 234
Prozac, 439
PRP (platelet-rich plasma), 344
prunes, 239, 240, 252
PSA screening, 314–16
psoriasis, 89, 447
psoriatic arthritis, 540
psyllium, 22, 250–52, 547
pterostilbene, 590
puberty, 201
pull test, 282
pumpkin pie spice, 196
pumpkin seeds, 260, 285–86
P value, 72
PVC plastics, 424–25
pyrithione zinc shampoo, 286

Q-tips, 289
quack remedies, 1, 3
quadriceps muscles, 348
quercetin, 41–42, 118, 521

radiation, 110, 508, 517, 551
radiation therapy, 113, 196, 302

radioactive products, 2
RAGE, 55–56
RAND Corporation, 338
rapamycin, 101–3, 107–8, 149, 510
raspberries, 391, 500–502, 516, 526
red blood cells, 313
red clover, 307
red meat, 125–26, 144, *153*, 228, 273, 277–78, 577
red rice, 188
red sage, 526
red tea (rooibos), 167–68
red wine, 34–35, 120, 131, 172
red yeast rice supplements, 270
refined foods, 143, 147, 152, 184, 207, 259, 292, 545, 572
religion, 198–99
Replens, 427
reproduction, 200–201
resistance exercise, 24, 108, 142, 316, 348, 405, 408, 411, 416, 521, 559, 567, 595
resistant starch, 547–48
respiratory disease, 90, 489, 493
respiratory syncytial virus, 327
resveratrol, 131–33, 136, 511
retina, 393, 471, 474–75, 504
Retin-A, 451
retinoids, 451–53
retirement, 214
Reynolds Risk Score, 269
rheumatoid arthritis, 20, 97, 98, 318, 355, 595
rhubarb, *495*
riboflavin, 211
rice, 64, 207, 413, 505, 525
rice milk, 27, 119
RNA, 518
Roberts, William Clifford, 263
Rochester Lifestyle Medicine Institute, 275
Rockefeller Foundation, 180
rooibos (red tea), 167
roots, 516
rose hips, 352, 513
rosemary, 98, 118, 239, 380–81, 444, 501, 515
rosemary oil, 287
rotator cuff surgery, 344
royal jelly, 47
Ruminococcus, 547–48
running, 142, 217, 243
Rush Memory and Aging Project, 392
Rush University Medical Center, 401

rye bread, 251–52
rye groats, 377

Sachs, Oliver, 399
saffron, 383–84, 438–39, 475
sage, 118–19, 195, 239, 381–82
salad, 31, 496–99
salad dressing, 119
salami, 497, 524
salicylic acid, 98–100, 101, 511
salmon, 93, 115, 441, 502–3
Salt Institute, 158
salt (sodium), 24, 89, 100, 119, 129, 130, 157–59, 182, 190, 240, 261, 266, 365, 388–89, 413, 465, 490, 538, 542–43, 598
salt substitutes, 159–60
Sanofi, 6
San Quentin State Penitentiary, 294
sarcopenia, 404, 406, 408, 414
Sardinia, 174, 180
SASP (senescence-associate secretory phenotype), 39, 43–44, 81, 100, 138
saturated fat, 18–19, 22, 24, 50, 58–59, 61, 84–86, 88, 92, 100, 106, 124, 129, 130, 141, 144–45, 157, 175–76, 186, 217–18, 221, 228, 238, 256, 263, 265, 267, 272–73, 293–94, 304, 317, 349, 369–72, 377, 388, 402, 406, 465, 468, 490, 497, 512, 580
sauerkraut, 34, 547
sausage, 144, 497, 524
saw palmetto berry, 260
scallops, 93
Scarborough Fair Diet, 239
schizophrenics, 144
sciatica, 355
Scripps Clinic Sleep Center, 226
scurvy, 114, 211, 512
sea buckthorn berries, 325
seaweed, 77, 190–91, 327–28
secondhand smoke, 95, 141, 152, 156, 165, 263, 372, 373
seeds, 66, 97, 152, *153*, 157, 337, 473
selenium, 94, 128, 134, 285, 384, 491
semen, 35, 199–200
senescent cells, 39, 40–42, 575
senility, 359–60
senna, 248
senolytics, 40–44
sepsis, 340
serotonin, 228, 357
sesame seeds, 97, 354, 514–15

Seven Countries Study, 180

Seventh-day Adventists (Loma Linda), 74, 105, 174, 197–202, 228, 394, 522, 563, 574

sex life, 12, 257–58, 308, 312, 313, 418–39, 555

sex toys, 425

sexual performance supplements, 436

sexually transmitted disease, 334

Shakespeare, William, 283

shark fins, 400

shingles, 80

shingles vaccine, 341–42

shoes, 461

short-chain fatty acids (SCFAs), 21, 61, 89, 91, 189, 332–44, 350, 532, 543–45, 548–49

shredded wheat, 63

shrimp, 93, 498

sigmoidoscopies, 254

silent infarcts, 365

Sinclair, David, 11, 560

sirtuins (silencing information regulators), 46, 130–36, *148*, 169, 188, 567, 584, 585, 587–89

skin, 12, 55, 81, 92, 97, 439–64

skin cancer, 26, 448, 454–59

Skin Cancer Foundation, 454

skin lotion, 81, 100, 450–51

skin treatments, 442–45, 450–54

sleep, 12, 28, 83, 84, 223–29, 316, 322–23, 372, 374–75, 444–45, 555, 559

sleep apnea, 225

sleeping pills, 226

smell, sense of, 287

smoking and tobacco, 19, 49, 50, 53, 57, 66, 75–76, 83, 95, 115, 120, 122, 124, 135–37, 141, 147, 151–52, 154, 156, 158, 161, 165–66, 170, 174, 213–14, 216, 229, 233–34, 263, 266–67, 282–83, 291, 348, 372–73, 419, 433, 440–41, 471, 492, 494, 498, 505, 561, 597, 599

smoothies, 95–96, 196–97, 222, 503

snoring, 228

social ties, 174, 230–31

Society on Sarcopenia, Cachexia and Wasting Disease, 417

soda, 137, 141, 145, 147–48, 154, 161–62, 164–65, 168, 240, 256–57, 351, 467, 517, 545

sodium. *See* salt

sodium phosphate enemas (Fleet), 249

sorghum, 63, 292

souvenaid (Fortasyn Connect), 385

Soviet Union, 329, 377

soy, 33, 187, 189–90, 200, 240–41, 285, 304–7, 328, 351, 395, 429, 447, 516, 521–22

soybean oil, 182

soybeans, 30, 175–76, 189, 240–41, 285, 305, 516

soy lecithin, 538

soymilk, 27, 34, 95, 165, 189, 241, 259, 285, 306, 351, 390

soy nuts, 305

soy protein, 27, 74, 189, 408

Spanish fly, 436

spearmint tea, 351

Spence, J. David, 274

sperm, 46, 139, 199–201, 438

spermidine, 29–38, 196

spices, 44, 64–65, 97–99, 116, 118–19, 130, 134–35, 158, 382–84, 394, 438–39, 501, 513

spinach, 54, 95, 117, 118, 326, 327, 389, 393, 414, 420, 444, 472–73, 496, 502, 578

spinach powder, 118

spine, 39, 55, 80, 342

spine fractures, 234

spirulina, 400

Splenda, 62

split peas, 61, 89, 92, 111–12, 175–77, 582

sports drinks, 131

SPRINT MIND study, 364

SPRINT (Systolic Blood Pressure Intervention Trial), 364

SSRI drugs, 439

STACs (sirtuin-activating compounds), 131–34

Stadtman, Earl, 109–10

Stamler, Jeremiah, 180, 182

Standard American Diet (SAD), 84

staph infections, 537

starch, 63

STAT, 436

statins, 42, 127, 265, 268–70, 275, 318, 349, 363, 434, 587

stem cells, 2, 38, 50

stents, 271–72

steps, daily, 406

sterilization, 200

steroids, 344, 558

stevia, 62

stomach cancer, 84, 234, 542–43

stomach ulcers, 99, 343, 531, 587

Stone Age, 113–14, 157, 600–601

stool softeners, 248

stool tests, 253
strawberries, 43, 44, 117–18, 196, 351–52, 389–90, 418, 445, 500, 502, 510, 525
Strehler, Bernard, 9
strength training, 244, 405, 408, 409, 417
strep infections, 537
streptomycin, 291
stress, 83, 279, 281–82
stress hormones, 402, 445, 558
stress incontinence, 255–58
stress management, 141–42, 229–30
Stroke Prevention and Atherosclerosis Research Centre, 274
strokes, 5, 31, 99, 137, 144, 165, 171, 183–84, 189, 201–2, 213, 236, 241, 268, 274–76, 298, 320, 341, 489, 492–93, 512, 514
subcutaneous fat, 220
Successful Aging Index, 395
sugar, 18, 56, 129, 130, 141, 161, 168, 173, 175, 228, 292, 304, 318, 388, 465, 467–68, 538, 556, 562
sulfide, 538–39
sulforaphane, 107, 122–23, 327, 352–53, 392, 494, 511, 521–22, 526
sulfur, 538–39
sun, 440–41, 446, 455–57, 478, 487
sunburn, 114, 455
sunflower oil, 182
sunscreen, 440–41, 444, 451, 453, 455–59
superoxide dismutase, 51, 119
supplements, 6, 12, 146–47, 193, 285, 324–25, 335–38, 356–57, 369, 379–87, 417, 436, 473–74, 485–87, 494, 500, 514–15, 541–42, 581, 585–94. *See also specific types*
surgery, 335, 344–45
sweat glands, 47
Sweden, 175, 230, 237
Swedish Obese Subjects (SOS) trial, 320
sweet potatoes, 58, 119, 187–89, 196, 198, 444, 505
swiss chard, *495*
synergy, 515–16
syphilis, 283
Szent-Györgyi, Albert, 41

Tabasco sauce, 180
Tai Chi, 244
Taiwan, 209, 366
TAME (Targeting Aging with Metformin) trial, 17
tanning beds, 441, 456, 478
tannins, 550

taste, 465
T cells, 328, 331, 335
tea, 27, 98, 107, 116, 148, 162, *164*, 165, 167–68, 239–40, 394, 445. *See also specific types*
tea tree oil, 461
teeth, 12, 464–70
teff, 577
telogen effluvium, 281–82
telomerase, 139–47
telomeres, 48, 130, 136–48, *148*, 199, 219, 414
tempeh, 33, 36, 38, 191, 241
tendons, 103
tequila, 168
Terbinafine (Lamisil), 460
testicles, 139, 353
testicular hormones, 271
testicular implantations, 294
testosterone, 280–82, 308–19, 425–26, 430
Testosterone in Older Men (TOM) trial, 313
testosterone therapy, 311–14, 319
tetanus vaccine, 337–38
theanine, 331
thiamin, 210
3-MCPD, 184–85
thyme, 119, 239
thyroid, 191, 464
thyroid hormone replacement, 279, 281, 297
ticks, 194
tilapia, 93
time-restricted eating, 562–63
TMAO (trimethylamine oxide), 539–40, 546
TNF-α; (tumor necrosis factor alpha), 87, 92
toenails, 460–63
tofu, 187, 577
tolterodine (Detrol), 256
tomatoes, 107, 179, 239, 262, 469–70, 496, 502, 515–16
tomato juice, 34, 96, 101, 118, 120, 173, 239, 326
tomato paste, 96, 101, 117, 444, 469
tongue, 158–59, 460, 496–97
toothbrushing, 468, 470
tooth loss, 465–66
tooth surgery, 98
toxins. *See* pollutants and toxins
trade-off theory of aging, 102
transcription factor 7, 526
trans fat, 84, 85, 265, 272, 274, 388
trees, 321–22
tretinoin, 451–52

triglycerides, 19, 20, 21, 36, 65, 135, 172, 194, 208, 220, 269, 275, 281, 317, 503, 555, 562, 582–83

tropical oils, 273

True Health Initiative, 600

Tru Niagen, 593

tryptophan, 73, 105, 228, 357, 411, 585–86, 588, 593

T-scores, 235

Tsimane men, 259, 267

tuberculosis, 82

tumor necrosis factor (TNF), 351–53

tumors, 69–71, 73, 137

tumor suppressor gene, 51

TUMT (transurethral microwave thermotherapy), 259

tuna, 93, 126, 278, 283, 502–3

TUNA (transurethral needle ablation), 259

turkey, 124, 498, 501–2, 503

turmeric, 36, 44, 89, 97, 99, 101, 118, 122, 134, 193, 195–96, 353, 382–83, 447, 501, 513, 516–17

TURP (transurethral resection of the prostate), 259

TVP (textured vegetable protein), 259

Twain, Mark, 446, 560

twenty-five-diets mega-study, 571–72, 579

27-hydroxycholesterol, 125

twin studies, 13, 282

2-nonenal, 420

Tyson, Neil deGrasse, 530

Uganda, 250, 459

ulcerative colitis, 132, 504

ultraviolet light, 224

United Kingdom, 206, 288

University of Zurich, 40

unsaturated fats, 18

urinary incontinence, 28, 255–59, 358. *See also* bladder; prostate enlargement

urinary incontinence and, 255–56

urine, 163, 506

urolithins, 550

U.S. Army Rangers, 556

USC Longevity Institute, 569

U.S. Department of Agriculture (USDA), 208, 210, 472

U.S. Dietary Guidelines, 156, 187

U.S. Preventive Services Task Force (USPSTF), 233–34, 253, 269, 299–301, 314–15, 454–55

U.S. Supreme Court, 200, 280, 319

U.S. Tobacco Institute, 152

uterine cancer, 299

UV rays, 114, 123, 441, 444–46, 451–52, 456, 478

V8 juice, 222, 496

vaccines, 80, 320, 338–42

vaginal atrophy, 295

vaginal dryness, 297, 305, 426–30

vaginal fennel cream, 429–30

vaginal hormones, 428–29

vaginal lubrication, 423, 426–27

vagus nerve, 378

valine, 105, 579

vanillin, 418

varicose veins, 202, 247, 459–60

vascular dementia, 359, 370

vascular disease, 431

vascular inflammation, 465

vegans, 50–51, 77, 125, 200, 205–7, 211, 242, 334, 387, 447–49, 479–80, 522, 540, 545, 566, 569, 578, 582

vegetable oils, 85, 124

vegetables, 32, 34, 49–50, 56–57, 87, 89–90, 92, 99–100, 114, 116, 121, 124–25, 141, 147, 152, *153*, 156–57, 174–75, 179, 181, 187, 207, 209, 213–14, 238, 254, 259, 304, 323, 326–27, 388, 413, 443–45, 447–48, 489, 512, 517, 525–26, 546, 577, 597

vegetarians, 12, 51, 58, 82–83, 124–25, 198–212, 218, 229, 242, 274–76, 303, 333–34, 366, 387, 395, 399, 416, 448, 460, 468–69, 479–80, 490, 522, 545, 578, 582

veggie Viagra effect, 438

venison, 87, 89

Veterans Affairs, 459

Viagra, 313, 431, 433–35

Vilcabamba, Ecuador, 173–74

vinegar, 20–23, 64, 123, 459

viruses, 80

visceral fat, 83, 220–21, 555, 574–75

vision, 12, 137, 393, 470–80, 492, 499, 504

VITACOG study, 385

VITAL study, 488

vitamin A, 112, 126, 210, 285, 436, 487

vitamin B$_3$ (niacin), 436, 452, 584–87. *See also* nicotinic acid

vitamin B$_6$, 385–86, 436

vitamin B₁₂, 12, 106, 125, 210–12, 385–87, 448, 486

vitamin B₁₂ deficiency, 125, 211–12, 279, 358, 387, 448

vitamin C, 27, 41, 93–94, 114, 121, 128–29, 206, 210, 239, 284, 336, 350, 411–12, 436, 449, 453–54, 460, 478, 498, 503, 515–17, 540

vitamin D, 146, 148, 224, 235–36, 242, 260, 281, 336–37, 384, 410, 415, 436, 456, 487–89

vitamin E, 93, 112, 121, 126, 210, 285, 336–37, 384, 412, 436, 453

vitamin K, 212, 499

vitamin "P," 41

Voluntarily Stopping Eating and Drinking (VSED), 482–83

vulvovaginal atrophy, 426

wakame, 190–91, 328

Walford, Roy, 555

walking, 65, 141, 142–43, 213–14, 217–18, 231, 241, 498, 597

walnuts, 117, 154, 184, 186, 397, 490–91, 521

warfarin (Coumadin), 499

water, 162–64, 175, 211, 470

watercress, 118

water filters, 164

watermelon, 438

Waterpiks, 290

Wegovy, 548

weight, ideal, 222–23, 223

weight-bearing exercise, 242, 316

weight control, 202, 214, 218, 219–23, 544, 597

weight loss, 20, 49, 82, 94–95, 143, 176, 194, 206–7, 217, 218, 221–22, 234, 251, 255, 266, 275–76, 316, 320–21, 347, 552, 556, 558–59, 561

weight-loss diet, best, 220–21

weight-loss drugs, 548

weight-loss surgery, 83

Werner syndrome, 42

wheat, purple, 188, 505

wheat germ, 30, 35–36, 38, 196

wheat grass juice, 120

whey protein, 25, 105, 106, 318, 407–10

white blood cells, 80, 95, 117, 326, 331

white matter, 219

white meat, 125–26, 273, 278

white noise, 291

white tea, 167

white wine, 172

whole food, plant-based diet, 124, 141–45, 148, 174–75, 182, 186, 197, 207–8, 254–55, 263, 274–75, 402–3, 442, 459–60, 470, 560, 569

whole grains, 21, 37, 56, 61, 89–92, 96–97, 152, 153, 161, 174–75, 207, 213, 292, 304, 377–78, 395–96, 546, 548, 568

whole wheat, 31, 33, 35

wild game, 87, 144

Wilkins, Maurice, 46

Willett, Walter, 162, 236

Wilson, Robert, 297

wine, 120, 131, 164, 164, 172, 331

wineberries, 501

Women's Health Initiative, 168, 240, 297–98, 300, 304, 573

World Anti-Doping Agency, 16

World Health Organization, 163, 171–72, 288, 338, 367, 368, 388, 396, 398, 427, 428, 489, 493

World Heart Federation, 172

World Sleep Society, 227

World War I, 551

World War II, 104, 198, 230, 329, 551, 554–55, 563

wormwood, 513

wounds, 104, 448–49, 558

wrinkles, 441, 444, 446–49, 453

xenohormesis, 509–18

xeno-microRNAs, 522–24

X-rays, 467–68, 478

Yamanaka factors, 50

Yanomami tribe, 158, 546

yeast, 14, 583

yoga, 243, 258

yogurt, 34, 107, 333, 529, 542

Yohimbine, 436

zeaxanthin, 393, 471–74, 478–79

zinc, 146, 175, 284, 337–38, 385, 473, 478

Zoloft, 215, 439

zombie cells, 39–40

Zostavax, 341–42

zoster, 341

About the Author

A founding member and fellow of the American College of Lifestyle Medicine, Dr. Michael Greger is a physician, *New York Times* bestselling author, and internationally recognized speaker on nutrition. He is a graduate of the Cornell University College of Agriculture and Life Sciences and Tufts University School of Medicine. All of the proceeds he receives from his books and speaking engagements are donated to charity.